The Routledge Handbook of Language and Health Communication

The Routledge Handbook of Language and Health Communication consists of forty chapters that provide a broad, comprehensive, and systematic overview of the role that linguistics plays within health communication research and its applications.

The *Handbook* is divided into three sections:

- Individuals' everyday health communication
- Health professionals' communicative practices
- Patient–provider communication in interaction

Special attention is given to cross-cutting themes, including the role of technology in health communication, narrative, and observations of authentic, naturally-occurring contexts. The chapters are written by international authorities representing a wide range of perspectives and approaches.

Building on established work with cutting-edge studies on the changing health communication landscape, this volume will be an essential reference for all those involved in health communication and applied linguistics research and practice.

Heidi E. Hamilton is Professor and Chair in the Department of Linguistics, Georgetown University, USA.

Wen-ying Sylvia Chou is a Program Director in the Health Communication and Informatics Research Branch at the National Cancer Institute, USA.

Routledge Handbooks in Applied Linguistics

Routledge Handbooks in Applied Linguistics provide comprehensive overviews of the key topics in applied linguistics. All entries for the *Handbooks* are specially commissioned and written by leading scholars in the field. Clear, accessible and carefully edited *Routledge Handbooks in Applied Linguistics* are the ideal resource for both advanced undergraduates and postgraduate students.

The Routledge Handbook of Forensic Linguistics
Edited by Malcolm Coulthard and Alison Johnson

The Routledge Handbook of Corpus Linguistics
Edited by Anne O'Keeffe and Mike McCarthy

The Routledge Handbook of World Englishes
Edited by Andy Kirkpatrick

The Routledge Handbook of Applied Linguistics
Edited by James Simpson

The Routledge Handbook of Discourse Analysis
Edited by James Paul Gee and Michael Handford

The Routledge Handbook of Second Language Acquisition
Edited by Susan Gass and Alison Mackey

The Routledge Handbook of Language and Intercultural Communication
Edited by Jane Jackson

The Routledge Handbook of Language Testing
Edited by Glenn Fulcher and Fred Davidson

The Routledge Handbook of Multilingualism
Edited by Marilyn Martin-Jones, Adrian Blackledge and Angela Creese

The Routledge Handbook of Translation Studies
Edited by Carmen Millán-Varela and Francesca Bartrina

The Routledge Handbook of Language and Health Communication
Edited by Heidi E. Hamilton and Wen-ying Sylvia Chou

The Routledge Handbook of Language and Professional Communication
Edited by Stephen Bremner and Vijay Bhatia

The Routledge Handbook of Language and Health Communication

Edited by
Heidi E. Hamilton and Wen-ying Sylvia Chou

Routledge
Taylor & Francis Group
LONDON AND NEW YORK

First published 2014
by Routledge
2 Park Square, Milton Park, Abingdon, Oxon OX14 4RN

and by Routledge
711 Third Avenue, New York, NY 10017

Routledge is an imprint of the Taylor & Francis Group, an informa business

British Library Cataloguing in Publication Data
A catalogue record for this book is available from the British Library

Library of Congress Cataloging in Publication Data
The Routledge handbook of language and health communication /
edited by Heidi E. Hamilton and Wen-ying Sylvia Chou.
pages cm. – (Routledge handbooks in applied linguistics)
1. Communication in medicine. 2. Medicine--Terminology. 3. Applied linguistics.
4. Therapist and patient. I. Hamilton, Heidi Ehernberger, editor of compilation.
II. Chou, Wen-ying Sylvia, editor of compilation.
III. Title: Handbook of language and health communication.
R118.R68 2014
610.1'4--dc23
2013023481

ISBN: 978-0-415-67043-2 (hbk)
ISBN: 978-1-315-85697-1 (ebk)

Typeset in Times New Roman
by Saxon Graphics Ltd, Derby

Printed and bound in the United States of America by Publishers Graphics, LLC on sustainably sourced paper.

We dedicate this book to our parents

Claire and Jerry Ehernberger
Jen-Chang and Linna Chou

With love, gratitude, and respect for setting us on
strong, principled and joyful paths in life

Contents

Illustrations

Figures

Tables

Contributors

Claudia V. Angelelli is a Professor of Spanish Linguistics at San Diego State University, USA. She is the author of *Medical Interpreting and Cross-cultural Communication* and *Revisiting the Role of the Interpreter*, and the co-editor of *Testing and Assessment in Translation and Interpreting Studies*.

Paula K. Baldwin is an Assistant Professor of Communication Studies at Western Oregon University, USA. Her research examines health communication and palliative care at the end-of-life. She studies challenging interpersonal interactions among interdisciplinary healthcare teams, patients, and caregivers in hospice and hospital settings.

Judith C. Barker is a Professor of Medical Anthropology at the University of California, San Francisco, USA. Her major interests include the experience of illness and its day-to-day management by patients and their families. She has a particular interest in these issues in the context of chronic conditions and of health disparities.

Ellen Barton is a Professor in the Linguistics Program and Department of English at Wayne State University, USA. Her research interests are in the discourse analysis of medical communication and medical rhetoric in ethically charged communicative events.

Wayne A. Beach is Professor in the School of Communication at San Diego State University and Member of the Moores Cancer Center, University of California, San Diego, USA. He is the author of *Conversations about Illness*, *A Natural History of Family Cancer*, and the edited *Handbook of Patient–Provider Interactions*.

Elizabeth M. Bishop is a Fellow at the Agency for Healthcare Research and Quality (AHRQ) in Rockville, Maryland, USA. Her research and health policy work focuses on: the effectiveness of care for patients with chronic kidney disease and diabetes; communication in healthcare settings; and collaboration and knowledge management in health services research.

Benjamin (Jim) Blatt is Professor of Medicine and Medical Director of the Clinical Learning and Simulation Skills Center at the George Washington University School of Medicine, USA. Dr. Blatt's primary interest is healthcare communication and development of communication curriculum for medical students.

Brian Brown is Professor of Health Communication in the Faculty of Health and Life Sciences at De Montfort University, UK. He is the author of 13 books and around 60 journal articles, and is a Fellow of the Royal Society of Medicine. In recent years he has written widely on communication in healthcare contexts, language and narratives.

Richard F. Brown is an Assistant Professor of Social and Behavioral Health in the School of Medicine and is affiliate faculty in the School of Nursing, both at Virginia Commonwealth University, USA. Dr. Brown has a joint appointment at the Massey Cancer Center where he is co-director of the Patient-Centered Outcomes Core and chair of the center's PRMS Cancer Prevention and Control subcommittee.

Nancy J. Burke is Associate Professor of Medical Anthropology at the University of California, San Francisco, USA. Her research interests include bioethics and clinical trials, technologies of cancer care and therapeutic subjectivity, social inequalities in cancer treatment and survivorship, the Cuban health(care) system, Global Health, and Women's Health.

Carma L. Bylund is Associate Director for Medical Education at Hamad Medical Corporation in Doha, Qatar. Dr. Bylund's teaching and research is focused on improving healthcare communication. She has published widely on the implementation and evaluation of communication skills training for physicians.

Linda D. Cameron is a Professor of Psychology at the University of California, Merced, USA. Her research focuses on cognitive and affective processes influencing responses to health threats, and the implications of these processes for designing health communications and interventions.

Christopher N. Candlin is Senior Research Professor Emeritus in the Department of Linguistics at Macquarie University, Sydney, Australia, and an Academician of the UK Academy of Social Sciences. His research offers critical analysis of institutional discourses in the domains of health care and law. He co-edits the *Journal of Applied Linguistics and Professional Practice*. Recent publications include *Discourses of Deficit* (2011) and *Discourses of Trust* (2013).

Sally Candlin is a Senior Research Fellow in the Department of Linguistics at Macquarie University, Sydney, Australia. She is the author of *Therapeutic Communication: A Lifespan Approach* (2008) and the co-author of *Communication and Professional Relationships in Healthcare Practice* (2013). She is a Registered Nurse and Midwife and holds an MSc in Public Health Research.

McKenzie Carlisle is a doctoral candidate in the Social and Health Psychology Program at the University of Utah, USA. Her research interests include how social relationships influence health. She is currently examining how attitudes towards different types of friends influence cardiovascular reactivity during stressful interactions.

Rita Charon is a Professor of Clinical Medicine and founder of the Program in Narrative Medicine at Columbia University, USA. Her research examines the consequences of reflective clinical practice and healthcare team effectiveness. She is the author of *Narrative Medicine: Honoring the Stories of Illness* (2006) and co-editor of *Stories Matter: The Role of Narrative in Medical Ethics* (Routledge, 2002) and *Psychoanalysis and Narrative Medicine* (2008).

Elaina Chen is a 2012 graduate of the Indiana University School of Medicine, USA. She is currently a resident in plastic surgery at the University of Rochester Medical Center in Rochester, New York.

Wen-ying Sylvia Chou is a Program Director in the Health Communication and Informatics Research Branch at the National Cancer Institute, USA. She holds a PhD in Linguistics, a Master's in Public Health, and is a graduate of the NCI Cancer Prevention Fellowship. Her research interests include social media and health, patient–provider communication, health literacy, and mixed methods approaches in behavioral sciences.

Aaron V. Cicourel is Professor of Cognitive Science and Sociology at the University of California, San Diego, USA. He has worked on the ways in which knowledge is accessed or manipulated in a variety of contexts, including courts, educational settings, and medical settings. His research has integrated traditional micro-sociology with current thinking within psychology and anthropology on the origin of context-specific knowledge and memory.

Rosemary Clerehan is Associate Professor and Director, International Postgraduate Academic Support, Faculty of Medicine, Nursing and Health Sciences, Monash University, Australia. Her research interests are doctor–patient communication, Internet pedagogies, postgraduate student writing, and cross-cultural issues in teaching and learning.

Ulla Connor is Chancellor's Professor of English, the Zimmer Chair in Intercultural Communication, and Director of the Indiana Center for Intercultural Communication at Indiana University, USA. Her research expertise is on intercultural rhetoric and applied linguistics. She currently studies patient-centric communication strategies to improve patients' adherence to medication and healthy behaviors.

Paul Crawford is Professor of Health Humanities at the School of Nursing, Midwifery and Physiotherapy at the University of Nottingham, UK. He is also a Fellow of the Royal Society of Arts and Professor of the Institute of Mental Health. He co-founded the Health Language Research Group at the University of Nottingham, bringing together academics and clinicians to advance communication research in healthcare settings.

Boyd Davis, Cone Professor of Applied Linguistics and Professor of Gerontology at UNC-Charlotte, USA, studies Alzheimer's speech; narrative, pragmatics and stance; and digital archives of speech. She is Co-Principal Investigator (PI) of the National Institutes of Health (NIH)-sponsored Carolinas Conversation Collection, a digital portal including Alzheimer talk.

Lee Ellington is an Associate Professor at the University of Utah College of Nursing, USA, a clinical psychologist, and a Huntsman Cancer Institute Investigator. She has studied interpersonal health communication in multiple healthcare contexts and among diverse groups of providers, including family practice, genetic counseling, poison control, and hospice home care. Her focus is on the communication mechanisms that predict adherence, health behaviors, and psychosocial adjustment.

Richard M. Frankel is Professor of Medicine and Geriatrics at the Indiana University School of Medicine and Director of the Walther Center for Palliative Care Research and Education at the Indiana University Simon Cancer Center, USA. His research focuses on clinician–patient communication and its effects on quality and safety, the effects of exam room computing on physician–patient communication, and effective organizational change strategies.

Heidi Gilstad is an adviser at the Norwegian Research Centre for Electronic Patient Records (NSEP). She holds a PhD from the Department of Language and Communication Studies at the Norwegian University of Science and Technology (NTNU), and previously worked at the National Centre for Foetal Medicine at St Olav's Hospital in Trondheim for ten years.

Larrie Greenberg is Senior Adviser of the Office of Medical Education and Clinical Professor of Pediatrics at The George Washington University School of Medicine and Health Sciences, USA. He has maintained a leadership role in medical education as part of the Association of American Medical Colleges since the 1970s. Much of his research has been in doctor–patient communication.

Heidi E. Hamilton is Professor and Chair in the Department of Linguistics, Georgetown University, USA. Her discourse analytic research and consulting interests focus on issues of language and Alzheimer's disease, language and aging, genetic counseling, and physician–patient interaction. She has also taught at the University of Innsbruck and the Freie Universität Berlin as a Fulbright Distinguished Chair and DAAD *Gastdozentin*.

Uwe Hartung was trained in mass communication and political communication, and is now a senior researcher at the Institute of Communication and Health of the Università della Svizzera italiana, Lugano, Switzerland, working in areas such as media coverage of and public opinion on health-related issues.

Kevin Harvey is Lecturer in Sociolinguistics at the School of English Studies at the University of Nottingham, UK. He chairs the Health Language Research Group (HLRG) and contributes to the MA in Health Communication. He is also involved in the Nottingham Health Communications Corpus (NHCC) project.

Evelyn Y. Ho is an Associate Professor of Communication Studies and Asian American Studies at the University of San Francisco, USA. Her research intersects health, culture and communication with a primary focus on holistic medicine in the United States.

Rick Iedema is Research Professor and Director of the Centre for Health Communication at the University of Technology Sydney, Australia. A Fellow of the Academy of Social Sciences of Australia and Associate Editor of *Health Expectations*, his research explores how communication impacts on care organization, quality and safety. His most recent work focuses on clinical handover, incident disclosure and professional communication around risk and infection control.

Rodney H. Jones is Associate Head of the Department of English at City University of Hong Kong. His research interests include health communication, language and sexuality and computer-mediated discourse. He is author of *Health and Risk Communication: An Applied Linguistic Perspective* (Routledge, 2013), and co-author with Christoph Hafner of *Understanding Digital Literacies: A Practical Introduction.*

Ki-tae Kim is Assistant Professor of English Education at Keimyung University, Korea. He previously taught and directed English as a Second Language at the University of Minnesota, Crookston, USA, and Teaching Korean as a Foreign Language at the Intercultural Institute of California. His current research areas include medical discourse and health communication, discourse analysis, critical applied linguistics, and positioning theory.

Christopher J. Koenig is a Research Sociologist in the Department of Medicine at the University of California, San Francisco, USA. He specializes in ethnographic methods and audio- and video-recordings to examine the provider–patient relationship, active patient participation in treatment, and provider culture in medical visits.

Jennifer S. Kramer is an Assistant Professor of Communication at The College of St. Benedict/St. John's University, USA. Her research examines the communication between primary care providers and their patients who suffer from chronic pain in order to identify barriers to using communication as a therapeutic tool.

Joyce Lamerichs is an Assistant Professor at the Department of Language and Communication, VU University Amsterdam. She uses insights from discursive psychology and conversation analysis to study online support groups and professional–client interaction about mental illness, trauma and coping.

Kathryn Lauten is the Assistant Director of the Survey Research Center and an adjunct faculty member in the IU School of Liberal Arts in Indianapolis, Indiana, USA. She received her BA from Dartmouth College and her PhD from the University of Michigan. Her current research focuses on improving patient outcomes through tailored communication.

Peter A. Lichtenberg, a clinical psychologist, is Director of the Institute of Gerontology and the Merrill Palmer Skillman Institute, and the Founding Director of the Wayne State University Lifespan Alliance. He is also a Professor of Psychology and Physical Medicine and Rehabilitation, Wayne State University, USA.

Feng-hwa Lu is an Associate Professor in the Division of Family Medicine and Department of Medicine and chairperson of the Institute of Gerontology at the National Cheng Kung University, Taiwan. He is also a visiting attending physician in the Department of Family Medicine, National Cheng Kung University Hospital, Taiwan.

Mark R. Luborsky, a medical anthropologist, is Professor of Anthropology, Professor of Gerontology, Director of Aging and Health Disparities Research, Institute of Gerontology, Wayne State University, USA. He is also Foreign Professor, Department of Neurobiology, Care Science and Society, Karolinksa Institutet, Stockholm, Sweden. His research focuses on life reorganization and continuity of meaning and function in the areas of physical disability and mental health.

Margaret Maclagan recently retired as Associate Professor of Communication Disorders at the University of Canterbury, Christchurch, New Zealand. She studies sound change over time, focusing on New Zealand English and Maori, and language change over time in Alzheimer's disease.

Amy McQueen is an Assistant Professor in the Department of Medicine (Division of Health Behavior Research) at Washington University in St. Louis School of Medicine, USA. She studies psychosocial influences of health behaviors, including individual's defenses against personally relevant risk information.

Claudio Gruber Mann has an MA in Psychiatric Nursing and Specialization in Mental Health at the Federal University of Rio de Janeiro, Brazil. His research activities have focused on mental health and STD/AIDS prevention, working with issues of sexuality and stigma. Currently, he is the intervention coordinator in the *Interdisciplinary Project in Sexuality, Mental Health and AIDS* sponsored by the National Institute of Mental Health (NIMH).

Douglas W. Maynard is Conway-Bascom Professor, University of Wisconsin, Madison, USA. His research addresses ethnomethodology and conversation analysis, including testing and diagnosis for autism, end-of-life discussions in oncology, and survey interview recruitment. Publications include a co-edited volume, *Communication in Medical Care: Interaction between Primary Care Physicians and Patients* (2006), and the *Bad News, Good News: Conversational Order in Everyday Talk and Clinical Settings* (2003).

Emily B. Peterson is a doctoral candidate in Communication at George Mason University, USA. Her research focuses on health care, interpersonal and intercultural communication. She has published in *Patient Education & Counseling, Journal of Health Psychology* and *Journal of Drug Education.*

Alison Pilnick is Professor of Language, Medicine and Society at the University of Nottingham, UK. She has a longstanding interest in communication between healthcare professionals and their clients, with a particular focus on the giving and receiving of advice.

Diana de Souza Pinto is researcher and Associate Professor at the Social Memory Graduate Program at the Federal University of the State of Rio de Janeiro, Brazil. She has an MA in Applied Linguistics and a PhD in Mental Health. Her research activities have focused on the development of an interdisciplinary approach to the study of psychiatric patients' discourse.

Abby Prestin is a social scientist at the Center for Tobacco Products, Food and Drug Administration, USA. Her research focuses on the role of media and digital technology in the relationship between emotion and health. She explores the interplay between cognition and emotion in understanding the effects of health messages, and the implications of new media and technology for health promotion.

Vaidehi Ramanathan is a Professor in the Linguistics Department at the University of California, Davis, USA. Her research interests include areas of language and health, and literacy and teacher-education. Her most recent publications include *Bodies and Language: Health, Ailments, Disabilities* (2010) and *Language, Body and Health* (co-edited, 2011).

Maija Reblin holds her doctorate in Social and Health Psychology and is assistant research faculty at the University of Utah College of Nursing, USA. Her research focuses on the interplay between relationship quality and communication and its impact on physiological and psychological stress as a mediator for other health outcomes.

Branca Telles Ribeiro is Associate Professor at Lesley University, USA. Her research examines communication between healthcare providers and patients in clinical settings. She leads a project exploring intercultural communication and access to health care for Brazilian immigrants in the Boston area. In Brazil, she is Associate Researcher at the Institute of Psychiatry, Federal University of Rio de Janeiro.

Celia Roberts is Professor of Applied Linguistics in the Centre for Language, Discourse and Communication at King's College London, UK. Her research interests include institutional discourse, language and ethnicity and the methods of linguistic ethnography.

Felicia Roberts is Associate Professor of Communication at Purdue University, USA, and a faculty member of Purdue's Interdisciplinary Linguistics Program. Her scholarship explores how meanings and relational identities arise and are maintained through talk and embodied action.

Donald Rubin is Professor Emeritus of Communication Studies, Language and Literacy Education, and Linguistics at University of Georgia, USA, where he is also a research scientist at the Center for Health and Risk Communication. He is co-editor of *Health Communication and Faith Communities* (2011) and co-PI on 'Meals on Wheels Volunteers as Health Literacy Coaches', funded by the National Institute on Aging.

Srikant Sarangi is Professor of Language and Communication and Director of the Health Communication Research Centre at Cardiff University, Wales. His research interests are in applied linguistics and institutional/professional discourse studies. He is the editor of *Text & Talk* and founding editor of *Communication & Medicine*.

Karen S. Schaepe is a PhD candidate in Sociology at the University of Wisconsin-Madison, USA, specializing in the sociology of health and medicine. Her dissertation explores disclosures of bad news as a longitudinal phenomenon, following leukemia, lymphoma, and myeloma patients and their families from diagnosis until post stem cell transplant.

Peter J. Schulz is Professor for Communication Theories and Health Communication at the Università della Svizzera italiana, Lugano, Switzerland. His recent research and publications have focused on consumer health literacy and empowerment, argumentation in health communications, and the epidemiology of prescription drug misuse.

Dena Shenk is Director of the Gerontology Program and Professor of Anthropology at UNC Charlotte, USA. Her research interests are diversity within the older population based on gender, culture and environment with an emphasis on individual expectations and experiences of aging.

Noemi Spinazzi is a pediatric resident at the Children's Hospital of Oakland. Originally from Milan, Italy, she studied Biology and Psychology at Boston University and went to medical school at the University of Pennsylvania. Her research interests include medical education, palliative care, and global health.

Thomas Spranz-Fogasy is a researcher in the section 'Pragmatik' at the Institute of the German Language (IDS) and Associate Professor at the University of Mannheim, Germany.

His interests include conversation analysis, argumentation, rhetoric, and understanding and interaction in medicine.

Wyke Stommel, PhD, is Assistant Professor at the Centre for Language Studies of Radboud University Nijmegen, the Netherlands. In her research she applies conversation analysis to study interactional aspects of online health communication (forum discussions, chat and e-mail) in both professional and lay settings.

Deborah Swinglehurst is a general practitioner in Suffolk and a NIHR Academic Clinical Lecturer at Queen Mary, University of London, UK. Her PhD thesis was a linguistic ethnographic study of the electronic patient record in general practice.

Mei-hui Tsai is an Associate Professor at the National Cheng Kung University, Taiwan. She received her PhD in Linguistics from Georgetown University, USA. Her current research interest focuses on discourse analysis of doctor–patient communication and the application of her research to medical education in Taiwan.

Wendy Vaughon is a Research Coordinator at the City University of New York's School of Public Health at Hunter College, USA. She is also a doctoral student in Public Health at the Graduate Center, City University of New York.

Melinda M. Villagran is a Professor in the Department of Communication Studies at Texas State University in San Marcos, Texas, USA. Her research focuses on effective communication in health organizations, with a special emphasis on clinical interactions among clinicians and patients from diverse backgrounds.

Sherrie Flynt Wallington is Assistant Professor of Oncology at the Lombardi Comprehensive Cancer Center, Georgetown University Medical Center, USA. Her research focuses on using community-based participatory research approaches to explore the role of health communication in reducing and eliminating health disparities among minority and underserved populations.

Erika A. Waters is an Assistant Professor in the Department of Surgery (Division of Public Health Sciences) at Washington University in St. Louis School of Medicine, USA. She studies how risk perception and communication affect health-related decisions and behaviors.

Andrew Winckles is a PhD student in the Department of English at Wayne State University, USA. His research interests are in eighteenth-century literature, religion, and culture. He is a research assistant on the ethics-in-interaction project.

Christina Zarcadoolas is a Professor at the City University of New York School of Public Health at Hunter College, USA, and Founder of the New York Roundtable on Public Health Literacy. She is a sociolinguist and expert in health literacy and public understanding of science.

Olga Zayts is Assistant Professor at the School of English, the University of Hong Kong. She leads Health Communication Research Cluster at the Center for the Humanities and Medicine. She has published widely on genetic counseling communication.

Acknowledgments

First of all, we would like to thank our contributors for their immediate enthusiasm and openness to participate in this *Handbook of Language and Health Communication*. We have both learned immensely from all of you and are grateful for your cooperation, sustained efforts, and patience as the volume evolved over the past three years.

Our sincere gratitude goes to Louisa Semlyen, Publisher, and Sophie Jaques, Senior Editorial Assistant, Routledge English Language and Applied Linguistics, for inviting us to take on this project and for being so optimistic, professional, and encouraging throughout the process, and to Anna Callander, Production Editor, for so competently seeing this volume through to its publication.

A thousand thanks to our editorial assistants, Leslie Cochrane and Joshua Kraut, doctoral students in Georgetown University's Department of Linguistics, for their proactive nature, joyful outlook on life, diligence, and meticulous attention to detail. It's been an absolute delight working with you on this project!

We are both very fortunate to work with wonderful colleagues who create a highly energizing environment in which to work. Thanks to the faculty, staff, and students of Georgetown University's Department of Linguistics for surrounding us with support, creativity, and insights. Thanks also to the support of the talented colleagues at National Cancer Institute's Division of Cancer Control and Population Sciences, particularly Brad Hesse, Chief of the Health Communication and Informatics Research Branch. We both want to acknowledge members of our cross-disciplinary Health Discourse Research Group – thank you for being a constant source of ideas and positive energy. We enjoy exploring the myriad facets of this very exciting domain together with you.

And, finally, heartfelt thanks to both our families, particularly our spouses, Dan Hamilton and Paul Portner, for their constant support during these many months of conceptualizing, writing, and editing. Love to our children, Siri and Sean Hamilton and Noah and Ben Portner, for the joy and perspective they bring to our lives. We are grateful to all of you!

Introduction

Health communication as applied linguistics

Heidi E. Hamilton and Wen-ying Sylvia Chou

This *Handbook* is a reference work covering key topics at the intersection of health communication and applied linguistics. It builds on the strong foundation of seminal work by providing key contributions on the leading ideas, debates, topics, approaches, and methodologies by the field's top researchers, both established and up-and-coming. Each chapter provides an accessible overview and exemplary analyses to an area of the field. Our intended audience comprises several groups: undergraduate and graduate students in applied linguistics and social sciences broadly conceived; linguists who are interested in learning about their field as it relates to health contexts and issues; health communication scholars who are eager to engage with linguistic theories and methodologies; medical school educators; and practicing health professionals and medical researchers who would like to learn more about the role of language in their own areas of experience and expertise.

Background and motivation

Over the past decades, scholars have been applying linguistics in efforts to understand the myriad profound and complex interrelationships between language and health issues and contexts. As these undertakings have become more expansive, collaboration across disciplines and between research and practice has become increasingly common. The intricacies of the mutual effects between language and human health – how language use affects health as well as how health affects language – have encouraged linguists to reach across disciplinary boundaries in their examinations of public and private dimensions of health communication. Some of these projects have illuminated a variety of health-related issues (Gotti and Salager-Meyer 2006; Gwyn 2002; Ramanathan 2009; Sarangi and Roberts 1999), but most have focused attention on one context or type of communication. These areas of focus have included patient–provider interactions (Ainsworth-Vaughn 1998; Heritage and Maynard 2006; Roberts 1999); mental health and counseling (Capps and Ochs 1995; Ferrara 1994; Peräkylä 1995; Ribeiro 1994); narrative as related to cognition and illness experience (Hunter 1991; Mattingly 1998); the discourse of public health (Higgins and Norton 2009); and health and risk communication (Jones 2013).

Some of these scholars have focused their efforts primarily on furthering our understanding of language – illuminating, for example, how pronouns and questions are used in healthcare interactions; others have directed their work to individuals who are regularly involved in healthcare – for example, offering training materials to the physicians and patients who speak with each other in clinics. Still others have attempted to live in both worlds, shuttling between linguistics conferences and health and medical conferences, and working hard as part of interdisciplinary teams to translate one set of disciplinary assumptions and frameworks into another.

Concurrently, outside linguistics, communication and health services researchers have examined communication in clinical and public health contexts by applying theories and methods from diverse social science disciplines, most notably communication and psychology (Hornik 2002; Epstein and Street 2007). While language plays a central role in these investigations, it is commonly viewed as facilitating exchange of information or enabling researchers' content analysis, rather than being an object of study in its own right. Given the differing – but complementary – areas of focus, this diversity of disciplines illuminating health communication offers opportunities for fruitful discussions that transcend disciplinary and professional boundaries, one of the primary aims of this volume.

It is in pursuit of this transcendent conversation that we envisioned and carried out this *Handbook of Language and Health Communication*. In the selection of contributors, we sought out prominent scholars and practitioners whose work would facilitate the building of a multifaceted volume, one that would represent a breadth of fascinating perspectives and insights – rather than aiming for a coherent volume organized along theoretical or methodological lines. To that end, contributors represent diverse disciplinary backgrounds, including but not limited to: linguistics, anthropology, sociology, psychology, communication, and mixed methods approaches in health sciences. They carry out their work in a variety of institutional contexts, including academic departments in universities, medical centers and hospitals, government agencies, and private sectors. The paradigms associated with these varied disciplines and institutions necessarily shape decisions regarding what kinds of research questions are thought to be both answerable, useful and important, as well as how best to design studies to answer these questions. As a result, readers of this *Handbook* will find a variety of conceptual frameworks within its chapters, ranging from hypothesis-driven investigations, to fine-grained local examinations of turn-by-turn interactions, to grammatical analyses of written texts, to 'thick' ethnographic descriptions of communicative contexts.

In addition, the chapters in the *Handbook* utilize various types of language evidence, including linguistic excerpts extracted from recorded and transcribed clinical encounters, interviews, focus groups, and other naturally occurring spoken discourses; excerpts of written online communication, scientific publications and other authentic written texts; personal experience narratives; quantitative findings from linguistic corpora and survey databases; and research field notes. Beyond diversity of approaches and evidence, this volume represents research and data from a wide range of geographical regions. From Hong Kong, Korea, Taiwan, Australia, New Zealand, the United Kingdom, Germany, the Netherlands, Norway, Switzerland, Brazil, and South Africa to a number of locations within the United States, we have aimed to demonstrate health discourse in the diverse, global context. Finally, readers will be able to engage with a wide variety of healthcare professions, contexts, diseases and conditions, patient populations, and critical issues that are explored within the volume.

Handbook organization

Following this introductory chapter, the remaining 40 chapters are organized into three major parts that provide a systematic overview of the role of language and linguistics in health communication research.

Part I: Individuals' everyday health communication
Part II: Health professionals' communicative practices
Part III: Patient–provider communication in interaction

This progression allows us to begin with separate examinations of communication around health, starting with the perspectives of individuals going about their everyday lives far away from any healthcare institution and moving to the perspectives of healthcare professions as they interact with each other within institutional contexts. Following these separate explorations, we consider communication within interactions that involves both patients and professionals as they come together to discuss mutually important issues in healthcare.

This tripartite structure was inspired by foundational work in medical anthropology (Mishler 1984), institutional discourse analysis (Agar 1985; Heritage 1997), and interactional sociolinguistics (Gumperz 1982; Tannen 1984) which has convincingly shown in a wide variety of contexts that communicative problems can arise due to mismatches between speakers' intentions and listeners' inferences. Because listeners must 'go beyond surface meaning to fill in for what is left unsaid' (Gumperz 1999: 458) in assessing what is intended by speakers, differences in speakers' and listeners' backgrounds can get in the way of understanding, and can cause 'crosstalk'. A primary aim of interactional sociolinguistics is 'to show how [such] diversity affects interpretation' (Gumperz 1999: 459). In connection to this *Handbook*'s domain, 'crosstalk' in health contexts can certainly be attributed to ethnic, cultural, or linguistic backgrounds (as was the case in Gumperz's studies), but it can also be rooted in differences in (1) professional perspectives (e.g., between physicians and nurses); (2) levels of familiarity with institutional goals or access to knowledge (see Agar 1985 and Heritage 1997); or (3) types of education, training, and experiences of patients and healthcare professionals, what Mishler (1984) characterizes as the distinction between the 'voice of the lifeworld' and the 'voice of medicine' (see Hamilton 2004 and Hamilton and Bartell 2011).

Given the importance of these divergent perspectives to understanding possible 'crosstalk' within patient–provider interactions, we decided to start the *Handbook* off with chapters that illuminate relevant aspects of each. In Part I, readers will find chapters that explore issues ranging from differences across laypersons in terms of how they perceive risk or deal with numeric information, to how they construct and represent health in written or spoken discourses, to how they interact with others in health contexts in-person or online, to how they 'consume' written health messages designed by providers or pharmaceutical companies. Part II contains chapters that introduce readers to ways in which health professionals are socialized into the ways of seeing, speaking, writing, and acting that go along with the acquisition of the relevant 'professional vision' (Goodwin 1994) as they gain the competence, activities, practices, and shared repertoires of experiences that are associated with their chosen professional community of practice (Lave and Wenger 1991). Following the focus on the professionalization process, chapters explore a range of communication issues that arise from inter-professional interactions within healthcare teams of various types. In Part III, the focus turns to interactions between healthcare providers and patients, beginning with fine-grained examinations of particularities, including prediagnostic statements, news disclosures, hopeful moments, morality, and the impact of electronic medical records within the clinical encounter. Subsequent chapters explore a range of issues related to the management of cultural and linguistic diversity, including language interpreting, cultural health beliefs, and code-switching that have become both increasingly common and critical as migration and globalization impact the provision of healthcare. Part III closes with chapters that highlight ethics in action within a variety of contexts ranging from health disparities, clinical trial enrollment, end-of-life care, and solicitation of human tissue donations.

Despite the benefits underlying the logic of the *Handbook*'s organization into the three parts just described, it is important to keep in mind that no sharp boundaries actually exist within and across these groups. Sarangi and Candlin (2011: 16) argue that individual professionals and clients should be understood as occupying different positions on a continuum rather than assuming that lay and expert systems in themselves are homogeneous entities, and Jones (2013: 5) suggests that increased accessibility of health information is leveling the playing field: 'No longer solely the property of experts, medical information circulates freely through the print and electronic media, public discourse, and the everyday conversations of laypeople, being constantly reinterpreted and repackaged as it moves from scientific journals to newspaper reports to online social networking sites to dinner-table conversations.' Recent discussions in public discourse of 'peer-to-peer healthcare', 'crowdsourcing', and 'participative medicine' all illustrate the increasingly blurry line between laypersons and the professionals as the health communication landscape continues to evolve. In spite of these important trends, it is our view that most laypersons still experience health in fundamentally different ways than professionals do – both inside and outside healthcare systems – and it can be instructive (not only convenient) to illuminate them separately before exploring their interaction.

Linguistics as applied to health communication

Because this volume is part of the *Routledge Handbooks in Applied Linguistics* series, we turn now to a brief discussion of the place of applied linguistics within the larger field of health communication.

We begin with Brumfit's (1995: 27) conceptualization of applied linguistics, arguably the most frequently used definition in the field: 'the theoretical and empirical investigation of real-world problems in which language is a central issue.' Although at first blush this definition seems to cover the wide range of work represented in this *Handbook*, our consideration of interdisciplinary discussions we have both had over the years with colleagues in health research and practice leads us to problematize Brumfit's characterization of the *centrality* of language issues in these investigations. Indeed it is our view that we as linguists may identify language or communication issues as being *central* to a particular problem or context, when our colleagues in disciplines outside of linguistics may not perceive the central problem in that way at all; they often will, for example, identify the problem as being one of individual attributes (such as personality, skill, or intelligence) or system-level factors (such as institutional constraints on time and resources or policy impact).

Of course, applied linguists can provide a valuable complementary perspective and associated analytical toolkit to shed new light on healthcare problems that have been identified by others as non-linguistic in nature, but arriving at a place where this contribution is actively embraced and integrated is a challenge of what Sarangi and Candlin (2003) have characterized as 'jointly inspired reflexive research'. As applied linguists, we need to be cautious as we work toward this 'joint problematisation' lest we be judged as acting in a parochial way by assuming that others on the research team will quickly grasp the central importance of language to the project.

Following Cameron et al. (1992), linguists can conduct studies *on, for*, or *with* research subjects, as these scholars move along a continuum of doing ethical research (*on*) to advocacy research (*on* and *for*) to empowering research (*on, for*, and *with*) vis-à-vis their subjects. By extending this perspective on relationships with research subjects to relationships with other disciplines and professions (in the case of this *Handbook,* those related to health), we arrive at the influential recommendation by Sarangi and Candlin (2011: 36, 45) that we elevate 'our research gaze beyond the immediacy of the text or the transcript' and embody an applied linguistics perspective that

> not only builds on the cumulative insights gained from discourse studies and the vast body of literature in the sociology of professions and the sociology of work, but also foregrounds problem-orientation, deeply embedded in methodological and analytical challenges, so that research outcomes are made practically relevant.

In order to be in a position to 'make applied linguistics matter', as Sarangi and Candlin (2011: 45) argue, applied linguists must prepare themselves to be successful members of interdisciplinary teams. Wasson (2004: 122) highlights this hard work in the following way: 'Researchers who inhabit both academic and applied worlds not only need to become fluent in the codes of each context, they also need to develop the ability to translate each world's logic to the other one.'

Contributors to this *Handbook* represent the full spectrum in terms of research engagement *on, for*, and *with* the health communication subject matter; some contributors are members of interdisciplinary teams whose work exemplifies the kind of 'joint problematisation'; others work as linguists within health institutions who are responsible for translating what they know about communication into training curriculum and education materials; still others work as collaborators or consultants on a case-by-case basis to identify solutions to specific health communication challenges; and, finally, some individual scholars within linguistics departments apply relevant tools from their toolkit to analyze selected texts and transcripts in efforts to illuminate the goings-on within motivated healthcare contexts. In so doing, their analyses shed light on language in social interactions more broadly.

It is our hope that readers will seek out and engage with those chapters that fit their needs and interests most closely – and will take steps towards attaining this 'fluency' (Wasson 2004: 122) by connecting ideas across disciplines, professions, health conditions, healthcare settings, and geographic regions. Perhaps a spark of recognition or a new idea as to how to proceed will lead to greater understanding of a problem under consideration – whether or not anyone thought at first blush that language or communication was actually centrally involved.

Finally, it is important to consider the contribution of health communication to linguistics; i.e., health communication as applied *to* linguistics. As in most 'applied' disciplines, most effort is spent applying, translating, and transferring knowledge and approaches to a new context – in our case, applying linguistic knowledge and analytic tools to health. However, such applied research can also contribute to basic inquiries, theories, and frameworks related to language and interaction. As we carry out our applied work, our emerging in-depth understandings of health communication interactions (e.g., from media messages, to clinical encounters, to social media discussions about health) can inform and enrich our knowledge of linguistic structures and functions, as well as of the social interaction of which this language is a part and works to create. We encourage applied linguists to realize (in both senses of the word) the enormous potential in using health discourse data and interdisciplinary health communication approaches to shed new light on language and social interaction.

Towards complementary perspectives on language and health communication

Given the myriad ways in which applied linguistics can be understood and in which linguists can engage across disciplines, we offer brief descriptions of our own work to make transparent the personal experiences and professional visions we bring to this *Handbook*. We then follow with key considerations in moving towards cross-disciplinary dialogue in language and health communication research.

Personal and professional journeys in health communication

Our disciplinary training at the doctoral level was nearly identical although 15 years apart (we both studied discourse analysis from an interactional sociolinguistic perspective at Georgetown University's Department of Linguistics); since then our paths in health communication have diverged. These commonalities and differences in our academic backgrounds and professional experiences have not only shaped the kinds of linguists we have become, but have also influenced the kinds of contacts we have made at professional meetings and in collaborations on projects. In short, the communities of practice (Lave and Wenger 1991) in which we each feel comfortable have become somewhat different from each other. We consider this expanded worldview to be a key benefit in our work in health communication in general, and on this volume in particular.

Since her early longitudinal explorations of conversational language and Alzheimer's disease, Hamilton has straddled both worlds of linguistics and healthcare from her position as faculty member in Georgetown University's Department of Linguistics. She has participated as a linguist expert in interdisciplinary projects surrounding a variety of health concerns, including head injury, inter-professional communication, genetic counseling discourse, health literacy and chronic disease self-management, and the impact of the presenting concern on the shape of physician–patient discourse. Most recently, Hamilton has begun to uncover the role of linguistic discourse analysis in illuminating the therapeutic effects of community-based arts programs for individuals with early Alzheimer's disease.

While trained as a sociolinguist with a dissertation on end-of-life discourse, Chou gained additional training in behavioral science methods as a postdoctoral fellow. As the lone linguist at the National Cancer Institute (to her knowledge!), her research in the areas of social media and health, patient–provider communication, health literacy and cancer disparities has utilized quantitative (e.g., analysis of cross-sectional data), qualitative (e.g., discourse analysis), and mixed methods and she publishes in diverse venues in the health sciences. As a National Institutes of Health (NIH) Program Director, she guides investigators on proposal development and grantsmanship; this professional role has allowed for fertile cross-disciplinary interactions about study aims and methods towards the goal of improving health.

Cross-disciplinary dialogue in language and health communication

Our numerous conversations with linguist and non-linguist colleagues during the development of this volume have bolstered our conviction that the field of health communication could benefit from more rigorous collaboration across disciplinary and professional boundaries. This collaboration can be accomplished by bringing new perspectives into an existing paradigm (such as a linguist to a Cancer Center team) or by training individuals to become, in essence, multilingual, speaking multiple disciplinary languages to accommodate various audiences, including collaborators, journal reviewers, or study section reviewers. We believe that our complementary research experiences have contributed to a partial achievement of this goal. We hope that this *Handbook* will facilitate even more of these critical cross-disciplinary dialogues.

To those linguists interested in setting off on this journey by participating in endeavors that involve representatives of other disciplines, we offer the following modest cautionary tale. Whether your involvement will be in research on health disparities, health literacy, or clinical decision-making, to name a few possibilities, it will be in your best interest to consider thoughtfully at the outset of the project the ways in which language is defined, considered, and characterized within your own and your partners' disciplines – and to engage in explicit discussions centered on authentic language data with these fellow researchers. The time spent bringing underlying assumptions to the surface and working through resulting differences will help to reduce subsequent confusion and frustration.

While running the risk of overgeneralization, it has been our experience that researchers trained in fields outside what Bucholtz and Hall (2005) call 'sociocultural linguistics'[1] tend to consider language in a more static way than do scholars who were trained with this sociocultural approach to language. And since many health research teams comprise individuals who have disciplinary backgrounds in medicine, nursing, public health, psychology, and social work, it is likely that, as a linguist, your perspective on language (while arguably a key motivation as to your inclusion on the team) will be in the minority. Illustrations of this non-linguistic understanding of language include the identification of stable lexical meanings that are understood to reflect the world (including its events and interlocutor's attitudes and perceptions); the connection of single functions to individual grammatical structures (such as pronouns or adverbs); and a focus on standard language use (sometimes in a prescriptivist way, although not always) to the exclusion of regional, social, and stylistic variation.[2] These practices are in stark contrast to sociocultural language scholars' dynamic notions of lexical and utterance meaning with the accompanying theoretical interest in socially meaningful variation[3] and the conceptualization of discourse as being interactively co-constructed. In the dynamic view, language does not merely *reflect* the world but works to *create* it as well, along with its myriad meanings, social dynamics, relationships, and institutions.

These contrasting understandings of language, not surprisingly, are associated with different research paradigms. One finds, for example, that the more static understanding of language works most expediently with quantitative and positivist approaches to research, whereas the dynamic understanding of language is more philosophically aligned with qualitative research methods. Specifically, in hypothesis-driven scientific endeavors, replicability as well as internal and external validity characterize methodological rigor; in studies of this type, it is preferable to work with an understanding of language that has less 'wiggle room' in its definitions, so that language data can be coded and counted with a high degree of inter-rater reliability. Given the tighter operational definitions, such approaches can handle vastly larger datasets much more efficiently (see Chou et al. 2012).

The dynamic understanding of language, on the other hand, tends to work more smoothly with qualitative studies that seek to understand situated interpretation; i.e., how 'hearers infer speakers' underlying strategies and intentions by interpreting the linguistic cues which contextualize their messages' (Schiffrin 1987: 21). Because such researchers seek to understand 'joint efforts from interactants to integrate knowing, meaning, speaking, and doing' (Schiffrin 1987: 29) in interactional discourse, the datasets tend to be much smaller (to allow for such fine-grained and nuanced analyses) with ecological validity a primary aim. These differences in approach can be mind-boggling and highly challenging at times – thus the cautionary tale. But our experiences have also shown that a significant investment in time and effort to discuss relative values of each type of approach can lead to the desired outcome of moving beyond differences in assumptions toward a joint solution. Our collective efforts can then be focused on the important enterprise of improving health communication and the concomitant resolution of health-related issues (see also Hamilton 1993 and Robins et al. 2008 for practical solutions to this type of research challenge).

Cross-cutting themes in the volume

We are very grateful that our 68 authors readily and enthusiastically agreed to be part of this collection. Our work with them has provided us with a sustained and wonderful learning experience, one that has helped us to understand old questions more completely and has also opened our eyes to new ones. As we consider issues at the intersection of linguistics and health that are likely to continue to gain in importance, three key themes emerge, each of which has been explored by multiple contributors to this *Handbook*.

Impact and implications of changes in technology-mediated communication

As Web 2.0 and mobile platforms continue to facilitate rapid and interactive exchanges online, communication about health has become ubiquitous and health promotion efforts are increasingly leveraging social media (Chou et al. 2013). Adoption of technology-mediated communication in and outside of the clinical care context has many implications for research at the intersection of linguistics and health, as reflected in this volume.

First, online interactions such as blogs, listservs, and social media have afforded researchers new sources of health communication data through which to better understand perceptions, attitudes, and behaviors related to health. Indeed, linguists have been able to take advantage of publically accessible social media discourse in their investigations, whether using corpus-based, Natural Language Process (NLP)-assisted analyses, or qualitative discourse analyses. Extending beyond the understanding of these interactions in their own right, linguists can offer insights into the type of conversations, content, and structures of online communication to assist 'communication surveillance' endeavors such as tracking of conversations about disease outbreaks, drug side effects, or attitudes about certain health recommendations (e.g., mammography screening tests or human papilloma virus (HPV) vaccine). Second, these new and emerging accessible media have notable impact on healthcare and decision-making, as informational and social support is afforded through digital platforms (e.g., WebMD for medical information, mobile reminder systems for appointments and medications, micromedia and support groups for particular health concerns). Finally, communication technologies that are used during clinical care, such as laptop computers and electronic medical records, necessarily influence patient–provider interactions and present a subject of inquiry in efforts to characterize and improve clinical encounters.

Moving forward, we anticipate that social media will become even more relevant over time. Extending beyond the use of social media as data in observational studies and surveillance efforts, health communication interventions are beginning to utilize social networking sites and mobile platforms to promote health. Such efforts include the prevention of underage drinking and risky sexual behavior, weight management, tobacco cessation, and support for cancer survivors, just to name a few.

The narrative turn in health communication

As multiple chapters in all three parts of this volume demonstrate, narrative insights have been increasingly integrated into a variety of health communication research and practice endeavors; we see no signs that this productive integration will wane in coming years. Some of these enterprises follow Rita Charon's pioneering work in narrative medicine, highlighting the importance of 'medicine practiced with the narrative competence to recognize, absorb, interpret, and be moved by the stories of illness' (Charon 2006: vii) within medical and nursing school education and professional practice. Others examine textual and discursive details of personal experience narratives and the storyworlds they create as a way to gain closer understanding of narrators' perceptions, experiences, and evolving senses of self (Schiffrin 1996) – of both patients and health professionals. Through nuanced examinations of the discursive construction of these storyworlds, researchers can learn, for example, about the emotional toll on health professionals who work in intensive care units; how healthcare professionals position their work within multidisciplinary health teams; how individuals are coping with their diagnosis or connecting decisions regarding their treatment plan to their health beliefs.

Still others have focused on the activity of storytelling itself, seeing it as a 'social practice that both shapes and is shaped by institutional contexts' (De Fina and Georgakopoulou 2012: ix). The recognition of this mutual influence is an important step towards enhanced management of care within institutional encounters. Awareness of this two-way street can help healthcare professionals facilitate the emergence of storytelling within the four walls of the physician's office and within support group sessions, leading to enhanced attunement of interlocutors' perspectives. Discursive characteristics of the narratives that are subsequently told within these institutional settings can then serve as a barometer of the quality of the institutional setting and the relationships that are negotiated within it. Finally, personal narratives are increasingly being incorporated into health promotion interventions (e.g., storytelling videos to increase mammography screening test utilization) and their positive effect on behaviors and attitudes are being documented in the literature (see, e.g., McQueen et al. 2011).

Observation of health communication within authentic contexts

While linguists who work on real-life problems have had an ongoing concern with naturally occurring language in interaction, many studies in the area of health research have construed communication more abstractly and have relied on indirect approaches, including interviews, focus groups, and cross-sectional survey data, to understand the quality of communication. Recently, there has been increasing interest in examining authentic, real-life health communication contexts to shed light on critical issues in clinical care and public health. For example, key concepts and theories in health behavior research, such as risk perception and communication, health literacy, and bioethics, can be further explored within particular communicative contexts involving particular individuals, in contrast to being considered more generically. Applied linguistics and medical anthropology are particularly apt disciplines to offer insights into how people use language in everyday situations to assess their risks, display and enact their health literacy or health beliefs, and make ethical decisions within specific sets of circumstances. Such investigations, as illustrated in this volume, can be expected to enhance the ecological validity of our understanding of abstract constructs, even as the accompanying details may complicate our view.

Closing thoughts

Whether you are approaching this volume as a linguist, a social scientist, a communications expert, a medical educator, or a practicing healthcare provider, we anticipate that you will find chapters that pique your interest, surprise you with a new perspective, or even lead you in new directions. In cases where you would like to pursue specific topics in greater depth, each chapter ends with suggestions for further reading. We also welcome you to explore the wealth of publications contained within the reference sections of all our chapters. In closing, it is our hope that this *Handbook* will contribute significantly to the 'opening [of] the circumference'[4] (Scollon and Scollon 2004) of the field of applied linguistics as it intersects in myriad ways with the dynamic and critically important domains of health communication.

Notes

1 'By *sociocultural linguistics*, we mean the broad interdisciplinary field concerned with the intersection of language, culture, and society. This term encompasses the disciplinary subfields of sociolinguistics, linguistic anthropology, socially oriented forms of discourse analysis (such as conversation analysis and critical discourse analysis), and linguistically oriented social psychology, among others' (Bucholtz and Hall 2005: 586).

2 At this juncture, it is important to point out that this non-linguistic approach has been used very effectively by prominent scholars from outside the fields associated with sociocultural linguistics; see, for example, two of the most far-reaching frameworks in health behavior research, psychologist James Pennebacker's Linguistic Inquiry and Word Count (LIWC) for text analysis and health behavior scientist Debra Roter's Interaction Analysis System (RIAS). In these validated analytic schemes, words and utterances are categorized, coded, and quantitatively analyzed to shed light on issues in health and healthcare. Both frameworks have been very successful in uncovering important patterns in very large corpora of written texts and spoken language interactions.

3 'If structure is at the heart of language, then variation defines its soul.' See Wolfram (2006) for a concise discussion of important aspects of language variation.

4 We are grateful to Rodney Jones for reminding us of the Scollons' skillful metaphor and for connecting it first to his own provocative work on health and risk communication (Jones 2013).

References

Agar, M. (1985) 'Institutional discourse', *Text*, 5: 147–168.

Ainsworth-Vaughn, N. (1998) *Claiming Power in Doctor–Patient Talk*, Oxford: Oxford University Press.

Brumfit, C. (1995) 'Teacher professionalism and research', in G. Cook and B. Seidlhofer (eds) *Principles and Practice in Applied Linguistics*, Oxford: Oxford University Press.

Bucholtz, M. and Hall, K. (2005) 'Identity and interaction: a sociocultural linguistic approach', *Discourse Studies*, 7(4–5): 585–614.

Cameron, D., Frazer, E., Harvey, P., Rampton, M. B. H. and Richardson, K. (1992) *Researching Language: issues of power and method*, London and New York: Routledge.

Capps, L. and Ochs, E. (1995) *Constructing Panic: the discourse of agoraphobia*, Cambridge, MA: Harvard University Press.

Charon, R. (2006) *Narrative Medicine: honoring the stories of illness*, Oxford: Oxford University Press.

Chou, W-y. S., Han, P., Pilsner, A., Coa, K., Greenberg, L. and Blatt, B. (2012) 'Interdisciplinary research on patient–provider communication: a cross-method comparison', *Communication and Medicine*, 8: 29–40.

Chou, W-y. S., Prestin, A., Lyons, C. and Wen, K. (2013) 'Web 2.0 for health communication: reviewing the current evidence', *American Journal of Public Health,* 103: 9–18.

De Fina, A. and Georgakopoulou, A. (2012) *Analyzing Narrative: discourse and sociolinguistic perspectives*, Cambridge: Cambridge University Press.

Epstein, R. M. and Street, R. (2007) *Patient-centered Communication in Cancer Care: promoting healing and reducing suffering,* Bethesda, MD: National Institutes of Health Publication.

Ferrara, K. W. (1994) *Therapeutic Ways with Words*, Oxford: Oxford University Press.

Goodwin, C. (1994) 'Professional vision', *American Anthropologist,* 96: 606–633.

Gotti, M. and Salager-Meyer, F. (eds) (2006) *Advances in Medical Discourse Analysis: oral and written contexts*, Bern: Peter Lang.

Gumperz, J. (1982) *Discourse Strategies*, Cambridge: Cambridge University Press.

——(1999) 'On interactional sociolinguistic method', in S. Sarangi and C. Roberts (eds) *Talk, Work and Institutional Order*, Berlin: Mouton de Gruyter.

Gwyn, R. (2002) *Communicating Health and Illness*, London: Sage.

Hamilton, H. E. (1993) 'Ethical issues for applying linguistics to clinical contexts: the case of speech–language pathology', *Issues in Applied Linguistics,* 4: 207–223.

——(2004) 'Symptoms and signs in particular: the influence of the medical concern on the shape of physician–patient talk', *Communication and Medicine,* 1: 59–70.

Hamilton, H. E. and Bartell, A. (2011) 'Peering inside the black box: lay and professional reasoning surrounding patient claims of adverse drug effects', in C. Candlin and S. Sarangi (eds) *Handbook of Communication in Organisations and Professions*, vol. 3 of *Handbooks of Applied Linguistics*, Berlin: Mouton de Gruyter.

Heritage, J. (1997) 'Conversation analysis and institutional talk', in D. Silverman (ed.) *Qualitative Research: theory, method, and practice*, London: Sage.

Heritage, J. and Maynard, D. W. (eds) (2006) *Communication in Medical Care: interaction between primary care physicians and patients*, Cambridge: Cambridge University Press.

Higgins, C. and Norton, B. (eds) (2009) *Language and HIV/AIDS*, Bristol: Multilingual Matters.

Hornik, R. (2002) *Public Health Communication: evidence for behavioral change*, Mahwah, NJ: Lawrence Erlbaum.

Hunter, K. M. (1991) *Doctors' Stories: the narrative structure of medical knowledge,* Princeton, NJ: Princeton University Press.

Jones, R. H. (2013) *Health and Risk Communication: an applied linguistic perspective*, London and New York: Routledge.

Lave, J. and Wenger, E. (1991) *Situated Learning: legitimate peripheral participation,* Cambridge: Cambridge University Press.

McQueen, A., Kreuter, M. W., Kalesan, B. and Alcaraz, K. I. (2011) 'Understanding narrative effects: the impact of breast cancer survivor stories on message processing, attitudes, and beliefs among African American women', *Health Psychology,* 30 (6): 674–82.

Mattingly, C. (1998) *Healing Dramas and Clinical Plots: the narrative structure of experience*, Cambridge: Cambridge University Press.

Mishler, E. (1984) *The Discourse of Medicine: dialectics of medical interviews*, Norwood, NJ: Ablex.

Peräkylä, A. (1995) *AIDS Counseling: institutional interaction and clinical practice,* Cambridge: Cambridge University Press.

Ramanathan, V. (2009) *Bodies and Language: health, ailments, disabilities*, Bristol: Multilingual Matters.

Ribeiro, B. T. (1994) *Coherence in Psychotic Discourse*, Oxford: Oxford University Press.

Roberts, F. (1999) *Talking about Treatment: recommendations for breast cancer adjuvant therapy*, Oxford: Oxford University Press.

Robins, C. S., Ware, N. C., dosReis, S., Willging, C. E., Chung, J.Y. and Lewis-Fernández, R. (2008) 'Dialogues on mixed methods and mental health services research: anticipating challenges, building solutions', *Psychiatric Services,* 59: 727–731.

Sarangi, S. and Candlin, C. N. (2003) 'Introduction: trading between reflexivity and relevance: new challenges for applied linguistics', *Applied Linguistics,* 24: 271–285.

——(2011) 'Professional and organizational practice: a discourse/communication perspective', in S. Sarangi and C. N. Candlin (eds) *The Handbook of Communication in Organisations and Professions*, Berlin: Mouton de Gruyter.

Sarangi, S. and Roberts, C. (eds) (1999) *Talk, Work and Institutional Order: discourse in Medical, Mediation and Management Settings,* Berlin: Mouton de Gruyter.

Schiffrin, D. (1987) *Discourse Markers*, Cambridge: Cambridge University Press.

——(1996) 'Narrative as self-portrait: sociolinguistic constructions of identity', *Language in Society,* 25: 167–203.

Scollon, R. and Scollon, S. B. K. (2004) *Nexus Analysis: discourse and the emerging internet*, London: Routledge.

Tannen, D. (1984) *Conversational Style*, Norwood, NJ: Ablex.

Wasson, C. (2004) 'Review of *Linguistics, language and the professions: education, journalism, law, medicine, and technology*, J.E. Alatis, H.E. Hamilton, and A-H. Tan (eds)', *Language in Society,* 33: 121–124.

Wolfram, W. (2006) 'Language and variation: an overview', in K. Brown (ed.) *Encyclopedia of Language and Linguistics* II, Oxford: Elsevier.

Part I

Individuals' everyday health communication

1

Health communication 'noise'

Insights from medical anthropology

Nancy J. Burke and Judith C. Barker

Introduction

Health promotion and communication studies often focus on the message and the medium, with the intent of affecting some sort of individual-based behavior change. Relying on a variety of health behavior change theories, the assumption is that effective communication of information can change a person's intention, which will then lead to a change in behavior (Pasick et al. 2009; Pasick and Burke 2008). While behavioral science seeks to understand, explain, and often change human behavior through the adoption of healthier lifestyles, behaviors, and attitudes, the theories employed have an individual, cognitive focus, largely abstracted from social context (Frohlich et al. 2001; Singer and Weeks 1996; Williams 1995). Based on these theories, much health communication research places emphasis on cognitive and motivational variables including how individuals interpret information, how they value that information, and how capable they feel to use the information (Bandura 1984; Krumeich et al. 2001; Singer and Weeks 1996). Social, organizational, historical, political, and cultural influences upon individual behavior are often relegated to the position of background variables, acknowledged only insofar as they affect beliefs that are theorized to be a dominant influence, or comprise factors thought to facilitate or block behavior change. However, critics have highlighted the limitations of this approach. For example, Glass and McAtee state,

> The study of health behavior in isolation from the broader social and environmental context is incomplete, and has contributed to disappointing results from experiments in behavior change. The solution requires a shift in emphasis, a reorientation of theories and new methods.
>
> (Glass and McAtee 2006)

These broader social, cultural, and environmental contexts have been qualified elsewhere as the 'noise' that complicates health communication and behavior change research, and which requires attention for effective translation and implementation (Getrich et al. 2007; Hohmann and Shear 2002). Similar to factors often described as barriers to communication by psychologists and behavioral scientists, what we refer to as 'noise' is not peripheral in the sense of the background static you might hear between radio stations, but rather constitute key components of health communication. In contrast to this understanding, Dixon-Woods and colleagues outline how 'noise' is traditionally conceptualized in patient education research framed within what they call the 'stimulus-response sequence' (Dixon-Woods et al. 2007). According to this model, 'failure of the recipient to interpret the message as intended is attributed to "noise" or "interference" in the system, such as poor readability of the printed materials or (reading) incompetence on the part of patients' (Dixon-Woods et al. 2007). In other words, the onus is on the recipient – patient – to correctly apprehend the intended message. Patients, in this model, are characterized as passive; 'written information will "do" something' to them (Dixon-Woods et al. 2007). Misunderstanding is, in this model, constructed as a technical problem which can be resolved through the application of principles of clear writing, leaflet design, and full disclosure. 'Noise' in this case is constructed as something to be overcome, to be fixed through application of specific communication techniques. In the research presented herein, the aspects of 'noise' emergent from personal, community, and institutional contexts and converging in problematic health communications may also be viewed as opportunities; sites for reconstitution of the whole patient as they interact with and within their social contexts; and spaces for rethinking effective communication. This chapter, then, illustrates the importance of tending to the 'noise' generated in various contexts, and posits that this 'noise' is an essential component of health communication. The chapter draws upon research conducted by the two authors in oncology and dental settings to illustrate the value of ethnography for questioning and broadening assumed understandings of 'effective communication' and 'culture' in health promotion activities, widely construed.

Critical issues and topics

Ethnography and health communication research

The value of qualitative methods for the study of health communication and promotion is well established (Pasick and Burke 2008; Popay et al. 1998; Kiefer 2006). Depending on the scope of the research question, a range of qualitative research approaches can be employed, from broadly encompassing ethnography through successively constricted approaches such as interviews, focus groups, observations, or archival examinations. The funding, time, and staff available for research can often limit the scope of the study, sometimes with unfortunate results. The narrow focus of much qualitative health research (often restricted to focus groups exploring the beliefs and practices of lay persons, for example) limits findings to variations on, and explorations of, preconceived biomedical and social-psychological concepts. Such an approach seldom generates new insights because it fails to understand communication as a result of interaction between health provider and patient, or to question the assumptions underlying the research or the categories and concepts employed; in other words, it does not 'reconfigure the boundaries of the problem'(Lambert and McKevitt 2002). Much qualitative health research also fails to examine the diversity of beliefs and practices encountered in the study populations or settings, which frequently are insufficiently identified, and to understand the degree to which provider-side behaviors help create and sustain barriers to patient participation in various healthcare decisions, as discussed below (Burke 2010; Butani et al. 2008).

Ethnography, however, takes as its starting point the questioning of categories and the critical analysis of the social and historical contexts in which a particular issue has emerged or in which a particular research topic has become acceptable. Ethnographic research questions the assumed normative and universal nature of biomedical categories, and takes a holistic approach to studying phenomena. For example, in a study of clinical communciaton, all actors and stakeholders are included (patients, providers, clinic staff, family members, etc.). Both lay and expert knowledge are explored, juxtaposed, and examined, each within its own context (Fetterman 1997; Lambert and McKevitt 2002; Mitteness and Barker 1995; Popay et al. 1998; Spradley 1979). Another key element that differentiates ethnographic study of health communication from many other qualitative health research and social behavioral approaches is that ethnographers do not limit their understanding to informant statements. As such, medical anthropology distinguishes between what people say should be the case (their opinions and beliefs), multiple perspectives on what is thought to be happening or has happened in the past (i.e., normative behaviors), and actual documented practices (Fetterman 1997; Lambert and McKevitt 2002; Spradley 1979). Ethnographic understanding is achieved through the combination of in-depth open-ended conversational and semi-structured interviews and participant observation. Participant observation involves observation of naturally occuring activities in the research setting and casual comments or informal conversations as well as more formally structured inquiry, through which the researcher identifies cultural norms, influences of socio-economic status and class on relationships and interactions in practice, and other cultural patterns that are not easily articulated or about which discussions are forbidden or difficult (Bernard 2006). The following two examples of ethnographic study of clinic-based communication highlight the different forms of data and consequent interpretations and understandings afforded by anthropologic approaches.

Current contributions and research

Clinical trials participation

Since the passage of the National Institutes of Health (NIH) Revitalization Act in 1993 in the United States, an inordinate amount of resources have been devoted to increasing the participation of minority participants in clinical trials. Approximately 20 percent of all adult cancer patients are medically eligible to participate in a cancer clinical trial, but only 2.5–9 percent of all adult patients do so. Accrual is even less for minority and medically underserved populations (Wendler et al. 2006).[1] Research conducted on the topic has documented barriers that individuals, ethnic groups, and communities face to clinical trial participation (Christian and Trimble 2003; Corbie-Smith et al. 2004; Cox and McGarry 2003; Ford et al. 2005; Noah 2003; Yancey et al. 2006). Research with African Americans, for example, has shown barriers to opportunity, acceptance (including perceived harms of clinical trials and mistrust of research, researchers, and the medical system), and awareness (Corbie-Smith et al. 1999; Ford et al. 2005; Freimuth et al. 2001; Gorelick et al. 1996; Stallings et al. 2000). Documented barriers to participation for Latinos include transportation, toxicity of treatment, and mistrust of research and the medical system (Borrayo et al. 2005; Ford et al. 2005). While cultural barriers such as 'fatalism' for Latinos and the legacy of Tuskegee experiments for African Americans have also been discussed in the literature, how these interact with system barriers associated with low health literacy is not understood (Davis et al. 2002). Despite insights gained from this research and resources dedicated to addressing the 1993 mandate, there has been little success in improving understanding of the issues facing participants or in increasing their enrollment in all phases of clinical trials.

Between 2008 and 2010, Burke, the first author, spent 18 months conducting participant observation in oncology wards in a public hospital. This included observation of clinic visits, treatment discussions, and clinical trials recruitment; participation in clinic rounds and staff meetings; attendance at tumor boards; and participation in patient education and support groups. In the course of the study, over 150 patient visits were observed and 37 patients of diverse ethnicities participated in in-depth interviews in which they recounted their understandings and evaluations of diagnosis and treatment experiences, decision-making processes, and challenges. All interview participants had been offered participation in a clinical trial. Their decision to participate or not, and their experience being part of a trial, if applicable, were also extensively explored. House staff (oncologists, nurse practitioners, fellows, residents) and social support staff (social workers, patient navigators) perspectives were gathered via ad-hoc conversational interviews conducted between patient appointments and at the end of clinic days.

While previous studies of clinical trial decision-making have focused primarily on informed consent processes, individual values, and cost–benefit analyses (Henderson et al. 2007; Lidz et al. 2004; McKay and Timmermans 2009; Probstfield and Frye 2011), analysis of field notes (written at the close of each participant observation session) and interview transcripts revealed the complex and multifaceted nature of the clinical trial decision-making process for public hospital cancer patients. Specifically, these data showed that participant understanding of research and clinical trials, and their decision-making processes were intimately linked to the different social contexts in which they found themselves. As Figure 1.1 illustrates, these contexts fell into three primary and overlapping spheres (Burke 2010; Burke et al. 2009):

- Personal (unpredictable employment, transnational connections/expectations, unstable living conditions, family expectations and constraints, healthcare coverage concerns);
- Community (migration context, neighborhood environment, poverty, experiences of discrimination); and
- Institutional (teaching hospital, lack of resources, physical structure/space, professional culture of providers, culture of medicine, communication between providers, availability of trials and their types, and provider role in research).

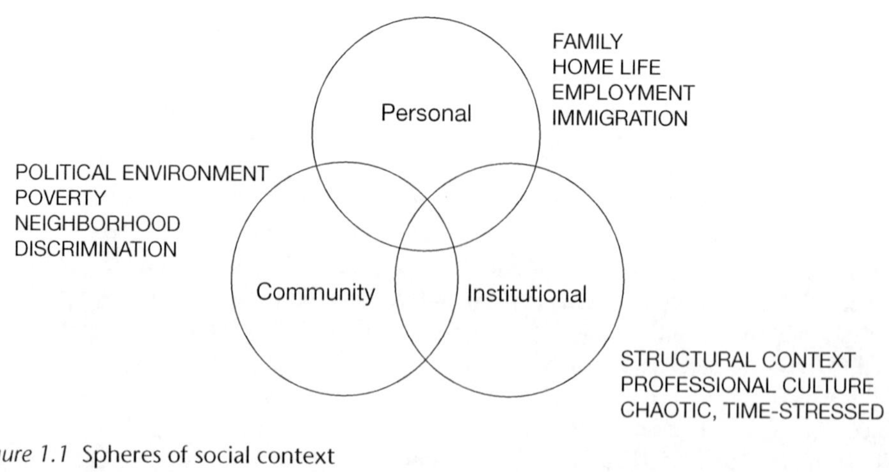

Figure 1.1 Spheres of social context

Personal sphere

The home lives of many of our participants were stressful and unstable, even chaotic. Many patients lived in multi-generational households, and were poor. As one participant said

> I really was a little bit more than paycheck to paycheck, but this crisis [cancer diagnosis], I had run out of all my savings and everything. I had no place to move to. I had no cash. I had no health insurance.

Friends and family were consistently involved in clinical trial participation decisions and often tried to dissuade patients from participating in trials. As one older woman stated

> She [the oncologist] said, you know 'you need to read it [the consent form] and go over it and think about it, talk about it.' And I didn't read it, but I did talk about it with my daughter. And I asked her opinion.

Another related

> A friend of mine was like, 'well, you should actually talk, see if you can talk to some other doctors about it [clinical trial] because they might have presented it to you in a slightly biased way'.

These findings resonate with the general literature on clinical trials recruitment, as they reflect patient barriers and concerns about participation. Our study also documented, however, how these concerns and variable understandings intersected with clinic procedures to produce misunderstandings and misconceptions. For example, one observation of a clinical trial recruitment discussion included the Clinical Trials Coordinator (CRC), the anthropologist, and the patient, a young Latina mother of a 12-month-old girl. The patient spoke English well, having moved to the United States from Mexico in her teenage years. She had come into the clinic that day to discuss problems she was having with her PICC[2] line (the port through which she received chemotherapy). It was bothering her at night when her young daughter wanted to breast feed and snuggle with her. The oncologist discussed these concerns with her, scheduled an appointment for her to go to another floor to have the PICC line adjusted, discussed her current birth control use (and made another appointment for her to change her birth control due to concerns about hormone use), and introduced the idea of participating in a clinical trial. She then left the room, giving instructions to the CRC to follow-up and explain the trial in more detail. The CRC proceeded to go through the consent form, using complicated technical language about various study 'arms' and randomization. Throughout, the young mother nodded her head and smiled, indicating understanding and agreement. As the conversation continued, however, she started looking down more often at the papers in her hands (consent form) and touching her arm which had the PICC line. Finally, after the CRC introduced the idea that the study would be 'blinded' and that they wouldn't know until the end whether the patient had received the trial drug or not, the young mother smiled sheepishly and asked 'Do I have to wear the blindfold the whole time?' Such a statement illustrates a clear disjunction between the goals of the trial recruiter, the clinic, the style of communication, and the patient's ability to grasp so much information in such a short time while experiencing physical discomfort.

Community sphere

Experiences of discrimination and exclusion from healthcare systems, coupled with histories of institutional racism and community experiences conveyed through inter-generational storytelling, can generate mistrust and low expectations. The impact of these expectations on follow-up and treatment adherence became apparent one morning in clinic when a young lung cancer patient (in his forties) was seen. He had been in clinic six months previously, scheduled for radiation treatment, but was then lost to follow-up. When he returned on the day observed, he told his provider he had made the appointment because he seemed to be getting worse. After a discussion of symptoms and physical examination, the clinician asked why he had disappeared, why he hadn't gone to his radiation appointment. The patient responded that he couldn't because he had had no way to pay for the treatment (which would have been administered at a nearby academic hospital) and couldn't face 'getting those huge bills in the mail.' For him, the burdens of debt, shame and powerlessness were strong enough deterrents to keep him from continuing his cancer treatment. The clinician informed him that the social workers had signed him up for Medicaid, so he wouldn't have had to pay for the treatment. The patient's face dropped. The fact that someone else would pay for him to get well was so far from his experience and imagination that it hadn't entered his mind. Somewhere, somehow, communication of this vital piece of information had broken down; either he hadn't heard/understood/accepted that he had been approved for Medicaid or he had never been informed. The result, unfortunately, was advanced disease.

Such feelings of hopelessness and lack of options were often expressed in interviews when patients recounted clinical trials decisions. A young breast cancer patient stated, 'I realize this is the only place to go in the city. If you're poor, or if you don't have insurance, this is where you're at.' Another clarified how her experiences of poverty and difficulty of access to medical care shaped her expectations: 'Truthfully, I felt obligated, like I should always participate in studies ... I think I should help because I've been helped so much.'

Institutional sphere

The research reported here took place in two different oncology clinics in a public teaching hospital, in a women's clinic and a general oncology clinic. Fellows rotated through the general oncology clinic every six months, and residents and students rotated in and out on a sometimes weekly basis in the women's clinic. Patients were often unaware of the distinctions among attending physicians, fellows, residents, and medical students, regarding them as equally and completely knowledgeable clinicians. Patients thus became uneasy when differing opinions or information were presented by various doctors, let alone by clinical trial coordinators. This was compounded by the work flow organization in diverse clinics. In the general oncology clinic, patients had an assigned provider whom they saw regularly until s/he rotated out of the clinic. In the women's clinic, however, patients never knew which provider they would see as charts were picked up in the order of appointment by whichever provider was available. Such disruptions and expectations of discontinuity in care impacted patient feelings of trust and confidence in their care. As one women's clinic patient stated 'but all of these different doctors, it's like a little confusing for me to figure out who I'm supposed to be talking to.' Other patients shared that they were overwhelmed by the experience of being in the clinic and trying to understand their treatment. 'And then when they talked to me about the clinical trials, well they told me that, how did that even go? That went really, I mean, there was so much.' The amount of information and the manner in which it was communicated also caused problems in these somewhat chaotic clinics. As another patient stated 'the information they gave me was like this, and then what I was reading was like this ... If I don't look for the information myself, I won't really get it from the doctors.' Another clarified the relation between this information overload and clinical trial recruitment. 'She did say that it was, uh, hormone, a hormone positive cancer – whatever that means. And that they, and then she told me about a study.' The structures of the clinics – the relatively short time clinicians spent with patients, long waiting time for appointments, lack of consistency of provider, and availability of clinical trials – impacted the kinds of communications that occurred about the precise nature of the patient's condition as well as about trials and how patients felt about these communications. These structural aspects, then, impacted patient decision-making about clinical trial participation.

This ethnographic study of cancer treatment and clinical trials communication highlights the importance of viewing clinical trial recruitment as a process that occurs over time and of recognizing that decisions change in response to many different factors. Conversations about clinical trials occur in many contexts and divergent opinions influence patient decisions. Professional staff in the clinics, whose jobs entail knowing about the technical aspects of diagnosing and treating disease and of conducting and managing clinical trials, often know little about the personal, institutional, and community influences on patients, and underestimate the impact of these on patients' decisions and behaviors. While the majority of research with patients regarding clinical trials understanding and participation barriers identifies patient barriers such as mistrust, low health literacy, fear, and logistical concerns, this ethnographic study clearly highlights the role of structural issues, such as those found in the institutional sphere, as equally powerful yet largely unexplored barriers. The interplay of these structural issues with personal and community issues constitute 'noise' that impinges upon and shapes communication about clinical trials participation in this setting.

Oral health disparities: early childhood caries

Outside of the clinical trial arena, personal, community, and institutional contexts also play seminal roles in oral health care communication and outcomes (Barker and Horton 2008). The Latino immigrant population is the fastest-growing and largest minority group in the United States, numbering 35.3 million in the 2000 census. During the California Smile Survey, conducted in 2005, over 21,000 kindergarten and 3rd grade students were assessed with comprehensive dental screenings. Over half of the children examined were Latino – 72 percent of whom had some caries, while 26 percent had rampant caries or decay in seven or more teeth. These results were nearly twice the determined rates for the non-Hispanic white population (Dental Health Foundation 2006). Young Latino children, those aged 5 or under, especially those of Mexican origin, in low-income families, or in rural locations, have higher rates of early childhood caries (ECC) than any other ethnic/racial group (Nurko et al. 1998; Stewart et al. 2002; Surgeon General 2000; Vargas et al. 1998). Despite this demonstrated need for dental care, Latinos of all ages have the lowest dental utilization rate of all ethnic/racial groups, with Mexican-Americans having the lowest utilization rate of all Latino groups (Newacheck et al. 2000; Scott 2005; US Department of Health and Human Services 2005). These findings persist even after controlling for factors such as age, income, education, sex, and dental insurance coverage (Wall and Brown 2004). The 2000–2003 National Health Interview Survey reported that 16.7 percent of Latino children ages 2–17 years, and 17.7 percent of Mexican American children, had never seen a dentist (US Department of Health and Human Services 2005).

Since 2005, Barker, the second author, has worked with a team of bilingual bicultural researchers conducting ethnographic inquiries into the personal, community, institutional, and macro-structural factors that influence the onset of ECC, a particular form of dental decay that adversely affects preschool children. The consequences of extensive ECC (also known as 'baby bottle tooth decay'), an infectious disease, can be severe and long-lasting – ECC can interfere with permanent tooth formation and jaw development; cause pain, abscesses, and chewing difficulties; create speech and communication deficits; interfere with learning/leisure activities, psychological well-being; and is associated with caries at later points in life (Peretz et al. 2003). Preschool age children are dependent on their parents for help with oral health care, for example, to establish regular practices such as tooth brushing. Research has shown that low-income Latino parents need assistance to learn about the causes of ECC, how to prevent it, how to guide children to develop good oral health habits, and to develop abilities to seek out dental services for their children (Swan et al. 2010).

More than 30 dentists whom we interviewed, in both urban and rural locations in Central California, discussed their encounters with low- income Mexican-origin Spanish-speaking mothers of young children. Over 100 parents, including 35 fathers, talked to us about their experiences of seeking and receiving oral health care for their preschool children (Barker and Horton 2008; Swan et al. 2010). While the oral health knowledge, beliefs, and experiences of parents in urban and rural areas proved to be fundamentally similar, we present here results from our studies with a focus mainly on the rural situation because the impact of communication issues is particularly evident there.

Personal sphere

While few dentists were Spanish-speaking, all had at least one staff member, often a receptionist or billing clerk, who was able to communicate with monolingual Spanish speakers. This communication was fraught with difficulties and inadequacies, and often had undesired consequences, from both the professional and the patient/parent view. The front desk/reception staff or billing clerks called upon to interpret in these clinics were not trained in medical interpretation, nor necessarily familiar with the technical terms embedded in the tiny print on the many forms parents had to sign in order to get treatment for their children. Interpreting was often a perfunctory affair as staff were too busy with their regular duties to do more than tell a parent that the forms allowed the child to be treated and where to sign it (Barker and Horton 2008). Many parents were not literate in Spanish, so providing printed translations would not facilitate better communication. Parents complained that they did not really know what else the forms said and so were unhappily surprised by some outcomes – when, for example, they were excluded from the treatment rooms, or found their child underwent an oral sedation procedure, or was strapped into a 'papoose' to control the child's movement. Children, too, were upset and distressed by the unexpected and unpleasant nature of such experiences and frequently developed dental fears. As a result, some parents refused to return to a dentist who strapped a child down without first receiving permission and so children received incomplete treatment. Similarly, parents thought they were taking children to have their 'stained' teeth cleaned only to discover that the child actually ended up having teeth extracted or receiving restorations because their teeth were carious (Horton and Barker 2008).

Most dentists simply did not appreciate the degree to which parents lacked basic oral health knowledge – of why, for example, primary teeth matter, of the role of diet in dental decay, of how to teach and help a child brush his or her teeth correctly, of why caries prevention mattered or how it could be undertaken. Dentists who were aware of this situation were often pessimistic about the outcome of trying to educate parents about these matters during the child's visit, and so did so rather perfunctorily. Oral health professionals seemed unaware that the majority of Mexican immigrant adults had little interaction with dentists throughout their lives: surveys of recent adult Mexican immigrants, especially those in rural areas, consistently report 20 percent or more of the adult population – especially the male population – has never seen a dentist. Some parents had not owned a toothbrush until they were 10 or 12 years of age. Those from rural areas of Mexico ate a far less cariogenic diet than did their children in the US, and so parents were not familiar with seeing or recognizing tooth decay among children (Hoeft et al. 2010; Hoeft et al. 2009; Horton and Barker 2008).

Community sphere

Two distinct yet interconnected community spheres exist, each with their own consequential communication patterns and habits. One sphere concerns that of the healthcare provider and actions in the clinic, for which some communication activities have already been noted above. The other comprises the wider social and civic setting within which patients and providers live and work.

In the clinic setting dentists described several kinds of 'challenging patients' whom they frequently avoided accepting as patients. Many times the level or nature of decay in young children's teeth was beyond a community dentist's skill set. Most general or community dentists are simply not trained in how to manage the behaviors of young children who cannot sit still for long in a dental chair or who cry, yell, or squirm. Children from low-income families often also have a need for extensive treatment, but dentists will receive only the low Medicaid reimbursement rate that rarely covers adequately the extra time and effort such patients require. Inability or refusal to treat certain children in general dental clinics is liable to be interpreted by parents as embarrassing, stigmatizing, or discriminatory regardless of the practitioner's intent.

Refusing to accept such 'problem cases' necessitates referral to a pediatric specialist so the child could have work performed under general anesthetic, a far more risky, costly, and traumatic undertaking. In the rural areas, the nearest specialist was 50 or more miles away. Moreover, the wait time for a consultation was often between three and four months, especially for a child with Medicaid insurance. No public transportation services were available so the family had to arrange their own access to a car and driver (Barker and Horton 2008). By the time the child was seen, his or her oral health had deteriorated considerably. Because of these financial and access barriers and communication issues, many children simply were not taken to specialists, but ended up as emergency cases where tooth extraction was sometimes the only option.

Dentists seemed unaware of how their treatment decisions could affect a family's well-being, or interface with their patients' personal and community circumstances. In rural areas, dentists generally work in federally qualified health centers and are reimbursed per visit rather than per completed episode of treatment. Rural dentists often asked parents to bring the child back for continued treatment at very short intervals, but seemed unaware that this jeopardized the financial welfare of the entire family. Mothers accompanying their children to frequent dental visits risked and sometime did lose their farmwork jobs for excessive absences. This loss of income in a family already likely to be earning less than $15,000 per year is a severe penalty (Barker and Horton 2008).

Outside the clinic, water consumption practices, community level water access, and understandings of the relationship between fluoridated water and caries prevention combine to further influence childhood oral health disparities. Fluoridation of a municipal water supply is an established, cheap, and effective preventative for dental caries. Most small rural towns, however, lack the resources to provide a centralized water supply, let alone the technical or fiscal resources to successfully fluoridate it. Wells installed on individual properties tap into underground aquifers vulnerable to pollution or contamination by agricultural chemicals and other environmental hazards, making citizens hesitant to consume the water. Moreover, Latino populations whether in rural or urban locations generally eschew consumption of municipal water supplies in favor of purchased bottled or filtered water which is mainly unfluoridated (Hobson et al. 2007; Scherzer et al. 2010), thereby reducing their children's access to an effective means of preventing caries.

Institutional sphere

Documented low-income families were able to sign up for Medicaid insurance. However, during the summer and harvest season with both parents working, the family's monthly income was too high for the children to qualify for health services. Thus, the family would wait until winter when the family had minimal income to enroll their children with a dentist, again, resulting in a delay to accessing care (Barker and Horton 2008). Few oral health professionals realized or made accommodations to this economic situation. Fluctuating seasonal eligibility for public health insurance intersected with a limited community infrastructure and civic amenities, including lack of public transportation, exacerbated difficulties in access to care.

Children's dental fear and poor provider–parent communication were compounded by a scarcity of dentists willing to serve rural (low-income) populations (Mertz and Grumbach 2001). Many healthcare professionals, including dentists, serving in rural areas are doing so under government schemes that enable them to significantly reduce or pay off educational loans if they serve in designated short supply areas for two or more years. This makes it hard for families to establish a trusted 'dental home' and continuity of care for their children. Stringent state fiscal reimbursement policies further complicated the situation. In order to receive Medicaid reimbursement, the state required dentists to provide radiographic (X-ray) evidence of the need for tooth restoration; good quality radiographs are difficult to obtain on young children who cannot sit still (Barker and Horton 2008). Yet another reason why referral occurs to practitioners with advanced training and the technical supports to handle young children.

Several societal sectors or contexts of care significantly intersected to produce or sustain poor oral health care for (rural Latino) children (Barker and Horton 2008; Castañeda et al. 2010; Horton and Barker 2008, 2010). Parental beliefs and practices, leading for example to delay in seeking care, were compounded by lack of key community or economic resources, and by the organization and delivery of professional dental services. In the context of state-mandated policies and procedures, these forms of 'noise' all worked to militate against children receiving timely care that would considerably reduce oral health disparities among this highly disadvantaged population. All of these intersecting processes were intimately linked to communication inadequacies between oral health professionals and their patients.

Conclusions and recommendations for practice

In their innovative work on community-based mental health research, Hohmann and Shear (2002) described clinic 'noise' as unanticipated factors such as patients' own perceptions of mental illness and treatment, primary care providers' non-adherence to guidelines-based treatment, and the social dynamics of the clinic site itself. Such noise, they argued, can impact the implementation and quality of treatment. Within the clinic, Hohmann and Shear identified issues including patient flow, staff organization, personnel disruption, and organizational culture and climate as exerting potential impacts on interventions. Getrich and colleagues (2007) identified three areas of clinic-based 'noise' – the clinics' physical ability to absorb the intervention, the challenges of co-worker instability and interpersonal relationships, and balancing extra workplace demands – in their ethnographic study of community-based mental health interventions in New Mexico. They contend that their research 'highlights the conceptual and practical importance of the intervention sites' spatial and social environments' (2007: 327).

The examples provided herein highlight the conceptual and practical importance of clinic structure, social environment, and patients' interpersonal and community contexts to basic communication of clinic procedures, whether they be the description of a clinical trial protocol, the communication of Medicaid provision, or the meaning and content of pediatric dental care forms. The 'noise' generated by regulatory and institutional contexts within which patients live and healthcare practitioners work must also be recognized and managed for its role in creating, complicating, and magnifying communicative 'noise' in the patient–practitioner encounter. We posit 'noise' to be essential background aspects of interpersonal encounters that should be recognized, identified, and managed. With more mindful awareness, some of this 'noise' can be eliminated; some cannot. Each 'sphere' contributes multiple forms of 'noise' that coalesce, expand, influence, and impact the receipt, engagement with, and understanding of health communication. Rather than posing a straightforward obstacle in need of a technical fix, identification and acknowledgement of the impact of 'noise' on health communication demands complex forms of intervention that engage both the patient, as situated in their social context, and the clinic, as a site of organizational challenges. As such, health communication 'noise' serves as a productive site for rethinking effective communication and appropriate intervention.

Related topics

Ethnography, participant observation, processes of care.

Acknowledgments of funding

K07CA126999 National Cancer Institute, Cancer Prevention, Control, Behavioral, and Population Sciences Career Development Award (Burke, PI) and NIH/NIDCR U54 DE014251 (Barker, PI).

Notes

1 Recent research has highlighted the disproportionate number of minority (primarily Black and Latino men) economically vulnerable participants in Phase I Trials, those that pose the greatest risk to healthy volunteers. Participation of minorities in later Phase Trials (II–IV) is still lower than Whites, however (Fisher and Kalbaugh 2011).

2 Peripherally inserted central catheter.

Further reading

Burke, N.J., Joseph, G., Pasick, R.J. and Barker, J.C. (2009) Theorizing social context: re-thinking behavioral theory. *Health Education and Behavior*, 36(5 Suppl.), pp. 55S–70S. (This paper reviews current theory as mobilized in public health research and argues for the need to include concepts and theories stemming from the disciplines of anthropology and sociology due to their capacity to address social structural as well as individual factors influencing health disparities.)

Russ, A.J. and Kaufman, S.R. (2005) Family perceptions of prognosis, silence, and the 'suddenness' of death. *Culture, Medicine and Psychiatry*, 29(1), pp. 103–123. (Based on ethnographic study of family decision-making at the end of life in American hospitals, this paper focuses on family member understandings of and conversations about prognosis, and the burdens of responsibility and regret posed to families by the ways communication is both conceived and evaded by different players in the hospital setting.)

Shim, J.K. (2010) Cultural health capital: a theoretical approach to understanding health care interactions and the dynamics of unequal treatment. *Journal of Health and Social Behavior*, 51(1), pp. 1–15. (This paper introduces and defines the concept of cultural health capital to help account for how patient–provider interactions unfold in ways that may generate disparities in health care.)

References

Bandura, A. (1984) Representing personal determinants in causal structures. *Psychological Review*, 91(4), pp. 508–511.

Barker, Judith C. and Horton, S.B. (2008) An ethnographic study of Latino preschool children's oral health in rural California: intersections among family, community, provider and regulatory sectors. *BMC Oral Health*, 8, p. 8.

Bernard, H.R. (2006) *Research Methods in Anthropology: Qualitative and Quantitative Approaches*, 4th ed., Walnut Creek, CA: AltaMira Press.

Borrayo, E.A., Lawsin, C. and Coit, C. (2005) Latinas' appraisal of participation in breast cancer prevention clinical trials. *Cancer Control: Journal of the Moffitt Cancer Center*, 12 (Suppl. 2), pp. 107–110.

Burke, N. (2010) Contexts of clinical trials decision-making: a multi-method approach. Oral presentation, *Minorities in Cancer Research*. Miami, FL: American Association for Cancer Research (AACR).

Burke, N.J., Joseph G., Pasick, R.J. and Barker, J.C. (2009) Theorizing social context: rethinking behavioral theory. *Health Education and Behavior*, 36(5 Suppl.), pp. 55S–70S.

Butani, Y., Weintraub, J.A. and Barker, J.C. (2008) Oral health-related cultural beliefs for four racial/ethnic groups: assessment of the literature. *BMC Oral Health*, 8, p. 26.

Castañeda, H., Carrion, I.V., Kline, N. and Martinez Tyson, D. (2010) False hope: effects of social class and health policy on oral health inequalities for migrant farmworker families. *Social Science and Medicine*, 71(11), pp. 2028–2037.

Christian, M.C. and Trimble, E.L. (2003) Increasing participation of physicians and patients from underrepresented racial and ethnic groups in National Cancer Institute-sponsored clinical trials. *Cancer Epidemiology, Biomarkers and Prevention*, 12(3), pp. 277s–283s.

Corbie-Smith, G., Thomas, S.B., Williams, M.V. and Moody-Ayers, S. (1999) Attitudes and beliefs of African Americans toward participation in medical research. *Journal of General Internal Medicine*, 14(9), pp. 537–546.

Corbie-Smith, G., Miller, W.C. and Ransohoff, D.F. (2004) Interpretations of 'appropriate' minority inclusion in clinical research. *American Journal of Medicine*, 116(4), pp. 249–252.

Cox, K. and McGarry, J. (2003) Why patients don't take part in cancer clinical trials: an overview of the literature. *European Journal of Cancer Care*, 12(2), pp. 114–122.

Davis, T.C., Williams, M.V., Marin, E., Parker, R.M. and Glass, J. (2002) Health literacy and cancer communication. *CA: A Cancer Journal for Clinicians*, 52(3), pp. 134–149.

Dental Health Foundation (2006) *'Mommy It Hurts to Chew': The California Smile Survey: An Oral Health Assessment of California's Kindergarten and 3rd Grade Children*, Oakland, CA: Dental Health Foundation. Available at: http://www.dentalhealthfoundation.org/publications.html [Accessed July 25, 2012].

Dixon-Woods, M., Ashcroft, R.E., Jackson, C.J., Tobin, M.D., Kivits, J., Burton, P.R. and Samani, N.J. (2007) Beyond 'misunderstanding': written information and decisions about taking part in a genetic epidemiology study. *Social Science and Medicine*, 65(11), pp. 2212–2222.

Fetterman, D.M. (1997) *Ethnography: Step-by-Step*, Applied Social Research Methods Series, Volume 17, 2nd ed., Thousand Oaks, CA: Sage Publications.

Fisher, J.A. and Kalbaugh, C.A. (2011) Challenging assumptions about minority participation in US clinical research. *American Journal of Public Health*, 101(12), pp. 2217–2222.

Ford, J.G., Howerton, M.W., Bolen, S., Gary, T.L., Lai, G.Y., Tilburt, J., et al. (2005) Knowledge and access to information on recruitment of underrepresented populations to cancer clinical trials. *Evidence Report/Technology Assessment (Summary)*, (122), pp. 1–11.

Freimuth, V.S., Quinn, S.E., Thomas, S.B., Cole, G., Zooke, E. and Duncan, T. (2001) African Americans' views on research and the Tuskegee Syphilis Study. *Social Science and Medicine (1982)*, 52(5), pp. 797–808.

Frohlich, K.L., Corin, E. and Potvin, L. (2001) A theoretical proposal for the relationship between context and disease. *Sociology of Health and Illness*, 23(6), pp. 776–797.

Getrich, C., Heying, S., Willging C. and Waitzkin, H. (2007) An ethnography of clinic 'noise' in a community-based, promotora-centered mental health intervention. *Social Science and Medicine*, 65(2), pp. 319–330.

Glass, T.A. and McAtee, M.J. (2006) Behavioral science at the crossroads in public health: extending horizons, envisioning the future. *Social Science and Medicine*, 62(7), pp. 1650–1671.

Gorelick, P.B., Richardson, D., Hudson, E., Perry, C., Robinson, D., Brown, N. and Harris, Y. (1996) Establishing a community network for recruitment of African Americans into a clinical trial. The African-American Antiplatelet Stroke Prevention Study (AAASPS) experience. *Journal of the National Medical Association*, 88(11), pp. 701–704.

Henderson, G.E., Churchill, L.R., Davis, A.M., Easter, M.M., Grady, C., Joffe, S., et al. (2007). Clinical trials and medical care: defining the therapeutic misconception. *PLoS Med*, 4(11), p. e324.

Hobson, W.L., Knochel, M.L., Byington, C.L., Young, P.C., Hoff, C.J. and Buchi, K.F. (2007) Bottled, filtered, and tap water use in Latino and non-Latino children. *Archives of Pediatrics and Adolescent Medicine*, 161(5), pp. 457–461.

Hoeft, K.S., Masterson, E.E. and Barker, J.C. (2009) Mexican American mothers' initiation and understanding of home oral hygiene for young children. *Pediatric Dentistry*, 31(5), pp. 395–404.

Hoeft, K.S., Barker, J.C. and Masterson, E.E. (2010) Urban Mexican-American mothers' beliefs about caries etiology in children. *Community Dentistry and Oral Epidemiology*, 38(3), pp. 244–255.

Hohmann, A.A. and Shear, M.K. (2002) Community-based intervention research: coping with the 'noise' of real life in study design. *American Journal of Psychiatry*, 159(2), pp. 201–207.

Horton, S. and Barker, J.C. (2008) Rural Latino immigrant caregivers' conceptions of their children's oral disease. *Journal of Public Health Dentistry*, 68(1), pp. 22–29.

——(2010) Stigmatized biologies: *Medical Anthropology Quarterly*, 24(2), pp. 199–219.

Kiefer, C.W. (2006) *Doing Health Anthropology: Research Methods for Community Assessment and Change,* New York: Springer.

Krumeich, A., Weijts, W., Reddy, P. and Meijer-Weitz, A. (2001) The benefits of anthropological approaches for health promotion research and practice. *Health Education Research*, 16(2), pp. 121–130.

Lambert, H. and McKevitt, C. (2002) Anthropology in health research: from qualitative methods to multidisciplinarity. *BMJ (Clinical Research Ed.)*, 325(7357), pp. 210–213.

Lidz, C.W., Appelbaum, P.S., Grisso, T. and Renaud, M. (2004) Therapeutic misconception and the appreciation of risks in clinical trials. *Social Science and Medicine*, 58(9), pp. 1689–1697.

McKay, T. and Timmermans, S. (2009) The bioethical misconception: a response to Lidz. *Social Science and Medicine*, 69(12), pp. 1793–1796.

Mertz, E.A. and Grumbach, K. (2001) Identifying communities with low dentist supply in California. *Journal of Public Health Dentistry*, 61(3), pp. 172–177.

Mitteness, L.S. and Barker, J.C. (1995) Stigmatizing a 'normal' condition: urinary incontinence in late life. *Medical Anthropology Quarterly*, 9(2), pp. 188–210.

Newacheck, P.W., Hughes, D.C., Hung, Y.Y., Wong, S. and Stoddard, J.J. (2000) The unmet health needs of America's children. *Pediatrics*, 105(4 Pt 2), pp. 989–997.

Noah, B.A. (2003) The participation of underrepresented minorities in clinical research. *American Journal of Law and Medicine*, 29(2–3), pp. 221–245.

Nurko, C., Aponte-Merced, L., Bradley, E.L. and Fox, L. (1998) Dental caries prevalence and dental health care of Mexican-American workers' children. *ASDC Journal of Dentistry for Children*, 65(1), pp. 65–72.

Pasick, R.J. and Burke, N.J. (2008) A critical review of theory in breast cancer screening promotion across cultures. *Annual Review of Public Health*, 29, pp. 351–368.

Pasick, R.J., Burke, N.J., Barker, J.C., Joseph, G., Bird, J.A., Otero-Sabogal, R., et al. (2009) Behavioral theory in a diverse society: like a compass on Mars. *Health Education and Behavior*, 36(5 Suppl.), pp. 11S–35S.

Peretz, B., Ram. D., Azo, E. and Efrat, Y. (2003) Preschool caries as an indicator of future caries: a longitudinal study. *Pediatric Dentistry*, 25(2), pp. 114–118.

Popay, J., Rogers, A. and Williams, G. (1998) Rationale and standards for the systematic review of qualitative literature in health services research. *Qualitative Health Research*, 8(3), pp. 341–351.

Probstfield, J.L. and Frye, R.L. (2011) Strategies for recruitment and retention of participants in clinical trials. *JAMA: Journal of the American Medical Association*, 306(16), pp. 1798–1799.

Scherzer, T., Barker, J.C., Pollick, H. and Weintraub, J.A. (2010) Water consumption beliefs and practices in a rural Latino community: implications for fluoridation. *Journal of Public Health Dentistry*, 70(4), pp. 337–343.

Scott, G. (2005) Access to Dental Care among Hispanic or Latino subgroups: United States 2002–03: Centers for Disease Control Division of Health Interview Statistics, www.cdc.gov/mmwr/pdf/other/su6001.pdf

Singer, M. and Weeks, M.R. (1996) Preventing AIDS in communities of color: anthropology and social prevention. *Human Organization*, 55(4), pp. 488–492.

Spradley, J.P. (1979) *The Ethnographic Interview*, New York: Harcourt, Brace, Jovanovich.

Stallings, F.L., Ford, M.E., Simpson, N.K., Fouad, M., Jernigan, J.C., Trauth, J.M. and Miller, D.S. (2000) Black participation in the Prostate, Lung, Colorectal and Ovarian (PLCO) Cancer Screening Trial. *Controlled Clinical Trials*, 21(6 Suppl.), pp. 379S–389S.

Stewart, D.C.L., Ortega, A.N., Dausey, D. and Rosenheck, R. (2002) Oral health and use of dental services among Hispanics. *Journal of Public Health Dentistry*, 62(2), pp. 84–91.

Surgeon General, US Department of Health and Human Services, National Institute of Dental and Craniofacial Research (2000) *Oral Health in America: A Report of the Surgeon General (Executive Summary)*, Rockville, MD. Available at: http://www.nidcr.nih.gov/datastatistics/surgeongeneral/report/executivesummary.htm [Accessed December 19, 2013].

Swan, M.A., Barker, J.C. and Hoeft, K.S. (2010) Rural Latino farmworker fathers' understanding of children's oral health. *Pediatric Dentistry*, 32(5), pp. 400–406.

US Department of Health and Human Services (2005) *Access to Dental Care Among Hispanic or Latino Subgroups: United States, 2000–03. Advance Data from vital and Health Statistics*, Washington, DC.

Vargas, C.M., Crall, J.J. and Schneider, D.A. (1998) Sociodemographic distribution of pediatric dental caries: NHANES III, 1988–1994. *Journal of the American Dental Association*, 129(9), pp. 1229–1238.

Wall, T.P. and Brown, L.J. (2004) Dental visits among Hispanics in the United States, 1999. *Journal of the American Dental Association,* 135(7), pp. 1011–1017.

Wendler, D., Kington, R., Madans, J., Van Wye, G., Christ-Schmidt, H., Pratt, L.A., et al. (2006) Are racial and ethnic minorities less willing to participate in health research? *PLoS Medicine*, 3(2), p. e19.

Williams, S.J. (1995) Theorising class, health and lifestyles: can Bourdieu help us? *Sociology of Health and Illness*, 17(5), pp. 577–604.

Yancey, A.K., Ortega, A.N. and Kumanyika, S.K. (2006) Effective recruitment and retention of minority research participants. *Annual Review of Public Health*, 27, pp. 1–28.

2

Speaking your health

Self-appraised health, discourse, and culture

Mark R. Luborsky

Orientation: self-rate health and survey language and discourse

A puzzle for our time

A modern scientific puzzle is that we can neither predict which rating a person will select when asked to appraise their own health nor why the reply proves so consequential. Today a most powerful predictor of mortality and morbidity is a person's own report of their health when asked the innocuous question '*How would you rate your health today, excellent, good, fair, poor or bad?*' We now know that a reply of 'poor' confers a three-fold greater likelihood of dying relative to a reply of 'good' (Mossey and Shapiro 1982). Further, your own self-rated health (SRH) predicts health outcomes better than objective measures of the body from professional diagnosis and ratings, counts of diseases, gender, or normative constructs relative to the societal body such as age, socio-economic status, ethnicity (Idler et al. 2000). Stated bluntly, an individual's global self-rating of their health is the predictor of future adverse health and mortality, and we cannot predict how someone will appraise their health status based on the material or social conditions of their life.

Despite decades of extensive replication using gold standard probabilistic population-based epidemiological and clinical research, explanations remain elusive for the predictive power of this subjective viewpoint or for just what it is measuring! This puzzling phenomenon holds true for both the very healthiest elders, such as those being followed in the MacArthur Field Study of Successful Aging (Schoenfeld et al. 1994), and for persons with advanced terminal cancers (Shadbolt et al. 2002). The bulk of inquiries into SRH have explored ever larger samples, searched for underlying objective health facts, perhaps undiagnosed, to disconfirm the effect by showing it merely reflects other factors. Only limited success has been achieved. Perhaps it is time to envision newer questions, concepts, and methods.

Here I argue that answers may exist in the neglected but emerging realm of knowledge about SRH's linguistic, performative, and communicative dimensions. The aim of this chapter is to describe the self-rated health measure as a paramount puzzle in itself and an exemplar of more general health appraisal processes. The chapter is organized to first discuss the history and culture of health research studies on SRH (it is unintentionally among the oldest and most powerful survey items); then the discourse and co-production of health reports; and next the diverse units of time, experience, and values implicated despite the instructions to '*rate your health today.*' Finally, it describes a set of methods for studying health appraisal language and communication, and future research needs. Examples are drawn from recent National Institutes of Health (NIH) research and serve to show how the SRH measure illuminates more general health appraisal processes.

History and culture of self-rated health

Health surveys as social innovation, power, and justice

Health survey results are a popular media staple today. Yet the very notion of a survey to gauge the health status of a whole nation or community by means of personal questionnaires rather than direct medical exams is a recent social innovation. Of course, individual diagnosis and treatment stretches back in history (Porter 1999) to our early ancestors well before written evidence in the ancient Sanskrit Vedas circa 1500 BC, and globally across cultures where multiple philosophies of disease, illness, and healing practices continue today. But, the idea of a statistically representative profile of a population's health based on an individual's personal report of their conditions on a questionnaire instead of an objective professional exam is relatively new. Among the earliest was the 1957 US National Health Interview Survey (Linder et al. 1958) conducted annually now by the National Center for Health Statistics of the Centers for Disease Control (CDC). It determines the prevalence of major diseases and risk factors for diseases; findings are used to track our progress in achieving national well-being priorities.

Giving voice to the societal body: national data and social justice

The production of national-level appraisals of the public's health fomented social tensions because the findings revealed social justice issues beyond the raw data on the prevalence and distribution of disease and health (see Krieger 2011; Sweet 2011). For example, early surveys right after the great Depression documented that impoverished citizens incurred more illnesses and earlier death. Given our nation's growing economic capital, and our aspirations to democratic ideals of equality and the 'common' good, the hard evidence of health inequalities is a test of societal success. Surveys reveal unequal distribution of disease according to patterns defined by societal position such as residence, age, sex, income, education, and ethnicity, and regional locale. Raising awareness that health is socially distributed and reflective of basic social economic inequalities, highlights unresolved value dilemmas about how and where to invest funding in health promotion, disease prevention, and treatment.

A fascinating historical epoch is unfolding with lengthening lifespans, prevention and eradication of epidemic diseases such as polio, cholera, influenza, and advanced treatments that save lives after injury, infection, and once fatal conditions (HIV/AIDS) and chronic conditions. Clearly, accurate surveillance to record the existence and changes in presence of health and illness is critical to this progress. Even so, the rising tide of diabetes, cancers, and asthma show new challenges are ahead, not just known ones. This context is the backdrop to the advances discussed next.

Giving voice to the individual: physician exam vs. patient 'self-report'

Early in the emergence of health surveys a trade-off, or negotiation, was required to achieve large scale national data between the disciplinary standards of clinical medicine and epidemiology. Tensions linger today in arguments over subjective and objective measures. From the start health researchers struggled to balance competing demands, diagnostic certainty, and sample size. Objective physical exams conducted in-person by trained medical professionals is needed on a case-basis to accurately diagnose and evaluate an individual's health status. This strategy is costly in time and staff, and yields fewer cases but greater accuracy. Standardized questionnaires, research assistant or self-administered, serve as a proxy for such exams using measures whose limits regarding validity, reliability, and specificity are well documented. This strategy is portable, far less expensive, and provides large samples with greater generalizability. Readers should note that surveys relocate the source of authoritative knowledge from the exclusive realm of medical experts to include the citizen reporting their condition.

Birth of self-reported health: successful tools, socially dubious health discourse

Scientists laboring in the 1950s to create the National Health Interview Survey at the CDC developed a large pool of health interview questions and eventually reduced them to a small battery of items focused on the major organ systems (e.g., heart, lungs, and kidney) and physical function ability. As a tool this early survey showed good measurement properties. But field interviewers found it was socially awkward, even rude to abruptly start interrogating people about personal issues. Recognizing data collection interviews occur within a social event, the scientists decided to add a polite greeting, 'how are you today?' to build rapport prior to collecting the data (Schechter 1993). Of course, no scientific value was expected. Yet to conform to the other standardized questions the wording became 'In general, how would you rate your health today; would you say excellent, good, fair, poor or bad?' The original items were long ago replaced or refined; but the politeness strategy endures as an integral item in large and small studies.

Jumping forward to 1982 a startling article by Canadian epidemiologists (Mossey and Shapiro 1982) gave a new life to the SRH item. Working to locate who were the highest cost consumers of health care in the province of Manitoba (echoing a trend in public health surveillance from the 1930s focus on disease and mortality to the 1950s focus on health and chronic illness), they analyzed objective and subjective health data and actual health services used – and discovered that one question, 'how do you rate your health today?' best predicted death and morbidity. The risk for death for individuals reporting poor health was three-fold greater than those stating good or excellent health. This finding could not be explained away by other measures in the extensive survey using objective factors; SRH was a more powerful predictor than measures of disease, pain, or socio-demographics.

Of course skepticism met this result! How could the patient's own subjective opinion on a single simple question be so profound, and not the medical facts or cost data? An ensuing flood of articles examined SRH and reaffirmed the phenomenon in studies ranging from terminal patients to healthy persons (Shadbolt et al. 2002; Schoenfeld et al. 1994) and internationally. Eventually an ambitious meta-analysis of data consolidated from 27 epidemiological studies convincingly confirmed that self-assessed poor health conferred a roughly three times greater likelihood of death (Idler and Benyamini 1997) and SRH is largely independent from other factors. Now, 30 years later, the phenomenon remains largely

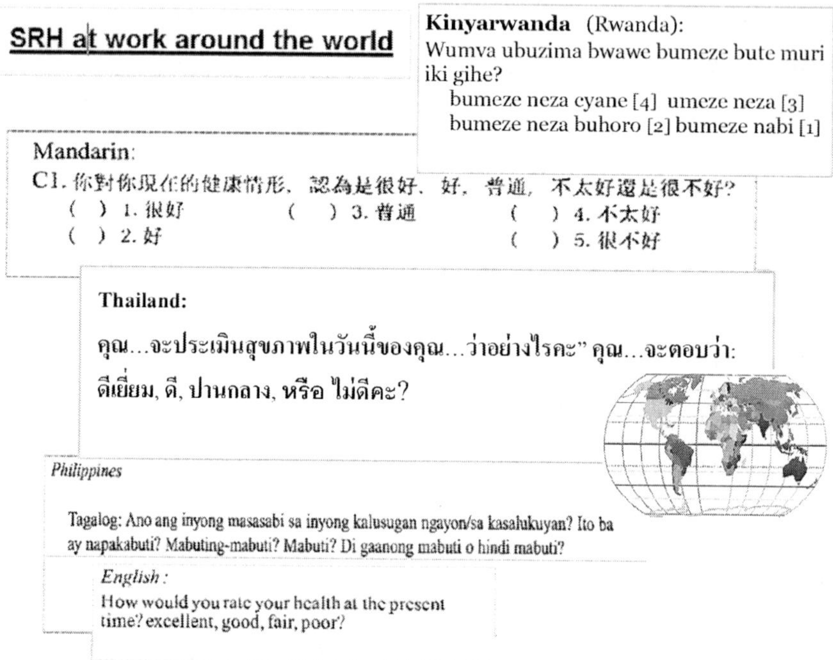

Figure 2.1 Self-rated health at work around the world

unchanged. It is replicated internationally and widely translated into, for example, Arabic, Mandarin, Tagalog, Thai, and Swahili. The World Health Organization annually along with many European countries now uses SRH for its national accountability report card on the legislative and political programs' success at producing 'good' societal health (see WHO 2010; Papanicolas and Smith 2013).

Facts, gaps, and critical issues

This section sketches the basic facts, gaps, and critical issues and serves to highlight where language and communication specialists can make needed contributions; it is not an in-depth review (interested readers can turn to core sources mentioned in the discussion below). It presents a basic portrait of the facts and then outlines instructive variations within and between regions.

Basic portrait of self-reported health

The cross-national view provided by Idler and Benyamini (1997; with added studies in Benyamini and Idler 1999, see also Jylhä 2009) from 27 highly rigorous studies conducted around the world, all using representative samples published in peer-review journals, will be condensed. Each study included adequate measures of physical health status as covariates and evaluated mortality by follow-ups 2 to 18 years later. Considering age, we see a steady shift from youth to old age whereby a declining percentage report excellent or good health and rates of poor SRH rise. Sex differences, though slender, show women report slightly lower health ratings; men's poor reported health is much more predictive of future death. Inexplicably women tend to rate their health worse but end up living longer. For income, every step-wise improvement confers incremental, although diminishingly, better SRH. In more social democratic countries, (e.g., Nordic countries) this effect is less profound. Considering ethnicity, an acute trend is for higher percentages of good to excellent health reports among non-Hispanic whites and markedly low rates among African-Americans and other minorities. Education has a very strong influence in promoting higher SRH across the scale.

Curiously from a language and discourse viewpoint, the putatively 'hard' objective socio-demographic variables actually are self-report items and seldom verified, such as age, sex, marital status, or income. Indeed variables such as chronological age or marital status are contingent social constructs rooted in specific historical periods and cultures, not universal objective tangible entities; some even are subjective such as ethnicity. This undermines criticisms that SRH is subjective.

Arguably the world's largest survey of its kind, the Behavioral Risk Factor Surveillance System random phone survey of over one million US residents, adds to the portrait. In 2008 the survey (CDC 2008) found 85 percent of adults reported good or better health but there is large variation by disability and race. Only one-third of adults with disabilities reported good to excellent SRH, compared to two-thirds without disabilities. Whites without disabilities had the highest rate of good or excellent SRH – about two-thirds versus just half of the black non-disabled respondents. Fair or poor health reports were most frequent among minorities but not among Asians. Readers seeking a detailed account of the design and findings for a highly regarded benchmark longitudinal study should refer to Idler et al. 2000.

Regional gradients adding to the puzzle of SRH across the globe (WHO 2010; Jen et al. 2009; Papanicolas and Smith 2013) are now well established and amplify Townsend and Davidson's (1982) landmark 'Black Report' revealing social class (and regional) health inequalities in the United Kingdom. An East–West divide in Europe exists which offers provocative settings to explore health changes after the former Soviet Republic dissolved. Andreev et al. (2003) combined WHO mortality data and the Russian Longitudinal Monitoring Survey to document the probability of death and poor health rises most sharply in the Russian Federation, with Eastern Europe in the middle, and the lowest probability in Western Europe; the split between Eastern Europe and the Russian Federation expands rapidly for older ages. As the field evolves, regional variations foster scientific debate about the magnitude, cause (speculations include duration since communism, and social capital), and study designs and analyses. Similar variability is observed in China, South Korea, Taiwan, and Japan (Hanibuchi et al. 2012), with Japan having modestly higher and South Korea lower self-appraised health. Data show the US rates of poor SRH have been continuing to rise for decades (Zack et al. 2004). But the pattern is unevenly distributed. The fastest rising poor SRH rates include the southern states such as Texas and Alabama with lower income and high income disparities, while northern states including Michigan and also Hawaii have stable or slowly rising rates of poor SRH with income at middle levels with smaller disparities in income (CDC 2010). In summary, a global view redirects attention beyond the body to societal forces driving down SRH (Kondo et al. 2009) and again illuminates its linkage to contextual and lived experiences.

Critical issues for interpreting the meaningfulness of self-reported health

Meaning-centered approaches to the self-reported health puzzle

Few researchers venture to explore the personal meanings and process of self-appraised health. Qualitative studies show that interpretive processes are essential to understanding self-rated health (Borawski et al. 1996; Idler et al. 1999; Jylhä 2009; Krause and Jay 1994; Silverman et al. 2000). For example, these studies suggest when a person is motivated to uphold desired identities and social values, higher health ratings may emerge as people transcend the biomedical criteria for health; and, this can be a strategy for holding a more positive view of health even when faced with health problems. Results generally parallel survey findings that physical function (e.g., walking) is a focal part of what people gauge when evaluating their SRH (Simon et al. 2005; Manderbacka 1998). Yet these studies use blunt qualitative methods. Specifically, they use a single open-ended question to ask why the reply was chosen, and very basic content coding analyses to generate a checklist of criteria or topics found across the whole sample rather than discerning how each person makes use of their own ideas in reasoning out a reply. Some limited success was provided by connecting generalized personality traits such as optimism or pessimism to a reply that is overly positive or negative given the medical condition (Borawski et al. 1996). Over a 19- year period better SRH was associated with Extraversion and Openness, and worse health to Neuroticism and Introversion (Löckenhoff et al. 2012). Limitations to answers about how personality types lead to expectable kinds of SRH (the notion of an enduring person-trait is not without contention among social scientists) may include questions about how SRH changes while personality traits are ideally stable. Personality traits may struggle to explain regional gradients described above, or the unique individual life history, age cohort, and community meanings shaping each person's interpretation. Fortunately, the next section exposes a host of observable discourse and cultural dimensions that add complexity and refute perspectives that condense the SRH reply to a stimulus-response fashion, even if mediated through a personality-style of attribution.

Even as a step in the right direction by capturing the participant's own words, these qualitative studies have design limitations. For example, personality-type approaches are insensitive to the particulars of an individual's living conditions, personal values, and the interactional discourse of the health interview. The designs ask relatively simple questions about SRH, have a narrow data collection focus, and analyze only spontaneous responses to an open-ended probe. Thus, these studies are tone deaf to the active meaning-making processes of individuals as they go about interpreting the immediate question, the setting, the interaction, and the interview, as well as their own earlier and future life. The methodologies do not aspire to capture the cultural rationales and individual explanations critical to understanding the logic instantiated and condensed by each SRH reply.

'He couldn't help me': a case example of data and limitations of the single open-ended probe

The excerpt below is from an article reporting on a project that conducted one open-ended probe. In it the researchers (Idler et al. 1999) describe their criteria for coding 'poor' SRH and illustrate with one female subject's reply when asked why she replied 'poor SRH'. The researchers argue their coding provides the most valid interpretation. What is your reading?

> The following response was given three initial codes; one for 'serious medical condition', although several conditions were mentioned; one for 'have symptoms', since pain is mentioned; and one for 'the doctor says':
>
> > Eleven years ago I had a mastectomy. I've had a very bad case of high blood pressure for many years. For 15 years, I've had diabetes. I have a sciatic nerve problem, which causes my legs to hurt when I walk. The last doctor I went to wanted to do surgery to remove the nerves around my spine. I refused and said I'd come back when I couldn't walk at all. He said if I didn't want surgery, he couldn't help me.
>
> This woman's response is also an example of a response that belongs in the first grouped coding category, because it contains only the purely biomedical criteria of physical health, diagnoses, and symptoms. Her reasons for rating her health are restricted to diagnosed illnesses and symptoms and to what her doctor says about them; she also rated her health as poor.
>
> *(quoted from Idler et al. 1999: 465)*

In brief, the researchers' identified only topic codes for physical problems and counted many such topics. An alternative interpretation starts by observing the convention used in the publication to display the transcribed talk. The paragraph format erases the naturally expressed language and idea units; rather it attends to conventions for sentence grammar and paragraphs. If we transform the quote by loosely chunking it into idea units following Chafe (1994) then a strikingly narrative mode of reasoning emerges in which the respondent constructs a nuanced cultural rationale and amplifies and intensifies it through repetition. The examples she gives weave a meaningful fabric of personal adversity and legitimate hopes for care, social actions by professionals, and unsavory results. We can see a very different interpretation for the listing of medical problems when I format the talk according to idea units as follows!

1 Eleven years ago I had a mastectomy.
2 I've had a very bad case of high blood pressure for many years.
3 For 15 years, I've had diabetes.
4 I have a sciatic nerve problem, which causes my legs to hurt when I walk.
5 The last doctor I went to wanted to do surgery to remove the nerves around my spine.
6 I refused and said I'd come back when I couldn't walk at all.
7 He said if I didn't want surgery, he couldn't help me.

Perhaps not just an enumeration of physical problems, we see the vigorous theme of a woman seeking needed care which damaged, rather than repaired, her body and capacity to live well. The 'poor' rating may be more about her low appraisal of her society and authority figures, and progressive loss of faith in legitimate expectations to be cared for, exemplified by being blamed (line 7) for her condition, than about her health as such. Approaching this complexly nuanced lifelong framework implicated in judgments about 'your health today' through brute coding or reduction to personality types is not adequate. This illustration is meant to show gaps in current research; a more recent study shows similar limitations (Simon et al. 2005). In this situation communication choices have dire real-world consequences. What you think and say matter!

To summarize, the contemporary rise of attention to self-appraisals marks a turn to legitimating the individual's own appraisal of conditions, in addition to objective medical factors. Historically, health appraisal research has moved several steps from a raw stimulus-response perspective that is uninflected by individual factors or settings. It is gaining a cognitive and more nuanced appreciation of multiple dimensions that inform a particular person's appraisal and production of answers as a combination of expectations and judgments about their health, meanings and consequences of those, and the conversational situations where data are collected.

Methods attuned to discovering self-reported health meanings and processes

Health appraisals are a ripe arena for contributions by language and communication researchers. To date, scant attention is devoted to the discourse context and the individual's own reasoning underlying a reply. Further, a simplistic qualitative method is used, a single open-ended probe, that merely asks people to explain their answer and replies are examined using basic topic coding. Predominantly, SRH studies employ standardized analyses befitting their focus on (exhaustive) replication across populations and conditions of life and the quest to explain it by reduction to correlations with other factors. Despite wide replication, SRH remains weakly explained by normative factors (e.g., age, race, health) or personality types. But these approaches have neither predicted the responses nor explained how people arrive at their own answer.

Expanding the conceptualization of the research problem

What is problematic about the survey questions and SRH in particular? Is it that the question raises issues beyond just bodily conditions and symptoms defined by medicine to include the person's own notions of health, identity, reasoning, and life settings? Yes, but there is more.

A key problem is that surveys demand cognitive effort, interpretive skill, and strategic action from respondents (Sudman et al. 1996). Subjects must work, for example, to understand what the question seems to ask, retrieve information, sometimes events from a distant time, organize and evaluate how to best fit personal experiences and ideas into predefined answer categories, and evaluate the implications in light of prior answers and the next questions. Phrases in questions and answers challenge people to discriminate between closely related concepts or feelings. The task of answering requires expertise at self-reflection about one's own experience. Some surveys expect you to keep the question stem or frame in memory and provide answers to variations in the time, events, or feelings. Readers likely now realize the impoverished nature of a single blunt open-ended probe. The one SRH open-ended probe question simply does not reach deeply enough into the social production in settings, moral reasoning, or experiential features shaping an individual's report on how they appraise and communicate their health with others.

Cognitive interview methods: reflective conversations on the interview itself

Cognitive Interview methods (CI) were developed in the 1980s when survey researchers realized that while standardizing the questions and answers could reveal variations in a population, variations in the actual data caused by individual differences in interpreting the survey were not controlled by standardization. New tools were needed to reduce these threats

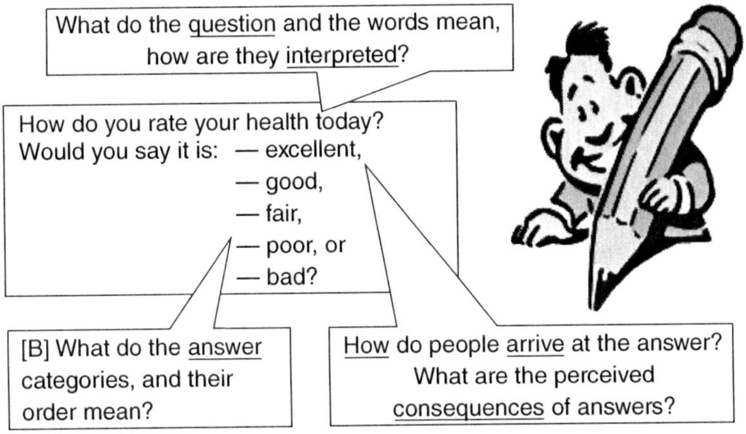

Figure 2.2 Unpacking the self-rated health enigma

to the validity of results. In a nutshell, CI methods enhance survey creation and evaluation by directly asking people how they understand the items, words, directions, answers, and interview process techniques (Willis 2005; Beatty and Willis 2007). These qualitative methods are structured (not standardized) to elicit verbal insights into respondents' cognitions, that is, reasoning and ideas about the survey questions and overall process. They build upon Tourangeau's (1984) four-stage cognitive model of survey response: comprehension of the question; retrieval of information; judgment about information and the adequacy of the answer; response where subjects work to fit their personal experience to the standardized answers categories.

CI employs two formats: (1) *concurrent methods* contemporaneous with the survey questions, and (2) *delayed methods* in a retrospective debriefing and also behavior analysis of conversations in transcripts. Each strategy has strengths and limitations. A benefit of concurrent probes is that memories about answering the question are fresh in mind, whereas for retrospective probes such memories may weaken given the delay between processing the question and the probe. A benefit of retrospective probing is that subjects can reflect on the whole interview without repeated interruptions. For self-administered surveys retrospective probing is preferable to allow completion of the questionnaire without interruption. Other CI formats, such as scientific expert panels or focus groups, are not discussed given the focus on the SRH question discourse with respondents. In brief, CI is widely used for detecting problems in surveys concerning health, labor, and other issues by private, public, and international agencies. It offers valuable tools for basic research on health language and communication and to deepen understandings of SRH.

This section presents a description of key cognitive interview methods I used in a series of studies. Note, the sequence of methods outlined here is not meant to suggest a standard order to follow. Sometimes multiple iterations of a method are used according to the goal and setting. I next describe the methods, some strengths and limitations, and illustrations from a longitudinal study of the meaning of self-rated health (Luborsky 1995; McMullen and Luborsky 2006; Rosso et al. 2008). An overview of the primary project is needed to contextualize my discussion of the methods.

Philadelphia-based Healthy Aging Study

The Philadelphia-based Healthy Aging Study (PHAS; NIH #R01AG15730) was a longitudinal project designed to learn what factors contributed to global SRH among community dwelling older individuals. To ensure adequate sex and race representation of persons for each of the distinct SRH ratings, a stratified quota sample was assembled. Individuals aged 65–74, who represent 'young elderly,' were targeted to increase the likelihood of a wide range across the health/illness continuum. Permission was gained to recruit subjects using the US Center for Medicare and Medicaid Services' computerized files of names of all Philadelphia County residents as the sampling frame. Before randomization, we divided the list of names into four files defined by race (African American/Caucasian) and gender, and the individuals in each subfile were randomly assigned a number. Roughly 25,500 people were contacted to yield the final stratified randomized sample of 241. Data were collected repeatedly for 12 to 14 months using home interviews starting with three extensive baseline interviews including measures of physical, mental, and cognitive health (self-report and performance measures), social and behavioral measures, and in-depth focused ethnographic interviews, life stories, and focused discussions about health, daily and social life, and values. Monthly phone interviews updated information. At the end the baseline measures were repeated. SRH was assessed on 14 occasions with each person.

Conducting cognitive interview methods

Concurrent cognitive interview methods: think aloud, and probing

Think aloud techniques are designed to capture a person's spontaneous reasoning without interruption by the researcher. Participants are instructed to speak their thoughts out loud as they go about interpreting the question, evaluating various considerations, and select their reply. We used the wording below to orient participants to the task and then asked the SRH question:

> Now we are going to do what's called a 'think-aloud' question. Please say out loud what is going through your mind from the time I ask the question until the time you pick and tell me the answer.
>
> For example, let's say the question is 'should you take an umbrella when you go out today?' As you hear my question, you begin speaking out loud what's going through your mind. So you might say, 'well, it looks sunny right now, but it's supposed to rain later. If I take my umbrella, well I might forget it somewhere while I'm running errands, yet my answer is that I should take an umbrella.'
>
> Remember – say out loud what you're thinking, even stuff you start thinking while I'm reading the question. *Okay*? Here's the think aloud question for you to answer: How do you rate your health today? Would you say it is excellent, good, fair, poor, or bad?

Results showed some expected criteria such as physical function, disease, or pain. But significantly 68 percent discussed influences on their answers related to managing the interview conversation, evaluations of the past (even though the question asks about present-day health), and comparisons with other people. Roughly 20 percent explained that regardless of their actual health they could never label themselves 'excellent' because that invites disaster or nothing is perfect, nor use 'poor' or 'bad' because it is morally pejorative. Thus, even though we observe that subjects did not use the full range of reply categories, statistical analyses would not discern this and would, therefore, depict results incorrectly as if the whole scale were used. In another example, reacting to the language of reply categories, two people with the same condition gave different replies.

> *Excerpt 1*
> Oh, I am thinking that, uh, basically I wouldn't ever use excellent, too extreme, and so I'm not suffering in any type of way, so I, my reaction would be, use the word good.
>
> *(female, age 66)*

> *Excerpt 2*
> Well, I rate it excellent because I can still do physical activities the same as I did years ago. And I don't have anything that handicaps me with eating, or working, or physical activities. I don't have any pains or aches on a daily basis.
>
> *(female, age 67)*

Comparative cultural rationales or reference points, neither medical facts nor only 'your health today' as the SRH question specifies, were used by about half of participants to arrive at a health rating. Three cultural rationales were used to frame their decision: *I am doing well considering my age, limitations, disease, or ethnicity or gender* (30 percent); *I could be better, could be worse* (12 percent); *others are worse off and I feel thankful* (15 percent).

> *Excerpt 3*
> At the age I'm at I'm pretty active and, I don't have any disabilities that I could. You know I have a few little aches and pains, but I don't have any disability. My eyesight is fair and everything else is fair. It's not as good as when I was younger. I don't feel like I'm that old but, so I would say I would be in between. I think I'm fair.
>
> *(male, age 72)*

Challenges to think aloud methods arise because subjects are put in an unfamiliar role. Typically survey instructions demand obedience to 'just answering the question' rather than to explain the question and answers to the experts! One strategy to ensure participants understand the goal is to capture the flow of their thoughts and also to acknowledge they may feel a bit awkward or self-conscious thinking aloud. Thus, time is needed to orient people.

Single question probe Immediately after a subject answers the survey question one can probe, 'why did you select that answer?' This technique is widely used to validate new or to refine existing measures to apply in a new population or setting. Analysis of the subject's talk is generally done by coding main topics, decontextualized, to enumerate all topics for the sample. The few qualitative SRH studies that inquired into the meaning of SRH answers (Krause and Jay 1994; Idler et al. 1999) did not conduct follow-up explorative discussion perhaps to enhance standardization. Findings from those studies are quite similar; the reply topics were health and disease conditions, physical function, pain, medications, and comparisons to oneself earlier or to others. An alternative strategy that we used during our longitudinal study of SRH was to repeat the probe at each monthly interview. This helped us learn if the topics or rationales for their health appraisal stayed the same or shifted over time, and how topics related to stability or change in the SRH reply.

Analyses must go beyond elementary topic summaries. The idiom and length of answers were illuminating in the Philadelphia SRH study (see excerpts above). Three response styles were observed: storied, listing conditions, and terse declaration of health status. Sharply differentiated by SRH, subjects explaining a poor or bad health rating deployed longer stories or narratives (mean 66 words) that provided evaluations and events directed to justifying the reasoning for low health ratings; in contrast, explanations for excellent or good were short (mean 40 words) terse statements of the SRH reply, or 'Good, that's just what it is.' The listing of conditions style (mean 49 words) featured inventories, 'I have diabetes, I can't walk' of problems without elaboration or story and was most associated with ratings of fair and less so with good. The roots of self-appraised misfortune, but not good fortune, are suited to narrative modes of reasoning and this is not preserved by methods that aggregate decontextualized topics statistically across a sample.

Limitations to the single open-ended probe include the brevity of responses and the lack of follow-up to clarify and amplify ideas in the reply. These limits constrain the capacity of analysts to develop rich interpretations. Further, as an open-ended qualitative method it limits rapport building needed to gain personal and deeper insights from the participant. Respondents work to figure out what information researchers want, and thus the open-ended probe is overly vague about the purpose or the right style of answer (Sudman et al. 1996). Overall, analyses that tell us what topics people mention cannot teach us how they use the topics to reason, evaluate, and construct an answer.

Multiple predefined question probes Strategically designed sets of probes can be prepared ahead to ensure systematic exploration of known key dimensions. One approach uses probes matched to each of Tourneau's four components of survey cognition. Thus questions address, respectively, comprehension, retrieval, judgment, and response fitting, in addition to suitability of the think aloud task. For example, in our study we began with the following question: 'Did you say things in the same order as you thought them, and, were there things going through your mind that you didn't have a chance to say out loud?' The following are samples of the probes we used. To gauge comprehension we asked 'What do you think that question is getting at? Did you already pick the answer before I finished asking the question?' To explore retrieval and reasoning, 'Did the answer just "pop" into your head, or were you thinking your way through it as you spoke? Were there things going through your mind that you didn't have a chance to say out loud? Was it hard to remember all the different choices?' To probe response fitting behaviors, 'Did you consider all of the choices or only two or three? Did you pick between opposites? Did you want to avoid any of the answers? What is the meaning of each answer category? What would it take for you to pick excellent, good, fair, poor?'

Briefly, multiple probes, such as asking about answers not selected, yield significant insights into the rating process and its salience, as displayed here in the case of a 67-year-old man.

> *Excerpt 4*
> It's difficult for me to think of myself in poor condition, but it's accurate.
> I was healthy so long and never could stand to be weak or having chronic conditions, it just isn't how I think of myself.
> There is some emotional aspect to saying poor,
> I'd rather not be seen as weak or really ill.
> It's hard for me to accept it and I am reluctant to admit it.

Other strategic probes can be tailored to the particular phenomena under study or to build on and critically examine existing concepts and knowledge. In the case of SRH a bedrock dilemma is the statistically high risk for death for those who report 'fair/poor' compared to 'good' health, and this raises an unanswered key question: do respondents themselves conceive of a serious chasm between 'fair' and 'good' or do they see each reply category as being equally distant from one another? To learn how the reply scale was conceptualized this question was asked:

> *Excerpt 5*
> Now, think of the different options – excellent, good, fair, poor, and bad – as points along a ruler. Imagine you are moving the points around on the ruler. Would there be equal spaces between excellent, good, fair, poor, and bad, or would some of the options get lumped together?

Unexpectedly, multiple opinions appeared which complicated interpretation of the scale but perhaps explained the robust mortality effects better than statistics alone. Among these are that subjects asserted: (a) core cultural moral judgments to explain that ratings of 'fair' and 'poor' are self-labeling as a personal failure similar to being financially poor, poor ability to cope or unwillingness to function, while ratings of good reflected morality and success; (b) a 'larger space' exists between 'good' and 'fair'; or, (c) their experience of SRH was one that perpetually fluctuated between the available reply categories so neither of those replies they give can reflect their personal self-rating. Further discussion is beyond the scope of this chapter, however the findings clearly highlight significant complexities in communication and language use and participants' interpretations and personal values during the interview. These kinds of findings should be viewed as offering the very information needed to decipher the SRH puzzle rather than as threats to survey standardization and biases to be minimized.

Delayed method approaches for cognitive interview techniques

Conduct of CI can be deferred until a questionnaire has been completed. Retrospective methods have benefits and limitations and may use the same probes and strategies outlined above. These are valuable when it is important to study the survey process in a naturalistic fashion as it would be conducted without the interruptions of probing after each item. Retrospective CI is also suitable for mixed methods designs that need data from both standardized and qualitative approaches concurrently (rather than at different times) from each person, to allow for meaningful comparisons between findings from each approach. Delaying the probes will protect the validity of the standardized scale data after which qualitative approaches can be used. Delayed methods are valuable in the final stage of survey refinement to evaluate the survey being conducted in its entirety, otherwise features such as effects of the question order are lost when interrupted in the item-by-item style. Also, deferred CI may be helpful when there is a need to minimize probes to responses from one question having an influence on responses to later items.

A protracted delay of one year for retrospective debriefing was used for our longitudinal SRH project to gain participants' insights and meanings of health ratings. During the final interview we probed by showing each person their year-long SRH data and asked, 'how accurately does this reflect your sense of overall health for the past twelve months, and were you aware of this pattern?' For language researchers such data adds a powerful authoritative voice of the participants to support (and complicate!) analyses. Charts were provided depicting each person's 12 monthly SRH replies, but in contrastive formats (e.g., bar graphs, pie chart, line graphs, spider web) for flexibility to learn if we gained different feedback from one or another format. Debriefing subjects by showing them their data facilitated a scientifically unique exploration of issues such as: awareness of SRH patterns; personal lifetime styles in SRH; relation between objective health events and change or stability in SRH; and explanations for multi-month chunks and shifts over time. Analyses showed roughly only 60 percent were aware of the pattern of their SRH replies, but 91 percent agreed it was accurate. Intriguingly, for those whose monthly profile was a regular shift alternating between the two or three answers (e.g., fair/good) subjects explained that the change was not a significant change in level of self-rated health but that the noted fluctuation was a stable personal norm for them. Discovery of these personalized concepts of SRH patterns further challenges interpretation of quantitative survey findings and heightens the epidemiological puzzle of SRH.

Conversation behavior analysis

Traditional methods for conversational analyses are well suited to the discourse of research interviews. Survey researchers use these to examine answers to each item across a sample, or longitudinally from each individual over time. Mishler (1991) argues that the research interview is both a context and narrative idiom and offers a still relevant critique of pervasive views of surveys as analogous to stimulus-response fact gathering neglecting vital discourse dimensions. Labov and Fanshel's (1977) historic comprehensive discourse analysis drew on one segment of a therapy session to examine speech across levels of analysis from phonology, to phrase, sentence, topic, and discourse level. Because these are well-known approaches and also presented in detail elsewhere in this volume, they are only briefly illustrated here in relation to SRH.

The construction of self-reported health and affect among elderly from a large standardized survey, conducted daily for 90 days using a five-point answer scale, was examined using discourse study of transcripts (Luborsky 1995) recorded on several sequential days at about halfway through the subject's participation. Results indicate that perceived health and positive affect is bolstered when a subject enmeshes their reply within side-talk of a life theme or value (e.g., 'I've always been a pusher' or 'the kind of person who tried to be active') compared to lower ratings on days when interviewers prevent side-talk. Self-reports were found to be influenced by the elderly monitoring of (1) prior and subsequent topics; (2) claims to a lifetime vs. at-the-moment self, (3) self-image management; and (4) researcher topic switches that break coherence, turn-taking, or juxtapose topics abrasively (e.g., following a subject's reply of depressed feelings with a researcher asking if the subject is happy). For example, Mr. K. only reported good health and little pain on the one occasion when he diverted and reframed questions about his 'at the moment' affect to answer in light of an idealized lifetime self-image of having always been healthy. In these texts reported positive health was situated in dialogic contexts framed by claims to lifelong personal themes which help instantiate resilience, but negative well-being occurred in talk about disability and social losses. Surely, one takeaway message for survey researchers is to train interviewers about the effects of side-talk; the message for language researchers is that much remains to be learned about the socio-cultural foundation of experiences of health and our scientific knowledge-base about elderly.

To summarize, cognitive interview methods are a powerful tool for the study of discourse and communication. They can provide basic scientific insights into the social foundations and production through language and communication of socio-politically authoritative scientific knowledge about citizens generated by modern health surveys. Further, the methods serve to illuminate a person's conceptions of health and moral reasoning and decisions about health status. Finally, CI methods are practicable and can be readily implemented on their own or in mixed methods approaches in a wide range of study settings and designs. This chapter focused on describing methods rather than detailed findings about SRH; description of patterns in replies, rationales, and their relation to health, gender, or ethnic differences are available elsewhere (Luborsky 1995; McMullen and Luborsky 2006; Rosso et al. 2008).

Recommendations for practice, and future directions

Seldom are the opportunities for language and communication approaches to make significant contributions clearer than to advance knowledge related to individuals' understandings of health and reporting health, particularly given the need for valid surveillance data about health and health disparities. Thus I present a range of recommendations to readers, both those guiding the programmatic development of your research expertise and those concerning your individual research projects.

At the level of the scholar–researcher–practitioner

Important advances in this field require disciplinary expertise and skills and expert knowledge of the numerous specialized tools and techniques for research measurement and study design. That is because the situations where language and communication is relevant span from pilot testing to refining measures to data collection for large-scale studies. At the same time this is necessary because there are many opportunities where such contributions are welcome and valued by collaborative multidisciplinary research projects.

Examples include in-depth historical knowledge and broader disciplinary expertise within your specialty area. First, become well educated about the history and course of the development of research on your topic from across the multidisciplinary working on the topic; this helps to minimize reinventing the wheel or raising questions and suggestions that might have been dealt with already. More fundamentally this work may help you reach deeper insights about long-standing limitations or blind spots. Second, become a specialist about the health condition under study to better understand the forms of knowledge, discursive practices, and settings of life relevant to the condition or health problem. In a similar fashion learn about the particular orientations, interests, and perspectives of the health professionals with whom you will collaborate on the one hand, but also treating them as potential research subjects on the other.

At the level of conducting specific research projects

First, work to become a scientific expert about your field rather than an automaton deploying the current tools. By this I mean: (1) undertake the effort to develop skills and comfort at presenting not just the strengths but also the limitations of the various approaches to gaining relevant information using your disciplines' tools, and (2) articulate potential ways to minimize problems with techniques and concepts in your field. Work to prepare several strong clear philosophical justifications for their use, as well as standard key references where the methods are developed and explained in detail. These are critical to helping you to promote and advance the body of knowledge in your own field, and, even more importantly, they are the calling cards for being a full participant in collaborative and multidisciplinary settings where it is widely understood that the questions and methods we have and our ability to gain data all remain in flux and are not yet adequate to meet the needs.

Second, avoid reflexively retreating to conventional dead-end arguments about qualitative versus quantitative methods (see Luborsky and Sankar 2006). Mixed and multiple methods have existed for a long time (the CI methods are an example) but now are gaining wider recognition. Thus, if you propose a mixed methods approach as a way to situate studies of language and communication, familiarize yourself with the specialized journals, debates and the wealth of other materials on this so that you can more effectively articulate the benefits and limitations in your own use of mixed methods.

Third, explore how other fields utilize approaches you may regard as the exclusive province of sociolinguistics, language, and communication. That is, this chapter showed that attention to language, performance, and meaning have a long tradition but under different names, such as cognitive interviewing, in the development of surveys. Every standardized scale had an early life as a pilot study and preliminary set of measures which were refined and tested using these kinds of methods.

In closing, you have learned about a strangely enduring puzzle and powerful tool for predicting future adverse health and death. The curious history of SRH and national health surveys, the basic facts of SRH and features of self-assessment of health more generally have been clarified. Hopefully it provided a vista onto how the SRH instructions to 'rate your health today' and associated reply categories provoke a vast landscape of concerns from biographical lifetime experiences, values, identities to active cognitive appraisals of the survey goals, meanings behind the language, and interactions in the interview setting. These add up to compelling evidence for much wider arrays of elements in SRH than just the body, even if this has been recognized by prior studies. You also were familiarized with the uses and limitations of some effective tools and illustrations to guide your thinking about how to pursue richer interpretations of health communication in your own work. A prominent concern should be to enhance those uniform check boxes for survey replies with approaches that unpack the rich narrative idioms by which each person appraises and reasons about their health. Finally, methods, analyses, and forms for writing up study results should be chosen to preserve rather than erase such idioms of thought and communication. Truly this is a case where what you think is important. I hope one takeaway message is that we urgently need scholars with expertise in language and communication not to just amass data with existing tools but to hammer away at posing critical new questions.

Related topics

Self-rated health; discourse of health surveys; social determinates of health; cognitive interview survey development methods; analysis of self-assessed health questions.

Acknowledgments

The research reported here is supported by NIH #R01AG13790 and SFO-V/Strategiska forskningsområdet vårdforskning, Sweden.

Further reading

Sudman, S., Bradburn, N., and Schwarz, N. (1996) *Thinking about Answers: The Application of Cognitive Processes to Survey Methodology*, San Francisco, CA: Jossey-Bass.

Tanur, J. (ed.) (1992) *Questions about Questions: Inquiries into the Cognitive Bases of Surveys*, New York: Russell Sage Foundation.

Tourangeau, R., Rips, L., and Rasinski, K. (2000) *The Psychology of Survey Response*, Cambridge: Cambridge University Press.

References

Andreev, E., McKee, M., and Shkolnikov, V. (2003) 'Health expectancy in the Russian Federation: a new perspective on the health divide in Europe', *Bulletin of the World Health Organization,* 81: 778–788.

Beatty, P., and Willis, G. (2007) 'Research synthesis: the practice of cognitive interviewing', *Public Opinion Quarterly*, 71(2): 287–311.

Benyamini, Y., and Idler E. (1999) 'Community studies reporting associations between self-rated health and mortality: additional studies, 1995 to 1998', *Research on Aging*, 21: 392–401.

Borawski, E., Kinney, A., and Kahana, E. (1996) 'The meaning of older adults health appraisals: congruence with health status and determinant of mortality', *Journal of Gerontology*, 51B: 157–170.

Centers for Disease Control (CDC) (2010) *Behavioral Risk Factor Surveillance System annual trend data by state 1993–2010, Percentage of adults reporting fair or poor self-rated health by state.* Available: www.cdc.gov/hrqol/surveillance.htm (accessed May 30, 2013).

Centers for Disease Control and Prevention (2005) 'Health-related quality of life surveillance – United States, 1993–2002', *MMWR: Morbidity and Mortality Weekly Report*, 54: SS-4.

——(2008) 'Racial/ethnic disparities in self-rated health status among adults with and without disabilities', *MMWR: Morbidity and Mortality Weekly Report,* 57(39): 1069–1073.

Chafe, W. (1994) *Discourse, Consciousness, and Time*, Chicago, IL: University of Chicago Press.

Hanibuchi, T., Nakaya, T., and Murat, C. (2012) 'Socio-economic status and self-rated health in East Asia: a comparison of China, Japan, South Korea and Taiwan', *European Journal of Public Health*, 22(1): 47–52.

Idler, E., and Benyamini, Y. (1997) 'Self-rated health and mortality: a review of twenty-seven community studies', *Journal of Health and Social Behavior*, 38: 12–37.

Idler, E., Hudson, S., and Leventhal, H. (1999) 'The meaning of self-ratings of health: a qualitative and quantitative approach', *Research on Aging*, 3: 458–476.

Idler, E., Russell, L., and Davis, D. (2000) 'Survival, functional limitations, and self-rated health in the NHANES I Epidemiologic Follow-up Study, 1992, First National Health and Nutrition Examination Survey', *American Journal of Epidemiology*, 152: 874–883.

Jen, M., Jones, K., and Johnston, R. (2009) 'Global variations in health: evaluating Wilkinson's income inequality hypothesis using the World Values Survey', *Social Science & Medicine*, 68(4): 643–653.

Jylhä, M. (2009) 'What is self-rated health and why does it predict mortality? Towards a unified conceptual model', *Social Science & Medicine,* 69: 307–316.

Kondo, N., Sembajwe, G., Kawachl, I., van Dam, R., Subramanian, S., and Yamagata, Z. (2009) 'Income inequality, mortality, and self-rated health: meta-analysis of multilevel studies', *British Medical Journal*, 339: b4471.

Krause, N., and Jay, G. (1994) 'What do global self-rated health items measure?' *Medical Care*, 32(9): 930–942.

Krieger, N. (2011) *Epidemiology and The People's Health: Theory and Context*, New York: Oxford University Press.

Labov, W., and Fanshel, D. (1977) *Therapeutic Discourse: Psychotherapy as Conversation*, New York: Academic Press.

Linder, F., Woolsey, T., Waterhouse, A., Simmons, W., Sagen, O., Lawrence, P., and Cunningham, M. (1958) *Origin and Program of the U.S. National Health Survey*. Series A-1. Public Health Service Publication No. 584-A1. www.cdc.gov/nchs/products/public_health.htm (accessed June 1, 2013).

Löckenhoff, C., Terracciano, A., Ferrucci, L., and Costa, P. (2012) 'Five-factor personality traits and age trajectories of self-rated health', *Journal of Personality,* 80(2): 375–401.

Luborsky, M. (1995) 'The process of self-report of impairment in clinical research', *Social Science & Medicine*, 40(11): 1447–1459.

Luborsky, M., and Sankar, A. (2006) 'Cultural forces in the acceptance of qualitative research: advancing mixed method research', in L. Curry, R. Shield, and T. Wetle (eds) *Improving Aging and Public Health Research: Qualitative & Mixed Methods,* Washington, DC: American Public Health Association.

McMullen, K., and Luborsky, M. (2006) 'Self-rated health as cultural and identity process: African-American elders' health evaluative rationales', *The Gerontologist*, 46(4): 431–438.

Manderbacka, K. (1998) 'Examining what self-rated health questions is understood to mean by respondents', *Scandinavian Journal of Social Medicine,* 26: 145–53.

Mischler, E. (1991) *Research Interviewing: Context and Narrative*, Cambridge, MA: Harvard University Press.

Mossey, J., and Shapiro, E. (1982) 'Self-rated health: a predictor of mortality among the elderly', *American Journal of Public Health*, 72: 800–808.

Papanicolas, I., and Smith, P. (eds) (2013) *Health System Performance Comparison. An Agenda for Policy, Information and Research,* New York: Open University Press.

Porter, D. (1999) *Health, Civilization and the State: A History of Public Health from Ancient to Modern Times*, New York: Routledge.

Rosso, A., Gallagher, R., Luborsky, M., and Mossey, J. (2008) 'Depression and self-rated health are proximal predictors of episodes of sustained change in pain in independently living community dwelling elderly', *Pain Medicine*, 9(8): 1035–1049.

Schechter, S. (ed.) (1993) *Proceedings of the 1993 NCHS Conference on the Cognitive Aspects of Self-Reported Health Status*. Cognitive Methods Staff Working Paper No. 10. Hyattsville, MD: National Center for Health Statistics.

Schoenfeld, D., Malmrose, L., Blazer, D., Gold, D., and Seeman T. (1994) 'Self-rated health and mortality in the high-functioning elderly – a closer look at healthy individuals: MacArthur field study of successful aging', *Journal of Gerontology: Medical Sciences*, 49(3): M109–115.

Shadbolt, B., Barresi, J., and Craft, P. (2002) 'Self-rated health as a predictor of survival among patients with advanced cancer', *Journal of Clinical Oncology*, 20(10): 2514–2519.

Silverman, M., Smola, S., and Musa, D. (2000) 'The meaning of healthy and not healthy: older African Americans and Whites with chronic illness', *Journal of Cross-Cultural Gerontology*, 15: 139–156.

Simon, J., De Boer, J., Joung, I., Bosma, H., and Mackenbach, J. (2005) 'How is your health in general? A qualitative study on self-assessed health', *European Journal of Public Health*, 15(2): 2000–2008.

Sudman, S., Bradburn, N., and Schwarz, N. (1996) *Thinking about Answers: The Application of Cognitive Processes to Survey Methodology*, San Francisco, CA: Jossey-Bass.

Sweet, E. (2011) 'Symbolic capital, consumption, and health inequality', *American Journal of Public Health,* 101(2): 260–264.

Tourangeau, R. (1984) 'Cognitive science and survey methods', in T. Jabine, M. Straf, J.N. Tanur, and R. Tourangeau (eds) *Cognitive Aspects of Survey Methodology: Building a Bridge Between Disciplines*, Washington, DC: National Academy Press.

Townsend, P., and Davidson, N. (eds) (1982) *Inequalities in Health: The Black Report,* Harmondsworth: Penguin.

Willis, G. (2005) *Cognitive Interviewing: A Tool for Improving Questionnaire Design*, Thousand Oaks, CA: Sage Publications.

World Health Organization (WHO) (2010) Portugal Health System Performance Assessment. WHO Regional Office for Europe. Copenhagen, Denmark.

Zack, M., Moriarity, D., Stroup, D., Ford, E., and Mokdad, A. (2004) 'Worsening trends in adult health-related quality of life and self-rated health: United States, 1993–2001', *Public Health Reports,* 119(5): 493–505.

3

Perceived risk and health risk communication

Erika A. Waters, Amy McQueen, and Linda D. Cameron

The multiple meanings of risk

Risk is a complex concept that has multiple meanings. The term *risk* can be used as a noun (e.g., 'Death is a risk of sky diving'), verb (e.g., 'I'll risk it'), adjective (e.g., 'Sky diving is risky'), or probability (e.g., 'The risk of death while skydiving is ##%'). Risk can refer to multiple topic domains, including financial, health, social, and legal hazards. *Perceptions* of risk are inherently subjective. Although it is possible to calculate a probability estimate of experiencing a particular outcome, the *meaning* of that outcome to an individual varies based on a variety of intrapersonal, interpersonal, contextual, and societal factors that include both cognitive and affective/emotional components (Slovic 2000; Pidgeon et al. 2003; Tversky and Kahneman 1974). It is also likely that linguistic features (e.g., word choice) and non-verbal cues (e.g., facial expressions) help shape risk perceptions. These factors and others make it exceptionally challenging to inform people about health risks in a way that persuades them to change their behavior (Weinstein and Klein 1995; Lerman et al. 1997).[1]

In general, people with higher perceived risk of developing a negative health outcome at one point in time are more likely to engage in health-protective behaviors in the future (e.g., Janssen et al. 2011). The size of the effect is highly variable and dependent upon multiple contextual factors, but for volitional and for new behaviors (e.g., not habitual and obtaining a newly available vaccine, respectively), people need to feel some minimal amount of personal risk in order to be motivated to act (see Figure 3.1). Adept communication of health risk information capitalizes on this relationship by changing risk perceptions in the appropriate direction and improving health-related behaviors.

Educating people about the characteristics (i.e., risk factors) that increase or decrease one's likelihood of experiencing a negative health outcome is one approach to health education, but finer-grained efforts can be more effective. One way to engage in more targeted efforts is to differentiate among the terms *absolute*, *comparative*, and *relative* risk (Ranby et al. 2010). *Absolute risk* is the likelihood of experiencing an outcome over a specific period of time. Absolute risk can be represented as probability estimates or as verbal qualifiers (e.g., Her absolute risk of developing heart disease within the next ten years is <u>2 percent</u>; He is at <u>moderate risk</u> of developing colon cancer in the next five years; It is <u>very likely</u> that he will experience side effects after undergoing treatment). *Comparative risk* is how likely one person is to experience a hazard compared to another person or compared to the average

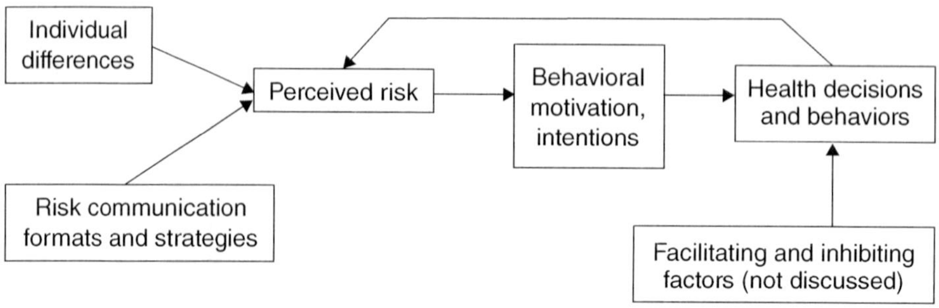

Figure 3.1 Broad conceptual framework of perceived risk, health decisions, and behavior

Source: Adapted from common theories of health behavior (e.g., Health Belief Model, Theory of Planned Behavior, Protection Motivation Theory). See Conner and Sparks (1995) for an overview of each of these theories.

person (e.g., She is at higher risk of developing osteoporosis than her mother, *vs.* His risk of developing prostate cancer is below average). *Relative risk* has a specific epidemiological meaning that identifies the extent to which a risk factor increases or decreases one's risk of developing a particular illness (e.g., She is 50 percent more likely to develop heart disease than someone who engages in daily physical activity). However, the term has also been used in non-epidemiological contexts interchangeably with the term *comparative risk*. We recommend careful use of these two terms; using them interchangeably may create confusion, especially for transdisciplinary research efforts.

This chapter will distill the risk perception and communication literatures into a document that is relevant for researchers and advanced students in linguistics and public health. The chapter emphasizes the challenges inherent in communicating risk and, rather than reiterating established guidelines for communicating probabilistic risk information to individuals, it refers readers to several excellent review articles. This enables the authors to focus on the newest, most innovative, and most promising directions in which the field is moving.

Evaluating comprehension of health risks

For many years, clinicians and researchers approached health risk communication by providing people with probability information. The expectation was that such information would motivate people to engage in appropriate health behaviors. Although such understanding might be helpful under some circumstances, true comprehension involves more than 'getting the numbers right' (Fischhoff 1995).

One reason true comprehension is not limited to the accurate estimation of risk probabilities is because risk perceptions often go awry. For example, many women vastly overestimate their risk of developing breast cancer when asked to provide a numerical probability estimate, but providing them with accurate information may only reduce – not eliminate – overestimation. The situation is somewhat different for comparative risk perceptions. With some exceptions, people believe that they are at lower risk of developing health problems than the average person their age and sex. However, not everyone can be at below average risk. This *unrealistic optimism* (also referred to as optimistic bias) reveals itself in many health hazards and populations (Weinstein 1987). Whether people overestimate their absolute numerical risk, underestimate their comparative risk, or make both errors simultaneously, 'fixing' these perceptions is difficult (Weinstein and Klein 1995; Lerman 1995; Lipkus et al. 2000).

One alternative to viewing risk comprehension as 'getting the number right' relies on a dichotomous conceptualization of perceived risk. According to this view, true comprehension of one's risk might be better understood as a 'gist' interpretation of a hazard as being risky or not risky. For example, one study examined how medical personnel triaged patients presenting to the emergency room with heart attack symptoms (Reyna and Lloyd 2006). Patients could be discharged, admitted for observation, or admitted to the intensive care unit. The most experienced personnel, cardiologists, drew sharp all-or-none distinctions and typically either discharged patients (i.e., the patient is not at risk) or admitted them to the intensive care unit (i.e., the patient is at risk). Less experienced personnel (i.e., non-cardiologists) were more likely to admit patients to a less intensive setting because they were less able to determine whether someone was or was not likely having a heart attack. They resolved this uncertainty by admitting patients for observation. A different study revealed that adolescents who adopted a gist-based view of risk were less likely to engage in risky behavior than adolescents who evaluated risks using a more quantitative likelihood approach (Mills et al. 2008). Specifically, adolescents who thought about the risks of engaging in sexual behavior probabilistically were more likely to engage in sexual behavior than those who endorsed gist-based statements such as, 'No risk is better than some risk.'

Another approach to evaluating whether people understand a risk is to define comprehension more broadly (Weinstein 1999). This approach includes several criteria. First, people should understand the nature of the risk, including its name, the approximate absolute and comparative likelihood of experiencing it, and the severity of possible consequences. People should also understand factors that can reduce one's susceptibility to experiencing harm (e.g., quitting smoking), and the difficulty of avoiding harm (e.g., nicotine is far more addictive than many smokers expect). Although this approach is more complex than inferring comprehension from accurate likelihood estimates, it highlights the fact that risk perception is a multidimensional construct.

Understanding theoretical and conceptual approaches to perceived risk

Health risk communication efforts have met with varying degrees of success. In part, this may be due to a lack of clarity among intervention developers about how laypeople think about health risk information. We briefly describe several theoretical approaches to understanding how people perceive risk.[2]

The *rational choice* approach to perceived risk asserts that people make decisions and engage in behaviors based on a *rational* evaluation of the risks and benefits of engaging (or not engaging) in a particular behavior. Many health communication interventions conceptualize risk in this way (Conner and Sparks 1995), but the approach is incomplete. It does not address habitual or addictive behaviors, and it relies upon a conscious, non-emotional, and rational deliberation and evaluation of outcomes. However, depending on the context, some individuals may not be willing or capable of making detailed calculations. In addition, emotions are integral to risk perceptions.

Another approach to understanding risk perceptions involves *heuristics*, or mental shortcuts (Tversky and Kahneman 1974). The *anchoring and adjustment heuristic* states that risk judgments can be influenced by prior information and any adjustment made based on new information is insufficient. Consequently, the revised risk judgment is still either excessively large or small. For example, a woman who knows she is at low risk of having a heart attack (the anchor) might misinterpret chest pain as intestinal discomfort and not call an ambulance (insufficient adjustment). The *availability heuristic* refers to the tendency that people judge events as more frequent when examples of those events are more easily brought to mind. For example, a woman who has several friends with breast cancer may perceive her risk as higher than a woman who does not have any friends with cancer. *Framing effects* occur when people perceive a hazard differently based on whether it is presented as a gain or loss. For example, presenting the consequences of health behaviors as gains (e.g., by eating a healthy diet you may live longer) or losses (e.g., by *not* eating a healthy diet you may develop cancer) may elicit different levels of motivation to change behavior (O'Keefe and Jensen 2007; Latimer et al. 2007). One manifestation of the *representativeness heuristic* involves judging the probability of an event according to the extent to which it resembles a category. For example, a woman who experiences sudden indigestion, weakness, extreme fatigue, and cold sweats might not realize she is having a heart attack because the symptoms do not resemble (i.e., are not representative of) typical heart attack symptoms. Health risk communicators can use these heuristics to design effective campaigns. For instance, the availability heuristic may be overcome by emphasizing that smoking causes not only lung cancer, but also macular degeneration and bladder cancer (Klein and Stefanek 2007).

Mental models or representations of health threats are another way to conceptualize risk beliefs. The Common-Sense Model (CSM) (Cameron 2008; Leventhal et al. 2003) proposes that cognitive representations of an illness (e.g., for skin cancer) are structured to include information about the label (e.g., 'skin cancer' or 'melanoma'), physical characteristics they associate with the risk (e.g., pale skin, abnormal moles), causes (e.g., multiple sunburns), a timeline of occurrence (e.g., in late adulthood), consequences (e.g., painful surgery, death), and control (e.g., via sunscreen use). These mental models stimulate fear or worry that motivates action, and they guide the selection of protective actions such as getting a skin exam and using sunscreen. By delineating the attributes of risk representations as is illustrated above, the CSM points to specific informational contents that can be used in communications to alter risk perceptions. For example, a communication aimed at enhancing risk perceptions can provide information about the identity, causes, timeline, consequences, and control measures rather than focusing solely on probability estimates. Unlike abstract probability estimates, when these contents are presented in a coherent 'common sense' manner, they are more likely to be encoded and retained in memory.

Despite their absence in many health behavior theories, *affect and emotions* provide information about health threats that is important and distinct from more cognitively oriented conceptualizations of perceived risk (Slovic et al. 2002; Loewenstein et al. 2001). *Feelings of risk* (e.g., 'If I don't get screened, I would feel very vulnerable to getting colon cancer sometime in my life') were more predictive of behavior and intentions than cognitive likelihood estimates (e.g., 'If I don't get screened, I think my chances of getting colon cancer sometime in my life are [almost zero – almost certain]') (Janssen et al. 2011; Brewer et al. 2007). As is evident in the fear appeal literature (e.g., Witte and Allen 2000), *fear* and *worry* are also important for motivating healthy behaviors (e.g., McCaul et al. 1996). In some cases, worry about the consequences of a behavior may be more effective than perceived risk in motivating people to consider changing their behavior. However, fear appeals that do not inform recipients about how to reduce their risk may be counterproductive and may inhibit behavior change.

The *Social Amplification of Risk Framework* (SARF) (Kasperson et al. 1988; Pidgeon et al. 2003) characterizes perceived risk according to a multilevel framework including psychological, social, and cultural factors. These factors act alone and in concert to amplify or attenuate perceptions of risk and to alter behavior related to a particular hazard. Behavioral responses at the individual or group level can produce ripple effects that may have wider societal and economic consequences. This constellation of effects is referred to as *social amplification*. *Social attenuation* occurs when the constellation of ripple effects results in reduced interest by the public. Risk amplification and attenuation may be especially relevant in the current environment, in which the Internet and social networking have important roles in educating and alerting people to health hazards (Chou et al. 2009; Viswanath et al. 2006). Linguists might use SARF to examine how the forms, structures, contents, and contexts of health risk communications affect people's perceptions within the context of social amplification and attenuation.

Individual and contextual differences associated with risk perceptions

As mentioned previously, the goals of many health risk communication interventions include encouraging people to engage in healthy behaviors by altering their perceptions of risk. However, often only modest and temporary changes in risk perceptions have been observed (Lerman 1995). Considering how individual differences and contextual features affect risk perceptions may explain why altering them can be so challenging.

Individual differences

Multiple studies have examined sociodemographic correlates of risk perceptions. In general, gender, education, age, and race/ethnicity are associated with perceived risk. However, the effects are not consistent. Being a woman or being younger is often associated with having higher risk perceptions, but some studies show the opposite relationship. The data are also equivocal for educational attainment and race/ethnicity. Several explanations exist for this heterogeneity. For example, each disease has unique characteristics, and these characteristics may be perceived differently by different population segments. The reason most relevant to linguists is that most studies conceptualized perceived risk according to the rational choice approach. However, risk may hold different meanings for different populations (Joseph et al. 2009). For example, one study reported that beliefs about breast cancer risk among African American women were influenced in part by the belief that 'dwelling' on a risk might cause it to happen (Salant and Gehlert 2008). Other women in the same study were influenced by past experiences of watching loved ones die of breast cancer due to a lack of treatment. These factors combined to prompt some members of the community to avoid discussing breast cancer risk entirely.

Numeracy, or the ability to understand and use numerical information, is another important factor influencing the extent to which health risk communications can change risk perceptions and, consequently, behavior. Low numeracy is prevalent in many countries, including the USA. One study of 500 female US military veterans reported that one-third of the sample believed that 1,000 flips of a fair coin would result in fewer than 300 heads (Schwartz et al. 1997). When provided with numerical information about the degree to which mammography reduces the risk of death from breast cancer, women with low numeracy were less likely than women with high numeracy to correctly calculate the number of women who were 'saved' by mammography. In other words, women with low numeracy were less able to use relevant health information to determine the extent to which a medical procedure was beneficial on a population basis. Low numeracy is also associated with higher risk perceptions, less understanding of the risks and benefits of medical tests and treatments, increased susceptibility to improper use of decision heuristics, poorer quality medical decisions, less ability to indicate health preferences, and lower engagement in health behaviors such as cancer screening (for a review, see Nelson et al. 2008).

It should be noted that numeracy is only one component of general health literacy, which has been defined as 'the ability to read, understand, and apply health-related information in English' (White 2008: viii). Limited health literacy is also associated with poorer health-related decisions and behavior. However, a full discussion of this issue is beyond the scope of this chapter. (For more information, see the Institute of Medicine 2004; White 2008.)

Contextual features

Numerical risk information can also be problematic because numbers alone *lack context*. What does having 'a 12 percent lifetime risk' mean? Should I attend to the hazard immediately? Can I ignore it in lieu of other concerns? People attempt to answer these questions by adding their own contextual interpretations, such as placing the number into discrete categories like 'at risk/not at risk' or 'low/moderate/high'. However, use of verbal qualifiers to interpret numerical risks can be quite variable. For example, some participants might rate an 8 percent risk as 'extremely small', whereas others rate it as 'extremely large'. Individuals may also interpret a wide range of probabilities, such as 30 percent to 80 percent risk, as reflecting a common discrete category such as 'moderate risk' (Cameron et al. 2009).

When people encounter personally relevant yet threatening health risk information, they may engage a variety of *defensive strategies* in an effort to reduce negative affect (McQueen et al. 2012). This can result in rejection of personal health risk information. Greater defensiveness has been associated with decreased risk estimates, increased beliefs that a risk behavior is normative or common, and increased likelihood of engaging in a risk behavior (Gerrard et al. 1996).

In an effort to expand a stage model of defensive information processing, McQueen and colleagues developed and tested measures of four defensive strategies: attention avoidance, blunting, suppression, and counter-arguing (McQueen et al. 2012). In this model, a *defensive* perception of risk is characterized as denial of vulnerability (i.e., suppression of risk information and implications). Identifying the stage at which individuals stop processing threatening health information may identify future targets for improved health communication interventions. Linguists might find it interesting to explore the characteristics of health risk messages and communication modalities that elicit defensive strategies. This information could then be used to devise communication techniques to avoid triggering defensiveness in message recipients.

Differences between *lay and expert views* of risk can also influence risk perceptions. For example, information that experts convey with the intention of reassuring the public may inadvertently alarm them (Levy et al. 2008). Conversely, experts may not understand the value of the experiential knowledge laypeople use to construct their personal understanding of a health risk. Successfully bridging the divide between lay and expert views of risk requires that researchers understand how and why lay and expert views differ. Linguists likely have much to contribute to this discussion, particularly with respect to the different meanings laypeople and experts draw from identical pieces of information.

Communication formats and strategies that affect perceived risk

Health risk communicators and medical personnel seek to improve public health by providing individuals with information about the risks and benefits of certain behaviors and/ or medical treatments. The ways in which risk is communicated can influence perceived risk and, to a lesser but still important extent, health behavior and medical decisions. The formats and strategies used to convey risk information can also obfuscate details and mislead the public. This raises two important questions for risk communicators and clinicians to consider. First, where are the lines dividing educational, persuasive, and coercive risk communications? Second, when, for whom, and under what conditions is it appropriate and ethical to use persuasive techniques? There are seldom easy answers to these questions, but we encourage readers to consider them carefully prior to embarking on their next risk communication effort.

Communicating risk can be daunting; there seems to be an infinite array of possible communication choices. For example, to communicate risk probabilities, one must choose a numeric format (e.g., proportions, percentages, natural frequencies, 1 in N, odds, number needed to treat, relative risk ratio); decide whether to include a visual display and, if so, which one (e.g., bar graph, icon array, pie chart, risk ladder, survival curve); and consider the merits and pitfalls of including verbal descriptors (e.g., unlikely, rare, common) and/or comparative risk information. Numerous studies have attempted to find the best way to communicate risk probability information. The optimal strategy depends on the specific task an individual is asked to perform, but no format will be effective if the information is not relevant and meaningful to the audience. For example, icon arrays may be useful in minimizing some cognitive biases such as denominator neglect, but people with low numeracy and high graph literacy might benefit more than those with low graph literacy (Garcia-Retamero and Galesic 2010).

Several excellent literature reviews describe various aspects of communicating probabilistic risk information (e.g., Lipkus 2007). Readers who need specific advice on communicating probabilities should refer to these comprehensive resources. The following section will focus on health risk communication issues that have received less attention in the literature.

Uncertainty

Uncertainty regarding health risk information takes many forms and affects people differently (Han et al. 2011), but less is known about how to communicate it effectively. Probabilistic risk information is inherently uncertain, both in terms of *whether* an event might occur and *whom* it might affect. A woman with an 80 percent risk of breast cancer might not become ill, but a woman with a 5 percent risk might. It is therefore unsurprising that many laypeople have trouble accepting the personal relevance of a calculated risk estimate. There is also uncertainty surrounding the precision of an estimate. Although an algorithm might provide point estimates for the risk of heart disease (e.g., 5 percent), those estimates are actually within a larger confidence interval (e.g., 3–7 percent). Another type of uncertainty is represented by conflicting expert opinions, as in the case of the recurring controversy in the USA surrounding the value of annual mammography screening for women 40 to 49 years of age.

Most people understand that uncertainty exists and want to know when and if it applies to them, but their responses to receiving such information are highly variable (Politi and Street 2011). Whereas some people respond by placing more trust in the information source (e.g., physicians), others are mistrustful. In the clinical context, acknowledging the uncertainty surrounding cancer treatment options may produce dissatisfaction with the decision process in some patients. People react differently to uncertain information based on their tolerance of ambiguity, other personality characteristics, and the situation or specific context.

More research is needed to develop formats and strategies that effectively communicate uncertainty. For example, one strategy to convey the sense of randomness inherent in probabilistic risk estimates utilizes *dispersed* pictographs in which the affected patients are identified as shaded figures scattered randomly within the display. Evidence regarding the efficacy of this strategy is mixed, with reports of dispersed pictographs having no effect on risk perceptions, increasing risk perceptions, and increasing inaccuracy in providing numerical risk estimates. Providing confidence interval information can heighten absolute risk perceptions if the range is presented as text (e.g., 5–13 percent), but not if the range is presented in the context of a bar graph. Whether confidence interval information is perceived as 'wishy-washy' or acceptable may be dependent upon the individual's level of formal education. There are several strategies that convey uncertainty in a more qualitative manner, such as letter grades and faces, but empirical evidence of their effectiveness is sparse. In a clinical setting, careful conversation can improve communication of uncertainty that results from conflicting expert opinion and insufficient evidence (Politi et al. 2011). Research that identifies specific formats and strategies for discussing uncertainty with patients and the public is critical. Linguists can contribute to this endeavor by examining how subtle differences in the structure and content of language, as well as non-verbal communication like body language, influence laypeople's responses to uncertain information.

Mental model consistency

Another communication strategy that may influence risk perceptions and health behaviors involves the provision of information that enhances the consistency between one's mental model of the health risk and one's mental model of the protective behavior. Mental models, or representations, of protective actions are formed through 'IF–THEN' contingency rules or links. For example, a common-sense link between a risk and action representations for skin cancer risk may be, 'IF sunburns cause skin cancer, THEN reducing sun exposure will reduce my risk of skin cancer.' Motivation to engage in health behaviors and to adhere to treatments may require having a clear representation of the IF–THEN linkages between the health risk and the protective action. That is, individuals may be more motivated to engage in a protective action if they have a coherent understanding of *how* the action will reduce risk.

Research has demonstrated the efficacy of a communication strategy that provides information designed to enhance comprehension of the links between a disease risk, protective action, and disease control. In one study, women smokers who were at increased risk for cervical cancer received either no information, information on the health benefits of smoking cessation, or risk-action link information about how smoking increases cervical cancer risk (Bishop et al. 2005). The risk-action link information explained how cigarette chemicals pass into the bloodstream and travel through the body to the cervix, and how they attack cells of the cervical lining, making them abnormal so that they can develop into cancer. This brief explanation increased perceived understanding of how smoking cessation reduces cervical cancer risk (i.e., representational coherence), which in turn led to greater intentions to stop smoking relative to the other conditions. In other words, representational coherence mediated the effect of risk-action link information on intentions to stop smoking.

More recently, the efficacy of this communication strategy was tested in the context of genetic testing for disease risk (Cameron et al. 2011). A wide range of genetic tests are now available on the market, and many of these tests are for illnesses for which risk can be reduced through protective actions. Yet individuals often have trouble understanding how a genetically conferred risk for a disease could be reduced through a lifestyle behavior such as eating a low-fat diet (Marteau and Weinman 2006). This lack of understanding may undermine the test's potential to motivate protective action. In one study (Cameron et al. 2011), adults received messages about a genetic test for colon cancer risk that either did or did not include risk-action link information about the physiological processes involving the genetic mutation, digestion of high-fat foods, and colon cancer development. Compared to participants who were told only that eating a low-fat diet was important for avoiding colon cancer, participants receiving the risk-action link information reported greater understanding of how a low-fat diet reduces risk, greater beliefs in the efficacy of low-fat diets to reduce risk, and lower appraisals of anticipated risk of developing colon cancer given positive test results. These findings provide further evidence that describing risk-action links may promote risk-related beliefs that motivate protective action. Linguists could have a role in better understanding the development and contents of laypeople's mental models, as well as the IF–THEN links driving protective behaviors.

Narratives

In contrast to informational and expository communications that present reasons and arguments in favor of a particular course of action, narratives use storytelling and testimonials to depict events and consequences for characters (Kreuter et al. 2007). Narratives that 'transport' readers/listeners into another world are more engaging than those that do not (Green and Brock 2000). Engagement and strong identification with a narrative's characters (message source) are expected to increase empathy and cognitive rehearsal, decrease counter-arguing, and influence attitudes, perceived risk, perceived norms, and behaviors (Hinyard and Kreuter 2007). Narratives may increase perceived risk through the identification with and vicarious learning from the characters and by activating self-referencing thoughts and emotions. For example, taking the perspective of a character who has a skin cancer scare after years of tanning may elicit empathy and self-reflection of one's own memories of tanning, thereby increasing perceived similarity to the character and perceived vulnerability to skin cancer. The visual images that are evoked and based on meaning from the story are expected to influence story-congruent beliefs, especially for text-based narratives.

Narratives appear to be a promising intervention strategy for addressing health disparities (Houston et al. 2011), but additional research should determine whether the use of narratives may have an undesirable influence on objective judgment and decision-making. More theory-based experimental research is also needed to elucidate the effects of health communications in narrative format (Hinyard and Kreuter 2007). Understanding the processes and mechanisms, including linguistic processes and mechanisms, through which stories influence health-related decisions and behaviors is critical to maximizing their effectiveness and developing appropriate applications for use in practice settings.

Technology and health risk communication

Technological advances make it possible to develop and implement novel health risk communication strategies. The challenge is to use technological tools judiciously and effectively. For example, placing computer kiosks in clinic waiting rooms may be useful in providing tailored health risk materials, but they may not be feasible if each patient needs 20 minutes to complete the preliminary survey materials.

The Internet provides a promising way to increase the reach of health risk information. Internet use is widespread, and cell phones have expanded its availability to many underserved populations (www.pewinternet.org). However, Internet-based health risk communication has many challenges. First, despite increased prevalence of use, there are still population segments that have limited access to the Internet (e.g., the elderly, those with low incomes). Second, legitimate websites must compete with thousands of other websites that vary in the quality of the information provided. In addition, many websites do not provide the information that users need to evaluate its quality and trustworthiness (e.g., purpose, funding organization), nor are they written in a way that enables users with low literacy to understand. Lastly, although social networking websites like Facebook and Twitter can reach many people, they can also increase the risk of widespread dissemination of misinformation.

Personalized health risk assessment tools provide the opportunity to learn one's objective likelihood of developing an illness. Many of these tools are brief, available online, and provide information about a variety of illnesses (e.g., cancer, heart attack, diabetes). One content analysis identified over 40 interactive cancer risk calculators that were available online (Waters et al. 2009). Unfortunately, many of these calculators did not convey information using effective risk communication formats or strategies. In addition, the literature evaluating the tools' effectiveness is sparse. There is some evidence that the tools can educate people about their risk factors, but oftentimes people are reluctant to believe the estimate provided. Their effectiveness in changing behavior may be also limited, unless they are supplemented by additional educational materials or embedded within a larger intervention (Soler et al. 2010).

Advances in computing technology have also led to increased experimentation in risk communication strategies. One approach capitalized on the power of imagery by showing participants simulated but realistic images of a heart and coronary arteries that had been exposed to a long-term healthy diet and physical activity regiment *versus* eating an unhealthy diet and not engaging in physical activity (Lee et al. 2011). The images changed multiple aspects of participants' risk representations and increased short-term intentions to eat a healthy diet and engage in physical activity. The images also improved consumption of healthy foods two weeks after the intervention. Another study communicated the idea of probabilistic randomness by using a dynamic, scattered icon array in which different figures 'blinked' on and off for a few seconds (Han et al. 2012). Other researchers attempted to convey randomness by asking participants to play a game that required searching for affected cases by clicking identical boxes in an array (Ancker et al. 2011). A very novel approach used virtual reality technology to convey health risk information related to gene-by-environment (GxE) interactions via an elevator metaphor, in which the elevator buttons represented the presence or absence of genetic and lifestyle risk factors (Kaphingst et al. 2009: 388): 'The interaction between genetic risk and exercise behavior was represented as greater downward movement of the elevator for someone at increased genetic risk than [for] someone at lower genetic risk, reflecting increased protective effects of exercise and greater decrease in disease risk.'

Although each of these technological approaches to communicating risk appears promising, several study authors noted that the complexity and/or novelty of the interventions may have impeded learning. Thus, any novel risk communication format or strategy should be thoroughly pilot-tested and implemented with the awareness that the effects may be unexpected or mixed. There may also be opportunities for researchers and/or students in linguistics to explore how different language features and characteristics act independently and in concert with technological innovations to facilitate or inhibit effective health risk communication.

Conclusions and future research

We hope readers finish this chapter with a better understanding of the importance and complexity of perceived risk and health risk communication. Although public health and psychology as academic fields have studied risk perception and health risk communication extensively, many questions remain. We hope that researchers and students of linguistics will find ways to use their fresh eyes and unique expertise to help solve some of the most pressing problems in the field. The following is a non-exhaustive list of topics in which additional research is needed and in which linguists may have a pivotal role.

- Conduct more longitudinal work on the relationships among health risk communication, risk perceptions, and health-related behavior and decisions. Specific focus should be placed on the clinical setting, on multiple health behaviors, and in a wide variety of patient populations and health domains (e.g., diabetes, treatment adherence).
- Identify which language and linguistic choices elicit the most beneficial changes in behavior, not only perceived risk.
- Explore the mechanisms driving IF–THEN linkages and narrative communications, and develop strategies that increase their effectiveness in facilitating health protective behaviors.
- Improve our understanding of the role of affect in risk perceptions, including the unique and combined effects of perceived risk and affect on health behaviors.
- Examine how ethnic and cultural differences in the perceived risk affect responsiveness to health risk communication efforts, including how these differences influence behavior.
- Explore how incorporating theoretical approaches from the field of linguistics might improve existing theoretical and conceptual approaches to perceived risk.
- Improve understanding and communication of uncertain risk information (e.g., what are the characteristics of individuals who are likely to respond negatively to uncertain information; what strategies can communicate uncertainty clearly and effectively).

Acknowledgments

Erika A. Waters was supported by the Barnes-Jewish Hospital Foundation and grant MRSG CPPB-1121401 from the American Cancer Society. Amy McQueen was supported by grant MRSG CPPB-113766 from the American Cancer Society.

Related topics

Risk perception; numeracy; technology; theory; health behavior; emotion.

Notes

1 The construct *risk perception* has many names, including *perceived risk*, *perceived susceptibility*, *perceived vulnerability*, *perceived likelihood*, and *feelings of risk*. For simplicity, this chapter will use the terms *risk perception* and *perceived risk*.

2 To the best of our knowledge, there are no theories of risk perception or communication that were developed by or for linguists.

Further reading

Behavioral Constructs and Culture for Cancer Screening, edited by M. Kagawa-Singer and K.M. Emmons, *Health Education and Behavior* (2009) 36 (5 Suppl.). (This supplemental issue critically evaluates the extent to which several constructs described in many theories of health behavior (including perceived risk/susceptibility) are useful for implementing cancer screening interventions in racially and ethnically diverse populations.)

Fagelin, A., Zikmund-Fisher, B.J. and Ubel, P.A. (2011) 'Helping patients decide: ten steps to better risk communication', *Journal of National Cancer Institute*, 103(19): 1436–1443. (This article describes ten specific strategies for improving risk communication in the healthcare setting.)

Lipkus, I.M. (2007) 'Numeric, verbal, and visual formats of conveying health risks: suggested best practices and future recommendations', *Medical Decision Making*, 27: 696–713. (This article reviews over 20 years' worth of research examining how different risk communication formats affect cognitions and behavior among laypeople.)

Politi, M.C., Han, P.K.J. and Col, N.F. (2007) 'Communicating the uncertainty of harms and benefits of medical interventions', *Medical Decision Making*, 27: 681–695. (This article summarizes the state of the literature on communicating uncertainty to laypeople.)

Slovic, P. (2000) *The Perception of Risk*, London: Earthscan. (This book is a compilation of 25 years' worth of research that seeks to understand how people conceptualize, perceive, and use probabilistic risk information.)

References

Ancker, J.S., Weber, E.U. and Kukafka, R. (2011) 'Effects of game-like interactive graphics on risk perceptions and decisions', *Medical Decision Making*, 31: 130–142.

Bishop, A.J., Marteau, T.M., Hall, S., Kitchener, H. and Hajek, P. (2005) 'Increasing women's intentions to stop smoking following an abnormal cervical smear test result', *Preventative Medicine*, 41: 179–185.

Brewer, N.T., Chapman, G.B., Gibbons, F.X., Gerrard, M. and McCaul, K.D. (2007) 'A meta-analysis of the relationship between risk perception and health behavior: the example of vaccination', *Health Psychology*, 26: 136–145.

Cameron, L.D. (2008) 'Illness risk representations and motivations to engage in protective behavior: the case of skin cancer risk', *Psychology and Health*, 23: 91–112.

Cameron, L.D., Sherman, K.A., Marteau, T.M. and Brown, P.M. (2009) 'Impact of genetic risk information and type of disease on perceived risk, anticipated affect, and expected consequences of genetic tests', *Health Psychology*, 28: 307–316.

Cameron, L.D., Marteau, T.M., Brown, P.M., Klein, W.M. and Sherman, K.A. (2011) 'Communication strategies for enhancing understanding of the behavioral implications of genetic and biomarker tests for disease risk: the role of coherence', *Journal of Behavior Medicine*, 35(3): 286–298.

Chou, W.Y., Hunt, Y.M., Beckjord, E.B., Moser, R.P. and Hesse, B.W. (2009) 'Social media use in the United States: implications for health communication', *Journal of Medical Internet Research*, 11: e48.

Conner, M. and Sparks, P. (1995) 'The theory of planned behaviour and health behaviours', in M. Conner and P. Norman (eds) *Predicting Health Behaviour*, Philadelphia, PA: Open University Press.

Fischhoff, B. (1995) 'Risk perception and communication unplugged: twenty years of progress', *Risk Analysis*, 15: 137–145.

Garcia-Retamero, R. and Galesic, M. (2010) 'Who profits from visual aids: overcoming challenges in people's understanding of risks', *Social Science Medicine*, 70: 1019–1025.

Gerrard, M., Gibbons, F.X., Benthin, A.C. and Hessling, R.M. (1996) 'A longitudinal study of the reciprocal nature of risk behaviors and cognitions in adolescents: what you do shapes what you think, and vice versa', *Health Psychology*, 16: 344–354.

Green, M.C. and Brock, T.C. (2000) 'The role of transportation in the persuasiveness of public narratives', *Journal of Personality and Social Psychology*, 79: 701–721.

Han, P.K., Klein, W.M. and Arora, N.K. (2011) 'Varieties of uncertainty in health care: a conceptual taxonomy', *Medical Decision Making*, 31(6): 828–838.

Han, P.K., Klein, W.M., Killam, B., Lehhman, T., Massett, H. and Freedman, A.N. (2012) 'Representing randomness in the communication of individualized cancer risk estimates: effects on cancer risk perceptions, worry, and subjective uncertainty about risk', *Patient Education and Counseling*, 86: 106–113.

Hinyard, L.J. and Kreuter, M.W. (2007) 'Using narrative communciation as a tool for health behavior change: a conceptual, theoretical, and empirical overview', *Health Education and Behavior*, 34: 777–792.

Houston, T.K., Allison, J.J., Sussman, M., Horn, W., Holt, C.L., Trobaugh, J., et al. (2011) 'Culturally appropriate storytelling to improve blood pressure', *Annals of Internal Medicine,* 154: 77–84.

Institute of Medicine (2004) *Health Literacy: A Prescription to End Confusion,* Washington, DC: National Academies Press.

Janssen, E., Van Osch, L., De Vries, H. and Lechner, L. (2011) 'Measuring risk perceptions of skin cancer: reliability and validity of different operationalizations', *British Journal of Health Psychology,* 16: 92–112.

Joseph, G., Burke, N.J., Tuason, N., Barker, J C. and Pasick, R.J. (2009) 'Perceived susceptibility to illness and perceived benefits of preventive care: an exploration of behavioral theory constructs in a transcultural context', *Health Education and Behavior,* 36: 71S–90S.

Kaphingst, K.A., Persky, S., McCall, C., Lachance, C., Beall, A.C. and Blascovich, J. (2009) 'Testing communication strategies to convey genomic concepts using virtual reality technology', *Journal of Health Communication,* 14: 384–399.

Kasperson, R.E., Renn, O., Slovic, P., Brown, H.S., Emel, J., Goble, R., et al. (1988) 'The social amplification of risk: a conceptual framework', *Risk Analysis,* 8: 177–187.

Klein, W.M.P. and Stefanek, M.E. (2007) 'Cancer risk elicitation and communication: lessons from the psychology of risk perception', *CA: A Cancer Journal for Clinicians,* 57: 147–167.

Kreuter, M.W., Green, M.C., Cappella, J.N., Slater, M.D., Wise, M.E., Storey, D., et al. (2007) 'Narrative communication in cancer prevention and control: a framework to guide research and application', *Annals of Behavioral Medicine,* 33: 221–235.

Latimer, A.E., Salovey, P. and Rothman, A.J. (2007) 'The effectiveness of gain-framed messages for encouraging disease prevention behavior: Is all hope lost?', *Journal of Health Communication,* 12: 634–649.

Lee, T.J., Cameron, L.D., Wunsche, B. and Stevens, C. (2011) 'A randomized trial of computer-based communications using imagery and text information to alter representations of heart disease risk and motivate protective behaviour', *British Journal of Health Psychology,* 16: 72–91.

Lerman, C. (1995) 'Effects of individualized breast cancer risk counseling: a randomized trial', *Journal of the National Cancer Institute,* 87: 286–292.

Lerman, C., Biesecker, B., Benkendorf, J.L., Kerner, J., Gomez-Caminero, A., Hughes, C. and Reed, M. (1997) 'Controlled trial of pretest education approaches to enhance informed decision-making for BRCA1 gene testing', *Journal of the National Cancer Institute,* 89: 148–157.

Leventhal, H., Brissette, I. and Leventhal, E.A. (2003) 'The common-sense model of self-regulation of health and illness', in L.D. Cameron and H. Leventhal (eds) *The Self-Regulation of Health and Illness Behaviour,* New York: Routledge.

Levy, A.G., Weinstein, N., Kidney, E., Scheld, S. and Guarnaccia, P. (2008) 'Lay and expert interpretations of cancer cluster evidence', *Risk Analysis,* 28: 1531–1538.

Lipkus, I.M. (2007) 'Numeric, verbal, and visual formats of conveying health risks: suggested best practices and future recommendations', *Medical Decision Making,* 27: 696–713.

Lipkus, I.M., Kuchibhatla, M., McBride, C.M., Bosworth, H.B., Pollack, K.I., Siegler, I.C. and Rimer, B.K. (2000) 'Relationships among breast cancer perceived absolute risk, comparative risk, and worries', *Cancer Epidemiology, Biomarkers and Prevention,* 9: 973–975.

Loewenstein, G.F., Weber, E.U., Hsee, C.K. and Welch, N. (2001) 'Risk as feelings', *Psychological Bulletin,* 127: 267–286.

McCaul, K.D., Branstetter, A.D., Schroeder, D.M. and Glasgow, R.E. (1996) 'What is the relationship between breast cancer risk and mammography screening? A meta-analytic review', *Health Psychology,* 15: 423–429.

McQueen, A., Vernon, S.W. and Swank, P.R. (2012) 'Construct definition and scale development for defensive information processing: an application to colorectal cancer screening', *Health Psychology,* 32(2): 190–202.

Marteau, T.M. and Weinman, J. (2006) 'Self-regulation and the behavioural response to DNA risk information: a theoretical analysis and framework for future research', *Social Science and Medicine,* 62: 1360–1368.

Mills, B., Reyna, V.F. and Estrada, S. (2008) 'Explaining contradictory relations between risk perception and risk taking', *Psychological Science,* 19: 429–433.

Nelson, W., Reyna, V.F., Fagerlin, A., Lipkus, I. and Peters, E. (2008) 'Clinical implications of numeracy: theory and practice', *Annals of Behavioral Medicine,* 35: 261–274.

O'Keefe, D.J. and Jensen, J.D. (2007) 'The relative persuasiveness of gain-framed loss-framed messages for encouraging disease prevention behaviors: a meta-analytic review', *Journal of Health Communication,* 12: 623–644.

Pidgeon, N., Kaperson, R.E. and Slovic, P. (eds) (2003) *The Social Amplification of Risk,* Cambridge: Cambridge University Press.

Politi, M.C., Clark, M.A., Ombao, H., Dizon, D. and Elwyn, G. (2011) 'Communicating uncertainty can lead to less decision satisfaction: a necessary cost of involving patients in shared decision making?', *Health Expect,* 14: 84–91.

Politi, M.C. and Street, R.L., Jr. (2011) 'The importance of communication in collaborative decision making: facilitating shared mind and the management of uncertainty', *Journal of Evaluation in Clinical Practice,* 17: 579–584.

Ranby, K.W., Aiken, L.S., Gerend, M.A. and Erchull, M.J. (2010) 'Perceived susceptibility measures are not interchangeable: absolute, direct comparative, and indirect comparative risk', *Health Psychology: official journal of the Division of Health Psychology, American Psychological Association,* 29: 20–28.

Reyna, V.F. and Lloyd, F.J. (2006) 'Physician decision making and cardiac risk: effects of knowledge, risk perception, risk tolerance, and fuzzy processing', *Journal of Experimental Psychology: Applied,* 12: 179–195.

Salant, T. and Gehlert, S. (2008) 'Collective memory, candidacy, and victimisation: community epidemiologies of breast cancer risk', *Sociology of Health and Illness,* 30: 599–615.

Schwartz, L.M., Woloshin, S., Black, W. and Welch, G. (1997) 'The role of numeracy in understanding the benefit of screening mammography', *Annals of Internal Medicine,* 127: 966–972.

Slovic, P. (2000) *The Perception of Risk,* London: Earthscan.

Slovic, P., Finucane, M., Peters, E. and MacGregor, D.G. (2002) 'The affect heuristic', in T. Gilovich, D. Griffin, and D. Kahneman (eds) *Heuristics and Biases: The Psychology of Intuitive Judgment,* New York: Cambridge University Press.

Soler, R.E., Leeks, K.D., Razi, S., Hopkins, D.P., Griffith, M., Aten, A., et al. (2010) 'A systematic review of selected interventions for worksite health promotion. The assessment of health risks with feedback', *American Journal of Preventative Medicine,* 38: S237–62.

Tversky, A. and Kahneman, D. (1974) 'Judgment under uncertainty: heuristics and biases', *Science,* 185: 1124–1131.

Viswanath, K., Breen, N., Meissner, H., Moser, R.P., Hesse, B., Steele, W.R. and Rakowski, W. (2006) 'Cancer knowledge and disparities in the information age', *Journal of Health Communication,* 11: S 1, 1–17.

Waters, E.A., Sullivan, H.W., Nelson, W. and Hesse, B.W. (2009) 'What is my cancer risk? Identifying how Internet-based cancer risk calculators convey individualized risk estimates to the public', *Journal of Medical Internet Research,* 11: e33.

Weinstein, N.D. (1987) 'Unrealistic optimism about susceptibility to health problems: conclusions from a community wide sample', *Journal of Behavioral Medicine,* 10: 481–500.

——(1999) 'What does it mean to understand a risk? Evaluating risk comprehension', *Journal of the National Cancer Institute Monographs,* 25: 15–20.

Weinstein, N.D. and Klein, W.M. (1995) 'Resistance of personal risk perceptions to debiasing interventions', *Health Psychology,* 14: 132–140.

White, S. (2008) *Assessing the Nation's Health Literacy: Key Concepts and Findings of the National Assessment of Adult Literacy (NAAL),* Chicago, IL: AMA Foundation.

Witte, K. and Allen, M. (2000) 'A meta-analysis of fear appeals: implications for effective public health campaigns', *Health Education and Behavior,* 27: 591–615.

4

If numbers could speak

Numeracy and the digital revolution

Christina Zarcadoolas and Wendy Vaughon

Introduction

> Pick a number, any number.
>
> No, this isn't a riddle lifted from the Internet.
>
> Now, assume your number is the amount of calories in one serving of 'krall'. If your doctor told you that you need to limit your daily caloric intake to 1500 calories, what percentage of your daily total does a serving of krall represent?
>
> So, you're thinking – 'One serving of krall has 555 calories. That's 37 percent of my 1500 calories, so if I eat this I'll blow around a third of all the calories I'm allowed for the day. Forget about the krall today.'

If you easily and confidently did the calculation, then you are in the minority of adults in the US who have adequate numeracy skills. The most extensive national assessments of literacy (which includes numeracy) (Kirsch et al. 1993; Kutner et al. 2006) report that less than half of the adult population in the US has adequate literacy.

To communicate health and risk information to patients we find ourselves relying heavily on numbers and talk about numbers (numerical meta talk) to tell our story (Nelson et al. 2009), such as monitoring weight, counting calories, tracking blood pressure and blood glucose level, reading prescription/medication dosing, reviewing our lab test results, trying to determine the medical evidence for choosing one cancer treatment over another.

Using the risk calculator on the National Heart Lung and Blood Institute (NHLBI 2013) website, a consumer is required to know and input their total cholesterol, HDL cholesterol, and systolic blood pressure. When they receive their risk, it appears both as a percentage and a proportional statement: 'Means 8 of 100 people with this level of risk will have a heart attack in the next 10 years.' Furthermore the consumer is told that, 'Your risk score was calculated using an equation.' Other NCEP [National Cholesterol Education Program] products, such as printed ATP [Adult Treatment Panel] III materials, use a point system to determine a risk score that is close to the equation score.

In our recent research studying the readability and usability of patient-accessible electronic medical records (EMR, patient portals), one of the highest barrier elements we have identified during usability testing with low educational level consumers are tables and graphs presenting important numerical information such as a patient's cholesterol levels, historical trends, and other representations of risk factors.

The following is a typical example of this high-barrier information. In the one-on-one usability sessions for this study, participants were asked to review a series of test results as presented across three different EMR systems. Using a hypothetical patient's 'cholesterol number', study participants were asked to identify whether the number was normal (OK) or not normal ('too high', or 'too low'). While almost all participants could locate the hypothetical patient's 'cholesterol number' only about two-thirds could correctly identify whether the values fell within the normal range. See example in Table 4.1.

Table 4.1 Reading a cholesterol table (A)

Name	*Value*	*Reference range*
Appearance	CLEAR	
Cholesterol	206	0–200 mg/dl
Cholesterol/HDLC ratio	3.9	0.0–4.5
HDL cholesterol	55	40–50 mg/dl
LDL	129	0–130 mg/dl
Triglyceride	111	10–160 mg/dl
VLDL	21	10–40 mg/dl

Historical perspectives

In this chapter we add our contribution to the rich and growing literature on numeracy and health communications. What we discuss comes from our work with health literacy load and task analysis of a wide range of other digital health communication tools, in particular patient electronic medical records. We will present the theoretical underpinnings and practical application of linguistics (language study) and semiotic (sign/symbol study) theory. We see these two areas as an addition to the computational models, information processing and cognitive models, and models of intuitive/affective thinking, or gist-based thinking that have enhanced our understanding of numeracy and health numeracy.

Critical issues and topics

A major challenge to individual and public health continues to be the low literacy and low health literacy of millions of adults in the US. Literacy (referred to often as fundamental literacy or general literacy) is the ability to read, write, and work with numbers (numeracy). Health literacy is defined as one's ability to seek out, understand, and use health information (Nielsen-Bohlman et al. 2004; Zarcadoolas et al. 2006; Nutbeam 2000). A health literate person is able to better engage with health information, improve health decision-making and thus benefit from healthier choices. Most health information for consumers is written at the 10th and 12th grade levels (Root and Stableford 1999), with web-based material having reading levels often much higher (Zarcadoolas et al. 2006). A health literate individual can better participate in the 'social, economic and environmental determinants of health, and be directed towards the promotion of individual and collective actions which may lead to modification of these determinants' (Nutbeam 2000: 264). Low socio-economic status is highly correlated with low literacy levels as well as low health literacy (Nielsen-Bohlman et al. 2004; Schwartzberg et al. 2005). Low health literate populations often cannot read and understand medical information.

Low health literacy in the US has been studied for over 20 years. Interest in numeracy is more recent and generally has been initiated from outside of the health literacy field (education, cognitive science, cultural criticism). While the interest and knowledge about the specific mechanisms of numeracy is rapidly evolving, most would agree that numeracy skills include doing straight arithmetic, processing quantitative information, understanding basic mathematical concepts such as probability (Nelson et al. 2008) and spatial cognition (de Hevia et al. 2008).

Health numeracy is defined as 'the degree to which individuals have the capacity to access, process, interpret, communicate, and act on numerical, quantitative, graphical, biostatistical and probabilistic health information needed to make effective health decisions' (Golbeck et al. 2005: 376). There are four functional categories of health numeracy: basic, computational, analytical, and statistical. Inadequate health numeracy has been identified across age groups (Woloshin et al. 2001; Lipkus et al. 2001; Sheridan and Pignone 2002). As is easy to imagine, low numeracy interferes with what people understand from all sorts of health information, and this ultimately influences their health (Morrow et al. 2006; Nelson et al. 2008).

Another concern about low numeracy is that it leaves a person more likely to be influenced by framing effects (Hibbard and Peters 2003; Peters et al. 2007). In other words, low numeracy is also linked to our susceptibility to pseudoscience. As Paulos states in *Innumeracy* (1989), the US public's poor numeracy skills often lead to a huge gap between expert and lay risk perception, a gap 'that threatens eventually to lead either to unfounded and crippling anxieties or to impossible and economically paralyzing demands for risk-free guarantees' (Paulos 1989: 5).

As a remedy to low health literacy, experts in the field of health literacy have historically focused on how to present language in simple and clear ways (Nielsen-Bohlman et al. 2004; Zarcadoolas 2011). A popular assumption is that simplification of words and sentences will lead to greater patient/public comprehension, improved health literacy, and thus improved health behaviors and outcomes (McGee 1999; Schwartzberg et al. 2005).

Far less attention has been paid to analyzing what individuals can and are actually doing with linguistic texts that include numbers. Nor has there been much effort to move beyond a simplification model to a more ecological understanding of the mechanisms of health literacy and health numeracy. It is our premise, in this chapter, that such efforts would assist us to develop better techniques to present numerical health information in understandable ways (Ancker et al. 2006; Cosmides and Tooby 1996).

Life on the grid: e-health and m-health and numbers

Over a decade ago, Eysenbach (2001) pronounced this the era of consumer health, empowering providers to manage care and share clinical information with patients using electronic tools. Back then, Eysenbach called *e-health* an emerging field in the intersection of medical informatics, public health and business, referring to health services and information delivered or enhanced through the Internet and related technologies' (Eysenbach 2001: 3). This term characterized not only a technical development, but a vision of networked, global thinking to improve health care locally, regionally, and worldwide through communication technology. E-health has been seen as a way to improve the health of patients, while controlling costs and improving the efficiency, quality, and safety of health care (Buntin et al. 2011; Hillestad et al. 2005). The seismic shift to Internet and mobile use in our daily lives has changed both how we access and make use of health information (Nelson et al. 2009) as well as expanded the role patients and consumers need to take in seeking out, finding, understanding, and using this health information to live healthier lives.

Patients have not been slow to dive in. Today, people regularly perform Google searches or check out WebMD when they have a health question or get a new diagnosis. Patients want online access to their personal health records (Wen et al. 2010). In their searches, no doubt, consumers may stumble upon a patient blog or a pharmaceuticals website. Their searches invariably bring them face to face with a world of numbers – numbers to talk about risk, probability, report health status, describe the prevalence of a disease, and much more. For example, a woman might go to a National Cancer Institute (NCI) website to calculate her breast cancer risk. As Nelson questions, 'exactly what do these numbers mean? Is a 9.2% lifetime risk of developing breast cancer reassuring or worrisome?' (Nelson et al. 2008: 2).

The use of mobile technology for health purposes (m-health) is projected to explode, growing from $1.7 billion in 2010 to $5.7 billion in 2015 (Kolesnikov-Jessop 2011). A recent Pew Internet report found that of the 85 percent of adults who own a cell phone 31 percent have used their phones to look up medical or health information (Fox 2012). In the context of mobile device health applications, 19 percent of US adult smartphone users have downloaded an application that assists them in tracking or managing their health (Fox 2012).

Most of the US public will be able to communicate with their providers, access health information, including their own electronic medical records, and learn about relevant health information online and via mobile devices in the coming decade.

As with other patient information, online health information via computer and mobile devices is written at a level well above the reach of the average American consumer (Graber et al. 1999). Pressure to transition a large portion of healthcare information and services to electronic and mobile without addressing the numeracy needs of the general population has the potential to exacerbate disparities by widening the digital divide for underserved populations (Sarkar et al. 2011; Volandes and Paasche-Orlow 2007).

Importantly, while the hardware becomes ever more user-friendly with faster, more touch-based, intuitive logic and design, we cannot say the same for the presentation of numerical information for health communication (Shneiderman and Plaisant 2010).

Current contributions and research

There is reason to believe that a narrow focus on numeracy as computation will not yield the types of understandings and solutions to the health numeracy problem that are needed.

Working with numbers in everyday life

The social life of numbers is rich and varied. So too are the ways people work with numbers. Figure 4.1 shows a message that most every driver in New York City learns to interpret, by necessity, quite accurately. But based on the linguistic and numerical presentation, we wouldn't imagine this to be as true.

A parking savvy driver says to me during an intercept interview:

> Look, it says you can't park here between 8:00 in the morning and 9:00 – they're cleaning the streets. You see anyone with a broom? … And then from 9:00 until at night you have to feed the meter every hour. Today's Tuesday, it's Tuesday and it's 11:00 in the morning, so I'm good here at least for an hour if I feed the meter. That's how you do it if you don't want a ticket. But you never know. Listen to this. My friend told me …

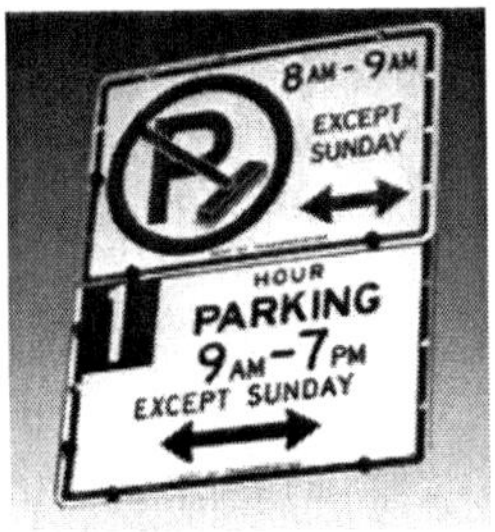
8AM - 9AM
EXCEPT SUNDAY
1
HOUR
PARKING
9AM-7PM
EXCEPT SUNDAY

Figure 4.1 New York City street parking sign

How do drivers do it?

The New Yorker has done what standard readability tests tell us is very hard to do: he's read and interpreted (decoded) an array of words, visuals, and numbers to make an informed decision. The array includes: directional arrows, a graphic of a letter 'P' and a less than obvious visual of a broom, the short exception phrase (Except Sunday), a time range represented with a dash; and the number '1' in a shaded square in the top left corner – which doesn't refer to the time of day, but the length of time, in total, you can park in this location. Lastly, based on a complicated across text deduction, the driver comprehends that he doesn't have to feed the meter on Sunday. In addition to all of the above, the driver needs a contextual understanding of what these signs mean for a driver in New York City. That the broom graphic on the upper sign represents 'street cleaning' (a.k.a. jockeying one's car around the block or alternate side of the street, while waiting out the arrival of the street sweeper), and that the lower sign refers to metered parking, not just legal parking.

This and countless other phenomena of people using numbers in everyday life has intrigued us and informed our interest in conducting research to better understand how to present health information in more relevant and understandable ways to patients and consumers.

Numeracy as a language

Elegant discussions of the political and cultural life of numbers have occupied anthropologists, linguists, and philosophers. For our purposes, in this chapter, the insights of these experts are condensed into a few tenets:

- Numeracy is the mathematical analog of literacy; numbers in arrays can be said to have their own grammar – rule-bound strings where each component has a structure and function.
- As with sentences, there is cohesive reference within and across a numerical display.
- Numeracy is semantically structured.
- Numbers are linguistic objects, often importantly tied to the specific language, culture, and social situation.
- Numerical text requires text level as well as sentence or utterance level skills.

Working with numbers depends on a range of competencies and mechanisms not all fully understood (Apter et al. 2008; Ancker and Kaufman 2007). Nelson sites four primary theories that have been used to describe numeracy processes thus far (Nelson et al. 2008).

Space does not permit elaboration of the four theories beyond naming them: computation, natural qualitative processing, intuitive/affective vs. analytical, and fuzzy trace theory/ gist-based. The bottom line is that different people use different processes for decoding numbers.

Ancker and Kaufman suggest that at least three domains of competency are needed: an individual's (1) linguistic competence, (2) competence interpreting visual representations of the numerical information, and (3) degree of engagement with the task. Identifying what skills an individual has and describing how numbers are represented are the two elements most commonly studied among numeracy experts (Ancker and Kaufman 2007). Additionally numeracy involves the degree of confidence an individual has.

Health contextualized numeracy skills

Researchers and health communicators have been manipulating the configuration of numbers trying to make them more comprehensible to patients. Apter and colleagues recommend the following in order to create more comprehensible numerical information: (1) simplifying the numerical concept, (2) removing non-essential information, (3) using visuals, (4) confirming comprehension (Apter et al. 2008).

Ancker and Kaufman draw upon a distributed cognition approach in their review of the literature, by elaborating the individual level quantitative skills integral to proficient health numeracy, namely, basic computation, estimation, and statistical literacy (Ancker and Kaufman 2007). They also name three skills: representational fluency, document literacy, and graphical literacy as key to a patient's ability to use information artifacts and suggest that well-designed information can help to bridge computational skill gaps and increase comprehension for low health numerate individuals.

What follows is our contribution of two additional constructs that can be added to the evolving understanding of people and their interpretation of numbers.

The linguistic integrity of numbers

In this section, we explore how aspects of both semiotic and linguistic theory can be used to advance our understanding of some of the synergistic mechanisms involved in numeracy skills, and contribute to a more understandable presentation of numbers.

Across our research, patient education, and evaluation of health communications, we have found, as others have, that individuals use different strategies to decode numerical information. Two of these are: (a) performing a straight calculation, and (b) decoding and interpreting the information by translating or recoding the numerical string into propositional statements. So, to return to our NYC commuter, the textual information, made up of words, icons (visuals), and numbers, is recoded into the statement he utters.

Through usability testing and think-aloud tasks in a range of studies with consumers, the majority of whom are low education level, low literate, and low health literate, we have collected and analyzed these verbalized propositional statements, as well as statements about the functional intent of arrays. We have done this to help us better diagnose the nature of the numeracy problem and to conceptualize better ways to present numerical information that would assist the decoder/consumer/patient to form more accurate propositional statements.

The following two models or theories, one derived from semiotics and one from linguistics, have informed our understanding of numeracy and health numeracy.

Semiotic theory: moving from the iconic to the symbolic

Semiotic theory, the study of signs and symbols, is useful in broadening the lens through which we see numeracy, in that numbers are a ubiquitous symbol system. When we work with symbols, rather than objects, meaning is not 'transmitted' to us – we actively create it according to a complex interplay of codes or conventions we know and understand about that symbol system. Becoming aware of such codes is inherently empowering. Sign theorists, semioticians, would explain our ability to work with numbers (and words) as highly 'contextually determined' (Hodge and Kress 1988; Hymes 1974).

Structuralist semiotic analysis involves identifying the constituent units in a semiotic system (such as a story or a numerical text) and the structural relationships between them (oppositions, correlations, and logical relations). It has long been understood that an individual element can only be fully decoded and understood in the context of the whole text. Developmental language studies have clearly shown the importance of context in comprehension. For example, passives, taken at face value, are a difficult transformation. However, they are understood when placed in context by children who could not comprehend them in isolation (Coleman 1964). Words, ambiguous alone, once embedded in a context, are laden with derivable, decodable meanings. The importance of context with numerical information is equally important.

As a symbol system the world of numbers is systematic, logical, and rule-governed, and thus we can talk about numbers as having a grammar of their own. When you are numerate you know that 12 is greater than 1; 5 to the 3rd power equals 125; or that the order in which you carry out addition or multiplication doesn't matter because both are commutative, but division and subtraction are different.

Simple math, or simple numbers, can be said to be 'iconic': '1' chair – the number can literally stand in for, or point, to a chair. When numbers move into greater degrees of abstraction or symbolism, people with poor numeracy run into difficulty. We can talk about '1 person in 10 is likely to develop diabetes' and, although not accurately representing the statistical risk conveyed in the proportion phrase, individuals can picture literally one person in a row of ten people (you've probably seen this type of silhouetted people chart before). But literally matching real-world counterparts quickly loses functionality in conveying larger or more abstract numbers. Working with numbers very quickly moves us from the iconic to the symbolic.

Linguistic theory

In addition to working with numbers symbolically, our ability to work with numbers is also linked to our metalinguistic abilities. By this we mean a person's abilities to objectify and talk about what they know and how they know it. Metalinguistic ability involves using language to talk about language.

Thus we can talk about the stock market going down, as well as what numbers we are using to forecast the market going back up; how our child's college tuition compares to when we went to school, and how much faith we have in those costs holding steady for a while; the fluctuations in our weight over time, and how many flights of stairs we have to climb to burn off that cream-filled donut.

In our patient portal usability study we observed two distinct types of approaches consumers used when faced with interpreting numerical information: (1) computational, and (2) propositional. We used talk-aloud as a method to gain insight to their thought processes while performing such decoding tasks with numbers. Recall, that for the example shown below, participants were asked to identify a hypothetical patient's 'cholesterol number', then to identify whether the number was normal or not normal. In contrast to the test results in Table 4.1, participants shown the example in Table 4.2 were more successful in accurately describing whether the test patient's numbers were normal.

Table 4.2 Reading a cholesterol table (B)

Component	*Your value*	*Standard range*	*Units*
Triglycerides	183	< 150	mg/dL
HDL	39	40–59	mg/dL
Cholesterol	240	100–199	mg/dL
LDL cholesterol	164	0–99	mg/dL

Three strategies for presenting numbers in health communication

Participant A: Vocabulary/linguistic approach

The following is a linguistic reading/decoding problem. The study participant tries to use the linguistic information to make meaning. However she is not familiar with the words 'value' and 'standard range'.

Tester: What is Mercedes' cholesterol number?

User: 24 and 164. That's her values. And her standard range. She has a value and a standard range. [said confusedly].

Tester: Does Mercedes know if her numbers are normal?

User: Hmmm. I would say they was abnormal [pensively] … cause I don't know if the value, the 240 means normal, or the standard range means normal. I don't know.

Participant B: Configurational knowledge approach

The following study participant uses a configuration/display strategy. Participant B identifies the cholesterol value (240) and moves across the chart and stops, at 100–200. He pauses and then concludes, 'It's too high'. The user is likely employing a configurational knowledge strategy – using skill in knowing how numbers are spatially and semantically related (Golledge and Stimpson 1987). In linguistic and semiotic theory the user is familiar with and is using the distinctive features of numerical information – numbers, numbers in various arrays (in this case numbers separated by a dash to indicate range, linear thread, columns, graphs, charts). We can say this is a syntagmatic approach to decoding. The syntagmatic analysis of a text involves assessing/sizing up the spatial and sequential relationships of the distinctive features (or 'syntagms') (Chandler 2010).

Participant C: Propositional statement approach

Participant C also starts by easily reporting 240 as the test patient's cholesterol number. This participant moves the cursor across the thread, then says, 'The patient's cholesterol is 240 but the standard range is 100–199, so she's above that. She's higher than 199.' In this case the reader linguistically recodes the numerical information, forming a coherent propositional statement. The reader embeds the numerical symbols into a sentence structure or mini–narrative and so is identifying and decoding the smallest structural narrative units (Barthes 1977; Kintsch and Vipond 1979).

The initial propositions are a list of statements derived from the text. Given the reader's abilities and the coherence of the text, these individual propositional statements are transformed into a connected, logical whole.

Recommendations for practice

As we stated earlier, our contribution to the discussion of both numeracy and rethinking presentation of health information using numeracy is derived from our work with patient portals and health literacy load and task analysis of a wide range of other digital health communication tools. The following are recommendations that we believe can inform the work of those who either review and/or assess health information or those who develop it.

Using propositional statements

One aiding tool we are pursuing is using propositional statements in the form of simple text language, co-located on the landscape of a chart or graph. These short simple statements could then be combined to yield a synthesized, coherent proposition. Where helpful, the propositional statements could refer to a specific character and thus form a short narrative that can serve as an analogy model.

For example: The cholesterol chart (Table 4.2) would also include companion language as follows:

> Is your cholesterol too high, too low, or just right?
>
> A healthy cholesterol number should fit between the numbers 100–199.
>
> For example, if your cholesterol number (value) is 120, 130, 140, … 180, etc., your cholesterol is OK.
>
> But if your cholesterol number is more than 199, your cholesterol is not OK.
>
> For example, if your cholesterol number is 210, 220, 230 … 300, etc., it is not OK.

Embedding numbers into narratives

In concordance with findings exploring narrative as a means to present complex information (Mazor et al. 2007), we recommend combining a narrative frame with a propositional frame. This would involve embedding propositional statements into a narrative structure. Narratives are the most primary and universal forms of communication and narrative texts are ubiquitous in our spoken lives. Whether a narrative is as simple as 'The king died and then the queen died of grief', or *War and Peace*, humans seem to be hardwired to encode and decode their world in narrative.

Mazor and colleagues have found a benefit in using narrative either along with or in place of some statistical information. We would like to further explore how design of the entire numerical–textual array (including language and numbers) can be designed to instigate or make it easier for the reader/user to translate the content into simple and understandable narrative structure.

User-centered research and design

Information design plays a critical role in user understanding and uptake of content (Nelson et al. 2009; Tufte 2001). An excellent and annotated discussion can be found in Nelson et al. (2009) in Further Reading at the end of this chapter. Thus far, the proclivity of researchers and educators working with underserved individuals has been to identify what people cannot do rather than what they can do. This has been very true, as we mentioned earlier, in the field of health literacy. Yet, as the NYC commuter demonstrates, each and everyday people are doing things with numbers. We strongly believe that more time should be spent identifying much more about what consumers/patients are actually doing with numerical information, how they are making meaning. For instance, what level of abstraction are they working with?; and do they have a numerical grammar, and, if so, how complex is it?

User-centered design involves an early and continual focus on users and an iterative approach to design whereby feedback from users (focus groups and pilot usability testing) is used to modify the design as appropriate. Optimally, target users should be involved in the process of designing and testing (Kirsh et al. 2008). It is well established in the human–computer interaction and information systems literature that involving stakeholders in the design and development of technology applications enhances the likelihood of developing more usable systems and ultimately of user acceptance and use of systems (Winkelman et al. 2005).

In order for e-health and m-health information to be comprehensible to a diverse population, writers and designers must adopt a user-centered design approach. User-centered design can lead to the development of linguistic and cognitive aids and tools that optimize the comprehension of important text elements such as: vocabulary and sentence construction, number arrays, cohesive ties, labeling, definitions. User-centered design is also essential in identifying the specific design elements that assist in navigation and making meaning – scanning/correcting, locating information, accumulating and interpreting information, referencing and decision-making.

Universal design

In addition to the abilities of the end-users, developers of e-health and m-health tools must consider the features available to the user. Regarding digital communications, developers must design highly plastic systems that convert across display sizes, mobile displays, languages, and support devices for disabled users. This is a component of the semantic web and refers to the possibility of making core components of online elements understandable across platforms. Much more work needs to be done to develop, user test, and then integrate certain universal design principles into the presentation of numerical information to communicate health information to patients.

Conclusion

In this chapter we have added our insights to the evolving discourse about what constitutes numeracy by discussing the symbolic characteristics of numbers and the specific linguistic function of propositional statements. We will continue to pursue how these two domains can be used to improve the way we communicate numerical health information to patients and consumers, particularly those who are low literate and underserved.

Space has not permitted us to discuss each of the four functional categories of health numeracy: basic, computational, analytical, and statistical, however we believe that the elements we have identified play a role in both representations and decoding across a wide range of numerical information and formats.

It is clear to us that no one theoretical model or approach will be adequate to the task. Rather we argue that adopting inter-disciplinary, ecological models of human competencies, including literacy and numeracy, are needed. This would include cross- disciplinary work in cognition, linguistics, health communication, human factors engineering, and universal design to name just a few fields.

Design of health information informed by empirical evidence, using theoretical principles of various domains of knowledge, reading, linguistics, cognitive science, and anthropology, to name a few, are needed. Ongoing empirical evidence demonstrating the efficacy of innovations in presentation of numeracy-based health information is likely to result in enhanced patient use of health information, greater engagement in health, and ultimately improvements in health status.

Future directions

More evidence-based approaches to developing and evaluating health communications across modalities are needed. Models that offer more than simply a focus on readability scores and writing to a certain grade level (adjusting word and sentence length) are gaining traction (Freedman et al. 2009; Zarcadoolas et al. 2006; Pleasant and Kuruvilla 2008). The use of health literacy models that take a more inclusive and ecological stance show much promise for revealing the mechanism of an individual's health literacy as it interacts with rich psycho-social and cognitive drivers.

Additionally, we stress the need to better understand the phenomenon, literally right under our noses, the ubiquitous use of emerging communication technologies by people across demographic categories. In 2013, there are more than 13,000 smart phones and tablet apps relevant to health, with many more likely in the pipeline. There are apps today for WebMD, apps to help you take medications, to monitor your exercise, to track your progress in physical therapy, to help you calculate your blood glucose readings throughout the day, as well as apps for eating healthily at restaurants, and more.

This society-changing phenomenon, that pulls consumers into choosing, learning, using, and talking about new tools, new apps, and newer, faster, and more fun ways to do just about anything, can provide us with some of our richest insights. We believe, going forward, more focus should be placed on learning how consumers are interacting with these technologies and what implications this has for how we design and present health information, including all those ubiquitous numbers.

Related topics

Linguistics, semiotic theory, numeracy, health numeracy, e-health, health literacy.

Further reading

Chandler, D. (2010) Semiotics for beginners. Online. Available: <http://www.aber.ac.uk/media/Documents/S4B/sem04.html> (accessed 11 November 2012).

Hymes, D. (1974) *Foundations of Sociolinguistics: An Ethnographic Approach*, Philadelphia, PA: University of Pennsylvania Press.

Nelson, D., Hesse, B., and Croyle, R. (2009) *Making Data Talk: Communicating Public Health Data to the Public, Policy Makers and the Press*, New York: Oxford University Press.

Nelson, W., Reyna, V. F., Fagerlin, A., Lipkus, I., and Peters, E. (2008) 'Clinical implications of numeracy: theory and practice', *Annals of Behavioral Medicine*, 35(3): 261–274.

Zarcadoolas, C., Pleasant, A., and Greer, D.S. (2006) *Advancing Health Literacy: A Framework for Understanding and Action*, San Francisco, CA: Jossey-Bass.

References

Ancker, J. and Kaufman, D. (2007) 'Rethinking health numeracy: a multidisciplinary literature review', *Journal of the American Medical Informatics Association,* 14(6): 713–721.

Ancker, J.S., Senathirajah, Y., Kukafka, R., and Starren, J.B. (2006) 'Design features of graphs in health risk communication: a systematic review', *Journal of the American Medical Informatics Association,* 13(6): 608–618.

Apter, A.J., Paasche-Orlow, M.K., Remillard, J.T., Bennett, I.M., Ben-Joseph, E.P., Batista, R.M., et al. (2008) 'Numeracy and communication with patients: they are counting on us', *Journal of General Internal Medicine,* 23(12): 2117–2124.

Barthes, R. (1977) *Image, Music, Text,* London: Harper Collins.

Buntin, M.B., Burke, M.F., Hoaglin, M.C., and Blumenthal, D. (2011) 'The benefits of health information technology: a review of the recent literature shows predominantly positive results', *Health Affairs (Millwood),* 30(3): 464–471.

Chandler, D. (2010) *Semiotics for Beginners*. Online. Available: <http://www.aber.ac.uk/media/Documents/S4B/sem04.html> (accessed 11 November 2012).

Coleman, E. (1964) 'The comprehensibility of several grammatical transformations', *Journal of Applied Psychology,* 48: 186–190.

Cosmides, L. and Tooby, J. (1996) 'Are humans good intuitive statisticians after all? Rethinking some conclusions from the literature on judgment under uncertainty', *Cognition*, 58: 1–73.

de Hevia, M.D., Vallar, G., and Girelli, L. (2008) 'Visualizing numbers in the mind's eye: the role of visuo-spatial processes in numerical abilities', *Neuroscience and Biobehavioral Reviews*, 32(8): 1361–1372.

Eysenbach, G. (2001) 'What is e-health?', *Journal of Medical Internet Research,* 3(2): E20.

Fox, S. (2012) *Mobile Health 2012*. Pew Internet and American Life Project. Online. Available: <www.pewinternet.org/~/media//Files/Reports/2012/PIP_MobileHealth2012.pdf> (accessed 5 December 2012).

Freedman, D.A., Bess, K.D., Tucker, H.A., Boyd, D.L., Tuchman, A.M., and Wallston, K.A. (2009) 'Public health literacy defined', *American Journal of Preventive Medicine,* 36(5): 446–451.

Golbeck, A., Ahlers-Schmidt, C., Paschal, A., and Dismuke, S. (2005) 'A definition and operational framework for health numeracy', *American Journal of Preventive Medicine,* 29(4): 375–376.

Golledge, R.G. and Stimpson, R.J. (1987) 'Learning and spatial behavior', in *Analytical Behavior Geography*, London: Croom Helm.

Graber, M.A., Roller, C.M., and Kaeble, B. (1999) 'Readability levels of patient education material on the World Wide Web', *Journal of Family Practice,* 48(1): 58–61.

Hibbard, J.H. and Peters, E. (2003) 'Supporting informed consumer health care decisions: data presentation approaches that facilitate the use of information in choice', *Annual Review of Public Health,* 24: 413–433.

Hillestad, R., Bigelow, J., Bower, A., Girosi, F., Meili, R., Scoville, R., and Taylor, R. (2005) 'Can electronic medical record systems transform health care? Potential health benefits, savings, and costs', *Health Affairs (Millwood),* 24(5): 1103–1117.

Hodge, R. and Kress, G. (1988) *Social Semiotics*, Cambridge: Polity.

Hymes, D. (1974) *Foundations of Sociolinguistics: An Ethnographic Approach,* Philadelphia, PA: University of Pennsylvania Press.

Kintsch, W. and Vipond, D. (1979) 'Reading comprehension and readability in educational practice and psychological theory', in L.G. Nilsson (ed.) *Perspectives on Memory Research,* Hillsdale, NJ: Erlbaum.

Kirsch, I., Jungeblut, A., Jenkins, L., and Kolstad, A. (1993) *Adult Literacy in America: A First Look at the Results of the National Adult Literacy Survey (NALS)*, Washington, DC: U.S. Government Printing Office.

Kirsh, S., Lawrence, R., and Aron, D. (2008) 'Tailoring an intervention to the context and system redesign related to the intervention: a case study of implementing shared medical appointments for diabetes', *Implementation Science,* 3: 34.

Kolesnikov-Jessop, S. (2011) *Do-It-Yourself Health Care With Smartphones,* Online. Available: <http://www.nytimes.com/2011/03/01/technology/01iht-srhealth01.html> (accessed 10 October 2012).

Kutner, M., Greenberg, E., Jin, Y., and Paulsen, C. (2006) *The Health Literacy of America's Adults: Results from the 2003 National Assessment of Adult Literacy,* Washington DC: National Center for Education Statistics.

Lipkus, I., Samsa, G., and Rimer, B. (2001) 'General performance on a numeracy scale among highly educated samples', *Medical Decision Making,* 21(1): 37–44.

McGee, J. (1999) *Writing and Designing Print Materials for Beneficiaries: A Guide for State Medicaid Agencies* (HCFA Publication Number 10145), Baltimore, MD: Centers for Medicare and Medicaid Services, U.S. Department of Health and Human Services.

Mazor, K.M., Baril, J.L., Dugan, E., Spencer, F.A., Burgwinkle, P., and Gurwitz, J.H. (2007) 'Patient education about anticoagulant medication: Is narrative evidence or statistical evidence more effective?', *Patient Education and Counseling,* 69(1–3): 145–157.

Morrow, D., Clark, D., Tu, W., Wu, J., Weiner, M., Steinley, D., and Murray, M. (2006) 'Correlates of health literacy in patients with chronic heart failure', *Gerontologist,* 46(5): 669–676.

National Heart Lung and Blood Institute (NHLBI) (2013) *Risk Assessment Tool for Estimating Your 10-year Risk of Having a Heart Attack.* Online. Available: <http://cvdrisk.nhlbi.nih.gov/calculator.asp> (accessed 19 December 2013).

Nelson, D., Hesse, B., and Croyle, R. (2009) *Making Data Talk: Communicating Public Health Data to the Public, Policy Makers and the Press,* New York: Oxford University Press.

Nelson, W., Reyna, V.F., Fagerlin, A., Lipkus, I., and Peters, E. (2008) 'Clinical implications of numeracy: theory and practice', *Annals of Behavioral Medicine,* 35(3): 261–274.

Nielsen-Bohlman, L., Panzer, A.M., and Kindig, D.A. (eds) (2004) *Health Literacy: A Prescription to End Confusion,* Washington, DC: National Academies Press.

Nutbeam, D. (2000) 'Health literacy as a public health goal: a challenge for contemporary health education and communication strategies into the 21st century', *Health Promotion International,* 15(3): 259–267.

Paulos, J.A. (1989) *Innumeracy: Mathematical Illiteracy and its Consequences,* New York: Hill and Wang.

Peters, E., Dieckmann, N., Dixon, A., Hibbard, J.H., and Mertz, C.K. (2007) 'Less is more in presenting quality information to consumers', *Medical Care Research and Review,* 64(2): 169–190.

Pleasant, A. and Kuruvilla, S. (2008) 'A tale of two health literacies: public health and clinical approaches to health literacy', *Health Promotion International*, 23(2): 152–159.

Root, J. and Stableford, S. (1999) 'Easy-to-read consumer communications: a missing link in Medicaid managed care', *Journal of Health Politics, Policy and Law,* 24(1): 1–26.

Sarkar, U., Karter, A.J., Liu, J.Y., Adler, N.E., Nguyen, R., López, A., and Schillinger, D. (2011) 'Social disparities in Internet patient portal use in diabetes: evidence that the digital divide extends beyond access', *Journal of the American Medical Informatics Association,* 18(3): 318–321.

Schwartzberg, J., Van Geest, J., and Wang, C. (eds) (2005) *Understanding Health Literacy: Implications for Medicine and Public Health,* Chicago, IL: AMA Press.

Sheridan, S.L. and Pignone, M. (2002) 'Numeracy and the medical student's ability to interpret data', *Effective Clinical Practice (ECP),* 5(1): 35–40.

Shneiderman, B. and Plaisant, C. (2010) *Designing the User Interface: Strategies for Effective Human–Computer Interaction,* Boston, MA: Pearson.

Tufte, E. (2001) *The Visual Display of Quantitative Information,* 2nd edn, Cheshire, CT: Graphics Press.

Volandes, A.E. and Paasche-Orlow, M.K. (2007) 'Health literacy, health inequality and a just healthcare system', *American Journal of Bioethics,* 7(11): 5–10.

Wen, K.Y., Kreps, G., Zhu, F., and Miller, S. (2010) 'Consumers' perceptions about and use of the Internet for personal health records and health information exchange: analysis of the 2007 Health Information National Trends Survey', *Journal of Medical Internet Research,* 12(4): e73.

Winkelman, W., Leonard, K., and Rossos, P. (2005) 'Patient-perceived usefulness of online electronic medical records: employing grounded theory in the development of information and communication technologies for use by patients living with chronic illness', *Journal of the American Medical Informatics Association,* 12(3): 306–314.

Woloshin, S., Schwartz, L., Moncur, M., Gabriel, S., and Tosteson, A. (2001) 'Assessing values for health: numeracy matters', *Medical Decision Making,* 21(5): 382–390.

Zarcadoolas, C. (2011) 'The simplicity complex: exploring simplified health messages in a complex world', *Health Promotion International*, 26(3): 338–350.

Zarcadoolas, C., Pleasant, A., and Greer, D.S. (2006) *Advancing Health Literacy: A Framework for Understanding and Action,* San Francisco, CA: Jossey-Bass.

5

Corpus linguistics and evidence-based health communication

Paul Crawford, Brian Brown, and Kevin Harvey

Introduction and definitions

In this chapter we present a critical overview of the state of play for Corpus Linguistics (CL) in health care. CL involves computational analysis of a corpus (or corpora, pl.) which is typically a large body of electronic text, sometimes running into millions of words, with the help of special software such as Wordsmith Tools or AntConc (see below). The corpus approach to linguistic analysis integrates both quantitative (computational analysis, frequency counts) of large or smaller datasets and qualitative techniques (discourse analysis, concordance analysis, and the like), affording a reliable means of identifying trends and patterns in communication. This is a major development in language analysis because it increases the scope of what can be investigated. Consider for a moment how long it might take an individual researcher to read and interpret a 10-million word text. Now, by using software we are able to 'diagnose' the key patterns and word frequencies in such large bodies of text, assisting the individual researcher in their overall interpretation.

Typically, at an early stage in analysis, the pattern of word frequencies can be used to establish the 'genre' or 'register' of communication in any context, it is then possible to adopt the recommendations of Orpin (2005) and Conrad (2002) to follow up particular terms in a more fine-grained fashion. In essence, the analysis of corpus material allows a process of 'drilling down' to address progressively more detailed and contextualized levels of analysis once the main features of any text have been apprehended. Concordance analysis, for example, a more qualitative approach to language study, enables researchers to examine every occurrence of a particular word or phrase in context and thus identify its situations and patterns of use. Concordance analysis enables a systematic interrogation of the content.

By examining diverse health language, be it that of policy, media, advertising, clinical consultations and interventions, or informal carers, service users and the public, CL has achieved an important shift in the status of applied language analysis in evidence-based healthcare communication (Brown et al. 2006).

Historical perspectives

Dominated by a positivist, biomedical ambit, modern healthcare organizations and cultures of research and clinical practice have been largely closed to purely interpretive investigations.

Funding agencies and review boards have tended to favor investigations planned in the manner of an experimental trial. CL offers a 'trojan horse' to such mentality, leading to innovative, mixed method and fundable work. More tellingly, it is proving a subversion point to traditional, anti-intellectual hierarchies of knowledge formation which are strongly marked in health care, where randomized control trials have been seen as the 'gold standard' (Timmermans and Berg 2003) and more highly valued than qualitative or interpretive investigations. As in other contexts, qualitative research is often framed as merely providing the groundwork for subsequent quantitative approaches. CL in health care promotes a different frame – with quantitative research (computational analysis) acting as a diagnostic for richer qualitative investigation.

The study of communication in health care has been dominated by investigations of doctor–patient interaction, which have a relatively long history. By the mid-1990s studies of the language and interaction of less powerful allied health professionals, such as nurses (Crawford et al. 1998), pharmacists (Pilnick 2003), physiotherapists (Wallin et al. 2009), occupational therapists (Vegni et al. 2010), and indeed patients, began to attract interest. This spread of focus not only opened up the kinds of health language that scholars might investigate but arguably led to a diversification of methodology. Indeed, the confluence of different professionals and different linguists at key research groups such as the Health Language Research Group (HLRG) based in the UK's East Midlands over the last 10 years, for example, led to the pursuit of new knowledge in the field of healthcare discourse, and opened up a distinctive multimodal style of inquiry, which embraced both quantitative and qualitative elements.

Critical issues and topics

Over recent years various scholars have highlighted a mixed method approach featuring CL in combining both a quantitative and qualitative approach (see Adolphs et al. 2004; McCarthy and Handford 2004; Simpson 2004; Orpin 2005; Baker 2010; McEnery and Hardie 2011; Cheng 2011; Harvey and Koteyko 2012). Indeed, multimodal CL analysis has now reached a 'tried-and-tested' status in health care, incorporating any or all of the following: Corpus Linguistics (CL), Discourse Analysis (DA), Critical Discourse Analysis (CDA) and Metaphor Analysis (MA) (see Adolphs et al. 2004; Harvey et al. 2007; Koteyko and Nerlich 2007; Brown et al. 2008; Crawford and Brown 2008; Crawford et al. 2008; Koteyko et al. 2008a; Koteyko et al. 2008b; Harvey et al. 2008; Brown and Crawford 2009a, 2009b; Crawford et al. 2010).

Applied linguistics in health care has thus accrued a substantial portfolio of multimodal research, bringing together new alliances in terms of method, most strikingly in combining corpus linguistics with various approaches to discourse, conversation or metaphor analysis. Alongside methodological innovation we have seen a strengthening international network of a diverse body of researchers in medical and health discourse with a number of complementary journal, conference and clinical practice initiatives emerging globally. In addition, there has been a good deal of trans-disciplinary working across academic and clinical disciplines as science, social science and humanities researchers join with clinicians in appreciating the value of sharing insights and theory, not least developing insider/outsider communities to generate and answer relevant questions. The confluence of applied linguists interested in or experienced in health care and clinicians interested in or schooled in applied linguistics will be the alchemy required to advance health language research as part of the broader field of health communication studies and practice. But this axis will need to explore and pursue new partnerships with a range of other relevant disciplines and their technologies in order to deliver increasingly nuanced and applicable findings.

Current contributions and research

Corpus linguistic studies of health communication, for example, Skelton et al.'s (2002) corpus linguistic study of the metaphoric expressions used by general practitioners and patients, utilize extensive datasets. Skelton's study grounds its findings in a collection of 373 consultations, and provides revealing insights into the figurative expression of psychological unease, combining both quantitative and qualitative approaches and thus providing a scope and reliability of linguistic analysis not otherwise possible (Biber et al. 1998). CL analysis of datasets is most readily managed through the application of purpose-built software such as WordSmith Tools (Scott 2004) or the freely available AntConc package on the website of Laurence Anthony (Anthony 2010). However, though popular in other branches of linguistics, corpus linguistics is still a relatively novel approach in healthcare communication studies and despite the growing number of studies we mentioned earlier, has yet to be extensively adopted by researchers working in the field of health. In mental health, Crawford et al.'s (1999b) early corpus-driven investigation of the language practices of trainee and qualified mental health nurses characterized them as 'profoundly rooted in everyday language' and consequently 'very ordinary' (1999b: 339). The linguistic insights generated by this corpus linguistic analysis led Crawford et al. to contend that nursing language needs to be 'addressed comprehensively in all forms of nurse training' (337). In raising awareness about the difficulties, uncertainties and conflicts of mental health nursing language, the authors advocate that professionals need to become aware of the power of language they use and consequently 'become as cautious about it as they are about registering blood pressure' (338). This was reiterated in a call to reflective practice in relation to language use in mental health care (Crawford et al. 1999a). But more recently, this approach has begun to develop in new and exciting ways. Further corpus linguistic analyses have been conducted that are directly or indirectly relevant to mental healthcare delivery, for example, in terms of adolescent email language on psychosexual matters (Harvey et al. 2007) and MRSA infections (Crawford et al. 2008; Brown and Crawford 2009a). In addition, a number of other corpus-driven empirical studies have been completed at the Health Language Research Group including a genealogy of the term 'personality disorder', the representation of mental illness in fiction, the language of depression in adolescent emails, language of health blogs, language of compassion, language of pain and so on.

In this section, we will outline a number of cases of research we have been involved in using CL applied to health care: adolescent health advice email language; cleanliness talk in health; and the language of compassion in mental health.

Adolescent health advice-seeking emails

Over recent years, there has been increased interest in the mediating role of the Internet in health interactivity or the exhange of health-related information and new websites have emerged that address the communication needs of young people in distress (Jones et al. 1997; Aynsley-Green et al. 2000; Biddle et al. 2008), not least perhaps because of the anonymity it affords (Rogers and Mead 2004; Lou et al. 2006; Rice 2006). The new electronic media and particularly email offer clear opportunities for adolescents to communicate their mental distress in a frank or candid way (Harvey et al. 2007; Harvey et al. 2008).

Email is the most widely known form of computer-mediated communication (Hewings and Coffin 2004) and has significant potential for the delivery of health care (Mandl et al. 1998; Spielberg 1999; Kleiner et al. 2002; Car and Sheikh 2004a, 2004b; Waldren and Kibbe 2004). The use of email in a range of healthcare settings and contexts has been examined, including physician–patient relationship (Mandl et al. 1998; Car and Sheikh 2004a, 2004b), pediatric triads (doctor, parent, child) (Kleiner et al. 2002), as well as unsolicited requests for physician advice (Eysenbach and Diepgen 1998). The work of Kevin Harvey and other scholars in the HLRG has focused on CL investigations of messages sent by adolescents to the Teenage Health Freak website (http://www.teenagehealthfreak.org), a popular doctor-led source of confidential health advice and information in the UK (McPherson and Macfarlane 2000).

Between February 2000 (the year of its launch) and January 2007, the Teenage Health Freak website received 60,000,000 visits, an average of 52,864 hits a day. The website receives and responds to messages that are communicated anonymously and in confidence by adolescents seeking health advice and information. These messages do not constitute emails in the traditional sense – contributors submit their requests for advice via an interface on the website rather than from their personal email accounts – but the communicative characteristics of the messages (i.e., high levels of personal disclosure) are very much similar to those found in traditional email forms (Baron 1998).

Since its inception the site has received over 120,000 emails from young people. While we cannot make precise demographic claims about adolescent health or the nature of teenagers' concerns in their entirety from this information, the experience it represents is not inconsiderable and merited inquiry in its own right in the light of the growing role of interactive Internet-based health advice. Whilst the study of the messages is ongoing, the data in Harvey et al. (2007) and Harvey et al. (2008) is based on an analysis of the messages anonymously posted to the website between January 2004 and December 2005. Comprising 62,794 messages, these linguistic data provide a considerable snapshot of the health concerns routinely communicated by young people.

The key findings from this study of the Teenage Health Freak corpus were that in their health advice messages young people felt able to communicate candidly about areas of health that ordinarily they might struggle to discuss in face-to-face interaction with figures of authority (e.g. teachers or general practitioners), such as sexual and mental health concerns (Harvey et al. 2007, 2008). In relation to the former, people writing in were candid in the use of sexual terminology. Key word analysis revealed the recurring presence of 'orthophemisms' (Allan and Burridge 2006), that is, language that is direct and neutral (i.e., non-euphemistic), e.g., *sex*, *penis*, *vagina*, *masturbate*, *erection*, as well as terms that denote precise anatomical detail, such as: *glans*, *scrotum*, *labia*, *vulva*, *clitoris*. Research into sexual health communication in face-to-face settings has described the defining presence of euphemism and circumlocution (e.g., Weijts et al. 1993; Stewart 2005). For example, both patients and professionals collaborate in referring to 'it', 'down there', 'that' and so forth, while terms like 'the event itself' and 'afterwards' are used to describe sex, without the nature of the 'event' being specified very closely (Weijts et al. 1993).

This corpus-based research into adolescent health highlights the role, and value, of corpus analyses of web-based fora as a means of eliciting the sexual health problems of a group who have often been reluctant to engage with terrestrial services and who frequently appear reticent in encounters with health practitioners, counsellors and educators. It was this corpus of data that first highlighted for us the possibility of corpus-based learning activities which can be deployed in getting students to understand the issues in healthcare encounters with underserved groups. In educating health professionals, corpus material can be utilized in data-driven learning (DDL) approaches which encourage learners to engage with the corpus via research tasks.

Cleanliness talk in health

A second example that illustrates the usefulness of corpus-based approaches is a study we undertook in 2005–2006 to examine the way in which healthcare-associated infections were talked and written about in policy discourse, mass media reporting and in the language of infection control specialists. In Crawford et al. (2008) we attempted to map the patterns in mass media coverage over the period 1995–2005. The study identified a shifting media narrative that involves changes in *dramatis personae* over the decade. First, personified forces of nature (in the form of the MRSA bacterium), doctors and hospitals are engaged in a battle of evil against good, but also intelligence over stupidity. Later, in 2000, the press presented the stories of victims of personified bacterial forces, and doctors and hospitals were cast as perpetrators of crimes of omission by not cleaning their hands or their wards, while bacteria were depicted as deploying ingenious strategies to thwart the action of antibiotics. Finally, in 2005, which was a general election year, MRSA became a party political issue, with the term increasingly collocated with the names of parties and politicians. With the publication of a number of key policy documents in the early twenty-first century, such as the Matron's Charter (Department of Health 2003) the 2005 corpus of press coverage highlighted the emergence of a new actor, the modern matron, to mediate between the doctors and the potential victims of MRSA, who was given political and symbolic power. Thus, corpus linguistics can provide a valuable indicator of the concerns of health discourse and how they change over time, and, with some contextual knowledge, the fluctuations of terms and collocations can make sense in terms of political and social events.

The language of compassion

In a recent corpus linguistic study, Crawford et al. (Crawford et al. 2013) examined the language of compassion in acute mental health. Gilbert (2009) notes that compassion is commonly defined as 'sensitivity to the suffering of others with a deep commitment to try to relieve it'. Yet little is known about how a 'compassionate mentality' is represented in health professional language. Curiously, in a corpus linguistic analysis of 20 acute mental health practitioner interview narratives on compassion, there was striking absence of what can be considered major attributes of a 'compassionate mentality' despite the congruent topic focus. Instead, the language used by these practitioners reveals a dominant 'production-line mentality' with a prominent focus on meeting care targets and processing patients – all set against a culture of threat, not least the demands of the clock.

By combining the frequencies of lexical variants of 27 attributes of 'compassionate mentality' as derived from Gilbert's (2009) seminal work, the study provides a fairly robust index of compassionate discourse (Table 5.1) in the interview narratives. Although words that aren't in themselves intrinsically compassion-related could still be used in structures that communicate compassionate meanings (structures that corpus frequency measures of individual lexical items are unable to apprehend) one would expect fair use of a lexicon related to the major attributes of 'compassionate mentality'.

Table 5.1 Lexical frequency of 'compassionate mentality' words in Acute Mental Health Practitioner (AMHP) Corpus (32,556 word tokens). The frequencies are combined for all lexical variations of the listed attributes specific to the context of compassion as identified through concordance analysis.

Attribute	*Frequency (n) of lexical variants*	*Total frequency*	*Attribute*	*Frequency (n) of lexical variants*	*Total frequency*
Kind	kind (7) kindness (1)	8	Concerned	n/a	0
Gentle	gentle (2) gently (4)	6	Empathic	empathy (10) empathetic (2)	12
Warm	warm (1) warmth (1)	2	Friendly	Friends (1) Friendly (1)	2
Loving	love (1)	1	Tolerant	n/a	0
Affectionate	n/a	0	Patient	patience (1) patient (1)	2
Caring	care (19) caring (28) cared (1)	48	Supportive	support (20) supported (2) supportive (3)	25
Sensitive	sensitive (1)	1	Encouraging	encourage (1) encouragement (1)	2
Helpful	help (24) helping (4) helpful (5)	33	Non-judgmental	non-judgmental (4)	4
Considerate	considerate (1)	1	Understanding	understand (7) understanding (12) understandable (1)	20
Sympathetic	n/a	0	Giving	give (20) giving (11)	31
Comforting	comforting (1) comfortable (3)	4	Soothing	n/a	0
Reassuring	n/a	0	Validating	n/a	0
Calming	n/a	0	Respectful	respect (3) respected (1) respecting (1)	5
Open	open (9) opened (1) opening (1)	11			

The most prominent of 27 attributes of compassionate mentality in the interview transcripts are: caring, helpful, giving, supportive and understanding. Yet we are able to identify only 218 lexical variants for all attributes, that is, 0.67 percent of total language used, a seemingly small percentage. This potentially reveals a limited use of language relevant to a 'compassionate mentality'. Indeed, the mean frequency of 'compassionate mentality' words used by interviewees is only 10.95, suggesting only modest evidence of compassionate language in this corpus. To see this relative lack of compassionate discourse more clearly, we can compare the interview corpus with a 10 million collection of general spoken English from the British National Corpus, producing a set of keywords as per the mechanism described in the adolescent health study outlined above. Comparing the two corpora using the corpus software WordSmith (Scott 2004) generated a list of 150 keywords. These salient items appear in Table 5.2 (although for the sake of space only the top 50 are reproduced).

Table 5.2 Top 50 keywords in compassion corpus (as compared with BNC spoken)

N	*Key word*	*Frequency*	*%*	*Keyness*
1	S	725	2.22	3,308.56
2	VE	281	0.86	2,907.55
3	WARD	202	0.62	1,743.61
4	T	345	1.06	1,652.54
5	RE	238	0.73	1,471.96
6	DON	154	0.47	1,332.93
7	PATIENTS	148	0.45	1,077.43
8	ERR	83	0.25	885.14
9	STAFF	136	0.42	644.58
10	PATIENT	78	0.24	554.90
11	ERM	604	1.85	527.48
12	COMPASSIONATE	48	0.15	513.40
13	COMPASSION	44	0.13	401.86
14	TIME	265	0.81	362.52
15	CARE	90	0.28	343.61
16	LL	35	0.11	324.03
17	THINK	387	1.19	320.42
18	PAPERWORK	41	0.13	303.38
19	KNOW	467	1.43	301.95
20	SOMETIMES	88	0.27	291.19
21	YEH	25	0.08	272.74
22	ISN	25	0.08	263.74
23	WE	548	1.68	251.36
24	ACUTE	25	0.08	205.70
25	CARING	29	0.09	198.10
26	M	77	0.24	190.20
27	MORE	182	0.56	183.94
28	D	72	0.22	182.10
29	TEAM	46	0.14	158.24
30	DOESN	15	0.05	155.98
31	STAFFING	23	0.07	149.08
32	HAVEN	18	0.06	147.26
33	THEY	429	1.32	138.24
34	REALLY	166	0.51	135.11
35	THINGS	124	0.38	126.98
36	SPEND	41	0.13	125.78
37	UNDERSTANDING	29	0.09	125.13
38	ROOM	57	0.17	125.11
39	CLINICAL	17	0.05	123.89
40	ENVIRONMENT	35	0.11	123.25
41	WARDS	19	0.06	123.08
42	SMOKE	30	0.09	121.51
43	NURSING	23	0.07	120.56
44	I	1,118	3.43	119.32
45	FEEL	66	0.20	113.68
46	STRESSFUL	14	0.04	112.73
47	PEOPLE	171	0.52	112.61
48	SOMEBODY	65	0.20	111.74
49	SUPERVISION	16	0.05	110.88
50	ROOMS	25	0.32	109.67

The keywords in Table 5.2 provide insight into the propositional content of the compassionate interviews. Although a number of 'compassionate mentality' related words (*compassion, compassionate, care, caring, understanding*) appear as key (i.e., appearing with a significant higher frequency than they do in spoken English), words pertaining to the clinical environment and work routines predominate. Given the interview focus on compassion, the keywords 'compassion' and 'compassionate' would be anticipated. Moreover, even the words that *prima facie* relate to compassion do not, when examined in context, typically communicate compassionate meanings or ideals. For example, occurences of *care*, one of the lexical variants of the most prominent attribute of caring (n = 48), reveal that the term is more to do with a process, a product or a system – that is, the work of hospitals – as it is the description of anything concerning positive emotional or affective engagement with the patients.

The general paucity of 'compassionate language' is perhaps related to the dominance of a 'production-line mentality' (Crawford and Brown 2011) in the language used by practitioners. A simple word list for this corpus has lexical items salient to the idea of compassion ranked lower than *paperwork* (127). The word *need* seems to be being used in a bureaucratic or actuarial sense. Interestingly, terms that are prominent in Gilbert (2009) such as *kind, gentle, warm* and *friendly* are rarely used. The absence of reference to friendship, bar one instance of *friendly*, is very revealing. In addition, despite the emphasis given in counseling and health communication down the years on being *warm, concerned, empathic, sympathetic, open, non-judgmental, calming, reassuring, respectful* or *validating*, these attributes and their lexical variants are barely visible. Overall, we might consider an emotional thermometer for how the practitioners in this current study talk about compassion and their work would register a low reading.

From this study, we can make a few preliminary observations based on our analysis of the AMHP corpus about the presence of a language of compassion versus a production-line, instrumental or institutional language that indicates a pervasive culture of threat in health care. First, there is little description of compassion in the interviews despite the topic focus on compassion and compassionate working. Second, a production-line mentality appears to dominate the discourse of practitioners, with heightened concern for managing and processing people to reach targets amid personnel or other resource shortages.

Main research methods

We have already described some of the techniques involved in corpus linguistics in this field in the process of laying out the ground and presenting examples of the work. However, now that the reader is familiar with some concrete examples of the approach, it is valuable to reflect on some of the overall methodological features of this approach. First, as we have seen, corpus linguistics typically involves working with large textual datasets and may involve exploring generalizations or abstractions grounded in a variety of methodological and theoretical perspectives (Barlow 2011). The insistence of this approach on using real life language examples has encouraged many corpus linguists to question the meaningfulness of a number of theoretical constructs, even such basic notions as parts-of-speech categories. A degree of skepticism is evident concerning the suitability of some of the established categories deriving from the Chomskyan tradition of language analysis (Barlow 2011: 5).

Aside from this preoccupation with real empirical language phenomena, there is a great deal of heterogeneity within the field of corpus linguistics. There is not a single agreed upon research method nor a common set of research questions (Thompson and Hunston 2006: 3) and, as Mahlberg (2005: 17) notes, there is no single unifying theory running through corpus linguistics analyses, apart from a commitment to do what Sinclair (2004) describes as 'trust the text'. In this way, as Barlow (2011) points out, a concentration on actual usage yields patterns that differ markedly from the kinds of material found in traditional cognitive theories of language, and are often more complex in that they are specific and actual, rather than general and idealized.

In the field of corpus linguistics, the bodies of language in question have often been specifically optimized for empirical study, compiled with regard to the ideals of 'true balancedness, representativity, machine-readability' (McEnery and Wilson 2001; McEnery et al. 2006; Kendall and Van Herk 2011).

Despite the diversity in corpus approaches there are some features of corpus analysis that appear in a number of different corpus analyses. From the very early days of corpus work, there was a good deal of interest in collocations (Firth 1957; Pawley and Syder 1983; Sinclair 1991; Kjellmer 1994) and similar syntagmatic units with a lexical component such as lexical frames (Renouf and Sinclair 1991). These collocated features have been called chunks, multiword units, lexical phrases, prefabricated units or lexical bundles (Moon 1998; Biber and Conrad 1999; Wray 2002). Researchers have investigated both their formal properties such as frequency or recurrence as well as their deployment in language as a meaningful unit (Sinclair 1991; Biber 2009).

A second characteristic of the aproach taken by many corpus linguists is the terndency to be guided by frequency information, and consequently a focus on *typical* forms of expression rather than on the range of *possible* forms of expression. Tognini-Bonelli (2001: 87) describes the goal of corpus-based approaches as being to 'derive linguistic categories systematically from the recurrent patterns and the frequency distributions that emerge from language in context'.

Third, another key aspect of the corpus approach is its focus on quantifying the variability found in language. In contrast to many theoretical and cognitive approaches to language that have typically concerned themselves with abstract idealized sentences, it is often far removed from the difficult and convoluted patterns of variation inherent in actual language use. Corpus studies have brought new aspects of variation into perspective, including the study of register and text types (Biber 1988; Stubbs 1996), local grammars (Barnbrook and Sinclair 2001), and variation in lexicogrammatical expressions (Wasow 2002; Nesselhauf and Römer 2007; Cheng et al. 2009). These studies highlight that there is plentiful evidence of what Barlow (2011) calls 'semi-fixed, variable categories' and little evidence of a clear division into well-behaved regular forms and idiosyncratic irregular forms (Barlow and Kemmer 1994).

We will now consider the role of CL for practice by focusing on corpus linguistics and data-driven learning (DDL) in health care.

Recommendations for practice

We would argue that corpus-based language study has a role as a tool for research and learning activities which can be deployed in getting researchers, practitioners and students to understand the issues in healthcare encounters. Indeed, it clearly supports a move towards data-driven learning (DDL). DDL encourages learners to engage with the corpus via research tasks, and is significant in that it is a pedagogical application of a research method, originating with Tim Johns's famous contention that 'research is too serious to be left to the researchers' (1991: 2). As Mishan (2004) describes it, the key feature of the methodology is this 'aura' of research, and this research agenda is what gives the sense of authenticity. In our work as educationalists, we have presented corpus data to health psychologists in training, nurses and counselors and there is generally a fascination with the data and a tendency to ask questions like 'How did they … ?', 'Did anybody say … ?' and 'Were there very many … ?' which are, of course empirical questions which they can then go on to investigate with the actual data. The research element confers a sense of the genuine discoveries that still remain to be made concerning the use of language in health care. Teaching and training sessions with these data can take a variety of forms. The authors have used the data to illustrate conventional lectures and presentations, and have implemented interactive sessions where students have explored all or part of the data themselves. This generates considerable interest and excitement among students who are often keen to share their 'findings' with the rest of the class in plenary sessions.

Despite such enthusiasm for the use of authentic examples and material from corpora in teaching about healthcare communication, it is important to note that there are some important differences between the material included in a corpus of language and the original. 'The texts which are collected in a corpus have only a reflected reality' (Widdowson 2000: 7), for 'Reality … does not travel with the text' (Widdowson 1998: 711–712). The reality, the authenticity, of text is tarnished by transposition (Mishan 2004). There is a need for pedagogic mediation and a willingness to extend the material under consideration over longer meaning units than individual concordance lines if the full value of corpus approaches is to be realized (Flowerdew 2009). In addition, there will be some research questions that it would be very difficult to address in this way without considerable further research to ascertain the demographic characteristics of the correspondents.

Yet, as we have argued, a data-driven learning approach might have a great deal to offer health services. Understanding the idiomatic expressions used to describe health problems, grasping the lay theories and folk ways used to interpret what has gone wrong and getting a grip on the rhythms of complaint might well be facilitated by the use of corpora of healthcare language. In the UK it is becoming increasingly urgent to come up with new ways of educating and training health service personnel, especially in the light of changes in the National Health Service (NHS) workforce and rapid demographic, epidemiological and linguistic changes in the population. There seems to be little support for non-native speakers of English in the NHS, despite the large number of such employees in the organization. For example it is estimated that 25 percent of doctors do not have English as a first language (Cangiano et al. 2009). At present the situation is addressed largely by means of third-party examinations in English such as the International English Language Testing System (IELTS), yet this is only a single point measure, and is only applied to speakers of non-European Union languages. Changes in European regulatory processes may relax this language requirement. Consequently, exploratory exercises like the ones we have described can be integrated into curricula and may have a role to play in educating practitioners and trainees in the idioms of particular kinds of healthcare work, over and above that offered by generic second language teaching.

As corpus research discloses, there is considerably more to health concerns and healthcare practice than simply being able to translate from one language to another and having the relevant professional qualifications. If we take the view that language is transactional, it is important to consider how the language of a healthcare encounter can be 'recipient tailored' (Brown and Fraser 1979). Indeed, it may well be that clients give different accounts of themselves in response to different healthcare professionals, even if the latter are following more or less the same assessment script.

Communication between health professionals and patients is a special type of institutional discourse where participants differ both in the stocks of knowledge and the linguistic resources available to verbalize this knowledge. In order for medical work to proceed successfully it is presumably necessary that the patients' knowledge about their body and complaints is adapted to the purposes of the medical institution through language in interaction. On the other hand it is also necessary that the professional knowledge of the health professionals is adapted to the lay knowledge of the patients. In this mutual exchange there may be a whole variety of speech actions, which each have their own functionality. A simple question such as 'how are you?' for example may be a conversation opener or a request for a display of symptoms, depending on the context (Coupland et al. 1994). Lindwall et al. (2003) describe the use of communication innovations in attempts to engage with the patient's feelings and thoughts and at the time they are scheduled for operations.

It is important to stress here that the overall methods of linguistic research can be applied flexibly and be used to address a whole variety of questions, topics and ideas. These aims will perhaps best be achieved by means of a willingness to work flexibly with partners in the education system, in health policy and in the commercial sector so as to explore topics of mutual interest and reach conclusions that lead to tangible benefits in terms that make sense to policymakers, patient groups, practitioners and commercial partners. We are not suggesting that the corpora presented in this chapter would be applicable to everyone. The point is rather to stress the value of educators collecting corpora from the kinds of setting and reflecting the kinds of problem that practitioners will be working with.

While it is clear that the compilation of corpora is expanding, the emphasis has hitherto often been on language collections with implications for commerce or language teaching. Accordingly, with the data here, and other research materials, we have begun to put together the basis of a corpus specialized in healthcare language, the Nottingham Health Communication Corpus. However, the popularity of health care as an arena for small-scale study means that a good deal of material must have already been collected on a 'cottage industry' basis. This affords some intriguing opportunities for data sharing if the healthcare research community could be convinced of the value of ethically sound compiling of the existing data into a larger corpus.

It is particularly important to examine the issue of health language closely via corpus-based research at present because there are some important changes afoot in the health communication field. For example the emphasis on taking clients' views into account has gained favor with policymakers. It is through careful attention to the language of healthcare encounters that we will be able to document and enhance the shift from older models of information-giving to more contemporarily modish approaches to 'working with the client'. Although linguists and language teachers have in the past been the main users of corpora, they certainly need not be the sole users in the future. Health scientists will increasingly require access to *naturalistic* data which cannot be reproduced in laboratory conditions, while at the same time they are under pressure to quantify and test their theories rather than rely on qualitative data.

By building a large corpus of interactions in treatment provision or advice, it becomes possible to perform an in-depth analysis of vocabulary, interactional structure and reality construction. We can thereby advance an understanding of the conversational practices of the interactants as they achieve their mutual understanding or even mutual miscommunications. Once these formulations are accomplished, it is clear from previous work that their implications can have far-reaching effects if they are put into practice (Crawford et al. 1995; Brown et al. 1999).

We would therefore argue that progress in the healthcare disciplines may best be served by taking a leaf out of the modern linguists' book and using a similar approach to deal with teaching and learning healthcare language. Moreover it might well be possible to link communicative styles, strategies and motifs to data concerning the effectiveness of healthcare interventions. In this way a more effective and evidence-based approach to healthcare language can be developed which will promote the best use of class time for trainees and scarce and expensive resources such as drugs and treatment facilities.

In the next section we will indicate possible future developments in the application of CL in health care.

Future directions

In this chapter we have attempted to highlight some new trends and possibilities in the learning of healthcare communication skills which have some promise to shift the envelope of debate about healthcare communication and the way in which it can be taught. Our account of corpus-based research and data-driven learning in health care, and the cases outlined, have shown how new ways of making sense of language have a place in the education of healthcare practitioners. These techniques can extend the work of educators and raise the consciousness of practitioners.

Since corpus linguistics has only recently been applied in the study of health communication it is difficult yet to know how to evaluate it. Moreover, once we detect sociolinguistic features in healthcare encounters it is an even more problematic task to decide whether they are desirable and whether they are features we wish to encourage in healthcare professionals in the future.

The data that many authors have so far collected concerning interactions between health professionals and clients are often the result of carefully staged investigations in specific research programs. Consequently, a wider use of more lifelike encounters for teaching purposes might be advantageous. Learning the skills of the clinical encounter is a little like learning a new language. In the same way that the use of corpus linguistics has revolutionized the study of language learning and has highlighted the way that some of what is taught in conventional curricula may well be actively misleading. This is why some contemporary scholars of language learning have been so keen to advocate a data-driven learning approach. We wish to make a similar plea for healthcare language and healthcare education.

Healthcare education is a long-term investment with multiple beneficiaries who are not always identified as stakeholders at the outset. As Shipengrover and James (1999) note, these vague and contradictory visions can lead to difficulty in characterizing and measuring the outcomes of education in health care.

It is vital that health language learning and practice advance beyond functionality and basic competence to an increasingly evidence-based and context-specific efficacy – in other words that it contributes to advancement of and not simply attunes to current health communication practices.

Corpus linguistics in health care has yet to achieve an application of advanced statistics or research trials design for determining the impact of particular language actions on clinical outcomes. Much of the work on health language using CL has been Western but there are clear signs that this approach is being applied in Asian contexts, for example Kang and Zayts (2010). The research outlined in Kang and Zayts's edited volume suggests that much more is to come from CL inquiries into Asian medical discourses in the future. While it is certainly good to see in this volume a number of studies that move beyond biomedicine (e.g. Bridges et al. 2010; Hussin 2010), it is to be hoped that health language research in the Asian context will focus much more on less explored contexts of non-doctor interactions relevant to healthcare practice and patient experience. Importantly, however, such work highlights the need to see medical discourses in ever-changing and ever-challenging contexts where global migration and mixed or multicultural ecologies of spoken and written language are not just increasingly prominent but thoroughly testing the boundaries of what can be achieved in interactions in 'fast health care' environments (Crawford and Brown 2011).

Related topics

Computational linguistics; corpus linguistics in health care; online health forums; quantitative linguistic analysis.

Further reading

Baker, P. (2010) *Sociolinguistics and Corpus Linguistics*, Edinburgh: Edinburgh Sociolinguistics. (This textbook outlines the possibilities and limitations in using corpus linguistics to study social phenomena.)

Brown, B., Crawford, P. and Carter, R. (2006) *Evidence-based Health Communication*, Maidenhead: Open University Press. (This book situates corpus-based and other strands of discourse analysis in the contexts of evidence-based health care.)

Cheng, W. (2011) *Exploring Corpus Linguistics: Language in Action*, London: Routledge. (This textbook introduces corpus linguistics using mini-projects to illustrate methods.)

Harvey, K. and Koteyko, N. (2012) *Exploring Health Communication: Language in Action*, London: Routledge. (This interdisciplinary book uses real life language data throughout, bringing together the different strands of health communication research.)

McEnery, T. and Hardie, A. (2011) *Corpus Linguistics: Method, Theory and Practice*, Cambridge: Cambridge Textbooks in Linguistics. (This book outlines basic methods of corpus linguistics and its development in relation to mainstream linguistics.)

References

Adolphs, S., Brown, B., Carter, R., Crawford, P. and Sahota, O. (2004) 'Applying corpus linguistics in a health care context', *Journal of Applied Linguistics* 1(1): 9–28.

Allan, K. and Burridge, K. (2006) *Forbidden Words: Taboo and the Censoring of Language*, Cambridge: Cambridge University Press.

Anthony, L. (2010) AntConc 3.2.1w. Available HTTP: <http://www.antlab.sci.waseda.ac.jp/software.html> (accessed 30 September 2011).

Aynsley-Green, A., Barker, M., Burr, S., Macfarlane, A., Morgan, J., Sibert, J., et al. (2000) 'Who is speaking for children and adolescents and for their health at the policy level?', *British Medical Journal* 321: 229–232.

Baker, P. (2010) *Sociolinguistics and Corpus Linguistics*, Edinburgh: Edinburgh Sociolinguistics.

Barlow, M. (2011) 'Corpus linguistics and theoretical linguistics', *International Journal of Corpus Linguistics* 16(1): 3–44.

Barlow, M. and Kemmer, S. (1994) 'A schema-based approach to grammatical description', in R. Corrigan, G. Iverson and S. Lima (eds) *The Reality of Linguistic Rules*, Amsterdam: John Benjamins.

Barnbrook, G. and Sinclair, J. McH. (2001) 'Specialized corpus, local and functional grammars', in M. Ghadessy, A. Henry and R.L. Roseberry (eds) *Small Corpus Studies and ELT*, Amsterdam: John Benjamins.

Baron, N. (1998) 'Letters by phone or speech by other means: the linguistics of email', *Language and Communication* 18: 133–170.

Biber, D. (1988) *Variation across Speech and Writing*, Cambridge: Cambridge University Press.

——(2009) 'A corpus-driven approach to formulaic language in English: multi-word patterns in speech and writing', *International Journal of Corpus Linguistics* 14(3): 275–311.

Biber, D. and Conrad, S. (1999) 'Lexical bundles in conversation and academic prose', in H. Hasselgard and S. Oksefiell (eds) *Out of Corpora: Studies in Honour of Stig Johansson*, Amsterdam: Rodopi.

Biber, D., Conrad, S. and Reppen, R. (1998) *Corpus Linguistics: Investigating Language Structure and Use*, Cambridge: Cambridge University Press.

Biddle, L., Donovan, J., Hawton, K., Kapur, N. and Gunnell, D. (2008) 'Suicide and the Internet', *British Medical Journal* 336: 800–802.

Bridges, S., McGrath, C., Yiu, C.K.Y. and Cheng, B.S.S. (2010) '"Reassuring" during clinical examinations: novice and expert talk in dentistry', *Journal of Asia Pacific Communication* 20(2): 185–206.

Brown, B. and Crawford, P. (2009a) '"Post antibiotic apocalypse": discourses of mutation in narratives of MRSA', *Sociology of Health and Illness* 31(4): 508–524.

——(2009b) 'Politeness strategies in question formulation in a UK telephone advisory service', *Journal of Politeness Research* 5(1): 73–91.

Brown, B., Crawford, P., Richards, K., and Nolan, P. (1999) 'Holding a mirror up to caring: language and reflective practice', *Mental Health Care* 4(3): 27–32.

Brown, B., Crawford, P. and Carter, R. (2006) *Evidence-based Health Communication*, Maidenhead: Open University Press.

Brown, B., Crawford, P., Nerlich, B. and Koteyko, N. (2008) 'The habitus of hygiene: discourses of cleanliness and infection control in nursing work', *Social Science and Medicine* 67: 1047–1055.

Brown, P. and Fraser, C. (1979) 'Speech as a marker of situation', in Scherer, K.R. and Giles, H. (eds) *Social Markers in Speech*, Cambridge: Cambridge University Press.

Cangiano, A., Shutes, I., Spencer, S. and Leeson, G. (2009) *Migrant Care Workers in Ageing Societies*, Oxford: Centre on Migration, Policy and Society.

Car, J. and Sheikh, A. (2004a) 'Email consultations in health care: 1 – scope and effectiveness', *British Medical Journal* 329: 435–438.

——(2004b) 'Email consultations in health care: 2 – acceptability and safe application', *British Medical Journal* 329: 439–442.

Cheng, W. (2011) *Exploring Corpus Linguistics: Language in Action*, London: Routledge.

Cheng, W., Greaves, C., Sinclair, J. McH. and Warren, M. (2009) 'Uncovering the extent of the phraseological tendency: towards a systematic analysis of Concgrams', *Applied Linguistics* 30(2): 236–252.

Conrad, S. (2002) 'Corpus linguistic approaches for discourse analysis', *Annual Review of Applied Linguistics* 22: 75–95.

Coupland, J., Robinson, J.D. and Coupland, N. (1994) 'Frame negotiation in doctor–elderly patient interactions', *Discourse and Society* 5: 89–124.

Crawford, P. and Brown, B. (2008) 'Soft authority: ecologies of infection management in the working lives of modern matrons and infection control staff', *Sociology of Health and Illness* 30(5): 756–771.

——(2011) 'Fast healthcare: brief communication, traps and opportunities', *Patient Education and Counselling* 82: 3–10.

Crawford, P., Nolan, P. and Brown, B. (1995) 'Linguistic entrapment: medico-nursing biographies as fictions', *Journal of Advanced Nursing* 22: 1141–1148.

Crawford, P., Brown, B. and Nolan, P. (1998) *Communicating Care: The Language of Nursing*, Cheltenham: Stanley Thornes.

——(1999a) 'Nursing language: uses and abuses', *Nursing Times* 95(6): 48–49.

Crawford, P., Johnson, A.J., Brown, B.J. and Nolan, P. (1999b) 'The language of mental health nursing: firing paper bullets?', *Journal of Advanced Nursing* 29(2): 331–340.

Crawford, P., Brown, B., Nerlich, B. and Koteyko, N. (2008) 'The moral careers of microbes and the rise of the matrons: an analysis of UK national press coverage of methicillin resistant staphylococcus aureus (MRSA) 1995–2006', *Health, Risk and Society* 10(4): 331–347.

——(2010) 'Nutritional altruism in lay discourse on probiotics', *Sociology of Health and Illness* 31(5): 1–16.

Crawford, P., Gilbert, P., Gilbert, J., Gale, C. and Harvey, K. (2013) 'The language of compassion in acute mental health care', *Qualitative Health Research* 23(6): 719–727.

Department of Health (2003) *A Matron's Charter: An Action Plan for Cleaner Hospitals*, London: The Stationery Office.

Eysenbach, G. and Diepgen, T. (1998) 'Towards quality management of medical information on the Internet: evaluation, labelling, and filtering of information', *British Medical Journal* 317: 1496–1502.

Firth, J.R. (1957) *Papers in Linguistics (1934–1951)*, London: Oxford University Press.

Flowerdew, L. (2009) 'Applying corpus linguistics to pedagogy: a critical evaluation', *International Journal of Corpus Linguistics* 14(3): 393–417.

Gilbert, P. (2009) *The Compassionate Mind*, London: Constable Robinson.

Harvey, K. and Koteyko, N. (2012) *Exploring Health Communication: Language in Action*, London: Routledge.

Harvey, K., Brown, B., Crawford, P., Macfarlane, A. and McPherson, A. (2007) '"Am I normal?": teenagers, sexual health and the Internet', *Social Science and Medicine* 65: 771–781.

Harvey, K., Churchill, D., Crawford, P., Brown, B., Mullany, L., Macfarlane, A. and McPherson, A. (2008) 'Health communication and adolescents: what do their emails tell us?', *Family Practice* 25: 1–8.

Hewings, A. and Coffin, C. (2004) 'Grammar in the construction of online discussion messages', in C. Coffin, A. Hewings and K. O' Halloran (eds) *Applying English Grammar: Functional and Corpus Approaches*, London: Edward Arnold.

Hussin, V. (2010) 'Indirectness in L2 Pharmacy Students' advice-giving role-plays', Paper presented at the 18th International Conference on Pragmatics and Language Learning (PLL18), Kobe University, Japan.

Johns, T.F. (1991) 'Should you be persuaded: two examples of data-driven learning', in T.F. Johns and P. King (eds) *Classroom Concordancing,* Birmingham: Empirical Language Research.

Jones, R., Finlay, N., Simpson, N. and Kreitman, T. (1997) 'How can adolescents' health needs and concerns best be met?', *British Journal of General Practice* 47: 631–634.

Kang, M.A. and Zayts, O. (2010) *Medical Communication in the Asian Context*, Amsterdam: John Benjamins.

Kendall, T. and Van Herk, G. (2011) 'Corpus linguistics and sociolinguistic inquiry: introduction to special issue', *Corpus Linguistics and Linguistic Theory* 7(1): 1–6.

Kjellmer, G. (1994) *A Dictionary of English Collocations Based on the Brown Corpus*, Oxford: Clarendon Press.

Kleiner, K., Akers, R., Burke, B. and Werner, J. (2002) 'Parent and physician attitudes regarding electronic communication in pediatric practices', *Pediatrics* 109: 740–744.

Koteyko, N. and Nerlich, B. (2007) 'Multimodal discourse analysis of probiotic web advertising', *Language, Society and Culture: The International Journal of Language Society and Culture* 23: 21–31.

Koteyko, N., Brown, B. and Crawford, P. (2008a) 'The dead parrot and the dying swan: the role of metaphor scenarios in UK press coverage of avian flu in the UK in 2005–2006', *Metaphor and Symbol* 23(4): 242–261.

Koteyko, N., Nerlich, B., Crawford, P. and Wright, N. (2008b) '"Not rocket science" or "no silver bullet"? Media and government discourses about MRSA and cleanliness', *Applied Linguistics* 29: 223–243.

Lindwall, L., von Post, I. and Bergbom, I. (2003) 'Patients' and nurses' experience of perioperative dialogues', *Journal of Advanced Nursing* 43(3): 246–253.

Lou, C., Zhao, Q., Gao, E. and Shah, I. (2006) 'Can the Internet be used effectively to provide sex education to young people in China?', *Journal of Adolescent Health* 39: 720–728.

McCarthy, M. and Handford, M. (2004) '"Invisible to us": a preliminary corpus-based study of spoken business English', in U. Connor and T. Upton (eds) *Discourse in the Professions: Perspectives from Corpus Linguistics*, Amsterdam: John Benjamins.

McEnery, T. and Wilson, A. (2001) *Corpus Linguistics*, 2nd edn, Edinburgh: Edinburgh University Press.

McEnery, T. and Hardie, A. (2011) *Corpus Linguistics: Method, Theory and Practice*, Cambridge: Cambridge Textbooks in Linguistics.

McEnery, T., Xiao, R. and Tono, Y. (2006) *Corpus-based Language Studies: An Advanced Resource Book*, New York: Routledge.

McPherson, A. and Macfarlane, A. (2000) *Teenage Health Freak website*. Available HTTP: <http://www.teenagehealthfreak.org/> (accessed 4 October 2012).

Mahlberg, M. (2005) *English General Nouns: A Corpus Theoretical Approach*, Amsterdam: John Benjamins.
Mandl, K., Kohane, I. and Brandt, A. (1998) 'Electronic patient–physician communication: problems and promise', *Annals of Internal Medicine* 129: 495–500.
Mishan, F. (2004) 'Authenticating corpora for language learning: a problem and its resolution', *ELT Journal* 58(3): 219–227.
Moon, R. (1998) *Fixed Expressions and Idioms: A Corpus-based Approach*, Oxford: Clarendon.
Nesselhauf, N. and Römer, U. (2007) 'Lexical-grammatical patterns in spoken English: the case of the progressive with future time reference', *International Journal of Corpus Linguistics* 12(3): 297–333.
Orpin, D. (2005) 'Corpus linguistics and critical discourse analysis: examining the ideology of sleaze', *International Journal of Corpus Linguistics* 10(1): 37–61.
Pawley, A. and Syder, F.H. (1983) 'Two puzzles for linguistic theory', in J.C. Richards and R.W. Schmidt (eds) *Language and Communication*, London: Longman.
Pilnick, A. (2003) 'Patient counselling by pharmacists: four approaches to the delivery of counselling sequences and their interactional reception', *Social Science and Medicine* 56(4): 835–849.
Renouf, A. and Sinclair, J. McH. (1991) 'Collocational frameworks in English', in K. Aijmer and B. Altenberg (eds) *English Corpus Linguistics: Studies in Honour of Jan Svartvik*, London: Longman.
Rice, R. (2006) 'Influences, usage, and outcomes of Internet health information seeking: multivariate results from the Pew Survey', *International Journal of Medical Informatics* 75: 8–28.
Rogers, A. and Mead, N. (2004) 'More than technology and access: primary care patients' views on the use and non-use of health information in the Internet age', *Health and Social Care in the Community* 12: 102–110.
Scott, M. (2004) *WordSmith: Software Tools for Windows*, Oxford: Oxford University Press.
Shipengrover, J.A. and James, P.A. (1999) 'Measuring instructional quality in community-orientated medical education: looking into the black box', *Medical Education* 33: 846–853.
Simpson, R. (2004) 'Stylistic features of academic speech: the role of formulaic expressions', in T. Upton and U. Connor (eds) *Discourse in the Professions: Perspectives from Corpus Linguistics*, Amsterdam: John Benjamins.
Sinclair, J. (1991) *Corpus, Concordance, Collocation*, Oxford: Oxford University Press.
——(2004) *Trust the Text: Language, Corpus and Discourse*, London: Routledge.
Skelton, J.R., Wearn, A.M. and Hobbs, F.D. (2002) 'A concordance-based study of metaphoric expressions used by general practitioners and patients in consultation', *British Journal of General Practice* 52(475): 114–118.
Spielberg, A. (1999) 'Reply to Gurwitz', *Journal of the American Medical Association* 282: 730.
Stewart, M. (2005) '"I'm just going to wash you down": sanitizing the vaginal examination', *Journal of Advanced Nursing* 5: 587–594.
Stubbs, M. (1996) *Text and Corpus Analysis: Computer-assisted Studies of Language and Culture*, Cambridge, MA: Blackwell.
Thompson, G. and Hunston, S. (2006) 'System and corpus: two traditions with a common ground', in G. Thompson and S. Hunston (eds) *System and Corpus: Exploring Connections*, London: Equinox.
Timmermans, S. and Berg, M. (2003) *The Gold Standard: The Challenge of Evidence Based Medicine and Standardization in Health Care*, Philadelphia, PA: Temple University Press.
Tognini-Bonelli, E. (2001) *Corpus Linguistics at Work*, Amsterdam: John Benjamins.
Vegni, E., Mauri, E., D'Apice, M. and Moja, E.A. (2010) 'A quantitative approach to measure occupational therapist–client interactions: a pilot study', *Scandinavian Journal of Occupational Therapy* 17(3): 217–224.
Waldren, S. and Kibbe, D. (2004) 'Email in clinical care: best as part of an electronic record', *British Medical Journal USA* 329: 503–504.
Wallin, M., Talvitie, U., Cattan, M. and Karppi S.L. (2009) 'Interaction between clients and physiotherapists in group exercise classes in geriatric rehabilitation', *Advances in Physiotherapy* 11(3): 145–153.
Wasow, T. (2002) *Postverbal Behavior*, Stanford, CA: CSLI Publications.
Weijts, W., Houtkoop, H. and Mullen, P. (1993) 'Talking delicacy: speaking about sexuality during gynaecological consultations', *Sociology of Heath and Illness* 15: 295–314.
Widdowson, H.G. (1998) 'Context, community and authentic language', *TESOL Quarterly* 32(4): 705–716.
——(2000) 'On the limitations of linguistics applied', *Applied Linguistics* 21(1): 3–25.
Wray, A. (2002) *Formulaic Language and the Lexicon*, Cambridge: Cambridge University Press.

6

A linguistic analysis of diabetes patients' talk

Reported adherence to healthy behaviors

Ulla Connor and Kathryn Lauten

Introduction

Non-adherence to prescribed medication and healthy behaviors is a pressing issue in today's healthcare system. Much research has been conducted in this area under a variety of labels, including *compliance, disease management* and, most recently, *adherence.* In an effort to better understand adherence, researchers have examined a wide range of variables, including psychological characteristics, health beliefs, and demographic information. The extensive literature is summarized in several excellent review articles. Rather than offering an additional review of the adherence literature in this chapter, we refer readers to van Dulmen et al. (2007).

In spite of the extensive research, factors related to predicting and explaining adherence remain elusive. Several possible explanations exist for this lack of powerful predictors. A frequently expressed concern is that research typically examines adherence from the perspective of healthcare professionals rather than from the perspective of people living with a particular health issue. In response to this concern, van Dulmen et al. (2008) have called for patient perspectives to be included in future research.

In this chapter, we present a study in which linguistic analysis was applied to patient life stories to provide a better understanding of patient-level factors related to adherence. Over the past four decades, researchers have examined a wide range of variables in an effort to better understand adherence. Drawing from health literacy and adherence research, we base our linguistic analysis on three psychosocial constructs consistently included in the literature: *control orientation*, based on locus of control research (Wallston et al. 1978); *agency*, based on self-efficacy (Bandura 1977); and *affect* or attitude and emotion (Martin and White 2005). By transforming these constructs into linguistically definable features and developing analytic systems to describe them, we offer researchers and caregivers new ways of understanding patient narratives. Through the analysis of patient talk, our research addresses the need to connect psychosocial constructs of adherence defined through a linguistic methodology and extensive research on health literacy and outcomes. In the rest of the chapter, we will discuss the state of the research in health literacy, as well as in adherence, followed by our research methods and analysis of patients' life story data.

Health literacy

Healthcare researchers are using multiple methods to investigate a variety of health literacy topics. A significant boost to the study of health literacy in the US came from the Institute of Medicine (IOM) 2004 Health Literacy report, which defined health literacy as 'the degree to which individuals have the capacity to obtain, process, and understand basic health information and services needed to make appropriate health decisions' (32). This is based on an individual's skills with health contexts, the healthcare system, and the education system, as well as social and cultural factors at home, work, and in the community.

Edwards et al. (2009) provide a meta-synthesis of the literature and propose a model of information seeking/giving that leads to an empowered patient. Their model points to the importance of other types of literacy beyond functional literacy, namely *interactive health literacy* and *critical health literacy*. Interactive health literacy involves the social and personal skills that enable individuals to derive meaning from different kinds of communication and apply it. Critical health literacy entails advanced skills used to critically analyze information and to control life events. According to Edwards et al. (2009), poor health literacy is associated with decreased ability to participate in shared decision-making.

Numerous studies have documented the difficulties that patients with low health literacy levels have reading labels on pill bottles, understanding patient information leaflets, reading educational materials, and understanding informed-consent forms (e.g., Ad Hoc Committee on Health Literacy for the Council on Scientific Affairs 1999; Doak et al. 1996; Gazmararian et al. 1999; Mayeaux et al. 1996). Research has also shown that poor health literacy is more common among patients who have low educational levels, as well as among immigrants and older patients (Ad Hoc Committee on Health Literacy for the Council on Scientific Affairs 1999). Functional health literacy has been related to poor oral comprehension among patients, particularly in the technical, explanatory dimensions of clinician–patient dialogue (Schillinger et al. 2004). Subsequent research has tested intervention strategies for more effective physician–patient intervention in communication by using regular comprehension checks (Schillinger et al. 2003).

In sum, the existing research points to a strong relationship between patients' literacy skills and how much they know about their disease; there is a clear connection between the ability to obtain information and turning that information into knowledge. This suggests a direct pathway for the development of literacy skills and health management. Patients who know how to access information about complex health issues should be better able to take care of themselves. Yet, research results indicate that additional skills, such as speaking and listening, need to be made part of health literacy.

Our linguistic discourse analysis of patient life stories contributes to an expanded notion of health literacy that considers speaking and listening and their complex interactions with certain psychosocial variables. These two foci – health literacy and psychosocial constructs – are charted in our health outcomes framework, known by the acronym PLAIN Health. The components of this working model are the *Process* of turning information into knowledge, *Literacy* (in its more common definition of reading and writing ability), the capacity to turn knowledge into *Action* (encompassing control orientation, agency, and affect related to health behaviors toward adherence and good health outcomes), *Intercultural/Interactive communication* with healthcare providers, family and friends, and *Numeracy*. The term PLAIN Health highlights factors with the most impact in this arena and reinforces the call to use more 'plain language' in communications with patients.

Adherence and psychosocial variables

To better understand both the *Process* of turning information into knowledge and the way that knowledge gets turned into *Action*, our team recognized the importance of integrating a linguistic system for coding psychosocial constructs of health behavior into the working PLAIN Health model, as psychosocial constructs have consistently proved relevant in other health behavior and adherence research. Linguistic indicators were thus identified for the three constructs that have been studied extensively in relationship to health behavior: *control orientation*, *agency*, and *affect* or attitude and emotion. Studies have shown that none of these constructs individually can account for adherence. Rather, their interaction must be studied within specific disease states (O'Hea 2003). By transforming these constructs into linguistically definable features and developing an analytic system to code them, caregivers will have new ways of understanding patient narratives, as well as an adaptive system to apply to open-ended questions about health management.

Control orientation

One of the most studied psychological constructs related to adherence in chronic diseases is locus of control (LOC). According to Rotter (1966), who introduced LOC as a psychological construct within his Social Learning Theory, a person who perceives an event as 'following some action of his own but not being entirely contingent upon his action' (1) is said to have *external* control, while a person who perceives an event as 'contingent upon his or her own behavior or relatively permanent personal characteristics' (1) is said to have *internal* control.

Rotter's seminal theories on LOC were later applied to healthcare and renamed Health Locus of Control (HLOC) (Wallston et al. 1978). In spite of the considerable research on HLOC and medical adherence, most studies report only moderately significant relationships between these two variables. Some suggest that the inconsistent findings may be, at least partly, the result of the surveys used to measure LOC.

One way to address these problems is to seek indicators of HLOC in the discourse of people with diabetes rather than through surveys. An inherent problem in survey research is the potential for social desirability bias; that is, respondents try 'to answer as "good" people "should" rather than in a way that reveals what they actually believe or feel' (Vogt 1999: 268). A patient's naturally occurring talk is less likely to be tainted by such bias. Thus, identifying specific linguistic features of control orientation that occur in responses to open-ended questions should provide an expanded framework for studying the relationship between control orientation and diabetes management.

Agency

Agency has been defined as the 'capacity to make a difference' (Castor and Cooren 2006: 573). Several researchers (e.g., Glasgow et al. 2001; Hadjistavropoulos and Shymkiw 2007) have attempted to identify the factors affecting individuals' health-related agency, or their ability to take actions that facilitate the self-management of chronic health conditions. Many have focused specifically on the management of diabetes (e.g., O'Hea et al. 2009; Wangberg 2007). Our use of the term agency, based on an individual's actual actions, is closely related but not identical to self-efficacy, which is based on one's *belief* in the ability to do what is needed to attain an outcome (Bandura 1977). Both agency and self-efficacy are concerned with a person acting positively in order to improve his or her health.

As with control orientation, the most common measures of agency and self-efficacy have been surveys (e.g., Anderson et al. 2000; Bandura 1977). We maintain, however, that the actual words of patients living with diabetes may contain more accurate indicators. Therefore, identifying specific linguistic features of patients' actions can provide a useful framework for expanding the study of the relationship between agency and diabetes management.

Affect

The expression or suppression of affect or emotions in relation to coping with illness, especially terminal illness, has been studied from numerous perspectives, perhaps most frequently in psychology (e.g., Keeling et al. 2012; Boinon et al. 2011; Schuettler and Kiviniemi 2006; Petticrew et al. 2002). While this research suggests that there is indeed a relationship between the expression of emotion and disease management, there have been relatively few studies that focus specifically on the role affect plays in adherence to treatment and self-care recommendations for chronic diseases such as diabetes.

To our knowledge, there has not been a systematic linguistic analysis of affect, although a subcategory of Martin and White's (2005) Appraisal Theory provides a linguistic system for its analysis. Because of the comprehensiveness of Martin and White's Appraisal Theory and its validation through empirical testing in other discourses (e.g., Hood and Forey 2008), we place it as the foundation of our analysis of the role of affect in patient accounts about living with diabetes.

Research methods and data

The data on which we report here came from an investigation of adherence among people with diabetes that was conducted by an interdisciplinary research team at the Indiana Center for Intercultural Communication (ICIC) at Indiana University-Purdue University Indianapolis (IUPUI) consisting of linguists, communication studies specialists, sociologists, and an endocrinologist. In-depth interviews were conducted with 43 English-speaking subjects and 22 Spanish-speaking subjects living with diabetes in the Indianapolis area. The data presented here are for the English-speaking interviews only. Of those, 21 were male and 22 were female. Twenty-three were non-Hispanic white, 15 were non-Hispanic black, one was Hispanic, and four classified themselves as Other. The mean age was 51.2 years, and the mean duration living with diabetes was 7.6 years.

The interviews had two sections. The first consisted of several questions asked to elicit life story information from the patients. Subsequent segments of the interview included questions about medication adherence, information sources and use, and health literacy level, as well as basic demographic information. The length of the transcribed interviewee talk on the open-ended questions section ranged from 608 to 11,274 words. The mean number of words was 3,055 (standard deviation 2212.03) words.

The three psychosocial constructs (control orientation, agency, and affect) were identified through analysis of patients' responses to 14 questions about diabetes and its management such as, 'In what ways has your thinking changed regarding diabetes since you were first diagnosed?' 'What do you do to manage your diabetes?' and 'Have you ever had any difficulties communicating with your provider? If so, please explain.' In addition, there were four questions about life decisions at the time of high school graduation, such as 'How did you end up doing what you did after high school?'

The initial coding systems for control orientation and agency were developed using six randomly selected transcripts. The coders carefully read the sample transcripts, making gestalt assessments of the variable that had been assigned to their team (i.e., high, medium, or low agency; internal vs. external control orientation) and highlighting specific phrases in the transcript that represented their assessments. The coders compared the individual coding of the six sample transcripts. The degree of agreement among individuals on the gestalt coding was computed as an indication of intercoder reliability. The percentage of agreement was 87.5 percent for agency and 94.5 percent for control orientation. This level of intercoder reliability was deemed acceptable, and coders then turned their attention to the linguistic instantiations of each construct. The system developed by the research team was applied to the remaining transcripts.

The affect analysis started from an existing framework and took a slightly different path. Six coders analyzed sample transcripts using the coding guidelines from Martin and White's (2005) Appraisal Theory. The group then came together and discussed the appropriateness of the guidelines for this dataset, as discussed in the 'Coding analysis of affect' section below.

Coding analysis of control orientation

After the gestalt assessment of internal vs. external control orientation, a linguistic feature system was compiled to distinguish internal and external patient talk. These linguistic features include semantic roles (i.e., agent for internal; patient, recipient, and beneficiary for external), metaphors, idioms, characterizations of self, claims of knowledge or ignorance, and the use of vague vs. detailed language. These particular features were found to be the most prominent linguistic factors between subjects with internal and external control. A list of features appears in Table 6.1 with relevant examples extracted from the data. A detailed explanation of each feature category is given in Connor et al. (2012).

Coding analysis of agency

The linguistic realizations denoting a subject's agency were also identified. Agency was operationalized as the degree of action the patient reported taking vis-à-vis adherence to current diabetes regimen recommendations.

In the first round of analysis, a subject's gestalt agency was analyzed (i.e., without consideration of the type of action taken or not taken). In this preliminary analysis, the subject received one agency score in a tripartite system of *high*, *moderate*, or *low* agency. Managing diabetes is complicated and involves adherence to medications and medical procedures, as well as adherence to lifestyle behaviors such as diet and exercise. After completing the first round of open coding, agency talk was found to differ, sometimes greatly, depending on the domain of diabetes management (e.g., exercise). Therefore, in the final analysis, agency was coded across six domains for each subject: Medication Adherence, Information and Support Seeking Behavior, Food Management, Exercise Management, Medical Management, and General Diabetes Management. In the final system, a subject's agency could fall into one of four categories for each domain: *high*, *moderate*, *low*, or *not articulated* for when nothing was said about his or her actions in a particular domain.

A subject's level of agency was determined by particular linguistic cues used to describe action or inaction with regards to managing diabetes. The language of agency is manifest in specific lexical and grammatical categorizations; however, agency can be understood in broader terms as well. Specifically, coders considered the ways in which subjects expressed action (i.e., behaviors subjects reported actually engaging in), stance (i.e., attitudes toward or assessment of their actions), and intensity (i.e., degree of intensity or commitment with which subjects reported performing an action or the degree of intensity of subjects' assessment of their actions). The linguistic realizations of agency and examples from the data can be found in Table 6.2.

Table 6.1 Prominent linguistic realizations of control orientation

Linguistic features coded as external control orientation	*Linguistic features coded as internal control orientation*
Semantic role	*Semantic role*
"she [wife] had me keep a little where I took my blood sugar every day" (Patient) "My daughter fixes my food." (Beneficiary)	"I check my feet every night before I go to bed." (Agent)
Metaphor	*Metaphor*
"It [diabetes] was hid back there and like hid out something [...] then it jumped on me and said I'm here now."	"I can whoop it and fight it [diabetes]." "If you work out diabetes gets mad [...] it hurts diabetes when you working out."
Idiom	*Idiom*
"If that's [manage diabetes] what I am kinda meant to do [...] if god wants me to do it then alright I'll do it." "That's [low blood glucose levels] just the way it happens sometimes."	"I'm really on my Ps and Qs." "The idea is to stay with it [managing blood glucose levels]."
Characterizations of self	*Characterizations of self*
"Unfortunately I'm a sweetaholic I love sweets [...] if they didn't make sweets I probably wouldn't be a type two." "I'm not like a real exercise person."	"I'm the type of person that's willing to learn things." "I'm the type of person who will go from one extreme to the other [i.e. able to change habits quickly]."
Claims of ignorance or forgetfulness	*Knowledge of diabetes*
"I don't really know what it [diabetes] is." "When I go out I forget to bring the medicines with me."	"I know everything it takes to get healthy [...] I know the right foods to eat [...] I know the exercise I need to do." "I'm fairly well educated from the outset on the disease."
Vague language in relation to medicine and diabetes	*Detailed/descriptive language and/or medical jargon*
"I'm taking two medications and things like that." "It's [blood glucose levels] up to two hundred or two fifty or whatever."	"There's type one [...] which is the autoimmune reaction where the body basically decides uh pancreas or the islets of langerhans are a foreign body and decides to destroy them."

Table 6.2 Prominent linguistic realizations of agency

	High agency	*Moderate agency*	*Low agency*
Propositions	"I exercise." (domain: exercise management) "I also keep track of you know how much portions I'm suppose to have." (food management)	"I do try to exercise." (exercise management) "I try to eat well." (food management)	"It's [exercise] stopping." (exercise management) "I went on an eating binge." (food management)
Intensity and stance			
Single adverbs of extent/degree and manner; Adverbial clauses of time	"I've been taking my medications constantly." (medication adherence) "I've been seeing him [doctor] *quite frequently*." (medical management)	"I took medicine *occasionally*" (medication adherence) "I've had it [blood glucose level] as low as sixty when I'm watching it." (medical management)	"I didn't take it [medication] *anymore*." (medication adherence) "I crave sweets *constantly*." (food management) "I used to have problems *consistently* [with low blood sugar]." (medical management)
Premodifying stance adverbs	"I *really* started managing it [diabetes]." (general diabetes management)	"I *pretty much* follow a 1500 to 1800 calorie diet." (food management)	"It's *very hard* for me to avoid it [sweet food]." (food management)
Hedges *(we found that hedges suggest moderate agency thus examples for high and low do not appear)*		"I see my doctor *kind of* on a regular basis." (medical management)	

Coding analysis of affect

In order to determine linguistic realizations of emotion, the subcategory 'affect' of the attitude meaning system was adopted from Martin and White's (2005) work on Appraisal Theory. Our modifications of Martin and White's system are described in detail in Connor et al. (2012).

In our transcripts of patient accounts, we were interested in the emotions of subjects toward their disease and its management, as well as toward their healthcare providers. All instances of affect were coded within one of four domains: *diagnosis*, *state of being diabetic*, *management of disease*, and *providers/system*. Each instance of affect was then coded for one of the following categories: *unhappiness*, *happiness*, *insecurity*, *security*, *dissatisfaction*, *satisfaction*, *disinclination*, or *inclination*. Instances of affect were further coded using a subcategory, as recommended by Martin and White (2005). Table 6.3 lists all of the categories (in italics) and subcategories (in parentheses) used in this study.

With refinements to the system, transcripts were coded and recoded accordingly as changes were made. Coded linguistic evidence for expressions of affect included nouns, verbs, and adjectives, as well as multiword phrases within the context of the utterance and agreed upon on a case-by-case basis as to whether or not they expressed affect according to the coding guidelines. Examples of multiword phrases include 'not another thing' and 'that's a bunch of baloney'. Each coder analyzed the transcripts independently, and then came together to discuss and compare results and to establish inter-rater reliability. Each case of affect was coded, categorized into domains, and counted. The total instances of affect in each transcript were divided by the total number of subject words in the transcript and multiplied by 1,000. If the two coders did not have the same counts, their results were averaged, which resulted in some fractions. Table 6.3 provides examples of each affect category. The domain used for coding is indicated before each example.

Table 6.3 Linguistic realizations of affect

Unhappiness (misery)	(diagnosis) "I was really -- I don't use the word depressed but I was you know I was *mad* you know..." (state) "I'm *just in constant* pain."
Unhappiness (antipathy)	(provider) "... I mean I got some of the clinics over [there] that I *don't like* going to because some of the people over there some with <u>attitude</u>..."
Happiness (cheer)	(management) "...when my sugar is lower ... it makes you *feel good.*"
Happiness (affect)	(provider) "I really *like* her."
Insecurity (disquiet)	(diagnosis) "I was *mad.*" "We didn't know how to deal with it." "It was a *disaster* for me to find out." (state) "...for me to tell people, it was kind of *embarrassing.*" (non-medication management) "I'm *scared* of needles."
Insecurity (surprise)	(diagnosis) "It's kind of *shocking.*" "It *threw me for a loop.*" (state) "I *never realized* how bad or how uh drastic uh diabetes can be."
Security (confidence)	(state) "I'm *alright.*" (collective management) "I'm doing *really well.*"
Security (trust)	(providers/system) "... science and medicine have a *better understanding* of how to control it [diabetes]."
Dissatisfaction (ennui)	(state) "I've been very *frustrated* by the whole thing." (diagnosis) "I was goin' to say maybe the first time when I first found out about it I was *kinda aggravated.*"
Dissatisfaction (displeasure)	(management) "'cuz it's *hard* when you have kids and you have to go home and cook them a meal and then you're trying to have a salad..." (provider) "...which if she's an endocrinology doctor she *shoulda known* that to begin with."
Satisfaction (interest)	(management) "I'd go through spurts where I'd *REALLY try.*" "...that's when I really started managing it *like I should.*"
Satisfaction (pleasure)	(provider) "The doctor made me feel real *comfortable.*" "He was *really good* at his job." (non-medication management) "It's *really about the healthiest diet* you can have."
Disinclination (fear)	(state) "The one thing that probably *frightens* me more than anything is losing my eyesight as a result of [diabetes]."
Inclination (desire)	(management) "I'm *extremely motivated.*" (management) "*I'll pick it back up* in the summer."

Analysis and results

In this section, we provide examples of coded excerpts from the transcripts. Then, we describe the quantitative results of the application of the three linguistic systems to our dataset and the correlations of results with self-reported adherence.

Examples of transcript coding

Guidelines for transcription were adopted by the team based on Jefferson (1979, as cited in Schiffrin 1994). In the following excerpts, a plus sign indicates a pause of less than a second; a number in parentheses indicates the length of a pause in seconds if more than one second; a colon indicates that a word was drawn out; non-verbal utterances are inserted within double parentheses; all capitals are used for extra loud words; 'I' stands for Interviewer; and all subject names have been changed to pseudonyms.

The following examples illustrate the application of the coding system to transcript excerpts. In each example, a complete coding of the excerpt is presented. However, these are only short excerpts from much longer interviews. A complete transcript analysis would show many more linguistic features being expressed in each interview. The second example provides the longest excerpt and gives an idea of the richness of the complete dataset.

The first two examples are both coded as internal control, but present the contrast between high vs. low agency coding and positive vs. negative coding. In the first example, Cory, diagnosed eight months before the interview, was coded overall as internal control, high agency in most domains, and positive affect. As the coding in Table 6.4 shows for this excerpt, his language is very specific in terms of what he does to manage diabetes, using phrases that indicate moderate to high agency for actions that adhere to recommended health behaviors. His outlook presents a positive 'can-do' attitude.

Excerpt 1

Interviewer (*I*):	What are you supposed to do to manage your diabetes?
Cory:	oh + they did give me a medication metformin I think it's called metformin my doctor game me metformin and I take it once a day thousand milligrams once a day in the evening. I try to anticipate that at some point in time I'll never have to take anything because I intend to lick this thing with my diet and exercise and I think that at the time I start a nice exercise regimen
I:	uh huh
Cory:	that the medication won't even be necessary.
I:	[...] What do you think about your ability to manage your diabetes [...]?
Cory:	Absolutely I absolutely think that I can manage it.

Table 6.4 Analysis of transcript excerpt for Cory

Coding	*Example from transcript excerpt*
Control orientation coding	
Metaphor	"I intend to lick this thing [diabetes]" (Internal)
Detailed/descriptive language and/or medical jargon	"my doctor gave me metformin and I take it once a day thousand milligrams once a day in the evening" (Internal)
Agency coding	
Propositions	"I take it once a day" (High)
Single adverbs of extent	"I absolutely think" (High)
Affect coding	
Inclination – desire	"I intend to lick this thing" (Positive); "the time I start a nice exercise regimen" (Positive)
Satisfaction – interest	"I absolutely think that I can manage it" (Positive)

In this second example, Delores, diagnosed six years before the interview, was coded overall as internal control, low agency in most domains with instances of high agency, and negative affect. As Table 6.5 shows, she assumes a controlling role over her disease management, using high agency direct propositions when describing her actions, but often qualifying her actions with hedges and adverbs that indicate lower agency. The majority of her expressions of affect are negative as she dwells on her fear and unhappiness of having diabetes.

Excerpt 2

I: What do you think about your ability to manage your diabetes?

Delores: […] it's hard when you have kids and you have to go home and cook them a meal and then you're trying to have a salad and a plain chicken breast […] It's just hard to um + like I said get home at six and have a meal on the table we don't get home to nine ten o'clock at night and you know by then it's fast food ((laughs))
[…]
o:::hhh I don't know + um >I just think like I said the fear of it at the beginning< made me want to do the right thing + and follow + and lose this weight and not be diabetic and not be on insulin

I: right

Delores: and you know not have all these horrible things happen because I'm diabetic you know as far as my um (   ) but putting that with reality in real life is two different things

I: yeah

Delores: and it worked for awhile because my kids were also panicked too you know and like I said just as time went on + and + so I don't care if I drink this pop + ((high pitched stylized voice for next two words)) it's bad + but + I ((next word stylized)) exercise and whenever I drink coffee I make myself drink a glass of water ((laughs)) the same you know and it just I just kinda played with it and make excuses so I can have something that I want ((laughs loudly)) so you know like at Thanksgiving I didn't eat the roll and the +

	dressing and the + sweet potatoes and the + mashed potatoes but I wanted a piece of that pie so + I had a little sliver of pie and I had my green beans and I- I was pretty happy with that you know I didn't have to have the whole + meal even though I cooked the whole meal for everybody else ((laugh)) so I- you just kinds + you know play games with yourself I guess
I:	yeah
Delores:	if I have this I won't have that
I:	yeah what other types of games ((Delores laughs)) do you play with yourself regarding the management of your diabetes ((I laughs))
Delores:	((laughing)) we::ll ++ that's basically it with the food and a- again + with the exercise I- I start out strong I may exercise two weeks steadily and then something – ((stylized nasal voice for the next two words)) it rains so – I have to pick my daughter up and I just totally forget it and then three four days later I go I was walking ((next two words stylized)) what happened and you start over you know.

Table 6.5 Analysis of transcript excerpt for Delores

Coding	*Example from transcript excerpt*
Control orientation coding	
Semantic role	"I make myself drink a glass of water" (assuming role of Agent – Internal)
Agency coding	
Propositions:	"You're trying to have a salad" (Moderate); "I exercise" (High); "I didn't eat the roll" (High); "you start over" (High)
Single adverbs of extent hedging	"I may exercise two weeks steadily" ("steadily" suggests High however "may" suggests Moderate due to hedging)
Premodifying stance adverbs	"I just totally forget it" (Low); "I just kinda played with it and make excuses" (Low); "it's just hard to um + like I said get home at six and have a meal on the table" (Low)
Affect coding	
Dissatisfaction – displeasure	"it's just hard to um + like I said" (Negative)
Insecurity – disquiet	"the fear of it" (Negative)
Inclination – desire	"made me want to do the right thing"; "and follow"; "and lose this weight" (Positive)
Disinclination – fear	"and not be diabetic"; "and not be on insulin"; "not have all these horrible things happen" (Negative)
Dissatisfaction – displeasure	"I don't care if I drink this pop"; "it's bad" (Negative)
Satisfaction – interest	"I was pretty happy with that" (Positive)

The third and final example is much shorter to show the contrast between internal and external control coding. Table 6.6 will only present the control orientation coding. In this example, Pam, who was diagnosed less than two years before the interview, was coded overall as external control, moderate agency in most domains, and negative affect. As Table 6.6 shows, she characterizes herself as being the recipient of diabetes due to her genetic make-up, showing no evidence that she had any role in getting the disease nor control over her craving for sweets.

Table 6.6 Analysis of transcript excerpt for Pam

Coding	*Example from transcript excerpt*
Control orientation coding	
Characterization of self	"it's been passed on uh gene-wise" (External); (sweets craving controls her) (External)

Excerpt 3

I: […] tell me how you were first diagnosed with diabetes and how you felt

Pam: […] it's hard to deal + with it for me because I know that it's been passed on + ((clears throat)) uh gene-wise

I: what do you think of YOUR ability to manage your diabetes?

[…]

Pam: […] the eating part is what I have a problem with and the craving for the sweets oh my GOD

[…]

Pam: sweets craving gets on my nerves.

The next section presents the results from the quantitative aspects of the mixed methods analysis.

Quantitative results

Control orientation

Coders applied the linguistic system of control orientation described in Table 6.1. Thirty-five of 43 (81 percent) were coded as external orientation, suggesting that the majority of interviewees talk about their diabetes as something beyond their control, while 8 of 43 (19 percent) were coded as internal orientation. Table 6.7 presents the frequency and percentage of individuals in each of the agency categories after coders had applied the linguistic system.

Table 6.7 Numbers and percentages of individuals in each coding category per agency domain

	High agency *N (%)*	*Moderate agency* *N (%)*	*Low agency* *N (%)*	*Not articulated** *N (%)*
Medication adherence	29 (67)	8 (19)	2 (5)	4 (9)
Information and support seeking behavior	21 (49)	8 (19)	9 (21)	5 (12)
Food management	16 (37)	19 (44)	8 (19)	0 (0)
Medical management	32 (74)	7 (16)	4 (9)	0 (0)
General diabetes management	10 (23)	26 (60)	4 (9)	3 (7)
Exercise management	12 (28)	12 (28)	9 (21)	10 (23)

Note: *The patient transcript contains no reference to this agency domain.

Agency

Generally speaking, the words of these interviewees indicated a moderate or high degree of agency. Of the interviewees, 32 of the 43 (74 percent) exhibited High Medical Management in their talk about scheduling and attending doctor's appointments, monitoring blood glucose levels, and checking skin and feet. Twenty-nine of 43 (67 percent) were classified as having High Medication Adherence. The domains in which the lowest agency was heard in patients' talk were related to managing diet (19 percent as Low Food Management), exercise (21 percent as Low Exercise Management), and information seeking (21 percent as Low Information and Support Seeking Behavior).

Affect

Instances of affect in each domain were counted by two coders who achieved high reliability. Those totals were then used in the quantitative analysis. Given the scope of that tabulation, we present only a synopsis of some of the more interesting results. Dissatisfaction (Displeasure) was expressed the most overall (524 instances). Dissatisfaction (Displeasure) for Non-medication Management received the highest overall instances (237 instances), suggesting predominant overall negative feelings about such things as diet and exercise. The second highest coding was Satisfaction (Pleasure) for Providers/System (208 instances). While Dissatisfaction (Displeasure) toward Providers/System (137.5 instances) was also relatively high, many examples referred to previous doctors. Once patients changed doctors, Satisfaction or an expression of Dissatisfaction with the insurance provider or healthcare system was reported. Security (Trust) was expressed the least overall (14 instances). Insecurity (Disquiet) was expressed most often in terms of diagnosis (81 instances) and the general condition of having diabetes (127 instances). These numbers were far greater than those for Security (Confidence) for diagnosis (3 instances) and general condition of having diabetes (23.5 instances). Overall, subjects expressed more negative emotions than positive ones about the management of diabetes, but expressed more positive emotions than negative ones about their healthcare providers.

Adherence to medication

After the quantification of the linguistic features, results were subjected to statistical analysis to better illuminate patient-reported adherence to medication. The linguistically identified constructs for each patient's control orientation, agency, and affect served as independent variables. The dependent variable was patients' self-reported medication adherence. Medication adherence was measured through a self-report response to the question 'How many times did you miss taking medications as prescribed during the previous month?' A subject was 'adherent' if the response was two times or fewer. In our dataset, 32 of 43 (or 72 percent) were 'adherent'. The Fisher's exact test (two-sided) was used to analyze the relationships between adherence and the independent variables. The following is a discussion of the statistically significant variables that are most relevant to the linguistic system presented in this chapter.

There was a statistically significant relationship to adherence for those who, through talking about living with diabetes, exhibited High Food Management according to our linguistic analysis system. This suggests that those who talk about controlling their diet (a critical component of Type 2 diabetes management) in an agentive manner also adhere to their medication regimen. An example of such agentive talk is, 'I also keep track of you know how much portions I'm suppose to have.' In contrast, those with less agentive talk (e.g., 'I try to eat well', with 'try' exemplifying the lower agency level) were less adherent to their medication regimen. Interestingly, since our model also examines the influence of health literacy on adherence, those who exhibited highly agentive talk with regards to seeking out information and support were also highly adherent.

We now turn to the expression of affect in these interviews. Of all the categories, expressing Dissatisfaction was the most significant variable when correlated with adherence. Thus, negative feelings are more likely to indicate lower adherence tendencies than positive feelings are to indicate higher adherence. While the former conclusion may seem intuitive (i.e., someone who is really dissatisfied with medication, care, diet, and exercise would be less inclined to follow a medication regimen), we suggest that the latter conclusion is less intuitive. To recognize that positive expressions do not necessarily indicate adherence is critical to understanding the patient and not assuming that positive affect means everything is going well.

Consistent with previously published LOC research, control orientation was not significant on its own in relationship to adherence. We believe, however, that understanding control orientation is critical when examining the interactions of these constructs and providing intervention recommendations through targeted communication, as described in the following section.

Recommendations for practice

Since daily self-care health behaviors are recommended to patients with a chronic illness like diabetes, it is important for healthcare providers to have a good understanding of the extent to which patients follow these recommendations. Providers also need clues to understand how to communicate effectively in a patient-centric manner. The coding system addresses both of these needs. It can be used to create profiles of patients that define their control orientation, agency, and affect. Once the profile of a patient is coded, providers can then provide patient-centric communication that has been tailored for that specific profile in a way the patient identifies with and responds to. For example, in its simplest form, a profile shows that a person displays external control, high agency and negative affect, or internal control, low agency and positive affect. More complex profiles give further information that breaks down agency and affect into domains so a person may show internal control, high agency in taking medication, but low agency in diet and exercise, or negative affect toward ability to manage diabetes, but positive affect toward healthcare providers. Tailored communication can be incorporated into face-to-face communication as well as written newsletters, emails, and text messages.

To train healthcare professionals to assess control orientation, several features of the system can be integrated into instruction about what to *listen* for when a patient speaks. For example: Are things described as happening to or for the patient (external), or is the patient a responsible initiator of the action (internal)? Do metaphors and self-characterizations reflect being dominated or relinquishing responsibility (external), or dominating and taking responsibility (internal)? Does the patient use vague language or claim to not know or forget what to do (external), or does the patient give detailed reports that show knowledge of diabetes and its care (internal)? (see Table 6.1).

To assess agency, healthcare professionals can be taught to listen for such things as: the use of 'try' with a verb, which indicates lower agency; adverbs that reveal intensity of an action;

and hedges like 'kind of' which show lower agency (see Table 6.2). Because the affect system is based more upon what is expressed rather than the linguistic manifestations of content, it requires less training than for control orientation and agency and is rather intuitive (see Table 6.3). Communication is then altered according to the results of the assessment for each patient.

Recommended strategies for people with an external control orientation include using the influence of important people in their lives and imposing an external authoritative structure. Based on results of this study, we recommend that phrases such as 'Your doctor holds the key to your health' or '9 out of 10 people with your health condition have benefited from this medicine' would resonate with those with external control orientation.

Recommended strategies for people with an internal control orientation include allowing them to take responsibility for their health and being clear about expected results to help avoid frustration with perceived failures. Phrases that focus on the individual being in control, such as 'You are in the driver's seat' or 'Consider these benefits of your medication and you may find they would address your concerns', would be appropriate for people with internal control orientation.

Agency has significant relationships with adherence and health outcomes. Thus, the goal of health improvement communication is to increase agency. This includes recommending 'Baby Steps' (DeWalt et al. 2009) and increasing exposure to others' experiences of success regarding the same behaviors. A recommended way to frame advice to increase agency would be, 'From this list of good food choices, pick just one you like. Next time you reach for a food high in carbs or sugar, eat this chosen one instead.'

Similarly, if negative affect is detected through linguistic cues – a variable shown to be related to poor adherence – then professionals could alter their tactics to better understand negative emotions and build up positive feelings by offering words of encouragement such as, 'You are not alone. Many people find it frustrating to watch everything you eat, but you'll feel the difference from just taking one step today to eating better.'

We believe that understanding how the three constructs interact in order to create communication recommendations that address all three states is an effective communication approach. Future intervention studies are needed to test these recommendations.

Future directions

While strictly qualitative research in patient discourse provides valuable insights to the patient experience, the strength of the multi-method approach presented in this chapter is that the qualitative data from the open-ended interview questions can be transferred into quantitative results. Thus, we were able to study the relationships between patient-reported adherence and their talk patterns. In future studies, we will use this approach on longitudinal data to identify trends that emerge in patient behavior over time. Additionally, we will use the quantitative results from this study to design research with larger numbers of subjects to better understand how the constructs interact in a health outcomes model. Finally, the linguistic features presented in this study need to be integrated into intervention strategies for healthcare professionals' use.

Summary

In this chapter, we have described an interdisciplinary, multi-method approach to understanding and explaining patients' own accounts about their health and their relation to health outcomes – adherence, in this case. Our working model, PLAIN Health, guided this linguistic research by forging close connections with praxis/process literature, health literacy, and patient adherence.

Through patient talk and the linguistic analysis of life stories, we identified patient profiles based on key psychosocial variables found in the literature on patient behaviors. Through a qualitative analysis, we first operationalized the linguistic features. These features were then quantified, enabling us to conduct statistical analyses to determine the relationships between discourse and behavior. In the field of health discourse, a great deal of previous research has presented qualitative case studies. The approach presented here provides an analytical system that we believe has important practical implications for translational intervention work.

Acknowledgments

This project was supported by a grant, 'Project for Health Literacy and Patient Adherence,' from the Eli Lilly & Company Foundation, 2007–2010.

Related topics

Diabetes; adherence; self-care; locus of control; agency; affect; applied linguistics.

Further reading

Davis, B., Pope, C., Mason, P., Magwood, G. and Jenkins, C. (2011) '"It's a wild thing, waiting to get me": stance analysis of African Americans with diabetes', *The Diabetes Educator*, April: 1–10.

Hamilton, H.E. (2001) 'Patient's voices in the medical world: an exploration of accounts of noncompliance', in D. Tannen and J.E. Alatis (eds) *Round Table on Languages and Linguistics. Linguistics, Language, and the Real World: Discourse and Beyond,* Washington, DC: Georgetown University Press.

Martin, J.R. and White, P.R.R. (2005) *The Language of Evaluation: Appraisal in English*, New York: Palgrave Macmillan.

O'Hea, E.L., Moon, S., Grothe, K.B., Boudreaux, E., Bodenlos, J.S., Wallston, K. and Brantley, P.J. (2009) 'The interaction of locus of control, self-efficacy, and outcome expectancy in relation to HbA1c in medically underserved individuals with type 2 diabetes', *Journal of Behavioral Medicine*, 32(1): 106–117.

van Dulmen, S., Sluijs, E., van Dijk, L., de Ridder, D., Heerdink, R., Bensing, J. and the International Expert Forum on Patient Adherence (2008) 'Furthering patient adherence: a position paper of the international expert forum on patient adherence based on an internet forum discussion', *BMC Health Services Research*, 8(1): 47.

References

Ad Hoc Committee on Health Literacy for the Council on Scientific Affairs, American Medical Association. (1999) 'Health literacy: report of the Council on Scientific Affairs', *Journal of the American Medical Association*, 282: 525–527.

Anderson, E.S., Winett, R.A. and Wojcik, J.R. (2000) 'Social-cognitive determinants of nutrition behavior among supermarket food shoppers: a structural equation analysis', *Health Psychology*, 19(5): 479–486.

Bandura, A. (1977) 'Self-efficacy: toward a unifying theory of behavioral change', *Psychological Review*, 84(2): 191–215.

Boinon, D., Charles, C., Dauchy, D. and Sultan, S. (2011) 'Effects of emotional expression on adjustment to cancer: a systematic review of research', *Psycho-onchologie*, 5(3): 173–190.

Castor, T. and Cooren, F. (2006) 'Organizations as hybrid forms of life: the implications of the selection of agency in problem formulation', *Management Communication Quarterly*, 19(4): 570–600.

Connor, U., Antón, M., Goering, E., Lauten, K., Roach, P., Balunda, S. and Hayat, A. (2012) 'Listening to patients' voices: linguistic indicators of diabetes self-management', *Communication & Medicine*, 9(1): 1–12.

DeWalt, D.A., Davis, T.C., Wallace, A.S., Seligman, H.K., Bryant-Shilliday, B., Arnold, C.L. and Schillinger, D. (2009) 'Goal setting in diabetes self-management: taking the baby steps to success', *Patient Education and Counseling*, 77(2): 218–223.

Doak, C.C., Doak, L.G. and Root, J.H. (1996) *Teaching Patients with Low Literacy Skills*, 2nd edn, Philadelphia, PA: Lippincott.

Edwards, M., Davies, M. and Edwards, A. (2009) 'What are the external influences on information exchange and shared decision-making in healthcare consultations: a meta-synthesis of the literature', *Patient Education and Counseling*, 75(1): 37–52.

Gazmararian, J.A., Baker, D.W., Williams, M.V., Parker, R.M., Scott, T.L., Green, D.C. and Koplan, J.P. (1999) 'Health literacy among Medicare enrollees in a managed care organization', *Journal of the American Medical Association*, 281(6): 545–551.

Glasgow, R.E., Toobert, D.J. and Gillette, C.D. (2001) 'Psychosocial barriers to diabetes self-management and quality of life', *Diabetes Spectrum*, 14(1): 33–41.

Hadjistavropoulos, H. and Shymkiw, J. (2007) 'Predicting readiness to self-manage pain', *Clinical Journal of Pain*, 23(3): 259–266.

Hood, S.E. and Forey, G. (2008) 'The inter-personal dynamics of call-centre interactions: co-constructing the rise and fall of emotion', *Discourse and Communication*, 2: 389–409.

Institute of Medicine (IOM) (2004) *Health Literacy: A Prescription to End Confusion*, Washington, DC: National Academic Press.

Jefferson, G. (1979) 'A technique for inviting laughter and its subsequent acceptance/declination', in G. Psathas (ed.) *Everyday Language: Studies in Ethnomethodology*, 79–96. New York: Irvington.

Keeling, M., Bambrough, J. and Simpson, J. (2012) 'Depression, anxiety and positive affect in people diagnosed with low-grade tumours: the role of illness perceptions,' *Psychooncology*. Online. Available: onlinelibrary.wiley.com/doi/10.1002/pon.3158/abstract (accessed 9 November 2012).

Martin, J.R. and White, P.R.R. (2005) *The Language of Evaluation: Appraisal in English*, New York: Palgrave Macmillan.

Mayeaux, E.J., Murphy, P.W., Arnold, C., Davis, T.C., Jackson, R.H. and Sentell, T. (1996) 'Improving patient education for patients with low literacy skills', *American Family Physician*, 53(1): 205–211.

O'Hea, E.L. (2003) 'Adherence to medical regimens in low-income adults with type 2 diabetes: the influence of perceived control constructs', Doctoral dissertation. Online. Available: http://etd.lsu.edu/docs/available/etd-0729103-130157

O'Hea, E.L., Moon, S., Grothe, K.B., Boudreaux, E., Bodenlos, J.S., Wallston, K. and Brantley, P.J. (2009) 'The interaction of locus of control, self-efficacy, and outcome expectancy in relation to HbA1c in medically underserved individuals with type 2 diabetes', *Journal of Behavioral Medicine*, 32(1): 106–117.

Petticrew, M., Bell, R. and Hunter, D. (2002) 'Influence of psychological coping on survival and recurrence in people with cancer: systematic review', *BMJ*. Online. Available: <http://dx.doi.org/10.1136/bmj.325.7372.1066> (accessed 18 December 2013).

Rotter, J.B. (1966) 'Generalized expectancies for internal versus external control of reinforcement', *Psychological Monographs: General and Applied*, 80(1): 1–28.

Schiffrin, D. (1994) *Approaches to Discourse*, Oxford: Blackwell.

Schillinger, D., Piette, J., Grumbach, K., Wang, F., Wilson, C., Daher, C. and Bindman, A.B. (2003) 'Closing the loop: physician communication with diabetic patients who have low health literacy', *Archives of Internal Medicine*, 163(1): 83–90.

Schillinger, D., Bindman, A., Wang, F., Stewart, A. and Piette, J. (2004) 'Functional health literacy and the quality of physician–patient communication among diabetes patients', *Patient Education and Counseling*, 52(3): 315–323.

Schuettler, D. and Kiviniemi, M.T. (2006) 'Does how I feel about it matter? The role of affect in cognitive and behavioral reactions to an illness diagnosis', *Journal of Applied Social Psychology*, 36(11): 2599–2618.

van Dulmen, S., Sluijs, E., van Dijk, L., de Ridder, D., Heerdink, R. and Bensing, J. (2007) 'Patient adherence to medical treatment: a review of reviews', *BMC Health Services Research*, 7: 55–67.

van Dulmen, S., Sluijs, E., van Dijk, L., de Ridder, D., Heerdink, R., Bensing, J. and the International Expert Forum on Patient Adherence (2008) 'Furthering patient adherence: a position paper of the international expert forum on patient adherence based on an internet forum discussion', *BMC Health Services Research*, 8(1): 47.

Vogt, W.P. (1999) *Dictionary of Statistics and Methodology: A Nontechnical Guide for the Social Sciences*, 2nd edn, Thousand Oaks, CA: Sage.

Wallston, K.A., Wallston, B.A. and DeVellis, R. (1978) 'Development of the multidimensional health locus of control (MHLC) scales', *Health Education & Behavior*, 6(2): 160–170.

Wangberg, S.C. (2007) 'An internet-based diabetes self-care intervention tailored to self-efficacy', *Health Education Research*, 23(1): 1–10.

7

Health risks and mediated discourse

A case study of 'AIDS in action'

Rodney H. Jones

Introduction

Despite years of health promotion campaigns, the wide availability of condoms, and high levels of knowledge about how to prevent transmission, HIV continues to spread. At the end of 2010, 34 million people were living with HIV worldwide (UNAIDS 2011). Sadly, the group in which the virus is spreading most quickly is the one in which it was first detected in 1982, and the one with arguably the most knowledge about preventing transmission: men who have sex with men (MSM). In the United States, between the years 2005 and 2008 the number of new diagnoses among MSM increased by 17 percent (CDC 2010), and in Europe the rate of transmission for MSM more than doubled in the same time period (van Griensvena et al. 2009). The same upward trend has been documented in Asia, Australasia, South America, and Africa (Roehr 2010). After two decades of efforts to 'de-gay' the epidemic, circumstances have made it necessary to 're-gay' prevention efforts (Kitzinger and Peel 2005).

Many reasons have been suggested for this resurgence of HIV transmission among MSM – a growing complacency that has come as a result of new anti-retroviral treatments, the fact that this generation of gay men have not gone through the trauma of seeing their friends fall sick and die, the popularity of drugs like ecstasy in some MSM communities, and, of course, the Internet, which makes meeting partners for casual sex easier than ever before. None of these explanations, however, can account for the countless episodes of unsafe sex by men who are not complacent or unaware or high on drugs, who did not meet their partners on the Internet and do not display other 'risk factors', men for whom unsafe sex was more of a matter of 'one thing leading to another', like the man who told the following story at a forum on HIV in San Francisco:

> So it was a weird thing, we're using a condom but we're talking about 'yeah, I'm going to come inside you and I'm gonna fuck you without a condom', that sort of thing. And it was just really hot and very compelling and then we pull off the condom, and we're actually doing it ...

> And you know I'm not high, I'm on no drugs. I am who I am. I know what's going on, and it's really hot, it's really compelling. He comes inside me, it's really brief, and it's all hitting me like 'How could I do this, what did I just do, oh my god. I just broke this intense barrier. I went on the other side'.
>
> *(Cotten et al. 1999)*

This chapter is about how 'one thing leads to another' when it comes to taking risks with our health. It introduces how concepts from *mediated discourse analysis* (Norris and Jones 2005; Scollon 2001a) can help us to understand how people negotiate risky activities moment by moment in their everyday lives. The context in which I will be exploring this issue is unsafe sex, but the principles I will be introducing are applicable to a wide range of risk behaviors from drug abuse to participation in extreme sports (see for example Jones 2005, 2011).

The perspective on risk that I'll be taking is based on the proposition that risk is a matter of the concrete social actions that people take. At first this may seem like a rather obvious statement, but, as I will explain, the connection between risk and what people actually *do* on the level of concrete, situated actions is surprisingly under-represented in research about risk and health.

Out of the shadow of Framingham

The Framingham Heart Study, initiated in 1948, represented a milestone in the way people understood the concept of risk. The study demonstrated a statistical relationship between cardiovascular disease and a range of 'risk factors' including age, obesity, smoking, and hypertension (Dawber 1980). Today much of the clinical focus in cardiology and many other medical specialties is not so much on treating diseases or conditions but on treating 'factors' (like high cholesterol) that put patients at risk for developing diseases or conditions, and mainstream preventative medicine has also come to focus on helping people to mitigate or eliminate 'risk factors'. For this we have Framingham to thank.

It was, in fact, in the Framingham Heart Study that the term 'risk factor' was coined (Kannel et al. 1964). Although the simple definition of a 'risk factor' is any variable that puts people at a higher risk for contracting or developing a disease or condition, what actually constitutes a risk factor is quite complicated. Risk factors may involve behavior, physical characteristics, membership in a particular social or ethnic group, or external environmental factors over which people have little control (Rothstein 2003). The variety of different kinds of things associated with risk is what makes the concept of the risk factor both such a powerful tool for epidemiologists, and sometimes a difficult tool to put into practical use for clinicians and health promoters.

When it comes to behavioral risk factors like smoking and drug use, attention is increasingly being paid not just to the way behavior influences vulnerability to various diseases, but the way other factors may influence vulnerability to certain kinds of behavior. A great deal of effort, for example, has been expended to identify the variables that influence unsafe sexual behaviors of men who have sex with men. Among the risk factors that have been associated with unprotected anal intercourse are: being alienated from the gay community (Herek and Glunt 1995), and being affiliated with the gay community (Flores et al. 2009); being in a committed relationship (Elford et al. 2001), and not being in a committed relationship (Rosenberg et al. 2011); feelings of invulnerability (Vieira De Souza et al. 1999), and a sense of the inevitability of becoming infected (Kalichman et al. 1997); meeting partners via the Internet (Benotsch et al. 2002), and lack of access to the Internet (McFarlane et al. 2005);

being younger (Mansergh and Marks 1998), and being older (Grossman 1995); being HIV positive (Halkitis and Parsons 2003), and being HIV negative (Shidlo et al. 2005).

The purpose of presenting this catalogue is not to undermine the value of such risk factors in predicating behavior among members of certain populations of gay men, but to illustrate the problems that arise when such findings are considered apart from their social contexts in which actual unprotected anal intercourse occurs between actual people. As Berg and Grimes (2010) put it, while such factors have predictive power, they often lack the kind of 'useful explanatory power' that might come from more qualitative research which takes into account 'unique local factors associated with unsafe sex'.

Finally, focusing on risk factors to understand risk behavior tends to obscure the role of individual agency as it unfolds over the course of a particular event or series of events. Actors are seen as more or less at the mercy of their demographic characteristics, their environments, or their attitudes and beliefs. This erasure of the individual as agent becomes complete when the isolation of 'risk factors' is translated into the identification of 'risk groups' for whom 'one size fits all' interventions are designed.

At the other extreme are approaches that overemphasize the role of individual decision-making in risk behavior, downplaying the importance of social and environmental factors. An example of this can be seen in a now famous article by systems analyst Ralph Keeney called 'Personal Decisions are the Leading Cause of Death' (2008) in which the author argues that the focus of public health be shifted from risk factors to the individual 'decisions' people take that lead to diseases. For those aged from 15 to 64, Keeney writes, 'about 55% of all deaths can be attributable to personal decisions' (1345). 'The inescapable conclusion of these results', he claims, 'is that individuals have a great deal of control over their own mortality.'

Although Keeney presents his approach as a radical 'reframing', this view of the risk-taker as a rational decision-maker is actually at the heart of many of the most influential models of health promotion, including the 'health belief model' (Becker 1974) and the 'theory of reasoned action' (Ajzen and Fishbein 1980; Fishbein et al. 1994). Of course, as both Keeney and others who subscribe to individualistic behavior change models are quick to point out, to say risk behavior is a matter of rational decision-making is not to say that individuals always make rational decisions. Nevertheless, the whole notion of a decision implies a process of conscious deliberation and 'assumes that the individual recognizes that he or she has a choice and has control of this choice' (Keeney 2008: 1136). From this perspective, the best way to change behavior is to provide people with information with which they can make more 'informed' choices.

It is not hard to see the limitations of such models when faced with sexual risk behavior, not just because sex is often associated with emotion rather than reasoned decision-making, but also because sex (at least the type which transmits HIV) never involves just one person, but is always a matter of 'joint decision-making' or negotiation between two or more parties, which is invariably affected by a host of 'social' factors like communication and power. The most persuasive argument against such models, however, is their poor track record in predicting behavior change (Van Campenhoudt et al. 1997). Countless studies of HIV-related risk have shown a wide discrepancy between knowledge and behavior (see for example O'Sullivan et al. 2006; Ratliff-Crain et al. 1999). Whatever the role played by deliberative decision-making in risk behavior, it is clear that more knowledge about HIV transmission and its dangers does not necessarily translate into safer sex. This is also true for a host of other high-risk behaviors like smoking and overeating.

This chapter aims to introduce a way of looking at risk behavior that avoids both the 'methodological individualism' of psychological models of behavior change and the environmental determinism implied by models based on 'risk factors', by focusing on the moment when psychological and environmental factors interact in the concrete observable *actions* that people take. When I speak of actions, I mean something rather different from 'behavior', which is often viewed as an abstract, essentialized phenomenon that can be considered independent of the context in which it occurs. 'Actions' – or, as I will be referring to them, *mediated actions* – are 'real-time, irreversible, one-time only' phenomena (Scollon 2001a: 5). Although it is the nature of mediated actions to produce and reproduce broader social practices (behaviors), social identities (such as group membership), and social structures, actions are best understood as taking place at particular *sites of engagement* in which particular social actors, social relationships, environmental conditions, and physical circumstances come together.

From this perspective, the question is not so much 'what are the factors associated with risk behavior?' as it is 'what is actually going on when somebody takes a risk?' It is a perspective that shifts our attention to the ways actions unfold under the influence of the various resources (social, psychological, and material) that are available to social actors and the negotiative processes they engage in when deploying these resources.

This approach is not meant to replace either of those I discussed above, but instead to provide a way in which risk factors and mental processes can be understood in the *context* of the interaction between social actors in particular situations. Understanding the 'causes' of risk-taking requires an understanding of risk as part of real-time social processes engaged in by 'real' people (Rhodes 1997; van Campenhoudt et al. 1997).

Such an approach is, of course, not without its own methodological difficulties, most central being the fact that it is hardly ever possible to observe first hand these real-time social processes, especially when it comes to things like unsafe sex. In my discussion below I rely for data on people's retrospective accounts of their sexual experiences taken from interviews and diary entries (Jones 2007; Jones and Candlin 2003), a reliance which naturally raises a host of issues regarding objectivity, memory, and the effect of the social occasion itself on the content of accounts. Epidemiological studies of behavior, however, also rely on self-reported data gathered through questionnaires, which have an even greater potential to distort what actually occurred by forcing it into predetermined behavioral categories. Qualitative accounts at least provide a window into the lived experiences of participants by allowing them to describe what happened in their own terms. While narrative accounts cannot be regarded as objective reflections of what actually occurred, they are reflections of how people *organize* their experiences retrospectively (Plumridge and Chetwynd 1999), and understanding how people organize past actions can give us important insights into how they anticipate future ones.

Risk and action

The theoretical framework on which this approach to risk is based is *mediated discourse analysis* (Norris and Jones 2005; Scollon 2001a, 2001b), a method of discourse analysis that focuses not so much on texts and talk as on the social actions that texts and talk make possible. Mediated discourse analysis has its roots in socio-cultural psychology, especially the work of Soviet psychologist Lev Vygotsky (1981), who attempted to explain the relationship between intramental (psychological) processes and intermental (social) processes through the concept of *mediation*. All actions, according to Vygotsky, are *mediated* through the cultural tools made available in our socio-cultural environments. These tools consist of two types. There are physical tools like screwdrivers, computers and, of course, in the context of 'safer sex', condoms. And there are what Vygotsky called 'psychological tools', which he defined as 'language and gestures, sign systems, reading and writing, mnemonic techniques, works of visual art, diagrams, maps and the like'. In the context of HIV prevention, we would want to include here the language and non-verbal codes that people use to negotiate the sexual act, 'sexual scripts' (Emmers-Sommer and Allen 2005; Laumann and Gagnon 1995), 'facts' about HIV transmission, slogans and directives from media and public health materials, and advice from people like friends, teachers, counselors, and parents.

All actions are social because they depend upon our access to and mastery of these shared resources. They are individual (psychological) insofar as individuals may adapt these resources to their own purposes. Actions, then, occur at the site of what Wertsch (1994: 205) calls the 'tension between the mediational means as provided in the sociocultural setting and the unique contextualized use of these means in carrying out particular concrete actions'.

From the perspective of mediated discourse analysis, there are three important things about cultural tools that affect the kinds of actions that people can take with them. The first is that all mediational means make some actions easier and other actions more difficult. In other words cultural tools have certain *affordances* and *constraints* associated with them. The second is that the appropriation of a mediational means always constitutes on some level the appropriation of one or more *social identities*. The third is that, even within the affordances and constraints of the mediational means available to take action, there are always opportunities for social actors to exercise *creativity* in adapting the mediational means to fit their particular circumstances and goals.

The affordances and constraints of mediational means might be inherent to the mediational means themselves (a hammer is inherently more useful for driving in nails than a screwdriver), or they might be the result of social conventions of use that have adhered to mediational means as a result of their histories within particular communities. Consider, for example, the account below (Excerpt 1) from the research diary of a 26-year-old gay man from Hong Kong in which he describes his sexual relationship with his partner:

> *Excerpt 1*
> When we are seized with a sudden impulse to have sex, I request him not to use a condom in order to have more intimate contact and he agrees. When he inserts his cock into my ass our sex and love are more substantial. Compared with using a condom, you can feel that sex without a condom is more exciting. Exempted from the worry of AIDS, sex is more enjoyable and exciting. When the intercourse is finished … I start to worry whether there is any probability of getting AIDS. In fact, under such romantic conditions, you don't really think about AIDS. Instead you feel safe to have sex with him because you believe he is faithful to you.
>
> *(Jones and Candlin 2003: 207)*

This example illustrates a fact observed in countless studies of condom use in intimate relationships (see for example Elford et al. 2001) that while condoms amplify the prevention of HIV transmission when regarded from a strictly technological perspective, in the context of actual relationships they often take on multiple complex meanings. In the situation described above, condoms are seen to *constrain* actions which may be just as important to this writer as avoiding HIV infection, actions like maximizing pleasure, establishing intimacy, and expressing love.

The second important thing about cultural tools is that their appropriation always involves claims and imputations of identity. As seen in the example above, not using a condom in the context of an intimate relationship has the effect of claiming for oneself and one's partner a particular relational status, and often the ratification of relational status is one of the primary *aims* of a sexual act. A participant interviewed for a study of AIDS prevention among gay men in China (Excerpt 2, Jones 2007) similarly resisted using condoms because he felt using them would result in claiming for himself and imputing on his partner 'spoiled identities' (Goffman 1963).

> *Excerpt 2*
> If I like my partner ... it feels strange to use this [a condom] ... it gives the feeling that you don't trust me ... you think I'm dirty ... and if you reverse it ... no ... you're not dirty ... I just want to protect you ... then I'm dirty ... this is the most important reason.
>
> *(Jones 2007: 107)*

The appropriation (or non-appropriation) of particular cultural tools does not just have the effect of communicating relational identity, but can also serve to claim or impute wider social identities. In the following quote (Excerpt 3), for example, an informant from China uses his refusal to use condoms as a way to claim heterosexual identity:

> *Excerpt 3*
> I only go to the fishing pond occasionally ... I'm not 'full-time' ... I've also got a girlfriend, so I'm not the same as most comrades ... right? ... so I really hate to use condoms ... and I don't need to use them.
>
> *(Jones 2007: 101)*

The third important thing about cultural tools is that their affordances and constraints are not determinant of the actions that can be taken with them. When we appropriate cultural tools, we always adapt them to our own purposes or, to use Bakhtin's (1981: 293) words, we 'populate' them with our 'own intentions', and so it is quite common for a tool which may have been intended for one purpose to end up being adapted to a different purpose altogether. This, unfortunately, seems to have occurred with the prohibitions on unprotected anal intercourse, so prevalent in public health discourse, which have ended up making this practice *more* rather than less attractive for many gay men. As the AIDS activist and educator Eric Rofes confessed:

> Sex has taken on new meanings for me derived specifically from AIDS prevention discourse. I have found that the idea of anal sex without a condom is a great turn-on for me, and have brought this fantasy into my sex life while refusing to engage in unprotected anal sex. To make the matter a bit more heretical, I have had sex with men who are uninfected, yet who enjoy the fantasy that I am HIV positive and about to have sex with them without a condom.
>
> *(Rofes 1998: 302)*

What such reflections, along with the growing popularity of intentional unprotected sex ('barebacking') among certain segments of the gay population reminds us is that the relationship between discourse and behavior is often complex and unpredictable, and that it is nearly impossible to 'read off' of a particular cultural tool the actions that people will take with it in particular social situations.

And so the first set of questions that mediated discourse analysts ask when it comes to risk behavior are: What is the relationship between the cultural tools available to people to avoid risk and the actions they are able to take? What is the relationship between these actions and the way people enact social identity in the context of particular relationships or particular communities? And, how do people adapt cultural tools to their own purposes?

Syntagms, paradigms, and the 'funnel of commitment'

In many of the accounts of unsafe sex I have collected, however, participants are much less clear about their reasons for not using condoms. Rather than reflecting on the affordances and constraints of the tools available to them or on the claims and imputations of social identity associated with these tools, participants explained episodes of unsafe sex as simply a matter of 'one thing leading to another'. Individuals may plan to refrain from unsafe sex or initiate sexual contact with the intention of using a condom only to be swept up in a chain of actions. In other words, what seemed to drive risk behavior was the sense of 'momentum' associated with the behavior itself. Scollon (2001b) calls this sense of 'momentum' 'the funnel of commitment'.

Sex, like all complex activities, is not a matter of discrete actions that can be considered separately, but is rather made up of *chains* of mediated actions, each following the other in predictable patterns based on all sorts of factors, including human biology, social convention, and the environment. Like language, these chains of mediated actions can be analyzed both syntagmatically and paradigmatically, both as a matter of 'one thing leading to another', and as a matter of behavioral *paradigms* or 'social practices' that over time have come to be conventionalized in particular social groups.

In analyzing accounts of unsafe sex syntagmatically, two things become apparent. First, people often arrange the actions in their accounts of unsafe sex in a way that each action is portrayed as creating the conditions for or 'inviting' subsequent actions, and providing evidence as to how the previous actions have been interpreted by partners, not very different from the relationship of 'conditional relevance' that conversation analysts (Sacks 1966; Schegloff 1968) have pointed out between utterances in conversations. Second, in assigning agency for these sequential actions, people often alternate responsibility for the actions between themselves and the other person so that the responsibility for unsafe sex is shared.

Both of these tendencies can be seen in the example below (Excerpt 4, Jones and Candlin 2003) in which the author of a diary entry relates an episode of unprotected anal intercourse between himself and 'Mr. A', a new acquaintance. As illustrated by the way I have arranged the sentences of the story into different columns, the account consists of sequential actions arranged in pairs, much like a conversation, each action by one particular actor portrayed as arising from the previous action of his partner, and as validating the meanings assigned to previous actions. Furthermore, agency for actions alternates between the narrator and his partner, Mr. A.

Analyses of such an account from the behavior change school of health communication would likely focus on the 'commentary' given by the storyteller (arranged in Excerpt 4 in the far left column) and conclude that it was primarily the storyteller's thoughts and feelings (for example, 'I felt so high that I didn't care') that drove this episode of unsafe sex. Mediated discourse analysis, while not discounting the role of thoughts and feelings, would focus more on the actions themselves and note the ways the storyteller makes himself accountable for these actions by arranging them in an orderly fashion, each action acting as a motivation for subsequent actions.

Excerpt 4

	ME	US	HIM
		Mr. A and I got very horny in the middle of the night, we therefore went into the toilet. We caressed, sucked.	
It lasted longer without a condom	I fucked him from behind and felt particularly high		
			Mr. A kept spitting on my penis and on his ass as lubricant.
I felt extremely comfortable. When I felt I was about to come, I felt so high that I didn't care	and shot in his ass.		Mr. A accepted it.

Source: From Jones and Candlin (2003: 206).

At the same time, the way people organize chains of actions is not just a matter of responding to previous actions. We also organize our actions with reference to socially recognized practices or 'scripts' (Emmers-Sommer and Allen 2005). Sexual encounters are more than just chains of actions: they are 'types' of activities, paradigms, and different sorts of paradigms allow certain elements to be introduced into them and don't allow other elements. The activity of 'making love' for example, as I noted above (see analysis of Excerpt 1), is a paradigm which resists the introduction of the element of a condom, whereas a casual sexual encounter in a bathhouse might more readily allow for such an element.

What Scollon (2001b) means by the 'funnel of commitment' is that the chains of action we engage in *themselves* play a role in our ability to resist or interrupt them. He gives the example of buying a cup of coffee, noting that the further along we progress in this chain of actions: entering the coffee shop, choosing a product, placing our order, paying, and accepting the coffee from the server, the harder it becomes to change or reverse this chain of actions. This is because of the dual force of the syntagmatic and the paradigmatic dimensions of the activity, the syntagmatic dimension driving the activity forward through the power of one action to constrain the kinds of actions that can follow it, and the paradigmatic dimension driving the activity forward by virtue of the expectations participants share about how this activity should be carried out. The same reasoning can be applied to a sexual encounter in which discrete actions 'open up slots' (Schegloff 1968) for subsequent actions and broader scripts about things like sex, love, and desire seem to push people into particular roles and particular actions.

From this perspective, rather than asking why a particular individual did or did not use a condom in a particular sexual encounter we might more productively ask: At what points in this encounter did using a condom become either more or less possible, and how was this affected by partners' shared expectations about how 'one thing follows another' in certain kinds of sexual encounters and certain kinds of relationships? The value of this way of thinking is that it gives researchers, counselors, and those who engage in risk behavior themselves a way to analyze what happened that avoids the fatalism implied in narratives of lost control ('I just couldn't help myself') and the self-blame implied in narratives of personal responsibility ('I should have known better'). It is a way of thinking that also has great practical value in helping people plan how future chains of actions can be altered and future expectations can be negotiated between partners in ways that unsafe sex can be avoided.

Actions, practices, and 'risk groups'

It is not enough, of course, from the point of view of public health, to confine our analysis to individual episodes of risk without asking how the chains of actions leading up to risky behavior come to constitute recognized social practices within certain communities. What are the mechanisms by which practices like 'safe sex' or 'barebacking' come to be regarded as 'community practices' (Watney 1990) in ways that they affect the paradigmatic dimension of people's actual sexual encounters?

The problem with traditional ways of regarding risk groups from an epidemiological perspective is that people are defined in terms of traits (such as age, ethnicity, and sexual orientation) rather than by the actions that they take together. In such approaches, even 'behaviors' are treated as traits rather than as phenomena. Mediated discourse analysts, on the other hand, define communities based on what people actually *do* together. Communities are communities *of practice* (Lave and Wenger 1991), or, as Scollon (2001a) calls them, *nexes of practice.*

Of course just because people engage in the same social actions this does not make them into a community; all of the gay men who engage in unsafe sex do not constitute a community in the same way 'barebackers' might. What separates groups of people who happen to engage in similar actions using similar cultural tools (what Wertsch (1998) calls 'implicit communities') from 'communities of practice' in which shared expectations about actions come to be regarded as emblems of group membership is what mediated discourse analysts call the 'technologization of practice' (Scollon 2001a; Jones 2002). The technologization of practice is the mechanism by which social actions themselves come to be regarded as cultural tools, which can be lifted out of their social contexts and appropriated into new contexts.

Like the mechanisms that drive social actions described above, the mechanisms that drive the technologization of social practices have both 'bottom-up' and 'top-down' dimensions. On the one hand it is a matter of active processes of 'imagining' (Anderson 1991) by members of particular groups accomplished through the circulation of texts and other semiotic tools. In the early days of the HIV epidemic among gay men, for example, texts like Michael Callen's 1983 pamphlet 'How to Have Sex in an Epidemic' helped gay men to see condom use in ways that affirmed rather than threatened the sex-positive values of the community. Similarly, websites, parties, and pornographic videos extolling the joys of 'barebacking' help men who engage in this practice to regard it as something more than just an individual proclivity. Sometimes the technologization of social practices can serve strategic purposes for communities, serving to distinguish them from other communities or to make them seem more 'normal'. In my analysis of unsafe sexual practices among Chinese MSM (Jones 2007), for example, I argued that one reason condom use had not been successfully technologized as a community practice is because it makes it harder for gay communities to portray themselves as conforming to traditional Chinese norms of sexual morality.

The circulation of texts and other semiotic tools, however, is not enough to drive the technologization of practice. If this were so, then the 'top-down' approaches of most health promotion would be much more successful than they actually are. The technologization of practices also takes place through the moment-by-moment claims and imputations of identity that occur in the kinds of situated sexual encounters I described above. In this regard, social practices come to be technologized in a kind of cyclical process by which sequences of actions are submerged into the habitus of individual members and then passed on to new members in subsequent encounters. Scollon (2001a), for example, shows how the social practice of 'handing' arises in the habitus of a child through the gradual accumulation of actions taken with family members over the course of several months, and my own analysis of gay men's narratives of early sexual encounters (Jones 2008) shows how habits of unsafe sex develop in individuals through the moment-by-moment negotiation of sexual encounters with other community members over time. In that study I relate the following story told by a gay man in Hong Kong:

> When I was studying at F3 or 4[1] I read a magazine article which mentioned about a homosexual got arrested because of his indecent behavior in the public toilet in Jordan. The article also reported on all the public toilets in Hong Kong which were very popular among gay people. After reading the article I could hardly wait and decided to go to the toilet in Shamshuipo on Saturday in the same week.
>
> I arrived there at 6pm, it took me quite a while to get there because I was unfamiliar with that area. I felt scared and excited. Scared because there might be bad guys, triad people, cops and I was only a 14–15 young man, you couldn't tell what others might think. Excited because of the unknown situation: I could meet a late teenager or someone at his early 20s, someone athletic with a sexy body.
>
> When I got there. I saw some men at the cubicles, some were at the urinal. I walked to the washing basin and started washing my hands and looked at the mirror as what the article described about how gay men cruise in the toilet.
>
> I saw a man in his 20s, he looked at me in the mirror and signaled us to leave together. I followed him. I was very nervous and also because it was my first time, I didn't really choose. When we were outside, this gay started to me questions about my name, age and my work ... I said to myself that he really had lots to say.
>
> We walked into a small park where there was a toilet. He went in first to check if there were other people around. He then took us in a cubicle and started to undress me and kissed me. He even used his mouth ... I was very excited then that I ejaculated in his mouth.
>
> Before we parted, he talked to me sincerely for a while: 'The gay circle is very complicated that you need to be careful. Police may come in at any time; play safe and use a condom, don't get an STD ...' He gave me his telephone number then left.
>
> On my way home, I was still recalling what had just happened. I asked myself if he would get AIDS because he had sucked my dick. But I didn't think he would.
>
> I kept wishing that I would have more similar experiences in the future. I want the thrill, the excitement. Since then, whenever I have time, I would look and cruise around.
>
> *(Jones 2008: 251–252)*

In this account we have both of the dimensions I mentioned working to technologize the practice of 'cruising around'. On the one hand it is technologized through the circulation of texts like newspaper articles and advice from older gay men to younger gay men. On the other hand, it is constituted through the moment-by-moment negotiation of discrete social actions such as gazing, signaling, following, and making certain uses of public spaces like toilet cubicles.

What is important to note in this example is that these two dimensions of the technologization of social practice are not always complementary: sometimes they exist in contradictory relationships. In this example, the way the older man characterizes sexual practices in his advice ('play safe'), for instance, contradicts the arguably unsafe practices the two partners have just engaged in.

The challenge of mediated-discourse oriented approaches to health communication is to come to a clearer understanding of how risk behaviors develop, both for the individual and for the communities of which they are a part, through attention to *both* broader processes of community practices and to the discursive negotiation of actions and identities in *situated* social encounters.

Applications and conclusion

In this chapter I have outlined how the principles of mediated discourse analysis can be applied to the analysis of risky behavior in ways that take us beyond the methodological individualism and environmental determinism of more traditional approaches. Simply giving people more information or belittling their risk behavior as 'irrational' is not very useful in helping them to change their behavior. An approach informed by mediated discourse analysis does not begin with the assumption that people's 'risky' behaviors are necessarily a result of 'deficiencies' in knowledge. Rather, it considers how behaviors arise from the ways individuals in actual interaction negotiate what they are *doing* using the discursive resources available to them, and also how these behaviors often have their own 'local logic', sometimes functioning as strategies for individuals or groups to accomplish important social goals.

The most important aspect of this approach, however, is its potential to inform interventions in which risk-takers can be made more aware of the moment-by-moment unfolding of their risk behavior through producing narratives, role plays, videos, and other artifacts of their experiences (see for example Jones 1997; Jones et al. 1998). The outcomes of such reflective accounts of risk can be an understanding of how certain tools might either constrain or amplify the avoidance of risk or how small alterations in behavior near the beginning of a 'funnel of commitment' can make a difference between risk and safety. Such reflective approaches to health behavior have already shown themselves effective in areas like drug abuse, exercise, diet and diabetes management (Frost and Smith 2003; Goetz 2010; Jones et al. 1998).

The principles laid out in this chapter argue for health promotion strategies that operate at the intersection between *actions* and the meanings through which these *actions* are apprehended and experienced, understanding the phenomenology of sexual experience rather than merely classifying actions to be condoned or prohibited. As Race (2003: 370) puts it, health promoters must 'attune themselves to the protective agency of individuals, the contexts in which embodied practice is worked out, and the concerns and systems of value that mediate practice'.

Related topics

Health promotion; HIV/AIDS; mediated discourse analysis; risk.

Note

1 F3 and F4 refer to Form 3 and Form 4, level of secondary education in Hong Kong which students normally engage in at ages 14 and 15 respectively.

Further reading

Jones, R.H. (2013) *Health and Risk Communication: An Applied Linguistics Perspective*, London: Routledge.

Norris, S. and Jones, R.H. (eds) *Discourse in Action: Introducing Mediated Discourse Analysis*, London: Routledge.

References

Ajzen, I. and Fishbein, M. (1980) *Understanding Attitudes and Predicting Social Behavior*, Englewood Cliffs, NJ: Prentice-Hall.

Anderson, B. (1991) *Imagined Communities*, London: Verso.

Bakhtin, M.M. (1981) *The Dialogic Imagination: Four Essays* (Trans. C. Emerson and M. Holquist), Austin, TX: University of Texas Press.

Becker, M.H. (ed.) (1974) 'The health belief model and personal health behavior', *Health Education Monographs,* 2: 324–508.

Benotsch, E.G., Kalichman, S., and Cage, M. (2002) 'Men who have met sex partners via the Internet: prevalence, predictors, and implications for HIV prevention', *Archives of Sexual Behavior,* 31(2): 177–183.

Berg, R.C. and Grimes, R. (2010) 'Do traditional risk factors predict whether men who have sex with men engage in unprotected anal intercourse? The need for locally based research to guide interventions', *Health,* 15(5): 517–531.

Callen, M. (1983) *How to Have Sex in an Epidemic*, New York: News From The Front Publications.

CDC (2010) 'HIV among gay, bisexual and other men who have sex with men (MSM)', Atlanta, GA: Centers for Disease Control and Prevention.

Cotten, P., Lustre, N., Schimel, S., Thomas, R., and Wagner, K. (1999) 'Speaking out about sex in silent spaces', Paper presented at the The Rubberless Fuck, May 8, University of California, Berkeley.

Dawber, T. (1980) *The Framingham Study: The Epidemiology of Atherosclerotic Disease*, Cambridge, MA: Harvard University Press.

Elford, J., Bolding, G., Maguire, M., and Sherr, L. (2001) 'Gay men, risk and relationships', *AIDS,* 15: 1053–1055.

Emmers-Sommer, T.M. and Allen, M. (2005) *Safer Sex in Personal Relationships: The Role of Sexual Scripts in HIV Infection and Prevention*, Mahwah, NJ: Lawrence Erlbaum.

Fishbein, M., Middlestadt, S.E., and Hitchcock, P.J. (1994) 'Using information to change sexually transmitted disease related behaviors', in R.J. DiClemente and J.L. Peterson (eds) *Preventing AIDS: Theories and Methods of Behavioral Interventions* (pp. 61–78), New York: Plenum Press.

Flores, S.A., Mansergh, G., Marks, G., Guzman, R., and Colfa, G. (2009) 'Gay identity-related factors and sexual risk among men who have sex with men in San Francisco', *AIDS Education and Prevention*, 21(2): 91–103.

Frost, J.H. and Smith, B.K. (2003) 'Visualizing health: imagery in diabetes education', Paper presented at the Designing For User Experiences Conference, June 5–7, San Francisco, CA.

Goetz, T. (2010) *The Decision Tree: Taking Control of your Health in a New Era of Personalized Medicine*, New York: Rodale.

Goffman, E. (1963) *Stigma: Notes on the Management of Spoiled Identity*, London: Penguin.

Grossman, A.H. (1995) 'At risk, infected, and invisible: older gay men and HIV/AIDS', *Journal of the Association of Nurses in AIDS Care*, 6(6): 13–19.

Halkitis, P.N. and Parsons, J.T. (2003) 'Intentional unsafe sex (barebacking) among HIV-positive gay men who seek sexual partners on the Internet', *AIDS Care,* 15(3): 367–378.

Herek, G.M. and Glunt, E.K. (1995) 'Identity and community among gay and bisexual men in the AIDS era: preliminary findings from the Sacramento Men's Health Study', in G.M. Herek and B. Greene (eds) *Aids, Identity, and Community,* Vol. 2 (pp. 55–84), Thousand Oaks, CA: Sage.

Jones, R.H. (1997) 'College students responses to AIDS education: a sociolinguistic approach', in Ho, B. (ed.) *Building New Hope Together: Proceedings of the Hong Kong AIDS Conference 1996* (pp. 107–119), Hong Kong: HK Advisory Council on AIDS.

——(2002) 'Mediated action and sexual risk: discourses of sexuality and AIDS in the People's Republic of China', Unpublished PhD dissertation, Macquarie University, Sydney, Australia.

——(2005) 'Mediated addiction: the drug discourses of Hong Kong youth', *Health, Risk and Society,* 7(1): 25–45.

——(2007) 'Imagined comrades and imaginary protections: identity, community and sexual risk among men who have sex with men in China', *Journal of Homosexuality,* 53(3): 83–115.

——(2008) 'Good sex and bad karma: discourse and the historical body', in V.K. Bhatia, J. Flowerdew, and R. Jones (eds) *Advances in Discourse Studies* (pp. 245–257), London: Routledge.

——(2011) 'Discourse, technology and bodies without organs', in C. Thurlow and K. Mroczek (eds) *Language in the New Media* (pp. 321–339), Oxford: Oxford University Press.

Jones, R.H. and Candlin, C.N. (2003) 'Constructing risk across timescales and trajectories: gay men's stories of sexual encounters', *Health, Risk and Society,* 5(2): 199–213.

Jones, R., Lin, A., and Tsang, W. (1998) 'Empowering at-risk teens in drug education', Paper presented at the 'Working Together for Better Health' International Conference on Health Promotion (sponsored by WHO), September 23–25, Cardiff.

Kalichman, S.C., Kelly, J.A., Morgan, M., and Rompa, D. (1997) 'Fatalism, current life satisfaction, and risk for HIV infection among gay and bisexual men', *Journal of Consulting and Clinical Psychology,* 65: 542–546.

Kannel, W.B., Dawber, T.R., Friedman, G.D., Glennon, W.E., and McNamara, P.M. (1964) 'Risk factors in coronary heart disease: an evaluation of several serum lipids as predictors of coronary heart disease; the Framingham study', *Annals of Internal Medicine,* 61: 888–899.

Keeney, R.L. (2008) 'Personal decisions are the leading cause of death', *Operations Research,* 56(6): 1225–1347.

Kitzinger, C. and Peel, E. (2005) 'The de-gaying and re-gaying of AIDS: contested homophobias in lesbian and gay awareness training', *Discourse and Society,* 16(2): 173–197.

Laumann, E. and Gagnon, J.H. (1995) 'A sociological perspective on sexual action', in R. Parker and J. Gagnon (eds) *Conceiving Sexuality: Approaches to Sex Research in a Post-Modern World,* New York: Routledge.

Lave, J. and Wenger, E. (1991) *Situated Learning: Legitimate Peripheral Participation,* Cambridge: Cambridge University Press.

McFarlane, M., Kachur, R., Klausner, J.D., Roland, E., and Cohn, M. (2005) 'Internet-based health promotion and disease control in the 8 cities: successes, barriers and future plans', *Sexually Transmitted Diseases,* 32(10): S60–S64.

Mansergh, G. and Marks, G. (1998) 'Age and risk of HIV infection in men who have sex with men', *AIDS,* 12: 1119–1128.

Norris, S. and Jones, R. (eds) (2005) *Discourse in Action: Introducing Mediated Discourse Analysis,* London: Routledge.

O'Sullivan, L.F., Udell, W., and Patel, V.L. (2006) 'Young urban adults' heterosexual risk encounters and perceived risk and safety: a structured diary study', *Journal of Sex Research,* 43(4): 343–351.

Plumridge, E. and Chetwynd, J. (1999) 'Identity and the social construction of risk: injecting drug use', *Sociology of Health and Illness,* 21: 329–343.

Race, K.D. (2003) 'Revaluation of risk among gay men', *AIDS Education and Prevention,* 15(4): 369–381.

Ratliff-Crain, J., Donald, K.M., and Dalton, J. (1999) 'Knowledge, beliefs, peer norms, and past behaviors as correlates of risky sexual behaviors among college students', *Psychology and Health,* 14(4): 625–641.

Rhodes, T. (1997) 'Risk theory in epidemic times: sex, drugs and the social organization of "risk behavior"', *Sociology of Health and Illness,* 19(2): 208–227.

Roehr, B. (2010) 'Closeted calamity: the hidden HIV epidemic of men who have sex with men', *Scientific American*, February 25. Retrieved January 16, 2012, from: http://www.scientificamerican.com/article.cfm?id=closeted-calamity-the-hidden-hiv-epidemic
Rofes, E. (1998) *Dry Bones Breathe: Gay Men Creating Post-AIDS Identities and Culture*, New York: Haworth Press.
Rosenberg, E.S., Sullivan, P.S., DiNenno, E.A., Salazar, L.F., and Sanchez, T.H. (2011) 'Number of casual male sexual partners and associated factors among men who have sex with men: results from the National HIV Behavioral Surveillance system', *BMC Public Health,* 11: 189–198.
Rothstein, W.G. (2003) *Public Health and the Risk Factor: A History of an Uneven Medical Revolution*, Rochester, NY: Rochester University Press.
Sacks, H. (1966) 'The search for help: no one to turn to', Unpublished doctoral dissertation, University of California, Berkeley.
Schegloff, E. (1968) 'Sequencing in conversational openings', *American Anthropologist,* 70: 1075–1095.
Scollon, R. (2001a) *Mediated Discourse: The Nexus of Practice*, London: Routledge.
——(2001b) 'Action and text: toward an integrated understanding of the place of text in social (inter) action', in R. Wodak and M. Meyer (eds) *Methods in Critical Discourse Analysis* (pp. 139–183), London: Sage.
Shidlo, A., Yi, H., and Dalit, B. (2005) 'Attitudes towards unprotected anal intercourse: assessing HIV-negative gay or bisexual men', *Journal of Gay and Lesbian Psychotherapy,* 9(3–4): 107–128.
UNAIDS (2011) *Global HIV/AIDS Response: Progress Report*, Geneva: UNAIDS.
van Campenhoudt, L., Cohen, M., Guizzardi, G., and Hausser, D. (eds) (1997) *Sexual Interactions and HIV Risk: New Conceptual Perspectives in European Research,* London: Taylor and Francis.
van Griensvena, F., de Lind van Wijngaardenc, J.W., Barald, S., and Gruliche, A. (2009) 'The global epidemic of HIV infection among men who have sex with men', *Current Opinion in HIV and AIDS,* 4: 300–307.
Vieira De Souza, C.T., Bastos, F.I., Lowndes, C.M., Landman Szwarcwald, C., Moreira Dos Santos, E., Ayres De Castilhl, E., and Stumoller, F. (1999) 'Perception of vulnerability to HIV infection in a cohort of homosexual/bisexual men in Rio de Janeiro, Brazil', *AIDS,* 11(5): 567–579.
Vygotsky, L.S. (1981) 'The instrumental method in psychology', in J.V. Wertsch (ed.) *The Concept of Activity in Soviet Psychology* (pp. 134–143), Armonk, NY: M.E. Sharpe.
Watney, S. (1990) 'Safer sex as community practice', in P. Aggleton, P. Davis, and G. Hart (eds) *AIDS: Individual, Cultural and Policy Dimensions* (pp. 19–33), London: Falmer Press.
Wertsch, J.V. (1994) 'The primacy of mediated action in sociocultural studies', *Mind, Culture and Activity,* 1(4): 202–208.
——(1998) 'Vygotsky and Bakhtin on community', Unpublished manuscript, St. Louis, MO: Washington University.

8

Contesting chemotherapy, amputation, and prosthesis

Insights from patient and caregiver accounts

Vaidehi Ramanathan

> In the intimate public space of the Breast Cancer waiting room … women held their heads at odd angles and fixed their gazes on distant points in a largely unsuccessful attempt to avoid seeing – and knowing – too much about those who waited on them … Although the flimsily tied hospital gown marked the site of the white-haired woman's vulnerability to the scrutiny of a public gaze that threatened to expose the contours of her body, the repeated visual marker of that distinctively patterned gown also signaled *a collective susceptibility to illness and death* not located on an individual body but diffused and projected throughout the waiting room.
>
> (Tanner: 79; my emphasis)

Introduction

The above quote captures some key themes that I wish to explore in this chapter. In particular, I wish to address what the 'collective susceptibility to illness and death' (italicized above) refers to in the context of breast cancer, and how probing narratives around it permits us to let go of the fear-instilled silence that we tend to participate in regarding this condition. While applied/sociolinguistic scholarship has addressed language in medical settings in a variety of contexts (Hamilton 1994; Davis 2005; Sarangi and Roberts 1999; Ramanathan 2010), areas relating to patient accounts of their bodily (dys)functions have tended to remain under-investigated. Particularly unexplored are patient and caregiver accounts of how the condition is lived with and managed. This bottom-up approach, wherein we pay attention to very local concerns, is crucial, since it gives us insights into how people cope with body conditions, the rationalizations that prompt them (or not) to take various actions in the medical world, and ways in which these emerge through particular language use.

The silences around some body conditions are more palpable than others and breast cancer is one such ailment. The veil of silence we have drawn over this domain can be accounted for by a variety of reasons (it is about cancer in a sexualized body-part; it is too 'female' a concern and so men 'cannot' talk about it; it is viewed as 'unclean' and 'messy' and very much in the domain of feminine concerns; it sometimes involves mastectomies and a woman with only one breast is viewed as not having a 'normal' body), and while it is not the purpose of this discussion to open them up, these tropes do provide a partial impetus for speaking/writing about it. Our understandings about 'normal bodies' are held in place by a variety of rationalizations (such as the above) and get constructed for us by a range of discourses including societal, biomedical, and poststructuralist ones. Nowhere is the sense of body norms felt more palpably than in the space around 'disabled', ailing bodies, whose functionings are deemed 'deviant'. Women who have had mastectomies and who do/do not choose to wear prostheses know this only too well.

Making language the primary way into this space, this chapter addresses the nuances of three key terms related to (breast) cancer (more on this presently). Taking as its point of entry the written, published autobiographical accounts of women with breast cancer, as well as accounts of their partners, I will focus on cancer's *metaprescriptive utterances*, terms that Lyotard (1984) partially defines as utterances whose power is legitimized by particular discourses (societal, medical, institutional), and whose effect is profoundly colonizing. The three metaprescriptive terms that I will address are: *chemotherapy*, *amputation*, and *prosthesis*. The central questions informing the discussion are: (a) In what ways do the patient accounts (auto-pathographies) and caregiver accounts (bio-pathographies) reveal the spillages and messinesses of chemotherapy, amputation, and prosthesis as they relate to breast cancer? And (b) In what ways do such pathographies allow us to directly address larger communal concerns about health policies and dis-citizenship?

Historical, current, and critical perspectives on health and health communication

Lennard Davis (1995, 2006) maintains that to understand the 'impaired'/'ailing' or 'disabled' body, one must return to the idea of the 'normal' body, since problems in issues around 'disabilities' have to do with the way 'normalcy is constructed to create the "problem" of the disabled person' (2006: 3). The cluster of words – 'normal', 'normalcy', 'abnormal', 'deviant', 'able', 'able-ism', 'disabled', 'disability' – emerged in the English language at a particular time, with the modern uses of 'normality' and 'normalcy' appearing in the mid-1800s, getting sedimented in all kinds of domains and acquiring legitimacy through the discourses of scientific rationalism. In relation to human bodies, the notion of a 'norm' emerges in a host of expectations, including having 10 fingers and 10 toes, to women having two breasts, and to having all of one's limbs and faculties.

Health- and medically related research in applied sociolinguistics has probed issues around 'norms' for at least a couple of decades now. Hamilton's (1994) ground-breaking research on interactions with an Alzheimer's patient partially addresses the extent to which psycholinguistic scholarship deems Alzheimer speech as 'non-normal' and 'deviant', and questions the prompts we use that elicits speech that then gets labeled this way. This theme also gets echoed in Davis (2006).

In the area of medical settings is research by Sarangi and Roberts (1999) wherein they address the language used in and by medical institutions, including language used by nurses, and non-medical personnel such as receptionists. Also in this realm is work by Angelelli (2004) who focuses on issues of interpretations between languages, and finds that interpreters must negotiate tensions around the policies that govern their work and have enormous power and responsibility as agents of information transfer, where they have to make quick decisions as 'gatekeepers' of health information, deciding how to transmit linguistic as well as cultural information.

The present exploration of breast cancer accounts situates itself amidst the partial sketch of scholarship such as the above. While some of my previous work has addressed interactions with patients (Ramanathan 1997) and health policies and their negotiations (Ramanathan 2010), the focus of this discussion is on the perspectives of people with breast cancer and their caregivers. This is an area that the medical sciences have already been paying attention to (Charon 2002). I will, in particular, be focusing on first-person written and published accounts of people with this 'disabling' condition and those of their caregivers, who are also dealing with the condition, albeit differently. Moving our attention to how and why patients and their partners view the ailment and bodies in the ways they do allows us to begin framing our discussions about health and citizenship differently.

Contextualizing metaprescriptive utterances

As mentioned earlier, this chapter explores ways in which key terms associated with cancer – chemotherapy, amputation, and prosthesis – are metaprescriptive terms that elide the lived and corporeal realities around living with the condition. The power of these terms in the context of (breast) cancer is total, with them becoming catch-all terms that in their singular nature mask a most heterogeneous and complex set of issues. According to Lyotard (1984), they are prescriptive statements that describe what the rules of language use or languaging must be in a given domain; in other words, they have the colonizing power to dictate what language use must be like.

It is these denotative statements – seemingly objective realities, 'facts', – that make up the power of metaprescriptive utterances. The power of medical experts and the authority vested in medical personnel mandate the 'visible', 'what can be seen' and thus what can be languaged. This visibility factor – what we see – and the harsh dynamics of what we see, where we would sooner construct unidimensional, simple pictures instead of addressing ailments as multiple, heterogeneous domains is part of our destructive gaze because we have bought into metaprescriptive utterances handed down to us by the medical world. The medical gaze, of course, exaggerates this tendency in its various contexts to where the person with the ailment (and in some cases their partners as well, as the present chapter will show) is pushed into assuming 'the speak' of medical practitioners, participating thereby in absenting themselves in their presence, speaking of their body parts in the language that is coming at them, thus denying the spillages around their bodies.

Lyotard offers *paralogy* – a focus on the local, the anti-method – to counter the rationality, deterministic orientation, and denotative statements of science. He says:

> The function of differential, or imaginative or paralogical activity of the current pragmatics of science is to point out these metaprescriptives (science's 'presuppositions') *and to petition the players to accept different ones. The only legitimation that can make this kind of request admissible is that it will generate ideas, in other words new statements.*
>
> *(Lyotard 1984: 65; author emphasis).*

As we will presently see, the power that suffuses metaprescriptive utterances finds articulation in patient and caregiver accounts that partially allow us to see the colonizing impact of the metaprescriptive utterances. It is making room for such (paralogical) accounts, opening them up for critical interpretation and insights, and then addressing the implications that arise from this endeavor that this chapter is devoted to.

Main research methods

My choice of first-hand written accounts of people with the condition and their caregivers is deliberate. My opting to focus on the written form stems partially from wanting the kind of reflection and retrospection that (on-the-spot) oral narratives may not engender. I was aiming for a comprehensive set of pathographies that would cover a range of issues relating to breast cancer, and towards that end picked the following:

1 Audre Lorde, *The Cancer Journals*, 1980.
2 Marcy Jane Knopf-Newman, *Beyond Slash, Burn, and Poison: Transforming Breast Cancer Stories into Action*, 2004.
3 Mark Weiss, *When Your Wife Has Breast Cancer*, 2006.
4 Barbara Stevens, *Not Just One In Eight*, 2000 (a collection of published oral narratives).
5 Segments of Jackie Stacey's *Teratologies*, 1997.

Between them, these published accounts offer perspectives of living with the condition from both the patient's point of view as well as caregivers'.

Metaprescriptive utterances and breast cancer pathographies

The various pathographies offer insights into a range of issues relating to lived realities around chemotherapy, amputation, and prosthesis. These include themes of sexuality, ethnicity, and gender, accounts by lesbian women dealing with prosthetic implants, male perspectives about their wives' reconstructed breasts, and female views about 'femininity' being heavily associated with one's breasts. They also include accounts of everyday negotiations with coming to terms with their changing bodies and relationships. The following section addresses each of these metaprescriptive terms.

Chemotherapy

The word 'chemotherapy' is a combination of 'chemo' and 'therapy' with the former being derived from '*chemo*' meaning 'chemicals' but specifically in this instance chemicals which have 'a toxic effect' and the latter from *therape* meaning 'treatment' or 'cure'. The juxtaposition of seeming opposites – a toxic compound that kills (chemo) with a treatment that cures (therapy) is reminiscent of Derrida's *pharmakon* wherein the remedy and the poison are part of each other; the term means both poison and cure. While Derrida (1981) views writing as a pharmakon, both a remedy to relieve overburdened memory and also a dangerous drug (in the Socratic sense), the idea that the opposite is already built into the term is relevant here. That is, the cure contains disease; it's not difficult to see why 'pharmakon' is both. In the following narrative excerpts, we see Susan and Robert Alexander wrestling with how chemotherapy sessions – intended to cure Susan's breast cancer – contributed to their relationship breaking down.

Susan's narrative

1. Chemotherapy is awful. I felt sick, like having the flu;
2. moreover, I felt as though I was being slowly, methodically poisoned.
3. I would lay in the dark in my bedroom, with a towel over my head feeling very nauseated.
4. Compazine, an antinausea medication was ineffective, because I still vomited.
5. In fact, all it did was make me tired.
6. The only thing that helped me was smoking a little marijuana given to me by friends.
7. When I looked at myself in the mirror I saw a woman with dark circles under her eyes.
8. Robert could not deal with my illness; consequently, he was never home.
9. As a result my two boys, Charlie, age ten at the time, and Matt age six would be running throughout the house, all the televisions would be on and junk food would be everywhere.
10. Robert and I have been together twenty-two years, twenty of them married.
11. The last five have been a challenge; this last year very rough.
12. My getting breast cancer put more of a strain on the relationship …
13. It is too scary for him to comprehend so he buries it, and escapes by going to the office …
14. We have made the decision to separate.
15. I feel good about this decision because now I can move forward as I need to for myself and for my children.

Robert's (Susan's husband) narrative

1. Although our communication wasn't great, I thought our friendship had been pretty strong until the time Susan got sick.
2. I had gone to all her doctor's appointments including the consultation with her oncologist.
3. I assumed we would go together for her first chemotherapy treatment.
4. Then she told me 'My mother's going with me.' I not only felt as though I had been kicked, but I felt left out.
5. A couple of other times I asked if she wanted me to come with her and I guess she must have said no.
6. So other than going with her to one radiation treatment, I never asked or went again.
7. It was not until later that I found out it had affected her that I hadn't gone with her to anything but by then it was too late.
8. Having the financial burden solely on my shoulders was frightening. Nobody ever talks about that or all the other things that have to be taken care of: picking up the kids after school, making meals, having someone come over in the evening for a few hours so that the partner can go out for a bit to do whatever …
9. That is why I think it is a good idea to sit down with family or friends, or whoever is part of your support system without your partner, and tell them that you need their assistance to help ease the pressure somewhat.
10. Sometimes a spouse is uncomfortable asking for help because they are not *his* family …
11. It's frustrating having 'to be the man', having to be strong.

16 I am in a state of self-awareness where I am striving to be happy and want to be fulfilled.
17 I don't want to live my life full of anger, resentment and hostility, which is how I feel after the way he treated me.
18 Robert is still running.

From: Susan Alexander's 'I thought I had a good marriage', in Stevens (2000: 33–34; author's emphasis).

12 Women have certain expectations about men and the way they think men should behave … Perhaps we need to take a deep breath and tell the woman 'I am just as fragile as you are.
13 I know that is not how I come across.
14 You might think I don't care, but maybe it is because I care so much, and am so afraid that I run'.

From: Susan Alexander's 'I thought I had a good marriage', in Stevens (2000: 35–38; author's emphasis).

Several issues emerge in both narratives around 'chemotherapy': Susan Alexander's frustration at her husband not being able to deal with the house and kids, her disappointment at his not taking care of insurance and policy claims, and her decision to separate because of the 'resentment and hostility' she feels against him (lines 8–13, 14–16). In Robert's case, issues around chemotherapy assume nuances around who was going to accompany Susan to the session (himself or her mother, lines 2–7, 8–9), picking up the responsibilities around the house and kids (lines 8–9), feeling frustrated at being locked into a 'male' role and his general inability to communicate his conflict (lines 12–14). These are issues that the metaprescriptive term of 'chemotherapy' draws a veil over and the radiating ripples around this term/event stay hidden.

Going back to my previous points about oppositions built into terms, in the case of 'chemotherapy' – a real drug administered to cancer patients – this opposition, or, as it turns out, non-opposition, is lived out: the 'therapy' patients actually receive makes them ill (as Susan points out in her narrative). I stress these issues around etymology and morphology here to highlight the rift or gap between these terms that otherwise go unnoticed. *Chemotherapy* has become a metaprescriptive utterance with particular associations and specific conceptual apparatus that begs to be texted and infused with new associations and meanings. As Culler points out (1983), this practice of relying on the terms of an opposition in one's argument (chemotherapy in the present case) while simultaneously seeking to displace that opposition permits the possibility of new meanings, a point that Derrida (1981) discusses in his sections on 'paleonymics', the retention of old names while grafting new meaning upon them. Opening up 'chemotherapy' and its various normative predicates to interpret it in the more grounded space of a narrative of a patient and her partner permits one to both resist the prior dominantly biomedical and societal associations around it while also opening doors for life's related messiness to float into our view (as in Susan's and Robert's narratives). To move from a linguistic taking apart of the elements of a word understood denotatively to the repercussions of the connotations it has acquired is to see more than just the body of the patient who suffers. The intensity and anxiety associated with the word itself, knowledge that the cure entails the death of one's tissue and the loss of one's hair and energy are connotations functioning in such a way as to threaten the social fabric of the family. The *chemo* (the toxic chemical) that is intended to cure the body, poisons familial relations, becoming thus the 'therapy' that isn't.

We need to ask whether these metaprescriptive terms require to be changed, or, if they cannot (seeing how completely dominant they are of bodies and ailments), what we can do to make room for paralogical – more localized, alternate – accounts that illuminate both the extent of these colonizing tropes while also making room for the messinesses and spillage they mask. Doing so would lead to the cultivation of a discourse that is at once more holistic and expressive, wholly antithetical to the kind of discourse demanded of scientists at the time of the founding of the Royal Society in Britain (Atkinson 1998). Scientists were then exhorted to use plain simple language and dispense with flourishes of rhetoric which feed the imagination rather than the cold observing intellect – the birth of the purely denotative. It was imperative to separate myth from empirical fact if science was to take the course it did; but there was an accompanying impoverishment, the loss of a richer more uncertain 'surround'.

Amputation

If metaprescriptive associations around *chemotherapy* are partially about the conjoining of opposites, amputation relies on another set of polarities, namely those relating to 'losing a part to save the whole'. Much of the language regarding amputation that we collectively have in place emerges from concerns regarding sites of amputation, infections that prompt it (gangrene, severe injury, a tumor), and rehabilitation after surgery (a theme often associated with soldiers losing body parts). In the case of breast cancer, where one or sometimes both breasts get amputated, the local articulations assume nuances relating to sexuality, sexiness, and one's public image (Manderson and Stirling 2007). Breast cancer patients and their partners seem to find themselves claiming particular subjectivities in the face of cancer's uncertain and onward march; while also resisting societal metaphors around 'attractive' sexual bodies, they seem to have little choice about the 'lose-a-part-to-save-the-whole' discourse of medicine, points that emerge in Barbara's and Bart's (Barbara's partner) narratives.

Barbara's line about not saying 'goodbye to her breasts' (line 1) coupled with Bart's articulations about 'getting used' to her scars (line 6) and regarding their removal as no 'big deal' (line 7) speaks of their need to *re-cog-nize* each and the other's body, a point that has significance for the complex intersection of bodily contingencies and identity construction. Lorde voices similar dilemmas in *The Cancer Journals* (1980) where she insists that 'any amputation is a physical and psychic reality that must be integrated into a new sense of self' (1980: 16) and writes: 'I would lie if I did not also speak of loss ... the absence of my breast is a recurring sadness, but certainly not one that dominates my life.' Lorde's line echoes a latent sentiment in Barbara's narrative: the tumult of having one's sense of self overturned by a dominant medical metaprescriptive utterance (of both being a cancer patient and having a body part removed) while also speaking agentively of trying to reconceptualize herself, and of coming to terms with losing a body part to save her life.

This point of 'losing one's breasts' raises concerns about bodies with amputated breasts being 'unattractive and asexual' (Bart above needing to convince himself that Barbara still looked sexy, for instance). Inextricably tied to male gazes (Hall and Bucholtz 1995) that view breasts as 'attractive' objects, issues around restoring a female body to its 'original' form can be seen to be tied to associations around personalized body horrors and 'ugliness' (Kristeva 1982). The following narrative of a husband whose wife underwent a mastectomy articulates his concerns about his wife not having two breasts and about his coming to terms with her not-so-beautiful-anymore body.

Barbara Stevens: Breast cancer really is a wake-up call!

1 Barbara: I have since thought, How odd I never said goodbye to my breasts.
2 It was a day of experiences and wonderful people.
3 … as I was being wheeled into the operating room one of the staff held my hand.
4 I cannot express how comforting that was.
5 I made terrible jokes to my medical team. Things such as never having breast pain again.
6 I was freezing when I woke up.
7 My chest hurt terribly. Not from surgery, but from the bandage that was wrapped so tightly around me.
8 My nurse was wonderful.
9 She rubbed my back because it hurt.
10 I was unable to lie on my stomach because of the surgery or my sides because of the drains.
11 When Bart came to visit early the next morning he crawled into bed with me and we went to sleep in one another's arms.
12 Neither of us had slept the night before.
13 My husband is the most wonderful, caring, gentle man I have ever known.

From: Stevens (2000: 5–7; author's emphasis).

Bart, her husband:

1 Barb does not remember her surgeon showing us pictures of women who had undergone mastectomies so that we could be prepared.
2 That is one of the reasons I went with her to all her doctor's appointments.
3 There were things both of us missed.
4 I agreed with her decision to remove her breasts.
5 Had she not done she would have lived her whole life wondering, 'When will I get it in the other breast?' I have no doubt she would have.
6 When her bandages were removed the day she was discharged from the hospital I knew the best way for me to handle it was to look directly at her scars and get used to them.
7 You know what? I looked and thought '*No big deal!*' She looked great. She just did not have breasts, and
8 I thought, *Barb still looks sexy*! After a while I no longer saw the scars.

From: Stevens (2000: 8–9; author's emphasis).

Mark Weiss's experience in a support group for partners

1 The guys for the most part talked candidly and emotionally about their experiences with chemo or with surgery.
2 One guy spoke about his wife's cancer being misdiagnosed at another hospital and his feelings of frustration and guilt for not questioning the doctor who initially screwed it up.
3 To my discredit, I didn't read the room correctly; this group was focused on the survival of their spouses, the acute issues and I should have respected this.
4 No one in the group really spoke about the private things that I felt only husbands in our situation could really feel.
5 Sexuality had to be one of those items, yet the discussions didn't go there.
6 When it was my turn, I took a chance and spoke about my desire to know what type of breasts my wife would end up having after the reconstruction process, thinking that this would start a discussion about the sexual consequences of cancer treatments.
7 The guy to my right began radiating hostility at me for initiating this type of discussion.
8 He was about sixty years old and probably thinking that I was a shallow, uncaring little SOB whose paramount and only concern should have been my wife's survival.
9 The guy actually interrupted me twice, stating that his love for his wife far outweighed something as petty as the appearance of her breasts. He seemed to hold sway with the room because I felt it was eleven (including Roz) against one.
10 … I also pointed out that every time I went to the reconstructive plastic surgeon's office and looked at his book of pictures of reconstructed breasts, I saw pictures of overweight, postmenopausal women with youthful looking breasts that didn't quite fit.
11 I wanted to see pictures of young, beautiful women with reconstructed breasts because my wife is young and beautiful.
12 I explained that if the new breasts weren't going to be beautiful, then I wanted to start coming to grips with that now and not be disappointed later.
13 It also validated my feelings that it was OK to hope to have an even more beautiful and happy wife at the end of the treatments and surgery.

From: Weiss (2006: 102–104).

Mark Weiss's open and honest articulation of his desire to have his wife's body 'restored' with reconstructive surgery (addressed in more detail in relation to prosthesis in the next section), evokes a mix of reactions. On the one hand we can intuit his (male) insistence that a woman's body have two breasts and be a certain way. On the other hand, though, his anxieties are bringing to the surface some key implicit assumptions about bodies, 'normality', and 'deviance' that we have collectively assembled. His utterances about 'overweight, postmenopausal women with reconstructed breasts' are an articulation of the 'horrors' that perhaps mark the significance of the various boundaries and orifices of the body, a key premise for discourses of abjection. Kristeva critiques the cultural, political, and historical conditions under which 'clean, obedient, law-abiding, decent bodies emerge' (1982: 89). Abjection for her, as for Longhurst is 'the affect or feeling of anxiety, loathing and disgust that the subject has in encountering certain matter, images, fantasies – the horrible to which it can only respond with aversion, nausea, and distraction' (2001: 28). The abject evokes fear and disgust because it exposes the border between the self and other; the abject threatens to disband the subject by melting the border.

For Weiss, his wife's body with only one breast renders her body abject and non-normal, and thus asexual and 'unattractive'. His hope that his wife's body might even be more beautiful after the surgery (line 13) might be partially seen to emerge from this sense of threat of the 'disfigured borders'/contours of his wife's body threatening his ability to relate to her sexually. Her beauty mattered to his sense of who *he* was, and to his sense of continued maleness ('I wanted to see pictures of young, beautiful women with reconstructed breasts'). Probing the metaprescriptive associations around the amputated body suddenly casts light on the assembled equations between 'two breasts, attractive, and sexual' and the polarities inherent in them. At this point, the amputated body is not so much about losing a part to save the whole, as much as it is about losing a part and replacing it to appear normal (to please men, not look 'deviant'; c.f. Goffman 1967).

If '*chemotherapy*' raised issues of language – its 'doubleness', the supremacy of the denotative in scientific discourse, '*amputation*' raises issues of the social construction of the norm and notions of the normal. A norm is based on statistical supremacy and it is worth pondering why exactly a woman needs two breasts. We have two kidneys, silently there, the other taking over if one is lost; but the visibility of breasts complicates the 'norm' in this case; it generates beauty myths and 'becomes' or is perhaps 'constructed' into being the site of sexual arousal. The essential function of lactation of offspring is completely overlooked till the moment a woman gives birth.

Prosthesis

Issues of amputation are, of course, intimately linked to concerns about reconstruction, and there are, as with the previous metaprescriptive utterances, some very complex views about this as well. The polarities around prosthesis play on absent (non-normal) breasts versus those bodies that are 'normal', polarities that exert pressure on women to present their public, body images (Grosz 1994) in specific ways. Lorde (1980) critiques prosthesis on four bases: that women who opt for it risk losing self-awareness and feminist visibility (particular statements that the bodies of a single-breasted or no-breasted woman can make); that this choice is complicit in the patriarchal culture's sexist politics of appearance; that there are dangers in reconstructive surgery, since cancerous breast tissue can form and be hidden under implants; and reconstructed women cannot be effective breast cancer activists. Lorde concludes that the cultural emphasis upon surgical prosthesis serves a 'way of avoiding having women come to terms with their own pain and loss, and thereby, with their own strength' (1980: 49), and swears to either love my body one-breasted now, or remain forever alien to myself (1980: 44). Since 'self-alienation is unthinkable, self-acceptance becomes essential. I refuse to have my scars hidden or trivialized behind lambswool or silicone gel' (1980: 60).

Some of these views find echoes in the following narrative of a young college student struggling with whether or not to have her body reconstructed:

Tania: a 21-year-old college student on 'Why I chose not to be reconstructed'

1 Initially, I didn't think about the aesthetics when I lost my breast.
2 I thought 'In order for me to live, it has to go! Wearing a prosthesis or having reconstruction didn't occur to me until I was recovering and was visited by a Reach for Recovery volunteer.
3 She brought me this silly little stocking thing with stuffing in it.
4 I became angry, because it was as though everyone would be much happier if I 'had a booby'.
5 It wasn't my fault I had lost my breast, and I didn't feel there should be any shame involved. At that point, I became adamantly against reconstruction.
6 I didn't wear a prosthesis for three years because I wanted to become comfortable with who I was, having only one breast.
7 I'm a lesbian and for me having only one breast was like 'coming out' all over again. When is it a good time to tell someone? Do I have to tell them?
8 Is it an issue or non-issue?
9 Most days I feel comfortable not wearing a prosthesis but it is easier having two breasts, because then it is a non-issue.
10 I wore my prosthesis to a job interview. Why? Because I didn't want to go through potential discrimination.
11 If I don't wear a prosthesis to work I wear baggy shirts, simply because I don't want to deal with it. I like having the option.
12 Sometimes though I do think about reconstruction, particularly when my clothes don't hang right.
13 I was fired as a camp counselor because I had only one breast.
14 When the director found out, he asked me what would I tell the girls when we were showering together.
15 I told him I would answer their questions and educate them.
16 Shortly thereafter I was fired with full severance.
17 Was the bottom line what would the children think?
18 What impact would that have on their parents? Or was it because I was gay?
19 I was discriminated against, but I've chosen not to think about it in those terms.

From: Stevens (2002: 229–230; author's emphasis).

While Tania above does not, like Lorde, articulate her desire to be adamantly single-breasted – she is after all only 21 at the time of this narrative – she does, like Barbara earlier, wrestle with her altered identity. Her body image (Grosz 1994) has changed and, as she points out, she didn't wear a prosthesis for three years because she wanted to become comfortable with her altered body. Her statement about 'coming out all over again' (line 7) in the light of her surgery underscores the agency with which she both confidently speaks of both her body and her sexuality. The notion of the abject body that we saw earlier in relation to Weiss's desire for his wife's body to have both breasts applies in this present context too, albeit differently. In the current case, Tania's (and Lorde's) desire to come to terms with their different bodies speaks of their resisting what McClintock (1995) refers to as the 'psychic processes of abjection' (fetishism, disavowal, the uncanny) to take up abjections as political stands that allows them to counter the metaprescriptive associations around prosthetic bodyparts.

The abject is intimately tied to powers of horror (Kristeva 1982), taboos, and collective ideas about repulsion, purity, and the sacred. In light of the present discussion, abject bodies may be simultaneously sites of internalized male gazes, where Tania's concerns about clothes hanging well for interviews dominate (line 10), as well as sites of agency, where she counters being discriminated against for being single-breasted.

Recommendations for practice and future directions

This chapter began with the assertion that the paralogical – the local, the ordinary, the everyday, the lived, the corporeal – is crucial to counter cancer's metaprescriptive utterances and as the above discussion pointed out one way to do so is to actively make room for various pathographies around the condition and to critically interrogate the social, political, and linguistic nuances that make up the nexus of issues. I turn now to addressing the importance of such engagements with the paralogical in the areas of health policies and citizenship.

Paralogy contesting 'normalcy'

A goal of critical disability theory is not to theorize disability to where its relevance to the larger world of engagement is lost, but to address issues of empowerment, of making room for alternate views about bodies, about countering dominant tropes from the medical worlds, and about creating contexts of equality (Devlin and Pothier 2006). A key point here isn't just to focus on impairments or functional 'inadequacies' but to attempt, among other things, to raise awareness about how patients' bodies get positioned and constrained by policies, how patients' voices and experiences with their bodies run counter to those held by the medical world, and how institutionalized discourses in the world of pharmacists, doctors, nurses, and medical personnel legitimize dehumanizing orientations to bodies and ailments (see Collins and Slembrouck 2006). Certainly, the various auto- and bio-pathographies call our attention to ways in which patients and their partners come to terms with the various contingencies that the condition brings on: whether it is Barbara waking up to having no breasts, or her husband wrestling with how to deal with her changed body, or Susan realizing that aspects of her marriage were disappointing or her husband attempting to negotiate his role around her and their children. Reading their pathographies, on the one hand, makes us take account of how viewing illness/disability in individualized ways runs the risk of framing it as personal bad luck, a risk that leans towards an orientation of charity and pity. On the other hand, their negotiations with this condition allows us to shift focus and view the ravages of cancer in terms of societal views about 'normalcy' or 'normal bodies' and in so doing bring difference, equality, and inclusion into the discussion, making us squarely face how we contribute to upholding collective notions of 'normal' bodies. Such a shift in our cognitions, perceptions, and attitudes is imperative if we wish for communal ideologies about bodies and ultimately about health policies to change.

The paralogical and citizenship

Central too are issues of citizenship and policies that partially dictate how bodies are policed, who is regarded 'normal', and lines of exclusion that determine insider status. I am using the term 'citizenship' here not in terms of the passport one carries, but very broadly to refer to the 'ability to participate fully' without constraints or clauses. Such a definition moves debates about citizenship away from its commonplace understanding of individual status to it being a practice that gains legitimacy from ideologies that perpetuate it and keep it circulating. As Devlin and Pothier point out such a view:

> raises questions of access and participation, exclusion and inclusion, rights and obligations, legitimate governance and democracy, liberty and equality, public and private, marginalization and belonging, social recognition and redistribution of sources, structure and agency, identity and personhood, and self and other.
>
> *(Devlin and Pothier 2006: 2)*

Devlin and Pothier (2006: 2) use the term 'dis-citizens' to speak to a disabling citizenship. Certainly, the various pathographies discussed here make us realize the extent to which our collective notions of 'normalcy' are dis-abling. The politics of and around who gets identified as 'normal' or 'disabled' as well as who identifies him/herself as such seems crucial to probe, since so much is at stake. As Wendell (1996) points out, it is important to keep in mind that some people who consider themselves 'ailing' or 'disabled' are not identified as such by everyone else, and not everyone who is identified by other people as 'ill' or 'disabled' (either for purposes of entitlement, discrimination, or any other) considers him/herself disabled. While on the one hand, the label of 'disability' is disabling, on the other the social/official/legitimized recognition of disability determines the practical help a person receives from doctors, government agencies, insurance companies, charity organizations, and often families and friends. Moreover, being identified by others as 'disabled' works to affirm disabling experiences, just as denial of particular conditions can cause stress, alienation, and despair in people (who seek validation, but do not get it; c.f. Wendell 1996). 'Dis-citizenship', then, is deeply entangled in issues around policies and recognition on the one hand with concerns about over-slotting and discrimination on the other.

Dis-citizenship issues also touch on concerns regarding auto- versus bio-pathographies. Can caregivers and partners speak for their ailing/'disabled' loved ones, or are they by doing so 'dis-abling' them, casting them into the shadows of dis-citizenship? From such a point of view, my speaking of my partner's serious chronic condition, or of my writing of breast cancer can be seen as questionable. But perspectives of family and caregivers are crucial to address as well, since, as we have just seen, they negotiate with the condition as well (albeit differently). Paralogical endeavors such as this one need to include their voices and concerns as well because frustrations of caregivers with larger communal inequities around condition can and is often the fuel that motivates societal change. From this point of view, making the paralogical as multiply laminated as possible is crucial.

Final summary

In conclusion, then, the rigor and strength of the paralogical in ailment-related writing makes us all – patients, caregivers, researchers, scholars in disability studies – take account of the fact that corporeal, material, and language-related issues around bodies (in this case, cancer) matter, that contesting the metaprescriptive language of ailments/disability experiences matters, that making room for the paralogical through multiple pathographies matters, and that countering societal views about 'normal' bodies and 'normal' language competencies matters perhaps most of all.

Related topics

Bodies; breast cancer; disabilities; sexualized body parts; gender studies.

Further reading

Davis, B. (ed.) (2005) *Alzheimer Talk, Text and Context*, London: Palgrave Macmillan.
Duchan and Kovarsky (eds) (2005) *Diagnosis as Cultural Practice*, Berlin: Mouton de Gruyter.
Hamilton, Heidi E. (2003) *Glimmers: A Journey Through Alzheimer's Disease*, Ashland, OR: RiverWood Books.
McPherron, P. and Ramanathan, V. (eds) (2011) *Language, Body and Health*, Berlin: Mouton de Gruyter.
Ramanathan, V. (2009) *Bodies and Language: Health, Ailments, Disabilities*, Clevedon: Multilingual Matters.

References

Angelelli, C. (2004) *Revisiting the Interpreter's Role*, Amsterdam: John Benjamin.
Atkinson, D. (1998) *Scientific Discourse in Sociohistorical Context: The Philosophical Transactions of the Royal Society of London, 1675–1975*, Mahwah, NJ: Lawrence Erlbaum.
Charon, R. (2002) *Stories Matter: The Role of Narrative in Medical Ethics*, New York: Routledge.
Collins, J. and Slembrouck, S. (2006) 'You don't know what they translate': language contact, institutional procedure, and literacy practices in neighborhood health centers in urban Flanders, *Journal of Linguistic Anthropology*, 16(2): 249–268.
Culler, J. (1983) *On Deconstruction*, Ithaca, NY: Cornell University Press.
Davis, B. (ed.) (2005) *Alzheimer Talk: Text and Context*, London: Palgrave.
Davis, L. (1995) *Enforcing Normalcy: Disability, Deafness and the Body*, New York: Verso.
——(2006) *The Disability Reader*, New York: Routledge.
Derrida, J. (1981) *Dissemination*, trans. Barbara Johnson, Chicago, IL: University of Chicago Press.
Devlin, R. and Pothier, D. (2006) Introduction: Toward a critical theory of Dis-citizenship, *Critical Disability Theory: Essays in Philosophy, Politics, Policy, and Law,* 1–22, Vancouver: British Colombia Press.
Goffman, E. (1967) *The Presentation of Self in Everyday Life*, New York: Pantheon.
Grosz, E. (1994) *Volatile Bodies: Towards a Corporeal Feminism*, St. Leonards: Allen and Unwin.
Hall, K. and Bucholtz, M. (1995) *Gender Articulated: Language and the Socially Constructed Self*, New York: Routledge.
Hamilton, H. (1994) *Conversations with an Alzheimer's Patient: An Interactional Sociolinguistic Study*, Cambridge: Cambridge University Press.
Knopf-Newman, M. (2004) *Beyond Slash, Burn, and Poison: Transforming Breast Cancer Stories into Action*, New Brunswick, NJ: Rutgers University Press.
Kristeva, J. (1982) *Powers of Horror: An Essay on Abjection*, New York: Colombia University Press.
Longhurst, R. (2001) *Bodies: Exploring Fluid Boundaries*, London: Routledge.
Lorde, A. (1980) *The Cancer Journals*, San Francisco, CA: Aunt Lute.
Lyotard, J. (1984) *The Postmodern Condition*, trans. Geoffrey Bennington and Brian Massumi, Minneapolis, MN: University of Minnesota Press.
McClintock, A. (1995) *Imperial Leather: Race, Gender, and Sexuality in the Colonial Contest*, New York: Routledge.
Manderson, L. and Stirling, L. (2007) The absent breast: speaking of the mastectomied body, *Feminism and Psychology*, 17(1): 75–92.
Ramanathan, V. (1997) *Alzheimer's Discourse: Some Sociolinguistic Dimensions*, Mahwah, NJ: Lawrence Erlbaum.
——(2008) Applied linguistics redux: a Derridean exploration of Alzheimer lifehistories, *Applied Linguistics*, 29(1): 1–23.
——(2010) *Bodies and Language: Health, Ailments, Disabilities*, Clevedon: Multilingual Matters.
Sarangi, S. and Roberts, C. (eds) (1999) *Talk, Work and Institutional Order: Discourse in Medical, Mediation, and Management Settings*, New York: Mouton de Gruyter.

Stacey, J. (1997) *Teratologies*, New York: Routledge.
Stevens, B. (2000) *Not Just One In Eight: Stories of Breast Cancer Survivors and Their Families*, Deerfield Beach, FL: Health Communications.
Tanner, L. (2006) *Lost Bodies: Inhabiting the Borders of Life and Death*, Ithaca, NY: Cornell University Press.
Weiss, M. (2006) *When Your Wife Has Breast Cancer: A Story of Love, Courage, and Survival*, New York: ibooks.
Wendell, S. (1996) *The Rejected Body: Feminist Philosophical Reflections on Disability*, New York: Routledge.

9

Alzheimer's diagnosis on trial

Ethical consequences at the intersection of health and law

Peter A. Lichtenberg and Mark R. Luborsky

Whether assigned rightly or wrongly, affixing the Alzheimer's label to an individual brings dire social and personal consequences. Distressingly, this remains true in professional contexts where our growing gerontological knowledge has not adequately infused the conduct of routine official processes. Here we seek answers, from the collaboration between a geriatric neuropsychologist and a medical anthropologist, to the questions: how are the standardized clinical, medical, and legal criteria for cognitive capacity enacted to apply to the particularities of individual cases during legal probate proceedings, and how do courts and attorneys seek and utilize information from healthcare professionals? Our purpose is to reveal performativity in the conduct of legal determinations of cognitive decision-making capacity when focused on *testamentary capacity* (financial decision-making). This is a nascent arena for scholarship on cognition, language, and communication, as well as science and society. Systematic knowledge of how legal practices produce judgments about older adults facing later life decisions is minuscule relative to gerontological knowledge from medicine, social and population sciences, or humanities. Our chapter draws on 15 years' work by first author Lichtenberg on over 75 probative cases (e.g., capacity to live alone, sign contracts, guardianship, capacity for sexual activity), writing assessment guidebooks for psychologists, and providing capacity assessment training to attorneys, judges, and health professionals.

Just what is at stake? Culture's foundational validation of one's full personhood! As we age from birth we accrue legal rights and duties and gain full adult personhood with rights to decide in voting for leaders, laws, parenting, or ownership. But personhood can be withdrawn for violating norms. We are held accountable for properly conducting affairs at home, supporting family, work, and order in the community. The legal system can strip away rights to child custody, a driving license, or holding office. In extreme cases, capital punishment can be death or life imprisonment in order to remove an offender in order to protect the social order. Today, awareness is growing of the erosion of full personhood and stigma from illness, disability (Luborsky 1994; Murphy 1990) and Alzheimer's (Hamilton 2008; Taylor 2008; Davis and Pope 2010). Thus, deep suffering from the social experience of Alzheimer's disease (AD) arises as it dissolves those abilities and memory needed to fulfill expected roles, tasks, or even recognize friends and family.

Arguably, AD diagnosis is akin to capital punishment (Luborsky and Lichtenberg 2012) by terminating an older adult's right as 'head' decision-maker about his or her own affairs. Notably, following, philosopher Giorgio Agamben's (2009) analysis of the State's sovereign exemption, the societal legal agents who enact this process are exempted from being held accountable for causing the harm as when, here, the medical and legal experts deploy the social apparatus of their authority (e.g., technologies of cognitive tests, diagnostic schemes). Simply, we lack systematic knowledge of the professional stakeholders, settings, and practices by which cognitive capacity determinations are formulated and legitimated. This chapter illuminates the formal clinical and legal processes that strip an adult person of control over her or his own affairs, finances, or right to will assets to heirs.

The confluence of a surging aging population, rising financial abuse and mistreatment of elderly combined with our era's large intergenerational transfer of wealth, and the publicity of salacious cases of sibling rivalry and probate cases together are heightening awareness of testamentary capacity in older adults in the legal and professional arenas. Leading elder law attorneys describe this crisis, costing families and the taxpayers hundreds of millions of dollars, as a failure to plan (Mayoras and Mayoras 2009); others view it as a natural consequence of sibling rivalry, evolutionary psychology, and emotional pain (Accettura 2011). The prevalence of AD is stable at roughly 11 percent in the United States (Herbet et al. 2010), affecting over 5 million adults and over 15 million unpaid caregivers caring for a person with AD or other dementias at a cost of $200 billion (Alzheimer's Association 2012).

Paternalistically, the very desire to protect elderly from financial exploitation and abuse tramples elders' well-being, and it does matter. Langer and Rodin's (1976) classic nursing home study demonstrated the power of personal control. Adults who could control their own schedules and activities were happier, exhibited fewer behavioral disturbances and less medical complications than those without control. Reich and Zautra (1990) and Lang and Heckhausen (2001) found personal control in older adults linked to depression and longevity. Thus, issues broader than legal protection of elderly enter the discussion and include social justice, loss of control, and health effects raising a tension between autonomy (individual choice) and paternalism (individual protection) in cases of cognitive capacity.

On the surface, testamentary capacity standards appear simplistic and easy to gauge. In Michigan, for example, only four legal standards must be met, does the individual know: (1) what is a will; (2) the nature and extent of their property; (3) their natural heirs; and (4) have a plan for distributing their property? A fifth requirement, not in the same legal standards, requires that wills be created by free choice without undue influence. Many challenges to wills succeed by producing evidence of undue influence.

The actual determination of testamentary capacity is a dialogical multi-stage process. It includes multiple stakeholders and complex sets of roles for the professional (clinical, legal, ethical) conducting the evaluation and providing a final determination. One major focus is the assessment process itself (record reviews, interviews with stakeholders, cognitive evaluation, and integrating clinical with legal standards), including the engagement, preparation and review, assessment and communication phases. While testamentary capacity builds from established scientific consensus principles, the conduct of the evaluation is socially shaped by practical and ethical concerns.

Challenging a will or trust successfully requires good information from three sources (Mayoras and Mayoras 2009). (1) Medical records must document an expert testamentary capacity assessment. These experts must have: (a) substantial geriatric knowledge of late life syndromes that affect cognitive and mental health functioning, including dementia, delirium, frailty, and how chronic diseases (e.g., diabetes, kidney failure) and disabilities (e.g., mobility loss) influence life and cognition; and (b) expertise in the life changes and vulnerability of elderly especially those with impaired cognition or function. (2) Witness testimony is needed attesting to inadequate cognitive and functional abilities, and (3) good independent expert medical evaluations of the presence of cognitive impairment, an individual's decisional abilities, ability to compensate for deficits, any undue influence, and how the individual's deficits align with the legal standards governing the legal transaction.

In this chapter, we first describe the history, current research, and clinical implications of cognitive competence. We then explore today's critical issues using an actual case, Mr. Stan Arnheim, to describe the course, discourses, and the dialogical performative process whereby clinical experts engage with those representing the legal system to assess, debate, and then formulate a competence determination. The firsthand descriptions of these discourses include the first author Lichtenberg, in his expert psychologist role with the multiple parties in testamentary capacity cases. We show the diametric opposition between clinical assessment and clinical care work. Finally, we discuss current conflicts and future directions.

Historical background

Competence is a legal construct, and officially determining incompetence can only be established through the judicial system. Mental health professionals are closely involved in these decisions since the courts rely heavily on expert witness evidence. Yet, only recently is specialized gerontological knowledge about later life language and behavior emerging, as well as systematic study of the conduct of the determination in legal cases.

Who participates and what issue is debated in court?

An early study (Iris 1988) directly observed guardianship evaluations performed in 141 courtroom proceedings and interviewed 11 attorneys. Findings were telling. First, the older adult was less likely to appear in court, less likely to contest a petition, and more likely to have a plenary guardian (having total control) of both the estate and the person appointed. Second, protests about guardianship for older adults focused not on *if* protection was needed but *who* should be the guardian. Subsequently, Keith and Wacker (1993) examined 1,160 court records of elderly guardianship hearings. Notably only 4 percent had their own private attorney, and again, few (13 percent) elderly attended the hearing. Both studies concluded that the healthcare professional role was pivotal in the hearings. Judges relied heavily on the expert's testimony. Historically, challenges to expert testimony were few, but the field itself began to discern ambiguities (Appelbaum and Grisso 1988) in basic definitions and their consequences.

Currently, *competency* defined as the capacity for self-determination (Moye 1999) refers to the capacity for self-care or property care (incompetence resulting in a guardian or conservator), and the capacity to consent to medical decisions. Key to competency is the perception of how well someone can perform self-care or financial decisions (Pruchno et al. 1995). In the US, each state's statutes require significant patient deficits in one or more areas: (1) disorders or disabilities, (2) decision-making/communication disability, and/or (3) functional impairment.

Today we know the mere presence of a mental disorder does not create legal incompetence (Grisso 1994). A diagnosis of a neurologic condition does not automatically render one incapable of self-care determination. A clinical disorder must be linked to disabilities. Second, as Grisso remarked, legal incompetence is not an all-or-nothing status. The question should be incompetent for what? Limited incompetency judgments may become more the norm as opposed to persons losing all competencies. Third, legal incompetence is not to be conceptualized as permanent. For example, delirium (due to a treatable fever, infection, or drug reaction) may produce an incompetency judgment but, when treated and cured, the person regains her or his capacity. Finally, there still is no single legal definition of incompetence, so a causal link must be established between cognitive deficits and the particular capacity in question.

Medical decision-making as an early focus in cognitive capacity research

Galvanized by advances in medical technology and dramatic news about young brain-injured persons in vegetative states, debates about how and who decides to start or stop life support led to patient consent procedures and to advance directives (e.g., stating your wishes for treatment before the need arises). It was soon realized that, rather than a few exceptional youth, now growing numbers of elderly with possible cognitive impairments dictated an urgent need to develop standards. Formal criteria emerged that professionals and healthcare researchers agree on as the key issues of consent to medical treatments. The central components (Roth et al. 1977; Appelbaum and Grisso 1988) include communicating choices, understanding relevant information, appreciation of the situation and consequences, and the ability to manipulate information rationally.

How is cognition related to decisional competence assessed?

This early question continues. New methods were required because a question–answer test approach proved ill-suited. A vignette approach was developed to provide naturalistic observation of the individual's reasoning processes while discussing fictional scenarios. To differentiate persons with Alzheimer's from healthy individuals, Marson et al. (1995) created two specialized vignettes tailored to competency to consent to medical treatment. Competency was assessed by expert raters across five domains: *Legal Standard 1*: evidence of choice; *Legal Standard 2*: reasonable choice; *Legal Standard 3*: appreciate consequences of choice; *Legal Standard 4*: rational reasons; and *Legal Standard 5*: understanding choice (interrater reliability $\underline{r} = 0.83$, $p < 0.05$).

AD patients differed significantly in three areas: Legal Standards 3, 4, and 5. All demonstrated compromise on Legal Standard 5. Whereas on Legal Standard 4 all the moderately impaired individuals displayed compromise, only 50 percent of the mildly impaired group did so. Next, extending this notable work these researchers explored the fit between cognitive performance and Legal Standards 1, 3, and 5, re-examining the same sample (Marson et al. 1996). The results were similar to their work on Legal Standard 4. Significant correlations ranged from 0.44 to 0.81. Overall, correct classifications ranged from 91–98 percent. Thus, creative work by Marson and colleagues added a new competency assessment tool and it correlated with performance-based cognitive measures.

In summary, the new specialty of geriatric financial cognitive competence determination is emerging within the neuropsychology of later life cognition. The need for progress is great in this new sparse literature; 'determining the point at which a cognitively impaired older adult is no longer capable of independent financial management poses an onerous task for family members and professionals. At present, no agreed-upon standard exists for evaluating financial capacity, and issues pertaining what level of impairment constitutes incapacity remain largely unresolved' (Pinsker et al. 2010: 333). Arising from early general work on guardianship and treatment decision-making, unique later life cognition processes and health that must be considered were revealed. New discoveries are needed given the growth of elderly, financial exploitation, and social tensions over transfer of assets from elderly, to help minimize elderly exploitation and premature loss of autonomy and independence as whole persons. Large gaps exist in our knowledge and critical skills beyond just attuning diagnostic tools to later life. Opportunities, especially for language and communication, are outlined next.

Critical issues and topics in the field

We next specify the structure that financial decision capacity determination follows. Then we identify challenges arising when textbook normative clinical and legal criteria are applied in the workings of actual legal determinations, and illuminate these issues using a forensic case history of Mr. Stan Arnheim from the first author's caseload.

Social justice and rights are at the core of competency issues. Losing control over financial or personal life decisions can have direct negative health effects (Lang and Heckhausen 2001). Yet, failing to detect diminished capacity has dire outcomes too, including victimization by theft, fraud, or self-neglect.

The discourses of cognitive capacity determination: a dialogic process

The capacity determination is not a single test, rather it is an extended dialogic communication process precipitated by a family member or care provider worried about how the older person is managing daily finances or changing their will. Often adult children (in conflict) or a spouse seek legal help to contest the division of assets. When this stage is set, episodically roughly six arenas of activity ensue. These include: (1) contacting and negotiating with an independent psychology expert. The expert (2) performs a comprehensive geriatric assessment; (3) reviews medical and other records; (4) interviews the older person (if alive), other experts, and perhaps family; and then (5) strategically crafts a master narrative from these multiple stories from diverse sources and stances on the person's capacity. The task is to transform these medical and social criteria to address the legal criteria for testamentary capacity. (6) This independent report narrative is deployed in court to arrive at a legal determination. Extensive narrative smoothing (Spence 1986; Luborsky 1990) is performed to craft a single clear, positioned, story. Next, we discuss each episode and practice-based suggestions.

Negotiating referral

An expert may be approached by a court representative or attorney advocating for one side. The expert must determine: (a) what capacity is in question? (b) is it a forensic assessment (medical records only as if the older person died) or will it require a new assessment? (c) what legal standards (i.e., state court case law) are germane to the specific capacity? (d) what is the time frame when the analysis is needed? (e) does the hiring party understand the impartial nature of the assessment – regardless of who hires the expert the assessment is independent and its conclusions are not mutable? and (f) that a fee is agreed upon.

Obtaining records and setting the evaluation

An expert often must persistently push in order to get both medical and legal records. These allow the expert to create a timeline of relevant events. The medical records serve as a fundamental source of unbiased information, often including notations about cognitive decline or dementia. Being able to view the progressive decline or lack thereof is essential to establishing the correct diagnosis. When scheduling the evaluation the expert must explain who will be involved (e.g., family caregiver or other informants interviewed). The expert must also clarify that no one except the examiner and the older person can be present.

Obtaining informed consent

Strikingly, *no patient confidentiality exists* for the medical facts collected unlike other medical evaluations. Thus, prior to the interview and formal assessment, the person must give informed consent or (if not possible) assent. The expert must explain to the older adult that unlike almost all health procedures, results of the capacity assessment are shared with all parties in the legal proceedings. This lack of confidentiality is a glaring, underappreciated, contrast between a clinical and a legal capacity assessment.

Preliminary discussion of results with older person and hiring party

After the assessment it is important to review with the older person how the results will be shared. Thank the older person for their cooperation and explain that the results will be shared with their attorney who can then share it with the older adult. If the court is the hiring party, then the judge and two attorneys have agreed to use the results of the assessment and so the formal report is prepared and shared. If the expert was hired by an attorney advocating for one side then it is crucial that the expert speaks to the hiring attorney first before generating a report. For example, in one case of Lichtenberg's an older woman changed her will (testamentary capacity), although her cognitive impairments were mild, she changed the will based on a paranoid delusion that her son was trying to get her money. But, in fact, a second son who lived with her was stealing the money while poisoning her relationship with the first son. The attorney accepted the feedback but asked that no report be produced.

Verbal detailed discussion of issues in report with hiring attorney

Once an attorney requests a report, germane facts are determined by the expert and then crystallized for *verbal* discussion with the attorney (see 'discoverable' below). An expert's conclusion is only as good as the accuracy of their assessment, understanding of the history, and integration with the legal standards. Verbally discussing findings allows the expert and the attorney to double check facts but also ensures the expert is addressing the capacity issue(s) in question.

Sharing report with hiring attorney

The report should be shared only with the hiring attorney. Factual errors can be detected (e.g., incorrect dates on historical documents in report) and corrected. Any other change, such as rewording the conclusion, is *discoverable*. That is, any written communications, including email, between attorney and expert can be subpoenaed by the opposing attorney. To find that opinion changes had occurred because of one attorney's comments would undermine the expert's credibility as an independent evaluator.

Sharing results verbally during deposition, hearing, or trial

Findings must be clear and concisely presented so the judge or jurors can understand what took place in the assessment and the expert's conclusions. Often, the expert will meet with the attorney earlier to discuss the questions and answers for the direct examination. The clinical expert must learn how to code-switch, that is defend his or her report upon cross-examination in an effective and responsive way. Questions asked must be answered, but learning to incorporate testimony given direct into the questions during cross-examination is critical.

Pragmatics shape the process. The content of what is communicated during the expert work and in the report is a related, but different matter. Experts differ on how scientific they want to appear, or how in-depth an assessment they can provide. Determining the different ways to use information in a clinical versus capacity assessment, and also understanding what to communicate to diverse stakeholders, varies considerably. The practitioner's art is in choosing which elements to emphasize in fitting diagnostic category groups to the legal criteria and the particulars of that case.

Stan Arnheim's trial and the case of (im)proper Alzheimer's diagnosis

Stan Arnheim (pseudonym), from the first author's forensic caseload, illuminates both the dialogic nature of capacity determination and also how the outcome is not automatically defined by medical and legal facts. Rather, it is complexly shaped by the contexts of the evaluation and how the particularities of the individual fit the normative clinical and legal categories. Readers may be interested to note that they will read from the official (redacted) final forensic expert report. Mr. Arnheim's case is described in the first person using quotes from the case records.

Misdiagnoses of older adults, even by experienced health professionals, are common, and powerfully shape questions of capacity. The following case is one of mistaken diagnosis of AD and the legal battle resulting in a jury trial to determine testamentary capacity. While there is no 'typical' case, Stan Arnheim was selected because he highlights key features across many cases when conflicts arose between stakeholders in the process.

Instigation of conflict over testamentary capacity

Mr. Arnheim, born in 1925 and nearing his eighties with increasing physical disability due to late effects from childhood polio (affects only muscles not the brain; Scheer and Luborsky 1991), was cared for primarily by one of his sons. Fifteen months before his death he altered his will giving more money to his caregiving son than other children. After he died, the three other siblings sued in probate court, claiming the final will was invalid due to their father's lack of testamentary capacity. Lichtenberg was asked by the caregiving son's attorney to review the medical records. The issue was his testamentary capacity on the date he changed his will, 21 February 2005.

As a retrospective evaluation of testamentary capacity (see ABA 2005: 85–87) the case required a thorough review of not just medical records, but also business and financial records, and personal letters, diaries, and videos. In this case, medical records existed contemporaneous with his changes to the will. A comprehensive review of these records allowed me (Lichtenberg) to analyze several years' worth of cognitive and physical functioning, disabilities, and other medical disorders to determine Mr. Arnheim's level of functioning as close as possible to 21 February 2005.

Review of medical records – assembling a chronology and expert geriatric profile

Stan Arnheim, twice married and a widower, retired senior supervisor, was born in 1925. By 2000, aged 75, he had suffered from several medical problems in life, including childhood polio, congestive heart failure, diabetes mellitus, hypertension, arrhythmia, gastric disorders, and post-polio syndrome; he used a pacemaker.

2000 and 2001. No cognitive difficulties were noted in any medical records.

2002. While hospitalized in March, April, May, July, and August, he consistently demonstrated intact cognition during bedside professional assessments. During March, May, August hospitalizations he presented Dr. Xavier, his longtime family physician, with symptoms of lethargy, weakness, and multiple falls. The cause was determined to be anemia. Highly reversible, his symptoms cleared when treated and he returned to his regular activities.

2003. In February he sought Dr. Xavier with multiple complaints, including pain and gastric distress. His daughter's voiced concerns about his mind were written in the Doctor's notes 'according to his daughter he is also having some short-term memory problems'. Diagnosed with gastroparesis he was given medication. He fell in May fracturing his right leg and was hospitalized. He underwent a medical rehabilitation exam and Dr. Yasker wrote he was 'alert and oriented times three' (oriented to person, time, and place). Later during a two-week medical rehabilitation stay he was again observed as 'alert and oriented times three' and 'able to follow commands without difficulty'. A social worker note stated he was 'dressing and bathing independently, doing some of his meal prep.'. During November and December he was seeing Dr. Xavier for ongoing cellulitis (bacterial skin infection).

2004. In January he presented complaints of worsening fatigue and lethargy, which was attributed to increasing renal insufficiency and cellulitis. By February, when hospitalized due to lack of response to treatment, Dr. Zerkov (a hospitalist) stated on 18 February 'patient is alert and oriented to time, place and person'. During March he sought Dr. Xavier for shortness of breath and coughing; returning later for continuing cellulitis in his leg. From April to May he saw Dr. Xavier for worsening weakness and mobility; a CT scan revealed mild cortical atrophy, but no acute stroke. From June to August he visited regularly for leg edema and cellulitis. From August to December he experienced leg ulcerations, shortness of breath, and multiple falls. Hospitalized in December for severe cellulitis, Dr. Zerkov wrote Stan is 'alert, awake, and oriented to time, place and person'.

2005. In January the severe swelling and shortness of breath continued due to congestive heart failure. His caregiving son took him to Dr. Xavier in February, reporting his father exhibited significant confusion and losing track of time. The doctor conducted the Mini Mental Status Exam (MMSE) cognitive screening exam and wrote, 'There is evidence for some diminished function, showing perhaps some degree of mild impairment, with a total score of 23 out of 30.' A CT scan on 3 February revealed chronic ischemic changes, but no acute stroke or other change. On 5 February Dr. Xavier diagnosed AD and started on Namenda, a drug for moderate dementia (MMSE 3-14). A 10 February exam by Dr. Xavier found improved breathing and cellulitis. On 16 February the confusion was cleared with treatment, as evidenced when Mr. Arnheim phoned Dr. X's office and instructed the nurse that '[Dr. Xavier] told me I need the IV antibiotics for one more month'. Dr. Xavier wrote down he was correct and ordered the antibiotics. In March Dr. Xavier noted improved cognitive functioning and attributed this to Namenda. During April the leg ulcerations from cellulitis worsened; by a May visit Dr. Xavier wrote the leg infection improved significantly. The doctor reassessed his mental status, concluding, 'I believe the patient is of clear mind to make assessments and judgments and there does not appear to be any concern or issues at this point in time with dementia or Alzheimer's.'

2006. Mr. Arnheim, on 10 January presented to Dr. Xavier with a syncopal episode (fainting), lethargy and increased confusion. A CT scan showed no acute brain changes. The same day, the caregiving son phoned stating his father was hallucinating and wandering outside; Stan was hospitalized. On 12 January, Dr. Xavier's evaluation found him agitated, restless, unable to follow directions, hallucinating, severely memory impaired, and 'not capable of focusing and completing any goal directed task'. January 16, he was too lethargic to complete any of the MMSE; and was diagnosed with pneumonia. On 23 January he was transferred to a nursing center, where staff observed cognitive symptoms, severe attentional and memory disorders. These eventually resolved. Several months later Mr Arnheim died at the nursing center.

Summary of expert conclusions

Dr. Xavier, his physician, diagnosed Mr. Arnheim with AD in 2005 but incorrectly applied the diagnostic criteria for dementia, and omitted a diagnostic examination for delirium. The DSM-IV American Psychological Association criteria for diagnosing *dementia* include: (a) memory impairment and one other area of cognitive decline; (b) significantly impaired functioning; (c) course characterized by gradual onset and continuing cognitive decline; and (d) deficits do not occur exclusively during an episode of delirium.

Evidence of delirium

The evidence supports neither criteria (c) nor (d); onset was not gradual and, more importantly, each episode of cognitive confusion was due to a delirium. Cognitive confusion was abrupt, and later resolved (i.e., no continued decline consistent with delirium). The DSM-IV criteria for diagnosing *delirium* due to medical infection include: (a) disturbance of consciousness (reduced attentional abilities); (b) change in cognition; (c) disturbance develops over a short period of time (hours to days); and (d) evidence of underlying medical condition.

Lethargy and new-onset cognitive dysfunction are common to delirium. When the source of delirium is treated the symptoms can quickly remit. Mr. Arnheim's medical record was not consistent with a diagnosis of dementia throughout 2002–2005, but of delirium causing the cognitive confusion. Records showed his cognition improved once treatment began for the cellulitis: on 16 February 2005 which was two weeks after seeing Dr. Xavier for confusion, he phoned to remind Dr. Xavier to order more antibiotics. In March 2005, Dr. Xavier noted improved cognitive functioning, and in May Dr. Xavier documented complete absence of cognitive dysfunction.

Evidence of dementia, delirium, or both?

No evidence for a progressive dementia appears in the records. Critically to his children's legal claims, he suffered no progressive dementia during 2003–2005, the period when he made a new will. Further, there was no evidence of an episode of acute delirium during any of these transactions.

Misdiagnosis by second psychologist

A second psychologist reviewed these same medical records and interviewed each child. He diagnosed AD because: (a) one daughter complained of her father's memory problems in 2003, and, when interviewed by the psychologist, stated he continuously declined over the three-year period determined solely on the daughter's report; (b) one CT scan showed mild cortical atrophy and white-matter changes; and (c) the family physician had diagnosed Mr. Arnheim with AD on 5 February 2005.

Legal communications and outcome: Mr. Stan Arnheim was cognitively intact

After finishing the review and report, Lichtenberg felt strongly there was no evidence of a dementia; none that met clinical standards. Lichtenberg communicated to the attorney who hired him that the opposing side should be asked to demonstrate any period of confusion not caused by a delirium before he agreed to assign Mr. Arnheim a dementia label.

A jury trial ensued. In court Lichtenberg testified and on cross-examination the opposing attorney failed to demonstrate to the jury evidence of clinical criteria for dementia. When the second expert testified they again were unable to document any cognitive confusion apart from episodes of delirium. *Verdict*: Mr. Arnheim's capacity and will was upheld.

Recommendations for practice with elderly

The forensic case of Stan Arnheim spotlights dilemmas in the current practice of capacity determination among elderly. A clear practical take-away is that the gaps in scholarship, and of trained experienced geriatric experts, leave us ill-prepared to humanely address coming social challenges. Four dilemmas confront practitioners. For clarity we present them as oppositions.

Strong support for a conclusion: nomothetic vs. idiographic approach to capacity determination

Nomothetic, or aggregate group data (see Marson et al. 1996, above) indicate how group-level features are related to cognitive assessments. Such nomothetic data depict typical patterns and between decision-making abilities and cognition. For example, Marson's research sample showed memory dysfunction significantly related to meeting legal standards for medical decision-making. Experts who favor this approach cite Marson's work as strong support for a lack of capacity in an individual with significant memory deficits. In contrast, an idiographic (case) approach focuses heavily on the particular details of a specific older individual. The shortcoming of the nomothetic approach which is generalized and decontextualized is critical; capacity assessments and discourse are never about a group, and are only about an individual in their own unique lifetime and daily circumstance. Two cases of older women illustrate this well. Marge whose real estate career made her accustomed to dealing with large amounts of money and making financial decisions changed her estate plan. Pam, in contrast, was a homemaker with no experience in budgeting or financial decisions. Both wanted to change beneficiaries to their wills and create joint accounts. Marge's case was straightforward while Pam was being unduly influenced by one of her children. Thus, cognitive impairment is just one piece of the puzzle. Employment, influence of others, ability to plan and initiate discussions are all vital elements in cases.

Cognitive assessment vs. cognitive screening

Many aspects of capacity are heavily reliant on cognitive abilities. In the medical professions, including neurology and psychiatry, cognition is assessed using very broad basic screening measures. The measure's value is brevity and detection of any degree of cognitive impairment. Their weaknesses, problematic for capacity work, are the large numbers of false negatives; people who appear normal on cognitive screening only to exhibit significant cognitive deficits on extended assessment. Indeed, thorough cognitive assessment assesses five domains of cognition: attention, language, memory, visuospatial disorders, and executive functioning. Cognitive assessment identifies a more complete pattern of strengths and deficits, and differentiates permanent states of cognitive impairment (dementia) versus more transient states of cognitive deficits (delirium) in addition to assisting with dementia diagnosis and staging the severity of a dementia.

Personal knowledge of the individual: family, clinical, and legal assessments

Family members are often a clinician's best information source. They can tell key life history details, lifelong personality traits and values which the person with dementia cannot. Similarly a family doctor is valuable as in Mr. Arnheim's case. The family informant, often, can more accurately describe symptoms than the older person. Family's descriptions may provide detailed insights which enable the clinician to know it is a progressive age-related dementia even before the examination. In contrast, during legal assessments the family play a minimal role.

However, family members are stakeholders with strong motives for making someone appear more or less impaired. The family disputing control of property are influenced by the result they seek and thus, detailed reports unsubstantiated by medical or other records are suspect. An expert must consider medical or other records as more reliable than family. Yet the family may have unique information an expert will not want to ignore. The expert should interview family where indicated, and unlike the clinical case, use their report as ancillary data given more weight when consistent with other independent records and independent evaluations.

Understanding who the stakeholders are

The expert must have a clear understanding of the many stakeholders involved. First there are the disputing parties. Often a child alleges their parent, due to dementia, no longer has capacity (to live alone, handle money). Next there are the two (or more) attorneys involved, who each advocate for their client's position. There may be other interested relatives (e.g., other children) not directly involved in the dispute, or relatives or friends with strong beliefs about the case. Finally, the court, through the judge, is directly involved in rendering the final decision. What does an expert communicate to whom? The expert should either be communicating with the hiring attorney or both attorneys when the court has ordered the evaluation. Above we described the communication process, and ultimately it is the expert's report which stands as the central communication from the expert. Experts in legal cases should not provide feedback to the parties or family; unlike a clinical case where sharing detailed feedback is right. The primary reason is to avoid confusion. Persons with vested interests in the case tend to hear only things supporting their position.

Future directions: quest to prevent misinterpretations

In Mr. Arnheim's case, at least three reasons explain why the physician and second psychologist misdiagnosed his delirium as progressive dementia. First, simplistic stereotypes about AD abound, in two ways. AD remains equated with cognitive dysfunction in older adults – yet many treatable medical conditions such as urinary-tract infections and cellulitis can cause transient cognitive problems. Indeed, a founding geriatric medicine discovery was that confusion is not normal but may signal undiagnosed yet treatable depression or infection (elderly do not 'spike' a fever when ill unlike youth). Here, no serious consideration was given to the multiple instances in which Mr. Arnheim's cognition returned to baseline. Stereotypes about AD disease are so pervasive that the other psychologist dismissed medical records showing good cognition and no symptoms of dementia, a reversal inconsistent with AD. Further, stereotypical misattributions equating visible physical disability (such as polio) with mental infirmities (Murphy 1990) continue to shape cases, and may do so as new medical technologies save more lives.

Second, both Dr. Xavier and the second psychologist failed to consider frailty syndrome. Repeated episodes of delirium can occur in cases of frailty, a common geriatric syndrome when multiple systems are failing, and is related to both disability and comorbidity (Fried et al. 2001). Frailty has its own set of symptoms, which include exhaustion, loss of weight, weakness, and gait and balance problems. Consistent with frailty syndrome, Mr. Arnheim had physically 'weathered' during his lifetime starting with childhood polio, and he now suffered significant multisystem difficulties including weakness due to post-polio syndrome, exhaustion during acute infections, gait problems, and multiple falls. During the period relevant to the will, Mr. Arnheim's medical records did not indicate a late stage of frailty, when cognition is often significantly impaired. The cause for cognitive difficulties in later-stage frailty remains unknown, but it is *not* typical of AD where memory disorders, once prominent, worsen as do executive, attentional, and language deficits.

Third, there was an over-reliance on family report. In geriatric memory assessment, collateral reports are valued and used. By that we mean, people familiar with the patient can provide details about that individual's (idiographic) lifelong habits, personality, and skills to help better interpret the meaning of the person's scores on standardized (nomothetic) tests. Capacity work differs crucially from clinical work, however, because those involved may be powerfully motivated which can color their perceptions and even lead to falsehoods. In Mr. Arnheim's case, the second psychologist relied heavily on the three siblings' statements about his memory decline over time, but none saw their father more than once a year. Finally, the psychologist ignored statements in the medical records that he functioned managing his affairs independently. Thus, an ongoing cultural dilemma is that, while recognizing 'personalized' data about the person from family and providers is valued, such information can be biased towards overestimating or underestimating competence.

Future language and communication researchers need to expand our knowledge of how the complex final expert narrative product is strategically evoked, crafted, and negotiated. For example, we see the expert's final product is a highly 'smoothed' narrative (Spence 1986; Luborsky 1990) in at least three ways incompletely recognized. First, these are crafted by mining the rich corpus of evidentiary materials to pragmatically reassemble a new medico-legal narrative intended to establish a compelling case for, or against, competence. Second, the component 'facts' originate from a diversity of discourse idioms and professional formats whose provenience dictate the script (e.g., families reconstructed life biographies of the patient; chronological medical chart notes; neuropsychology exam;

test scores and symptom diagnostic interviews; notes about family in medical records) each with its own standards for relevance, content, and discourse structures. Thus, third, critical epistemological labor is demanded by the forensic task in evaluating how a 'fact' (knowledge and conclusions) from any source is itself situated, not absolute, and shaped the contexts, practices, and knowledge of each stakeholder. The expert must not only reinterpret this corpus in light of his/her specialized expertise about geriatrics, but also understand how to recast and transform the clinical, medical, and family information to meet the specific legal criteria. Clearly, this is not simply database mining to fill a checklist that adds up to the answer.

Multiple complex chronologies and narrative frames were engaged as the idiom for the contest of professional discourses between the two teams of psychologists, lawyers, and care providers. These are grounded, and serve as discourse resources for both parties, in the legal debate over cognitive capacity. Among these are the biographic span of Mr. Arnheim's lifetime, the trajectory of each episode of care seeking and its outcome, the children's experience and views of each of these, the records of each contact with the family doctor, the case record file of the rehabilitation hospital, acute care facility, and the cognitive assessments. One narrative developed by Lichtenberg was cast into a chronological medical narrative of his conditions and care from an in-depth review of records from disparate episodes of medical, hospital, and provider contacts over years. Mr. Arnheim's medical story was one of increasing physical frailty, bouts of symptoms mostly reversed when treated, onset of chronic illnesses, treatment seeking, and then death. In contrast, the children's opposing attorneys and psychologist, using the same events, labeled him with Alzheimer's by selecting symptoms only at the start of each episode.

The need for improved specialized geriatric knowledge remains unmet as does the effective dissemination and implementation of this knowledge in wider realms of society, law, and medicine. Similarly, given the ever rising numbers of elderly, greater insight into the contexts, processes, socio-cultural biases, and conflicts in language and communication with and about the older family members is needed. Today, our empirical knowledge and our critical epistemological and interpretive guidelines remain rudimentary. Perhaps the largest gap, and an exciting frontier for discovery, is naturalistic knowledge of how a judgment transpires in real-world cases. Questions persist about the discourses among participants that lead to the judgment of 'incompetent' to decide who receives one's money or property. The determination does not occur mechanistically from medical 'facts' nor in a social vacuum, yet we lack systematic knowledge of its dialogic transactional nature. Research is needed on how the singular case narrative is constructed from sometimes conflicting authoritative facts about an older person's cognitive capacity, from the story of the patient developed by expert psychologists, the legal criteria and determinations from lawyers, family and spouse's own direct experiences with the person's daily life competences and own expressions. What social stereotypes and values about aging, disability, and AD infuse the discourse and outcomes of the authoritative neuropsychological, medical, legal, and family appraisal of the older person? Clinical diagnostic categories are generalizations about group-level data that gives general probabilities, but in an individual case, how are the characteristics and (dis)abilities of the person mapped, or erased, when cast in terms of a neuropsychological diagnostic group category or score? Ultimately, how can these insights be best provided to enable the coming generations of children and parents to share a more meaningful and positive experience of shared later life transitions?

Related topics

Legal discourse; elderly; diagnostic language; social justice; financial exploitation.

Further reading

Acierno, R., Hernandez, M., Amstadter, A., Resnick, H., and Kilpatrick, D. (2010) Prevalence and correlates of emotional, physical, sexual and financial abuse and potential neglect in the United States. *American Journal of Public Health*, 100: 292–297.

Goodale, M. and Starr, J. (2004) *Practicing Ethnography in Law: New Dialogues, Enduring Methods*. New York: Palgrave Macmillan.

Krasik, M. (1989) The lights of science and experience: historical perspectives on legal attitudes toward the role of medical expertise in guardianship of the elderly. *American Journal of Legal History*, 33(3): 201–240.

Marson, D.C., Earnst, K.S., and Jamil, F. (2000) Consistency of physicians' legal standard and personal judgments of competency in patients with Alzheimer's disease. *Journal of the American Geriatrics Society*, 48: 911–918.

References

ABA. (2005) *Assessment of Older Adults with Diminished Capacity: A Handbook for Lawyers*, Washington, DC: American Bar Association commission on Law and Aging and American Psychological Association.

Accettura, M. (2011) *Blood & Money: Why Families Fight over Inheritance and What To Do about It*. Farmington Hills, MI: Collinwood Press.

Agamben, G. (2009) *What Is an Apparatus?* Stanford, CA: Stanford University Press.

Alzheimer's Association. (2012) Alzheimer's disease facts and figures. *Alzheimer's & Dementia*, 8(2): 1–68.

Appelbaum P. and Grisso, T. (1988) Assessing patients' capacities to consent to treatment. *New England Journal of Medicine*, 319: 1635–1638.

Davis, B. and Pope, C. (2010) Institutionalized ghosting: policy contexts and language use in erasing the person with Alzheimer's. *Language Policy*, 9: 29–44.

Fried, L., Tangen, C., Walston, J., Newman, A., Hirsch, C., Gottdiener, J., and McBurnie, M. (2001) Frailty in older adults: evidence for a phenotype. *Journal of Gerontology: Medical Sciences*, 56A(3): M146–156.

Grisso, T. (1994) Clinical assessments for legal competence of older adults, in M. Storandt and G. VandenBos (eds) *Neuropsychological Assessment of Dementia and Depression in Older Adults: A Clinician's Guide*. Washington, DC: American Psychological Association.

Hamilton, H. (2008) Language and dementia: sociolinguistic aspects. *Annual Review of Applied Linguistics*, 28: 91–110.

Herbert, L., Bienias, J., Aggarwal, N., Wilson, R., Bennett, D., Shaw, R., et al. (2010) Change in risk of Alzheimer disease over time. *Neurology*, 75(9): 786–791.

Iris, M. (1988) Guardianship and the elderly: a multi-perspective view of the decision-making process. *The Gerontologist*, 28(suppl): 3945.

Keith, P.M. and Wacker, R.R. (1993) Implementation of recommended guardianship practices and outcomes of hearings for older persons. *The Gerontologist*, 33(1): 81–87.

Lang, F. and Heckhausen, J. (2001) Perceived control over development and subjective well-being: differential benefits across adulthood. *Journal of Personality and Social Psychology*, 81(3): 509–523.

Langer, E. and Rodin, J. (1976) Effects of choice and enhanced personal responsibility for the aged: a field experiment in an institutional setting. *Journal of Personality and Social Psychology*, 34: 191–198.

Lichtenberg, P. (1998) *Mental Health Practice in Geriatric Health Care Settings*. New York: Haworth Press.

Luborsky, M. (1990) Alchemists' visions: cultural norms in eliciting and analyzing life history narratives. *Journal of Aging Studies*, 4(1): 17–29.

——(1994) The cultural adversity of physical disability: erosion of full adult personhood. *Journal of Aging Studies*, 8(3): 239–253.

Luborsky, M. and Lichtenberg, P. (2012) Patients, persons, and sovereignty: adjudicating moral, legal and clinical authority in delegitimizing decisional competence. Baltimore, MD: Joint meetings of Society for Applied Anthropology and Society for Medical Anthropology.

Marson, D., Ingram, K., Cody, H., and Harrell, L. (1995) Assessing the competency of patients with Alzheimer's disease under different legal standards. *Archives of Neurology,* 52: 949–954.

Marson, D., Chatterjee, A., Ingram, K., and Harrell, L. (1996) Toward a neurologic model of competency: cognitive predictors of capacity to consent in Alzheimer's disease using three different legal standards. *Neurology*, 46: 666–672.

Mayoras, A.W. and Mayoras, D.B. (2009) *Trial & Heirs: Famous Fortune Fights!* Long Beach, CA: Wise Circle Books.

Moye, J. (1999) Assessment of competency and decision-making capacity, in P.A. Lichtenberg (ed.) *Handbook of Assessment in Clinical Gerontology*. New York: John Wiley.

Murphy, R. (1990) *The Body Silent*. New York: W.W. Norton.

Pinsker, D., Pachana, V., Wilson, N., Tilse, C., and Byrne, G. (2010) Financial capacity in older adults: a review of clinical assessment approaches and considerations. *Clinical Gerontologist*, 33: 332–346.

Pruchno, R., Smyer, M., Rose, M., Hartman-Stein, P., and Laribee-Henderson, D. (1995) Competence of long-term care residents to participate in decisions about their medical care: a brief, objective assessment. *The Gerontologist*, 35: 622–629.

Reich, J.W. and Zautra, A.J. (1990) Dispositional control beliefs and consequences of a control-enhancing intervention. *Journal of Gerontology*, 45: P46–P51.

Roth, L., Meisel, C., and Lidz, C. (1977) Tests of competency to consent to treatment. *Canadian Journal of Psychiatry*, 134: 279–284.

Scheer, J. and Luborsky, M. (1991) The cultural context of polio biographies. *Orthopedics*, 14(11): 1173–1181.

Spence, D. (1986) Narrative smoothing and clinical wisdom, in T. Sarbin (ed.) *Narrative Psychology*. New York: Praeger.

Taylor, J. (2008) On recognition, caring, and dementia. *Medical Anthropology Quarterly*, 22(4): 313–335.

10

Applied linguistics as a resource for understanding and advancing health literacy

Donald Rubin

Introduction

Health and disease are of course constituted of tissue and physiology. But health status is also in no small degree constructed and controlled by language. After all, agreeing on a name for a person's state of dis-ease is tantamount to a medical diagnosis (see, for example, Jason et al. 1997 for the case of chronic fatigue syndrome). Not infrequently, a patient's need for a name to signify her health condition is nearly as great as her desire for a cure (Chiong 2001). Thus linguistic signification is a first and crucial step in disease treatment and its counterpart, health promotion.

The burgeoning field of health literacy is a pragmatic movement aimed at understanding and improving discourse practices that will promote health and decrease disease burden, especially as that burden is disproportionately distributed among diverse cultural and ethnic groups in a society. The definition of health literacy is itself the subject of vigorous discussion (Berkman et al. 2010; Sørenson et al. 2012; Speros 2005). The conventional definition currently promulgated by United States healthcare agencies is the 'degree to which individuals have the capacity to obtain, process, and understand basic health information and services needed to make appropriate decisions' (Parker and Ratzan 2010: 20). (Note that the health literacy movement is hardly limited to the United States nor just to Anglophone nations. See, for example, Levin-Zamir and Peterburg 2001). That definition has been useful in directing research and practice that conceptualizes health literacy mainly as an attribute of patients/consumers, and mainly as a comprehension deficiency that needs to be remediated among those individuals. However the prevailing definition fails to recognize health literacy, for example, as a personal and social asset upon which individuals draw when making decisions about their health (Nutbeam 2008; Shim 2010). Current ferment in conceptualizing health literacy provides a far richer notion of the construct (e.g., Baker 2006; Berkman et al. 2010; Cohen 2006; Coleman et al. 2008; Freidman and Hoffman-Goetz 2008; Nutbeam 2008; Paasche-Orlow and Wolf 2007; Peerson and Saunders 2009; Pleasant and Kuruvilla 2008; Zarcadoolas et al. 2005). An emerging consensus positions health literacy with respect to each of the following dimensions.

Multiple levels of health literacy

Health literacy as a trait of patients/consumers

Certainly health literacy is an individual difference variable distinguishing among patients/consumers. Some patients, for example, are more able to decode prescription labels, and others less so (Davis et al. 2006). Toward that end, most measurement efforts have sought to index individuals' levels of health literacy (Pleasant et al. 2011). Given differences in patient competence, one controversy in health services concerns the advisability of 'screening' patients for health literacy at the point of the clinical encounter (Hahn et al. 2010). Because such screening might stigmatize patients, because all patients show deficient communication under stressful circumstances, and because it is by no means clear that physicians are able to adapt their own communication appropriately, many authorities recommend instead a 'universal precautions' approach wherein all patients receive messages tailored for low health literate individuals (DeWalt et al. 2011).

Health literacy as a set of behaviors in which healthcare providers also participate

Health literacy is not just a problem caused by uncomprehending patients/consumers. Rather, healthcare providers are also imbued with greater or lesser skill in communicating health information. Medical educators today devote considerable effort to training and assessing student physicians in generic as well as in specific clinical discourse skills such as establishing rapport, taking a medical history, and delivering bad news (Makoul 2001). Physicians who are attuned to conversation analysis in medical settings are best equipped to improve their own health literacy skills (Maynard and Heritage 2005). Training to improve provider health literacy is by no means limited to physicians. For example, allied health practitioners such as radiology technicians and physical therapists likewise require enhanced discourse competence (Brown et al. 2004).

Health literacy as an attribute of healthcare organizations and systems

Often times efforts for exchanging meaningful information between providers and patients/consumers are thwarted by the sheer complexity and impenetrability of the healthcare systems that they are attempting to navigate. Thus it is appropriate to refer to the health literacy of an institution, like a hospital or clinic, which might include signage, check-in and informed consent procedures, even accessibility to visitors (Brach et al. 2012; Dray and Papen 2004; Rudd and Anderson 2006). Health insurance plans can also be assessed for health literacy, one criterion being the degree to which they make information about member benefits accessible or opaque (Gazmararian et al. 2010). Indeed, the structure of an entire society's healthcare system affects health literacy (Paasche-Orlow and Wolf 2007), and only those who enjoy high levels of health social capital – yielding comfort and familiarity with how health professionals talk and otherwise comport themselves – are likely to attain anything close to optimal utilization (Shim 2010).

Health literacy as a property of discourse

Health literacy is often attributed to the discourse itself that links (or isolates) patient/consumers, providers, and organizations (Dray and Papen 2004; Street 2001). Indeed, most health literacy efforts to this point has been directed toward improving the comprehensibility of health materials such as hospital informed consent forms (Davis et al. 1998) and patient education materials (Badarudeen and Sabharwal 2010). Thus one encounters guides such as *The Health Literacy Style Manual* (Covering Kids and Families 2005). As this chapter discusses in greater detail in a later section, the single-minded obsession with short sentences and simple vocabulary in the name of health literacy often does a disservice to patient/consumer's need to understand complex information (Zarcadoolas 2010).

Health literacy as a process

Regarding health literacy as a *process* of information exchange and appraisal-for-use synthesizes all of the preceding perspectives on health literacy and comports with recent, more nuanced conceptions (e.g., Parker and Ratzan 2010). The health literacy process leading toward a health behavior choice is likely to entail multiple discourse events over time with multiple interlocutors in multiple contexts (Fox and Jones 2009; Zukoski et al. 2011).

Consider for example the health literacy process of Eloise, a pregnant woman who smokes cigarettes. At her intake with her obstetrical practice, a nurse practitioner educates Eloise about the particular dangers of smoking during pregnancy ('Baby can get weak lungs'), provides brief counseling, and refers her to a smoking cessation hotline ('A lot of moms can do it easiest when they're pregnant, cause sometimes you don't even feel like smoking that much'). The nurse practitioner provides clear information without shaming Eloise about her lack of health knowledge on this topic ('Not very many people know this, but the baby's little heart actually speeds up every time the Mom takes a puff'). In fact, the nurse practitioner asks Eloise to 'teach back' the most important point she has just learned ('So suppose your friend Jannette tells you it's ok to smoke a Marlboro Lite, just not a regular Marlboro. Let's pretend I'm Jannette. What are you going to be able to tell me now about why lite cigs are just as scary?' See Lamiani and Furey 2009). Eloise feels comfortable asking a few questions about the reversibility of maternal smoking on fetal health. Eloise leaves the office with two brochures about smoking cessation. She pays particular attention to a graphic (Houts et al. 2006) illustrating effects of smoking on birth weight. Later, while watching TV, Eloise sees a direct-to-consumer advertisement (Royne and Meyers 2008) about a nicotine replacement therapy chewing gum ('Sink your teeth into fast craving relief'). Eloise calls the billing clerk at her obstetrical practice to find whether her health insurance policy will cover the costs of nicotine replacement therapy. The answer: 'It depends.' Eloise is becoming increasingly 'activated' (Hibbard et al. 2004) regarding smoking cessation, and she browses some web pages about smoking and pregnancy. She encounters a video online (Hayanga and Kaiser 2008) in which a celebrity she recognizes urges women to quit smoking when pregnant. Finally, Eloise talks over the phone to her mother, still a smoker ('I always felt guilty about smoking when you kids were young. I guess it's one of the ways I could've been a better mom'), and then has coffee with her friend who is a former smoker (Dunn et al. 2003). At this point, Eloise resolves to give herself two weeks to see how it goes cutting back to 10 cigarettes per day, and then to call the quit line number she has been given.

This schematic illustration of one health behavior decision serves to highlight the variety and sheer number of discourse events and skills that are involved in health literacy conceived as process. These components include (a) the provider's skill in clinical communication, (b) the provider's use of a specific discourse strategy – teach back, (c) the patient/consumer's listening comprehension, (d) her willingness to engage in questioning routines, (e) the readability and usability of the brochures, including interdependencies between print and graphics, (f) persuasion – including visual persuasion – and information load in direct-to-consumer pharmaceutical advertising, and (g) the patient/consumer's media literacy inherent in her response to televised and online messages, (h) her navigation of the healthcare system evinced in her query about insurance coverage, (i) the opacity of that system evinced in the clerk's response, (j) and the conversational competence enabling the patient/consumer to draw upon her social support networks for health information and confirmation.

The importance of health literacy

Health literacy remains just a small fragment of the medical and public health knowledge imparted in professional education. But as the prevailing (or at least the ideal) Western health and medical models shift to become more patient-centered and more focused on quality of life as an expectation and a human right, health literacy looms in importance. In affirming the centrality of health literacy in health care, the US Surgeon General has said, 'As clinicians, what we say does not matter unless our patients are able to understand the information we give them well enough to use it to make good health-care decisions. Otherwise, we didn't reach them, and that is the same as if we didn't treat them' (Benjamin 2010: 784).

Health literacy as predictor of health status and health services utilization

Measures of health literacy have proven to be robust predictors of individuals' health status, and also their utilization of health services such as emergency department visits or dialysis. The major review on this subject was conducted for the US Agency on Healthcare Research and Quality, most recently updated in 2011 (Berkman et al. 2011; see also Cho et al. 2008). Evidence supports the conclusion that health literacy reduces hospitalizations and emergency care use. Because of the high expense of hospital-based services, the cost of poor health literacy to the US healthcare system is estimated to be hundreds of billions of dollars (Vernon et al. 2007). Health literacy increases the likelihood that an individual will obtain preventive healthcare such as mammography, and influenza vaccine. On the other hand, people with low health literacy have inadequate capacity to interpret medication labels and health messages. They are at risk of medication errors. Among older adults, health literacy means better overall health status and longer lifespan. Such is the impact of discourse competence in health.

Health literacy as key to reducing health disparities

Good health – and the quality of life for which it is prerequisite – is by no means equally distributed among all sectors of society. For example, the mortality rate among African Americans is about 50 percent higher than for white Americans – a disparity that has not budged in about 50 years (Smedley et al. 2003). The forces contributing to health disparities are varied and include intergroup differences in genetic predispositions for disease, economic stratification leading to differences in access to health care or access to healthy environments, cultural differences in lifestyle that may for example lead to disparities in diabetes rates, and also differences in cultural beliefs about trustworthiness and efficacy of medical interventions such as vaccination or surgery (American College of Physicians 2004; Applewhite 1995;

Gordon-Larsen et al. 2006; Noel et al. 1998). Certainly lack of proficiency in the mainstream language among minority language patients/consumers is a major cause of health disparities.

Providing health-related language services for non-native language speakers is a major issue in health literacy. Current gaps in health-related professional language services are easily documentable (Flores 2005; McDowell et al. 2011). Best practices for translating health materials and for medical interpretation can help address some of those gaps (National Council on Interpreting in Healthcare 2005). The subject of medical interpretation is beyond the scope of this chapter but is further explicated in Chapter 35 of this *Handbook*.

Notwithstanding structural sources of health disparities – several of which are frustratingly intransigent – evidence is mounting that to a significant degree health disparities are instantiated through the discourses of health communication. That is, many disparities in prevention and treatment are a function of communication practices – not biological factors like genetic susceptibility – and therefore more amenable to health literacy interventions. From an epidemiological perspective, compelling evidence for the relation of health literacy with disparities comes from studies that compare health outcomes of minority and mainstream patients who are otherwise matched in terms of (a) disease severity and (b) access to care (Ashton et al. 2003). For example, an African American man and a white man are both standing in a urologist's office, both presenting similar stages of prostate cancer. Yet the white man is more likely to be referred for aggressive, life-saving treatment. What has happened in that interaction between urologist and patient that resulted in those different courses of treatment? Perhaps the patient's discourse practices trigger negative stereotypes or otherwise fail to induce the physician to address the full menu of treatment options (Shim 2010). In a similar vein, troublesome racial disparities in self-care behaviors like medication adherence among people living with HIV/AIDS disappear when individual differences in health literacy are statistically controlled (Osborn et al. 2007).

What dysfunctions of discourse result in documentable population-based disparities in health outcomes? Most obvious are the barriers imposed on patients who are discordant with the physician's native language – in most cases the dominant language. These language discordant patients often leave medical consultations underdiagnosed and with ineffectual self-care instructions (Schenker et al. 2010). The level of participation (e.g., turn-taking) of minority language patients when interacting with providers is typically low (Cooper and Powe 2004). But even among majority language speakers who are ethnic minorities, depth of participation in medical consultations tends to be low (Katz et al. 2006). No doubt part of the cause for those low rates of participation lies in the racial and ethnic prejudices of mainstream providers who too often dismiss the symptomology (e.g., pain levels) of minority patients (Burgess et al. 2006). Another causal element lies in cultural discourse practices that are mismatched with the discourses of medicine (Schouten and Meeuwesen 2006). Shim (2010; see also Williams et al. 2002) captures some of this mismatch with her concept of 'cultural health capital'. Patients with high cultural health capital are familiar with efficacious behaviors for navigating the healthcare system. They are comfortable uttering such insider terms as 'metastisis' and 'tumor margins', and consequently they receive serious attention from providers, compared with individuals who talk about 'how big the cancer is'.

Because culturally related discourse behaviors apparently account for substantial intergroup disparities in health outcomes, communication training for providers and for patients alike may help mitigate those inequities. Accordingly, training in 'cultural competence' has become a staple in medical and public health education (Beach et al. 2005). The complementary training in discourse behaviors for patients/consumers has received some limited attention, but with mixed success to date (Harrington et al. 2004). Much of that patient training involves programs to encourage question-asking among patients during medical encounters (Cegala et al. 2001). In one such program, Hispanic parents in a pediatric clinic did increase their question-asking following training (Mika et al. 2007) but, not surprisingly, little impact was observed in other practices at which patients already displayed high levels of active participation (Galliber et al. 2010).

Health literacy is encoded in healthcare policy

In acknowledgment of the profound role of health literacy in improving health status across all strata of society, governmental bodies have adopted health literacy goals and metrics into policy (Koh et al. 2012). The World Health Organization (2005), for example, proclaims the need to build health literacy infrastructure in its *Bangkok Charter for Health Promotion in a Globalized World*. In the US, public health policy is guided by a document called *Healthy People 2020*, which includes a 'developmental' objective to 'improve the health literacy of the population'. Indicators for measuring achievement in that objective come from a national survey of Medicare recipients inquiring about provider communication practices (e.g., the provider gives easy-to-understand instructions). Recently, the US Department of Health and Human Services (2010) has promulgated a *National Action Plan to Improve Health Literacy*. The *Plan* envisions a society that (a) 'provides everyone with access to accurate and actionable health information', (b) 'delivers person-centered health information and services', and (c) 'supports lifelong learning and skills to promote good health'. Health agencies and entities throughout the country are encouraged to create their own plans for helping to implement the *National Action Plan*.

Health literacy and 'plain language'

The plain language movement ('plain English' movement in Anglophone nations) was born in the early 1970s mainly out of frustration with the exclusionary effect of legal writing (Dorney 1988; Mazur 2000). Even administrative court judges – who are supposed to run 'people's courts' – deliberately wrote their decisions in an opaque style (Rubin and Floyd 1992). The movement to reform public writing soon suffused to public documents such as tax forms, and eventually to medical documents such as informed consent forms (Davis et al. 1998) and patient discharge instructions (Williams et al. 1996).

Notwithstanding the portrait of health information exchange as multifaceted and socially embedded, much of the practice and training of health literacy devolves into a single-minded pursuit after plain language and – more specifically – readability scores at low grade levels. Text readability itself is a rich construct that embraces a wide range of discourse variables ranging from use of graphics that aid text comprehension to use of headings and other organizational sign-posting (Holland and Campbell 1982). However guidelines for health-related documents often focus on the short sentences and short words that drive conventional readability formulae. Thus, the Centers for Disease Control and Prevention (2010) *Simply Put* guide enjoins health communicators to '[u]se words with one or two syllables when you can. Keep most sentences, if possible, between eight to ten words and limit paragraphs to three to five sentences' (2010: 6). It is not uncommon to see health literacy training materials that completely ban the use of passive voice. Health literacy authorities recommend keeping materials at the 8th grade reading level or lower (Badarudeen and Sabharwal 2010; Covering Kids and Families 2005).

Prescriptive readability guidelines such as these encourage 'writing to the formula' rather than writing for optimal information transfer with audiences (Armbruster et al. 1985; Schriver

2000; Zarcadoolas 2010). Ironically the *Federal Plain Language Guidelines* (Plain Language Action and Information Network, n.d.) – which was created to support the US Plain Writing Act of 2010 (Public Law 111–274) – is a great deal more commodious. The *Federal Plain Language Guidelines* in fact expressly discusses exceptions to the active voice recommendation (e.g., use passive voice 'when the law is the actor') and flatly states that no one level of readability is best for all audiences ('Only write for 8th graders if your audience is, in fact, an 8th grade class'). Indeed, this authoritative style manual – unlike many health literacy guides – is much more concerned about assuring document *usability* (Dumas and Redish 1999) by intended readers rather than meeting some arbitrary reading level benchmark.

Whether viewed as language norms – short sentences and short words – for achieving benchmark readability scores, or viewed from a more nuanced perspective for easing readers' cognitive burdens, a plain language paradigm is central to health literacy as commonly implemented. Thus, for example, the Council of State Governments (n.d.) enumerated nine actions for state policymakers to ameliorate health literacy. The four most concrete recommendations were all items pertaining to plain language: simplifying enrollment forms, rewriting and reformatting written materials, requiring 6th-grade readability levels or lower, and attending to document design features such as white space and font size. Similarly, large health insurance and health maintenance plans have responded to the health literacy movement primarily by attending to the readability of their consumer documents, often making use of readability software such as *Health Literacy Advisor*™ (America's Health Insurance Plans 2011).

Beyond plain language: interactive health literacy

The ease with which readability formulae can be applied to written health documents is one reason why the field of health literacy has focused on the written word. But when one considers the complex ecology in which patients and consumers make health decisions, the salience of written documents must be questioned. For example, health literacy advocates may have effected improvements in the readability and usability of drug package inserts, but the impact of written information about medicines on patient behavior is negligible (Nicolson et al. 2009). Even well-conceived health promotion brochures delivered to patients' homes can end up unread and in the trash (Parvanta et al. 2011). Patients often fail to consult printed instructions they receive upon hospital discharge; verbal interaction facilitates patient recall more than take-home instruction sheets (Isaacman et al. 1992).

Indeed, interpersonal interaction lies at the heart of health information exchange. Face-to-face interaction remains the most trusted source of health information, though younger people are likely to turn to the Internet as their first-consulted information source (Hesse et al. 2005). In addition to browsing web pages for health information, health information seekers increasingly rely on multimedia platforms such as YouTube and social media sites (Hayanga and Kaiser 2008). Whatever the source of health information – print, face-to-face interaction with healthcare professionals or with laypersons, or Internet-based media – consumers and patients vet health information and recommendations through their social networks before attributing credibility or actionability to that information (Fox and Jones 2009; Longo et al. 2010). Thus recommendation that a patient receives from her obstetrician about prenatal care must pass muster with the patient's friends and family before the patient herself adopts it (Dunn et al. 2003).

The interactive health literacy perspective (Rubin et al. 2011; see also Dray and Papen 2004) takes as foundational that health information exchange for decision-making is embedded deeply in social matrices. The patient's capacity to recount a coherent medical history to a nurse, the physician's effort to check a patient's comprehension of medication instructions, the TV watcher's recounting to her pharmacist of a direct-to-consumer ad, the insurance counselor's agility with metaphors about health coverage – all these oral discourse events are at least as central to health literacy as is reading an informed consent document (Baker 2006; Paasche-Orlow and Wolf 2007; Rosenfeld et al. 2011). Health literacy is by no means silent.

The linguistics of health literacy measurement

New methods of assessing health literacy have begun to acknowledge the importance of oral interaction. First-generation measures of health literacy were essentially reading tests. The Test of Functional Health Literacy in Adults (Parker et al. 1995) – arguably the most frequently used measure in health literacy research – is a cloze test with supplied options for filling in each blank; many correct answers can be guessed on the basis of grammatical knowledge alone. The Rapid Estimate of Adult Literacy in Medicine (Davis et al. 1993) is comprised of a list of isolated words; health literacy is scored by the number of words pronounced correctly. A single-item health literacy 'screener' simply asks patients how often they need help reading documents and filling out forms at the doctor's office (Morris et al. 2006). In contrast, more recent measures present listeners with broadcast messages and with patient–provider interactions either on audio (Mazor et al. 2012) or video (McCormack et al. 2010) recordings. Listener responses reflect not only comprehension, but also capacity to use the information presented to evaluate health decisions. The Measure of Interactive Health Literacy (Rubin et al. 2011) is currently the sole effort to assess individuals' actual health interaction behaviors. Trained interviewers give a standardized health message over the phone. The messages deliberately contain information gaps and uncomfortably long pauses. They also contain probes for listener questions. Participants receive scores for engagement (percent of talk time), information seeking (frequency of prompted and unprompted information-seeking utterances and requests for clarification), and turn-taking.

With the closer attention being accorded to interactive health literacy, new work has emerged to provide health literacy practitioners with tools to analyze oral language and to thereby improve communication between patient/consumers and providers. Roter (2011; Roter et al. 2009) characterizes 'oral literacy demand' of health interactions in terms of four dimensions: (1) medical jargon, (2) general language complexity, (3) contextualized language, and (4) dialogue structure. Language complexity in this formulation is operationalized using conventional readability formulae. Contextualized language is essentially language cast in personalized terms – marked by high frequencies of second person pronouns rather than abstract nouns (e.g., 'You will control your blood sugar better if you eat several smaller meals throughout your day' as opposed to, 'Diabetics achieve better control of blood sugar by eating smaller meals throughout the day'). Dialogue structure is comprised of three components: (a) speech rate, (b) turn density or thought units per turn, and (c) interactivity or the rate of conversational turn turnover. In an empirical test of the oral literacy demand framework, Roter and colleagues (2009) found that for low literacy individuals listening to recorded genetic counseling sessions, discourse interactivity and information contextualization predicted learning. For high literacy listeners, none of these factors predicted learning.

In a similar conceptualization, Rubin (2012) proposes discourse 'listenability' as a tool for advancing health literacy. The listenability formulation (Rubin 1993; Rubin et al. 2000) is based on the notion that listeners are constrained by similar psycholinguistic and contextual factors that constrain speakers (e.g., a fast-fading medium that challenges short-term memory, efficiency of deictic reference). Thus listenability is informed by the findings of applied linguists who have explored the nature of spoken language (e.g., Biber and Conrad 2009; Chafe and Tannen 1987; Halliday 1987). The listenability perspective deliberately eschews any reductionistic listenability score associated with a chunk of discourse, but it does recommend that practitioners adopt four types of listenable features. (1) Oral-based sentence structures include high frequencies of coordinated clauses and low levels of nominalization. (2) Oral-based vocabulary encompasses high frequencies of personal pronouns and low lexical diversity. (3) Features that evoke conversationality include use of questions to introduce topic shifts and frequent tag questions. (4) Discourse considerateness (Armbruster and Anderson 1985) involves providing listeners with internal summaries and embedding information in narrative structures.

Rubin (2012) tested the aural comprehensibility of listenable prose in an experiment involving surgical discharge instructions. An excerpt of the highly listenable version, to which listeners (but not readers) responded most favorably, follows:

> Barry Thompson called us in the first days after his heart surgery to say he heard an occasional 'clicking noise' and a clicking feeling in his chest. Barry's clicking noise got less frequent each day, and it went away completely within the first couple of weeks. Don't worry if you hear the same clicking noise Barry heard. That's normal. But let's say you start hearing more and more clicking. Then you better call us.

Future directions for applied linguistics in advancing health literacy

The symbiosis between health literacy and applied linguistics is strong. Both are pragmatic disciplines. And health, after all, is at least in part linguistically constructed. Much health literacy practice already involves language modification (i.e., Plain Language modifications). Thus the argument can be made that advances in health literacy are highly dependent on new insights and tools from applied linguistics.

For example, great strides have been made in training and certifying medical interpreters and making them available either in clinical sites or via telephonic links. However, since bilingual status is hardly a dichotomous category, issues still remain stemming from patients and practitioners alike who overestimate their capacity to communicate about highly nuanced health issues in a common language. Much applied linguistic work remains to be done to establish screening procedures to determine when it is necessary to order medical interpretation services (Diamond et al. 2012). In a related vein, international mobility in healthcare providers will surely increase as health staffing needs rise in the near future. While the US medical licensing authority has put in place rudimentary screening procedures to assure a degree of English language proficiency among international medical graduates, little is known about the actual comprehensibility of non-native speakers in often tense medical treatment situations, or about patients' attitudinal responses to providers speaking non-native varieties of English. And virtually nothing is known about measuring second (L2) language skills that predict effective performance among allied health professionals such as phlebotomists and nurse's aides, who are in closest daily contact with patients from discordant cultures and language backgrounds.

One of the most profound revolutions in patient-centered health care arises from universal mandates to implement electronic medical records (EMRs). EMRS, in turn, enable personal health records (PHRs), tools which at least in principle should promote transparency in health information and empower patients and consumers to make well-informed choices about their health – the fundamental goal of health literacy. One concern about EHRs is that providers become so consumed with meeting the demands of computerized health information intake that interpersonal communication with patients suffers (Margalit et al. 2006). In addition, providers sometimes compose incoherent appointment summaries that confuse patients rather than enlighten them. Patients and consumers, for their part, need guidance in interpreting technical information in their PHRs, such as blood test batteries, so that they do not become unduly alarmed by out-of-range values. Applied linguists can assist in designing scripts for information exchange that take into account the new electronic landscape of EMRs and PHRs, so as to optimize them as tools for enhancing patient–provider communication and engaged decision-making.

Another far-reaching trend is the growing diversity of portals that patients and consumers can use to obtain health information. In addition to the prototypical examination room consultation with a physician, patients/consumers now also obtain health information by interacting with chronic disease coaches, patient navigators, lay health workers, and telenurses. Physicians and other providers increasingly engage in email communication with patients. Broadcast media such as WebMD radio network medical reporters are also important sources. Online patient portals have become digitally sophisticated, incorporating multimedia resources as well as conventional web pages that can be tailored to patient/consumer needs (Koonce et al. 2007). Surely the characteristics of messages across these diverse media and information sources cannot be uniform, and message complexity must be manifest in correspondingly diverse ways. For example, health literacy practitioners have devoted a great deal of attention to utilizing graphics as a means of reducing complexity and increasing comprehension, but graphics that do not cohere with accompanying prose actually increase overall complexity and do not improve comprehension (Clark et al. 1999). No single complexity index – and certainly not the simple word and sentence length criteria that underlie readability formulae – is applicable across all these modalities. Perhaps the most fundamental contribution that applied linguistics can make to health literacy is to offer modality- and context-sensitive parameters for characterizing and then mitigating *health message complexity.*

Related topics

Culturally and linguistically appropriate health services; patient–provider communication; medical interpreting; health disparities; readability; oral language.

Further reading

Angelelli, C.V. (2004) *Medical Interpreting and Cross-cultural Communication.* Cambridge: Cambridge University Press.

Nielsen-Bohlman, L., Panzer, A.M., and Kindig, D.A. (eds) (2004) *Health Literacy: A Prescription to End Confusion.* Washington, DC: Institute of Medicine. Retrieved March 30, 2010, from: http://www.iom.edu/Reports/2004/Health-Literacy-A-Prescription-to-End-Confusion.aspx

Osborne, H. (2011) *Health Literacy from A to Z: Practical Ways to Communicate your Health Message,* 2nd edn, Sudbury, MA: Jones and Bartlett Learning.

Roter, D.L. (2011) Oral literacy demand on health care communication: challenges and solutions. *Nursing Outlook*, 59(2): 79–84.

Smedley, B.D., Stith, A.Y., and Nelson, A.R. (eds) Committee on Understanding and Eliminating Racial and Ethnic Disparities in Health Care. (2003) *Unequal Treatment: Confronting Racial and Ethnic Disparities in Health Care*. Washington, DC: Institute of Medicine. Retrieved March 30, 2010, from: http://www.nap.edu/catalog/10260.html

Sørenson, K., van den Broucke, S., Fulham, J., Doyle, G., Pelikan, J., Slonska, Z., and Brand, H. (2012) Health literacy and public health: a systematic review and integration of definitions and models. *BMC Public Health*, 12(80). Retrieved February 11, 2012, from: http://www.biomedcentral.com/1471-2458/12/80

Zarcadools, C., Pleasant, A., and Greer, D.S. (2006) *Advancing Health Literacy: A Framework for Understanding and Action.* San Francisco, CA: Jossey-Bass.

References

American College of Physicians (2004) Racial and ethnic disparities in health care. *Annals of Internal Medicine,* 141: 226–232.

America's Health Insurance Plans (2011) *Health Literacy and America's Health Insurance Plans: Laying the Foundation and Beyond.* Retrieved December 8, 2013, from: http://www.ahip.org/HealthLiteracy

Applewhite, S.L. (1995) Curanderismo: demystifying the health beliefs and practices of elderly Mexican Americans. *Health and Social Work,* 20(4): 247–254.

Armbruster, B.B. and Anderson, T.H. (1985) Producing 'considerate' expository text: or easy reading is damned hard writing. *Journal of Curriculum Studies,* 17(3): 247–274.

Armbruster, B.B., Osborn, J.H., and Davison, A.L. (1985) Readability formulas may be dangerous to your textbooks. *Educational Leadership,* 42(7): 18–20.

Ashton, C.M., Haidet, P., Paterniti, D.A., Collins, T.C., Gordon, H.S., O'Malley, K., et al. (2003) Racial and ethnic disparities in the use of health services: bias, preferences, or poor communication? *Journal of General Internal Medicine,* 18(2): 146–152.

Badarudeen, S. and Sabharwal, S. (2010) Assessing readability of patient education materials: current role in orthopaedics. *Clinical Orthopaedics and Related Research*, 468(1): 2572–2580.

Baker, D. (2006) The meaning and measure of health literacy. *Journal of General and Internal Medicine,* 21: 878–883.

Beach, M.C., Price, E.G., Gary, T.L., Robinson, K.A., Gozu, A., et al. (2005) Cultural competence: a systematic review of health care provider educational interventions. *Medical Care,* 43(4): 356–373.

Benjamin, R.M. (2010) Surgeon General's perspectives for improving health by improving health literacy. *Public Health Reports,* 125(6): 784–788.

Berkman, N.D., Davis, T.C., and McCormack, L. (2010) Health literacy: What is it? *Journal of Health Communication*, 15(S2): 9–10.

Berkman, N.D., Sheridan, S.L., Donahue, K.E., Halpern, D.J., and Crotty, K. (2011) Low health literacy and health outcomes: an updated systematic review. *Annals of Internal Medicine,* 155(2): 97–107.

Biber, D. and Conrad, S. (2009) *Register, Genre, and Style.* Cambridge: Cambridge University Press.

Brach, C., Dreyer, B., Schyve, P., Hernandez, L.M., Baur, C., Lemerise, A.J., and Parker, R. (2012) *Attributes of a Health Literate Organization.* Washington, DC: Institute of Medicine. Retrieved February 15, 2012, from: http://www.iom.edu/~/media/Files/Perspectives-Files/2012/Discussion-Papers/BPH_HLit_Attributes.pdf

Brown, D.R., Ludwig, R., Buck, G.A., Durham, D., Shumard, T., and Graham, S.S. (2004) Health literacy: universal precautions needed. *Journal of Allied Health,* 33(2): 150–155.

Burgess, D.J., van Ryn, M., Crowley-Matoka, M., and Malat, J. (2006) Understanding the provider contribution to race/ethnicity disparities in pain treatment: insights from dual process models of stereotyping. *Pain Medicine,* 7(2): 119–134.

Cegala, D.J., Post, D.M., and McClure, L. (2001) The effects of patient communication skills training on the discourse of older patients during a primary care interview. *Journal of the American Geriatrics Society,* 49(11): 1505–1511.

Centers for Disease Control and Prevention. (2010) Simply put: a guide for creating easy-to-understand material (3rd edn). Retrieved December 22, 2011, from: http://www.cdc.gov/healthliteracy/pdf/Simply_Put.pdf

Chafe, W. and Tannen, D. (1987) The relation between written and spoken language. *American Review of Anthropology,* 16: 383–407.

Chiong, W. (2001) Diagnosing and defining disease. *Journal of the American Medical Association,* 285(1): 89–90.

Cho, Y.I., Lee, S-Y., Arozullah, A.M., and Crittenden, K.S. (2008) Effects of health literacy on health status and health service utilization amongst the elderly. *Social Science and Medicine,* 66(8): 1809–1816.

Clark, K.L., AbuSabha, R., von Eye, A., and Achterberg, C. (1999) Text and graphics: manipulating nutrition brochures to maximize recall. *Health Education Research,* 14(4): 555–564.

Cohen, S. (2006) 'Following the physician's recommendations faithfully and accurately': functional health literacy, compliance, and the knowledge-based economy. *Journal for Critical Education Policy Studies*, 4(2). Retrieved December 15, 2011, from: http://www.jceps.com/?pageID=article&articleID=74

Coleman, C., Kurtz-Rossi, S., McKinney, J., Pleasant, A., Rootman, E., and Shohet, L. (2008) The Calgary Charter on Health Literacy. Centre for Literacy of Quebec. Accessed December 8, 2013, from: http://www.centreforliteracy.qc.ca/sites/default/files/CFL_Calgary_Charter_2011.pdf

Cooper, L.A. and Powe, N.R. (2004) Disparities in patient experiences, health care processes, and outcomes: the role of patient–provider racial, ethnic, and language concordance. (Research Report #753). Washington, DC. The Commonwealth Fund. Retrieved December 12, 2011, from: http://www.commonwealthfund.org/programs/minority/cooper_raceconcordance_753.pdf

Council of State Governments (n.d.) *Health literacy tool kit.* Retrieved March 5, 2012, from: http://www.csg.org/knowledgecenter/docs/Toolkit03HealthLiteracy.pdf

Covering Kids and Families (2005) *The Health Literacy Style Manual.* Columbia, SC: Southern Institute on Children and Families. Retrieved December 20, 2011, from: http://www.coveringkidsandfamilies.org/resources/docs/stylemanual.pdf

Davis, T.C., Long, S.W., Jackson, R.H., Mayeaux, E.J., Murphy, R.W., and Crouch, M.A. (1993) Rapid estimate of adult literacy in medicine: a shortened screening instrument. *Family Medicine,* 25(6): 391–395.

Davis, T.C., Holcombe, R.F., Berkel, H.J., Pramanik, S., and Divers, S.G. (1998) Informed consent for clinical trials: a comparative study of standard versus simplified forms. *Journal of the National Cancer Institute*, 90(9): 668–674.

Davis, T.C., Wolf, M.S., Bass, P.F. III, Middlebrooks, M., Kennen, E., Baker, D.W., et al. (2006) Literacy and misunderstanding prescription drug labels. *Annals of Internal Medicine,* 145: 887–894.

DeWalt, D.A., Broucksou, K.A., Hawk, V., Brach, C., Hink, A., Rudd, R., and Callahan, L. (2011) Developing and testing the health literacy universal precautions toolkit. *Nursing Outlook*, 59: 85–94.

Diamond, L.C., Luft, H.S., Chung, S., and Jacobs, E.A. (2012) Does this doctor speak my language? Improving the characterization of physician non-English language skills. *Health Services Research,* 47 (1, pt 2): 556–569.

Dorney, J.M. (1988) The plain English movement. *English Journal,* 77(3): 49–52.

Dray, S. and Papen, U. (2004) Literacy and health: towards a methodology for investigating patients' participation in healthcare. *Journal of Applied Linguistics*, 1(3): 311–332.

Dumas, J.S. and Redish, J. (1999) *A Practical Guide to Usability Testing*. Westport, CT: Greenwood.

Dunn, C.L., Pirie, P.L., and Hellerstedt, W.L. (2003) The advice-giving role of female friends and relatives during pregnancy. *Health Education Research,* 18(3): 352–362.

Flores, G. (2005) The impact of medical interpreter services on the quality of health care: a systematic review. *Medical Care Research Review,* 62(3): 255–299.

Fox, S. and Jones, S. (2009) The social life of health information. Retrieved December 20, 2011, from: http://www.pewinternet.org/Reports/2009/8-The-Social-Life-of-Health-Information.aspx

Freidman, D.B. and Hoffman-Goetz, L. (2008) Literacy and health literacy as defined in cancer education research: a systematic review. *Health Education Journal,* 67(4): 285–304.

Galliber, J., Post, D., Weiss, B.D., Dickinson, L.M., Manning, B.K., Staton, E.W., et al. (2010) Patients' question-asking behavior during primary care visits: a report from the AAFP National Research Network. *Annals of Family Medicine,* 8(2): 151–159.

Gazmararian, J.A., Beditz, K., Pisano, S., and Carreón, R. (2010) The development of a health literacy assessment tool for health plans. *Journal of Health Communication,* 15: (Supp. 2): 93–101.

Gordon-Larsen, P., Nelson, M.C., Page, P., and Popkin, B.M. (2006) Inequality in the built environment underlies key health disparities in physical activity and obesity. *Pediatrics*, 117(2): 417–424.

Hahn, E.A., Garcia, S.F., Du, H., and Cella, D. (2010) Patient attitudes and preferences regarding literacy screening in ambulatory cancer clinics. *Patient Related Outcome Measures,* 1: 19–27. Retrieved January 10, 2012, from: http://www.dovepress.com/patient-attitudes-and-preferences-regarding-literacy-screening-in-ambu-peer-reviewed-article-PROM-recommendation1

Halliday, M.A.K. (1987) Spoken and written modes of meaning. In R. Horowitz and S. Jay Samuels (eds) *Comprehending Oral and Written Language* (pp. 55–82). San Diego, CA: Academic Press.

Harrington, J., Noble, L.M., and Newman, S.P. (2004) Improving patients' communication with doctors: a systematic review of intervention studies. *Patient Education and Counseling,* 52(1): 7–16.

Hayanga, A.J. and Kaiser, H.E. (2008) Medical information on YouTube. *Journal of the American Medical Association,* 299(12): 1424–1425.

Hesse, B.S., Nelson, D.E., Kreps, G.L., Croyle, R.T., Arora, N.K., Rimer, B.K., and Viswanath, K. (2005) Trust and sources of health information. *Archives of Internal Medicine,* 165(22): 2618–2624.

Hibbard, J.H., Stockard, J., Mahoney, E.R., and Tusler, M. (2004) Development of the Patient Activation Measure (PAM): conceptualizing and measuring activation in patients and consumers. *Health Services Research,* 39(4): 1005–1026.

Holland, V.M. and Campbell, L.J. (1982) Understanding the language of public documents because readability formulas don't. In R. Pietro (ed.) *Linguistics and the Professions* (pp. 157–171). Hillsdale, NJ: Erlbaum.

Houts, P.S., Doak, C.C., Doak, L.G., and Loscalzo, M.J. (2006) The role of pictures in improving health communication: a review of research on attention, recall, and adherence. *Patient Education and Counseling,* 61(2): 173–190.

Isaacman, D.J., Purvis, K., Gyuro, J., Anderson, Y., and Smith, D. (1992) Standardized instructions: do they improve communication of discharge information from the emergency department? *Pediatrics,* 89 (6 Pt 2): 1204–1208.

Jason, L.A., Richman, J.A., Friedberg, F., Wagner, L., Taylor, R., and Jordan, K.M. (1997) Politics, science, and the emergence of a new disease: the case of chronic fatigue syndrome. *American Psychologist,* 52(9): 873–983.

Katz, M.G., Jacobson, T.A., Veledar, E., and Kripalani, S. (2006) Patient literacy and question-asking behavior during the medical encounter: a mixed methods analysis. *Journal of General Internal Medicine,* 22(6): 782–786.

Koh, H.K., Berwick, D.M., Clancy, C.M., Baur, C., Brach, C., Harris, L.M., and Zerhusen, E.G. (2012) New federal policy initiatives to boost health literacy can help the nation move beyond the cycle of costly 'crisis care'. *Health Affairs,* 31(2): 1–10.

Koonce, T.Y., Giuse, D.A., Beauregard, J.M., and Guise, N.B. (2007) Toward a more informed patient: bridging health information through an interactive communication portal. *Journal of the Medical Library Association,* 95(1): 77–81.

Lamiani, G. and Furey, A. (2009) Teaching nurses how to teach: an evaluation of a workshop on patient education. *Patient Education and Counseling,* 75(2): 270–273.

Levin-Zamir, D. and Peterburg, Y. (2001) Health literacy in health systems: perspectives on patient self-management in Israel. *Health Promotion International,* 16(1): 87–94.

Longo, D.R., Schubert, S.L., Wright, B.A., LeMaster, J., Williams, C.D., and Clore, J.N. (2010) Health information seeking, receipt, and use in diabetes self-management. *Annals of Family Medicine,* 8(4): 334–340.

McCormack, L., Bann, C., Squiers, L., Berkman, N.D., Squire, C., Schillinger, D., et al. (2010) Measuring health literacy: a pilot study of a new skills-based instrument. *Journal of Health Communication,* 15(Supp. 2): 51–71.

McDowell, L., Messias, D.K.H., and Estrada, R.D. (2011) The work of language interpretation in health care: complex, challenging, exhausting, and often invisible. *Journal of Transcultural Nursing,* 22: 137–147.

Makoul, G. (2001) Essential elements of communication in medical encounters: the Kalamazoo Consensus Statement. *Academic Medicine,* 76(4): 390–393.

Margalit, R.S., Roter, D., Dunevant, M.A., Larson, S., and Reiss, S. (2006) Electronic medical record use and physician–patient communication: an observational study of Israeli primary care encounters. *Patient Education and Counseling,* 61(1): 134–141.

Maynard, D.W. and Heritage, J. (2005) Conversation analysis, doctor–patient interaction and medical communication. *Medical Education,* 39: 428–435.

Mazor, K.M., Roblin, D.W., Williams, A.E., Greene, S.M., Gaglio, B., Field, T.S., et al. (2012) Health literacy and cancer prevention: two new instruments. *Patient Education and Counseling,* 88(1): 54–60.

Mazur, B. (2000) Revisiting plain language. *Technical Communication,* 47(2): 205–211.

Mika, V.S., Wood, P.R., Weiss, B.D., and Trevino, L. (2007) Ask me 3: improving communication in a Hispanic pediatric outpatient practice. *American Journal of Health Behavior,* 31(Suppl. 1): S115–121.

Morris, N.S., MacLean, C.D., Chew, L., and Littenberg, B. (2006) The single item literacy screener: evaluation of a brief instrument to identify limited reading ability. *BMC Family Practice,* 7(21). Retrieved January 11, 2012, from: http://www.biomedcentral.com/1471-2296/7/21

National Council on Interpreting in Healthcare (2005) *National Standards of Practice for Interpreters in Health Care*. Santa Rosa, CA: author. Retrieved December 8, 2013, from: http://www.ncihc.org/assets/documents/publications/NCIHC National Standards of Practice.pdf

Nicolson, D., Knapp, P., Raynor, D.K., and Spoor, P. (2009) Written information about individual medicines for consumers. *Cochrane Database of Systematic Reviews 2009 (2)* (Article No. CD002104).

Noel, P.H., Larme, A.C., Meyer, I., et al. (1998) Patient choice in diabetes education curriculum. *Diabetes Care*, 21(6): 896–901.

Nutbeam, D. (2008) The evolving concept of health literacy. *Social Science and Medicine,* 67: 2072–2078.

Osborn, C.Y., Paasche-Orlow, M., Davis, T.C., and Wolf, M. (2007) Health literacy: an overlooked factor in understanding HIV health disparities. *American Journal of Preventive Medicine,* 33(5): 374–378.

Paasche-Orlow, M.K. and Wolf, M.S. (2007) The causal pathways linking health literacy to health outcomes. *American Journal of Health Behavior,* 31(Supp. 1): S19–S26.

Parker, R.M. and Ratzan, S.C. (2010) Health literacy: a second decade of distinction for Americans. *Journal of Health Communication,* 15(S2): 20–33.

Parker, R.M., Baker, D.W., Williams, M.V., and Nurss, J.R. (1995) The test of functional health literacy in adults: a new instrument for measuring patients' literacy skills. *Journal of General Internal Medicine,* 10(10): 537–541.

Parvanta, C., Myers, R., DiCarlo, M., and Burgh, D. (2011) This call is being recorded for quality and training purposes: a qualitative analysis of patient navigation for colorectal cancer screening in an urban setting. Paper presented at the National Conference on Health Communication, Marketing, and Media, August 10, Atlanta, GA.

Peerson, A. and Saunders, M. (2009) Health literacy revisited. What do we mean and why does it matter? *Health Promotion International,* 24(3): 285–296.

Plain Language Action and Information Network (n.d.) *Federal Plain Language Guidelines*. Retrieved April 17, 2012, from: http://www.plainlanguage.gov/howto/guidelines/FederalPLGuidelines/index.cfm?CFID=9366693&CFTOKEN=bdd743e45a0c509a-98B305F7-1372-4132-8DF6DDE68066D9FE&jsessionid=8830e517e0fc77f8a34134783a77475a859c

Pleasant, A. and Kuruvilla, S. (2008) A tale of two health literacies: public health and clinical approaches to health literacy. *Health Promotion International,* 23(2): 152–159.

Pleasant A., McKinney, J., and Rikard R.V. (2011) Health literacy measurement: a proposed agenda. *Journal of Health Communication,* 16(S3): 11–21.

Rosenfeld, L., Rudd, R.E., Emmons, K.M., Acevedo-Garcia, D., Martin, L., and Buka, S. (2011) Health literacy: beyond reading alone: the relationship between aural literacy and asthma management. *Patient Education and Counseling,* 82(1): 110–116.

Roter, D.L. (2011) Oral literacy demand on health care communication: challenges and solutions. *Nursing Outlook*, 59(2): 79–84.

Roter, D.L., Erby, L., Larson, S., and Elington, L. (2009) Oral literacy demand of prenatal genetic counseling dialogue: predictors of learning. *Patient Education and Counseling,* 75(3): 392–397.

Royne, M.B. and Meyers, S.D. (2008) Recognizing consumer issues in DTC pharmaceutical advertising. *Journal of Consumer Affairs,* 42(2): 60–80.

Rubin, D.L. (1993) Listenability = oral-based language + considerateness. In A. Wolvin and C. Coakley (eds) *Perspectives on Listening* (pp. 262–282). Beverly Hills, CA: Sage.

——(2012) Listenability as a tool for advancing health literacy. *Journal of Health Communication,* 17 (Supp. 3): 176–190.

Rubin, D.L. and Floyd, D.H. (1992) A functional approach to writing for trial court judges. *Journal of Teaching Writing,* 11(2): 187–202.

Rubin, D.L., Hafer, T., and Arata, K. (2000) Reading and listening to oral-based versus literate-based discourse. *Communication Education,* 49(2): 121–134.

Rubin, D.L., Freimuth, V., Parmer, J., Kaley, T., and Okundaye, M. (2011) Associations between older adults' spoken interactive health literacy and selected health care and health communication outcomes. *Journal of Health Communication,* 16(S3): 191–204.

Rudd, R.E. and Anderson, J.E. (2006) *The Health Literacy Environment of Hospitals and Health Centers.* Cambridge, MA: National Center for the Study of Adult Learning and Literacy and the Harvard Health and Adult Literacy and Learning Initiative. Retrieved December 8, 2013, from: http://www.hsph.harvard.edu/healthliteracy/files/2012/09/healthliteracyenvironment.pdf

Schenker, Y., Karter, A.J., Schillinger, D., Warton, E.M., et. al. (2010) The impact of limited English proficiency and physician language concordance on reports of clinical interactions among patients with diabetes: The DISTANCE Study. *Patient Education and Counseling,* 81(2): 222–228.

Schouten, B.C. and Meeuwesen, L. (2006) Cultural differences in medical communication: a review of the literature. *Patient Education and Counseling,* 64: 21–34.

Schriver, K.A. (2000) Readability formulas in the new millennium: What's the use? *ACM Journal of Computer Documentation,* 24(3): 138–140.

Shim, J.K. (2010) Cultural health capital: a theoretical approach to understanding health care interaction. *Journal of Health and Social Behavior*, 51(1): 1–15.

Smedley, B.D., Stith, A.Y., and Nelson, A.R. (eds) Committee on Understanding and Eliminating Racial and Ethnic Disparities in Health Care. (2003) *Unequal Treatment: Confronting Racial and Ethnic Disparities in Health Care*. Washington, DC: Institute of Medicine. Retrieved March 30, 2010, from: http://www.nap.edu/catalog/10260.html

Sørenson, K., van den Broucke, S., Fulham, J., Doyle, G., Pelikan, J., Slonska, Z., and Brand, H. (2012) Health literacy and public health: a systematic review and integration of definitions and models. *BMC Public Health,* 12(80). Retrieved February 11, 2012, from: http://www.biomedcentral.com/1471-2458/12/80

Speros, C. (2005) Health literacy: concept analysis. *Journal of Advanced Nursing,* 50(6): 633–640.

Street, R.L. (2001) Active patients as powerful communicators: the linguistic foundations of participation in health care. In W.P. Robinson and H. Giles (eds) *Handbook of Language and Social Psychology* (pp. 541–560). Chichester: John Wiley.

US Department of Health and Human Services, Office of Disease Prevention and Health Promotion. (2010) *National Action Plan to Improve Health Literacy.* Washington, DC: Author. Retrieved November 14, 2011. from: http://health.gov/communication/HLActionPlan/

US Department of Health and Human Services (2012) *Healthy People 2020: Improving the Health of America*. Retrieved August 9, 2012, from: http://www.healthypeople.gov/2020/default.aspx

Vernon, J.A., Trujillo, A., Rosenbaum, S., and DeBuono, B. (2007) Low health literacy: implications for national health care policy. Washington, DC: George Washington University School of Public Health and Health Services.

Williams, D.M., Counselman, F.L., and Caggiano, C.D. (1996) Emergency department discharge instructions and patient literacy: a problem of disparity. *American Journal of Emergency Medicine,* 14(1): 19–22.

Williams, M.V., Davis, T., Parker, R.M., and Weiss, B.D. (2002) The role of health literacy in patient–physician communication. *Family Medicine*, 34(5): 383–389.

World Health Organization (2005) *Bangkok Charter for Health Promotion in a Globalized World.* Retrieved December 11, 2011, from: http://www.who.int/healthpromotion/conferences/6gchp/hpr_050829_%20BCHP.pdf

Zarcadoolas, C. (2010) The simplicity complex: exploring simplified health messages in a complex world. *Health Promotion International*, 26(3): 338–350.

Zarcadoolas, C., Pleasant, A., and Greer, D. (2005) Understanding health literacy: an expanded model. *Health Promotion International,* 20(2): 195–203.

Zukoski, A.P., Thorburn, S., and Stroud, J. (2011): Seeking information about HIV/AIDS: a qualitative study of health literacy among people living with HIV/AIDS in a low prevalence context, *AIDS Care,* 23(11): 1505–1508.

11

Health disparities research and practice

The role of language and health communication

Sherrie Flynt Wallington

Introduction

This chapter provides a much needed primer particularly for applied linguists, scholars, and students who understand linguistics somewhat generally, but perhaps do not know much about the role of linguistics in health communication, health disparities, and public health inquiry in general. Although these fields have existed singularly for a while, scholars and researchers are now finding ways of converging the science of each to illuminate our understanding of each separately as a field of inquiry. The importance of linguistics to health communication in particular transcends the motivation for this book and provides an important, often lacking, perspective in understanding the role of our world's language-related issues within health communication and health disparities scholarship.

Fanon wrote, 'To speak a language is to take on a world, a culture' (1967: 38). This quote resonates today in the United States through diversity and interactions of myriad cultures. Kagawa-Singer et al. (2010) defined culture as life's fundamental, dynamic, responsive, adaptive, and relatively coherent organizing system. This system ensures its members' survival and well-being, promoting meaning, purpose, and communication. Language is part of this system; thus, cultural linguistic diversity is growing in American society. Coupled with this diversity is a groundswell of consumer and patient engagement and empowerment (Hibbard and Lorig 2012; McAllister et al. 2012), fueled by demand for health information, shifting medical paradigms, patient advocacy groups, and differential preferences for health communication channels (Blake et al. 2011; Weiss and Lorenzi 2008).

Hence, what is the effect of this growing diversity and patient engagement and empowerment? What is the role of culture and language in promoting health communication and disparities? Finally, how will cultural and linguistic research affect future health communication research and theory? Admittedly, health communication alone cannot solve issues that plague health disparities; however, Viswanath et al. (2007) contended that communication is one of the central threads contributing to and mitigating disparities. Thus, this chapter focuses on how health communication addresses health disparities while particularly emphasizing interrelationships of culture and linguistics. Relevant theories, models, and community-level approaches – both widely used and emerging – are presented. The chapter concludes with recommendations to bridge some of the cultural and linguistic gaps in health communication and health disparities research.

Historical perspectives

Health communication

Health communication is a broad, encompassing, intrapersonal, interpersonal, group, organizational, and societal communication (Kreps et al. 1998), defined as the 'art and technique of informing, influencing, and motivating individual, institutional, and public audiences about important health issues' (US Department of Health and Human Services [HHS] 2000). Furthermore, health communication includes disease prevention, health promotion, healthcare policy, and the business of health care, as well as enhancement of the quality of life and health of individuals within the community. Health communications draw heavily from social sciences literature and the field of medicine, particularly patient–doctor communication issues (Kreps et al. 1998; Korsch and Negrete 1972). The origin of health communication can be traced to the eighteenth- and nineteenth-century public health campaigns promoting hygiene and immunization, to persuasion studies during and after World War II, and on to development of communication campaigns in the 1970s (Lazarsfeld et al. 1948; Hornik 1988; Hovland et al. 1949; Paisley 1989). These origins and evolution of health communication legitimized today's field of inquiry (Nussbaum 1989), permeating many disciplines and influential in many healthcare, community, and public policy arenas.

This growing legitimacy is owed to milestones such as the establishment of professional organizations such as the Health Communication Division, established through the International Communication Association, the creation of influential health communication journals, such as the *Journal of Health Communication, Health Communication,* and the *Journal of Communications in Healthcare*, curriculum development for both undergraduate and graduate programs, and annual conferences, expanding the field (Kreps et al. 1998; Wright et al. 2007).

Health communication studies have recently amplified significantly, proportionate to the nation's diversity. Access to care, healthcare quality gaps, disparities in treatment and accessibility to new communication technologies, increased health communication research funding initiatives, and patient dissatisfaction with medical professionals have all contributed to this growth (HHS 2008; Viswanath et al. 2006). Interdisciplinary studies have fueled more complex research in health communication, and linguistics has played a large role in this inducement (Halliday and Webster 2006). Contributions of linguistics to health care created significant research across myriad health topics such as readability of hospice materials (Kehl and McCarty 2012); YouTube cancer narratives (Chou et al. 2011); patient-centered interviewing (Hesson et al. 2012); sociolinguistics and genetics discourse analysis (Babul-Hirji et al. 2010), and language and dementia (Hamilton 2008; Muller and Mok 2012). Too, several linguistic studies focused on the interrelationship of culture, language, and health disparities (Calderón and Beltran 2005; Lim 2010; Kagawa-Singer et al. 2010).

Critical Issues and Topics

Health disparities

The Institute of Medicine (IOM 2002: 32) has well documented the pervasive US health disparities and defines a disparity as a difference in treatment provided to members of different racial (or ethnic) groups that is not justified by the underlying health conditions or treatment preferences of patients. Health disparities are related to race, ethnicity, gender, income, education, sexual orientation, quality of care, or geography. Fortunately, health communication researchers began to recognize the important roles of health communication to address health disparities. Kreps et al. wrote:

> Health communication inquiry is becoming increasingly concerned with the role of culture on health and healthcare. We believe that communication scholars will work to end the prejudicial treatment of marginalized cultural groups within the modern healthcare system, such as prejudicial treatment of people with AIDS, the poor, minorities, women, and the elderly.
>
> *(Kreps et al. 1998:13)*

Indeed, health communication is now considered essential to national health disparities initiatives. In February 1998, President Bill Clinton announced a new initiative to eliminate racial and ethnic disparities by the year 2010, first launching Healthy People 2010 and now Healthy People 2020, the nation's 10-year national initiatives for improving the health of all Americans. The Healthy People 2020 initiative has more than 600 objectives – some still evolving – and 42 topical areas. The health communication area of this initiative has 13 objectives, designed to affect health, health care, and healthy equity. These national efforts draw needed attention to disparities (Berkman et al. 2004; HHS 2012).

Health disparities have been well documented, induced by many factors, including culture and language, both central to addressing health disparities and development of effective health communication (Calderón and Beltran 2005; Kagawa-Singer et al. 2010). Kagawa-Singer et al. (2010) posited that culture contributes persistently to health disparities. Further, language is also used as a proxy for culture (Lee 2003). Moreover, communication barriers have been increasingly recognized as contributors to health disparities (Collins et al. 2002).

The role of language and culture in health disparities

Study and application of culture and linguistics in health communication warrant investigation, particularly as a potential remedy for health disparities. Jaspal (2009) suggests that language and culture are often tailored for unique expression of smaller social groups or subcultures, creating hybrid identity without rejecting original identity. Subcultures personalize language to establish distinctive subcultural identity. Thus, to understand these variances is to understand diversity (Jaspal 2009). For example, Rodriguez et al. (2008) doubted existence of a common culture of Pan-Latino identity among Latinos. Many might not differentiate between Hispanic and Latino, opting for one label since each speak and use the Spanish language distinctly. Asians too are often generalized and stereotyped, despite significant distinctions in their subcultures (Huang 2010; Timberlake and Williams 2012). Subcultures within larger racial and ethnic groups produce an array of ideologies and identities. Because of ever-changing US demographics, researchers and practitioners must acknowledge the subcultures and socio-cultural importance of linguistic and cultural sensitivity (Betancourt et al. 2003).

Rapidly growing cultural diversity has led to significant language diversity. An increase in the percentage of racial demographics from non-English-speaking backgrounds correlates with an increase in languages spoken in the United States. In 2000, 82.1 percent of Americans reported speaking English at home, while 17.9 percent spoke another language – 10.7 percent spoke Spanish, 3.8 percent spoke other Indo-European languages, and 2.7 percent spoke Asian and Pacific Island languages (US Census Bureau 2002). As such, lack of English proficiency has been a major obstacle to accessing medical and social services (Mutchler and Brallier 1999). The US census' term 'linguistically isolated' categorizes individuals aged 14 or above not proficient in English. Strikingly, out of 97,454,100 total US households, a language other than English was spoken in 14,005,410, and 3,026,542 households were classified as linguistically isolated (US Census Bureau 2010).

Researchers are yet to ascertain the full effect of these trends on health and health care as well as the effect in health communication. Communication plays an essential role promoting prevention of disease and poor health (IOM 2002) and scholars argue that diversity and change necessitate effective communication, thereby broadening the scope of health communication scholarship (Thompson et al. 2008). Relevant too is the negative effect of poor health communication. Thomas (2006) pointed to these as 'failures in communications', leading to malpractice suits, misdiagnoses, patients incompliance, cross-cultural misunderstandings, and other concerns. Lack of health literacy compounds these issues.

Current contributions and research

An important dimension of health communication specifically is the need to ensure that information is available to all those who need it, regardless of their social economic status or cultural, linguistic, or geographical background. Thus, the importance of providing this information to both individuals and communities becomes ever so urgent to combat the profound health disparities seen in our nation's populations. As the evidence has well documented (IOM 2003), many health problems including health disparities are the result of many complex factors that are attributable to lifestyle and behaviors that are modifiable given the right opportunity structure, access to healthcare, and, above all, information (Emmons 2000). As such, many public health and health communication interventions seek to intervene on these modifiable risk factors at various levels – individual, group, systems, and community. There is an arsenal of theoretical frameworks that are used to guide these interventions, and some are outlined in the following section.

Theoretical frameworks, models, and approaches to health behavior and health communication

Myriad health communication theories prioritize effective ways to communicate health promotion and disease prevention by changing attitudes, beliefs, and behaviors (Thomas 2006; Glanz et al. 2008). The use of theory in constructing and applying health communication messages provides a lens for guiding research, practice, curriculum development, evaluation, and development of effective communication and educational strategies, and assessment of the effect of health behavior interventions in complex social settings (Grol et al. 2007). In this section, widely used and emerging frameworks and approaches are presented, though not an exhaustive review. See also Glanz et al. (2008), Hamilton (2008). Presented are individual, group, social, systems, community-level frameworks, and also the influence of linguistics at each level is described.

Individual level

The Health Belief Model (HBM; Rosenstock 1974) posits that health prevention behavior is influenced by an individual's perceptions of the health problem's threat level, benefits of avoiding the threat, and factors influencing the decision to act. The HBM suggests individuals engage in healthful behavior when they perceive possible reduction of threat (Glanz et al. 2008).

Social Cognitive Theory (SCT) proposes that human behavior is a synthesis of three factors: personal, behavioral, and environmental (Bandura 1994). SCT suggests that individuals must believe their capability to engage in recommended behaviors.

The Theory of Reasoned Action (TRA) seeks to understand the relationship between attitudes and behavior, and provide methodologies for health risk message development (Fishbein and Ajzen 1981). TRA has been applied to health-related behaviors such as violence prevention (Meyer et al. 2004) and nutrition intervention studies (Booth-Butterfield and Reger 2004). Fishbein and Ajzen (1981) noted that TRA identifies two conditions that must be altered prior to behavior change: (a) attitude: beliefs about certain behaviors' consequences and evaluation of those consequences, and (b) subjective norm: assessment of other beliefs, or social referents about the behavior and the individual's motivation to comply with those referents.

The Extended Parallel Process Model (EPPM; Witte 1997) suggests that health risk messages initiate two cognitive appraisals: one of the threat and the other of the efficacy of the recommended response. Generally, EPPM suggests that strength of threat perception is proportionate to fear and motivation to act. People then appraise the efficacy of the recommended response before deciding and executing a behavioral response.

Group level

The Transtheoretical Model (TTM), also known as Stages of Change (Prochaska 1979), targets specific groups to collect health information. TTM acknowledges that individuals in the process of changing should receive interventions that cater to their stage of behavior change. TTM characterizes change as a process involving progress through six stages (Prochaska et al. 2002): (a) precontemplation: the individual is unaware of the problem or has not contemplated change seriously; (b) contemplation: the individual considers change; (c) preparation: the individual plans to act and adjust before change; (d) action: the individual implements specific actions to modify behavior and/or environment; (e) maintenance: the individual continues change implementation while employing recommendations to prevent lapse or relapse; and (f) termination: the individual has instituted the new behavior with no possibility of relapse.

Social marketing is also pivotal and employs myriad communication methods, including mass media campaigns to increase awareness of health risks to elicit desired behavior change (Savitz and Umble 2002). Kotler and Roberto (1989) defined social marketing as a planning process that promotes voluntary behavior changes by offering benefits to group members, reducing barriers of concern, and using persuasion to motivate program participation. Social marketing seeks to market healthy behavior as a product, and, as Storey et al. (2008) posited, to apply marketing's Four Ps: (a) *product*: behavior the target audience must change; (b) *price*: the perceived physical, social, and psychological costs of the intended behavior change; (c) *promotion*: how the product or behavior can be represented or packaged; and (d) *place*: availability of information or products related to the intended behavior change.

Social/and social determinants level

Individual health outcomes are shaped not merely by individual motivation but also by higher-level social and structural factors (i.e., social determinants of health). Disparities in health communication outcomes via social determinants potentially lead to risky behavior, morbidity, and mortality. These potential gaps in information acquisition engender significant communication inequalities, potentially stifling individuals or the capacity of community groups to process and employ health information (Viswanath et al. 2006). Viswanath et al.'s (2007) emerging Structural Influence Model of Health Communication (SIM) calls attention to inequalities in communication and consequent inequalities in health, linking social determinants explicitly with health outcomes. Important dimensions of communication inequality include: (a) access to and use of information channels and services, (b) attention to and processing of health information, and (c) capacity and ability to act on information provided. SIM posits a connection between social determinants and health outcomes through mass media and interpersonal communication outcomes such as access, usage, and processing of health communication messages. Social determinants such as social class or environment influence mass and interpersonal communication outcomes.

Systems level

The Social Ecological Model (SEM) emerges from the social ecology perspective (Hawley 1950) and the early work of Bronfenbrenner (1977). SEM examines the multiple effects and interrelatedness of social elements in an environment and, more specifically, how behavior is affected by multiple levels of influence (Centers for Disease Control and Prevention 2011a, 2011b, 2011c; McLeroy et al. 1988). The individual-centered model is comprised of increasingly broad levels of community hierarchy – individual, interpersonal, organizational, community, and policy (Glanz et al. 2008). Moreover, SEM provides a lens for better understanding the influence of social and structural systems on the cultural norms of various groups. Smedley and Syme (2000) stated 'It is unreasonable to expect that people will change their behavior easily when so many forces in the social, cultural, and physical environment conspire against such change.' SEM helps unearth what individual, social/structural, cultural, and lingustic factors promote or impede involving health communication and health disparity factors. Sallis et al. (2008) suggested that SEM represents a promising approach not yet fully articulated, applied, and evaluated.

Community level

There is growing interest in community-based participatory research (CBPR) to address health disparities (D'Alonzo 2010). CBPR is often used with other frameworks and models to examine behavior change (Minkler and Wallerstein 2003). CBPR involves equal partnership between researchers and a diverse selection of community partners to yield a multifaceted, in-depth, and practical solution while securing sustainable relationships with the target population (Israel et al. 2010; Schulz et al. 2011; Katz 2004). The result is a research program capable of addressing health disparities and policy advocacy, significantly increasing validity and efficacy of this community-based research program (Israel et al. 2010). CBPR involves diverse community partners and, drawing on knowledge and expertise of research experts, helps facilitate capacity building and policy change (Israel et al. 2010) to enhance potentiality of positive community change. CBPR builds upon traditional public health research methods through involvement of many different perspectives, resources, and skills, and facilitates learning for the researcher as well as the community members (Schulz et al. 2011) to counteract historically problematic obstacles to community partnerships (i.e., skepticism, hostility, etc.).

Theoretical linguistic challenges, influences, and possibilities

Taken together, all of the selected theories and framework are influenced by linguistics. These theories, models, and approaches all offer unique and explanatory lenses through which to better understand certain constructs that may facilitate or impede factors related to health communication and health disparities research. However, with all the levels – individual, groups, systems, and community – some challenges remain, particularly as it relates to the important role that language plays in the communication and behavioral process. For many populations, standard constructs such as perceived risk, perceived susceptibility, intention, attitudes, self-efficacy, etc. may not mean the same, exist in the native language, or are culturally and linguistically irrelevant (Giuliano et al. 2000; Pasick et al. 2009). Also, languages have words with multiple English meanings and some English words might not have an equivalent word in other languages (Hodge et al. 1996). Further, communication styles differ (verbal vs. written, body language) for minorities and this affects overall understanding. However, emerging research on the cultural and linguistic relevancy of existing theories and the need for new and expanded consideration of cultural and linguistic factors has brought attention to this issue (Pasick et al. 2009). Theories such as the Social Ecological Model and the Structural Influence Model offer promising frameworks and models that emphasize the social, structural, cultural and linguistic factors of individuals, groups, and communities. Some approaches have included the convergence of theories and models such as combining the Health Belief Model with the Social Ecological Model (Glanz et al. 2008). More recent approaches such as community-based participatory research, also greatly enhance the understanding of the underlying and shared cultural assumptions and linguistic preferences and practices of a community.

Methodological diversity and integration in health communications

Kreps (2011) called for methodological diversity and integration in health communication to achieve powerfully relevant health communication research and this is also needed particularly in the reduction and elimination of health disparities. Part of this diversity should include methodological components that emphasize culture and linguistics and collaboration across disciplines. This is partially achieved through full examinations of methods that allow inspection of multiple health variables and influences across cultures and languages (Campbell et al. 2003). An important goal is not to assume that all theories and methodologies are not 'universal' but demonstrating equivalence of constructs and measures used with target cultures and minimizing bias that may threaten valid cross-cultural comparisons (Ægisdóttir et al. 2007).

There are several design approaches that are well grounded across disciplines. One is the randomized controlled trial which is considered the 'gold standard', and is often used in health communication and health disparities research. Health communication research in particular is increasingly utilizing a broad range of designs, methods, and theories, both experimental and quasi-experimental (Glasgow et al. 2004; Koelen et al. 2001; Concato 2004), such as surveys, qualitative and quantitative textual analyses, and ethnographies, mixed methods, and meta-analytic methods (Kreps 2011). Experimental research establishes causality through manipulation of independent variables and measurement of antecedent dependent variables (Oakley 1998), while quasi-experimental research eliminates random assignment and provides greater freedom in the use of control groups (Campbell and Stanley 1966; Cook and Campbell 1979; Shadish et al. 2002). Survey research examines attitudes, beliefs, and activities of groups of respondents (Thompson 2003). Textual analyses describe and interpret the characteristics of recorded or visual messages (Frey et al. 2000). Ethnographic research provides in-depth analysis of social events (Kreps 2008).

With these study designs and approaches as well as a host of others, there is a critical need to establish the cross-cultural generalizability of theories and methodological approaches to eliminate erroneous conclusions about similarities and differences between cultural groups and with different languages. Also, it is important that researchers not assume an instrument, for an example, a survey instrument, developed for one culture and in one language, is appropriate for and will yield valid findings about another cultural group. Further, the role of linguistics is especially key in looking at 'construct and item bias'. Construct bias refers to the question of whether the same underlying constructs are being measured in each ethnic group (Meiring et al. 2005). Essentially the construct being measured is not identical across cultures. Item bias refers to measurement at the item level (Ægisdóttir et al. 2007). Item bias in particular can be the result from poor translation or poor item formulation (i.e., complex wording) or because item content may not be equally relevant or culturally or linguistically appropriate (Meiring et al. 2005).

Further, multi-methodological methods, or mixed methods (i.e., the combination of different methods), help researchers ascertain complexities, particularly cultural and linguistic, of health communication processes through data triangulation (Johnstone 2004; Creswell et al. 2004). The National Institutes of Health (NIH; 2012) has championed use of mixed methods research to optimize dissemination and implementation of health interventions. Meta-analytic research methods pool and analyze data from similar studies created through similar research measures to synthesize findings and reach larger conclusions (Lipsey and Wilson 2001).

Research exemplars

The literature describes several successful research examples that have employed some of the approaches discussed earlier. Selections presented here reflect the integration of cultural and linguistic factors as part of an overall health communication strategy.

Communicating across the generation gap

Generational differences in knowledge, awareness, and communication create need for age-specific linguistic tailoring (Harvey et al. 2008; Ford et al. 2002; Doak et al. 1996). Corpus linguistics has proven instrumental in communicating with populations such as adolescents that may prefer media technology and modified language (Harvey et al. 2008). Findings from Harvey et al. (2008) suggest that email may promote communication between health professionals and adolescents who may not seek conventional healthcare services. Conducting a corpus linguistic analysis of 62,794 emails from adolescent health website *Teen Health Freak*, researchers dissected the language that adolescents use. With permission, researchers performed keyword, collocational, and concordance analyses that revealed adolescent anxiety about communicating health concerns to adults. Keywords such as 'GP' (general practitioner) and 'parents' were among the most used on the website. Communication keywords were also prevalent: 'tell', 'ask', 'talk', 'answer', 'advice', 'question', 'advise', and 'explain'. Common adjectives included 'afraid', 'scared', 'worried', 'embarrassed', and 'stressed'. The web entries were frank, and results of the analyses revealed that, although some adolescents dislike communicating in person, they proficiently articulate their health concerns online, potentially enabling health communicators to provide adolescents with a preferred platform wherein comfortable and confidential communication with health professionals is possible.

Cultural relevance makes the difference

Cultural relevance is also important for linguistic-centered health development. Studies revealed the importance of maintaining cultural relevance to achieve comprehension and acceptance of health communication among target populations. Messages have to appeal to the target audience's cultural background and to their lifestyles (Tanjasiri et al. 2007). In a 2007 study, Tanjasiri et al. examined breast health interventions for Asian-American women, whose high breast cancer death rates corresponded to low screening rates. To counteract this disparity, Asian-American men and women participated in workshops. A total of 302 women and 314 Asian-American men, with an average age in the late forties, participated over the course of the one-year intervention. Literacy (English and Hmong) was minimal among both genders. The study's intervention included development of educational materials – a flipchart, brochure, and video – that targeted female participants as well as their husbands and urged women to receive regular breast cancer screenings. The social aspect of the intervention, grounded in the social learning theory, was central to the intervention development, merging fundamental messages with existing cultural communication structures and health beliefs. Pre- and post-surveys revealed increased knowledge and positive attitudes about screenings and intent to follow through with breast health examinations.

The structure of language in the linguistic approach

Including members of the target population is an effective means of ensuring cultural quality and effectiveness (Bradley et al. 2006; Nelson and Hamilton 2007), and may help reveal other key factors such as low literacy, preconceived notions, or health concerns (Hill-Briggs and Smith 2008; Johnson et al. 2003) that help structure health messages for optimal efficacy. Pictorial representations, as well as the length of health communication messages, can effect reception and target behaviors (Houts et al. 2006; Rawson et al. 2010). In testing the efficacy of structural and technical linguistic matters, as did Rawson et al. (2010) in their evaluation of the Medical Term Recognition Test (METER), researchers can improve the mechanics of health messages. Although health literacy assessments have emerged as useful tools, Rawson et al. (2010) sought to explore issues such as length of completion time and practitioner involvement as direct effects of tool efficacy. METER, brief and self-administered, was developed and tested among 155 participants in an urban outpatient cardiology program: 76.5 percent male and 92.6 percent white, with a mean age of 62.7 years and a mean of 14.1 years of education. The assessment measured health literacy, neuropsychological function, psychological health, and self-questionnaires. The two-minute assessment was compared with the Rapid Estimate of Adult Literacy in Medicine (REALM) assessment. METER correlated significantly with REALM and initial findings revealed METER as prompt and practical in clinical settings.

Culturally tailored outreach and CBPR

Aitaoto et al. (2012) developed a culturally and linguistically appropriate breast cancer screening intervention to increase mammography among Micronesian women in Hawaii, among whom 26 percent of those 40 years or older reported breast cancer screening in 2005. The Micronesians are comprised of Marshallese, Chuukese, Pohnpeians, and Kosraens, and all self-refer as Micronesian, though each has a distinct culture and language. From 2006–2007, trust building, joint assessment, cultural tailoring, and skills transfer were used to train and evaluate female Micronesian lay health educators' implementation of breast cancer awareness intervention. Eleven lay educators from each of the four Micronesian subcultures provided both one-on-one and small group information sessions in their respective languages. A total of 567 Micronesian women between the ages of 18 and 75 years participated in the information sessions. Of the 567 women, 202 were aged 40 years or older and eligible for mammography screening and 166 (82 percent) had never had a mammogram. Screening appointments were arranged for the latter. After six months of outreach, 146 of the 166 (88 percent) had received a mammogram, an 18 percent to 90 percent compliance increase. Lay educators also reported an increase in their skills and self-esteem, along with desire to apply their skills to other health issues. Researchers believe that the model may work in other communities to reduce disparities in cancer screening.

Recommendations for practice

The intent of this chapter has been to emphasize the importance and appreciation of culture and language as necessary components of a multidisciplinary health communication approach. Although this may seem apparent and somewhat widely acknowledged more clear linkages between linguistics and health communication interventions is needed and more broadly in public health at all levels – individual, group, systems, and community. The focus and influence of culture and linguistics should not be a mere afterthought or something that is sometimes considered, but become a key component of any lens developing health communication strategies generally and those addressing health disparities.

Second, this chapter has sought also to elucidate important demographic, patient and consumer advocacy trends that further augment the importance of health communication in addressing myriad health disparity gaps. The ascendency of the science of health communication will continue to yield theoretical and methodological productivity, ripe for expansion, new ideas, innovative research, and collaboration in hopes of translating and disseminating health information to American citizens. Tried and true as well as emerging theoretical frameworks will be challenged to appropriately address the cultural and linguistic complexities of health communication, health disparities, and overall public health strategies.

In health communication practice and research it is important to recognize vast changes spurred by significant developments – chiefly, the consumer demands for better quality health information. Additional significant developments include shifts from doctor-centered paradigms to patient-centered models; acknowledgment and implementation of communication technologies (i.e., the Internet, email, texting, and social media for health information and in healthcare settings); and growing prominence of health issues on the public agenda. By virtue of these developments, many organizations are strategically integrating communication and linguistics appropriately. Also, with the growing diversity of the US population, the need to address these factors and other socio-demographic details is essential.

Health communication alone cannot solve all the public health and health disparities confronting Americans and, thus, communication efforts must be supported by additional services, programs, resources, and sustained leadership designed to reach and appeal to all populations (Viswanath 2005). Kontos and colleagues (2007) suggested that health experts also rigorously monitor any emerging communication inequalities and evaluate how best to leverage social media for health promotion and disease prevention initiatives, and, ultimately, assess their effect on health outcomes. Access to these technologies poses a different set of challenges related to communication inequalities. Although these technologies may amplify health communication efforts (Blake et al. 2011) they may also potentially further divide those with access to the latest information technologies and those without (DiMaggio et al. 2001). At minimum, programs should be expected to conduct appropriate audience testing for need, cultural and linguistic competence, comprehension, and receptivity (Thomas 2006).

Future research

A chief research concern in health communication is continued methodological rigor and evaluation. Kreps (2011) also has discussed the importance of methodological diversity and integration, moving towards a mixed methods approach to better develop health communication interventions to assist with the translation and dissemination of evidence-based findings, particularly as they relate to health disparities. Part of this methodological diversity should include a linguistic focus across the research continuum – from study design to dissemination of findings. Also, efforts to include language-concordant research staff and health providers in practice add to this methodological diversity (Giuliano et al. 2000). Existing, expanded, and new theories, models, approaches, especially at the community level, are all necessary to increase the chances of success of any health communication effort. Continued research is needed to develop health communication messages for diverse populations; particularly those that emphasize both culture and language. Some consideration should include an understanding that Pidgin English is commonly used, so comprehension of Standard English is lower (Da Pidgin Coup 1999), that sentence structure influences comprehension (Akina 1998), and that many immigrant populations rely on culture-specific newspapers for health-related information, so existing education strategies for the general public may not be reaching them (Kim et al. 1999).

Related topics

Corpus linguistics; health disparities; cultural appropriateness; multilevel, health promotion.

Further reading

Freimuth, V.S. and Quinn, S.C. (2005) 'The contributions of health communication to eliminating health disparities,' *American Journal of Public Health*, 94: 2053–2054.

Harvey, K. and Koteyoko, N. (2012) *Exploring Health Communication: Language in Action,* New York: Routledge.

Institute of Medicine (2002) *Speaking of Health: Assessing Health Communication Strategies for Diverse Populations,* Washington, DC: National Academies Press.
Viswanath, K. and Ackerson, L.K. (2011) 'Race, ethnicity, language, social class, and health communication inequalities: a nationally-representative cross-sectional study,' *PLoS One*, 6: e14550.

References

Ægisdóttir, S., Gerstein, L.H., and Cinarbas, D.C. (2007) 'Methodological issues in cross-cultural counseling research,' *Counseling Psychologist*, 36(2): 188–219.

Aitaoto, N., Braun, K.L., Estrella, J., Epeluk, A., and Tsark, J. (2012) 'Design and results of a culturally tailored cancer outreach project by and for Micronesian women,' *Preventing Chronicle Disease*, 9:E82 Epub.

Akina, C. (1998) 'Native Hawaiian Heart Disease Initiative.' Presentation at the Workshop for Physicians, Kaluako'i Hotel, Moloka'i, Hawai'i.

Babul-Hirji, R., Hewson, S., and Frescura, M. (2010) 'A sociolinguistic exploration of genetic counseling discourse involving a child with a new genetic diagnosis,' *Patient Education and Counseling,* 78: 40–45.

Bandura, A. (1994) 'Self-efficacy.' In V.S. Ramachaudran (ed.) *Encyclopedia of Human Behavior,* 4: 71–81, New York: Academic Press.

Berkman, N.D., Dewalt, D.A., Pignone, M.P., Sheridan, S.L., Lohr, K.N., Lux, L., et al. (2004) 'Literacy and health outcomes,' *Evidence Report/technology Assessment*, 1(87): 1–8.

Betancourt, J.R., Green, A.R., Carrillo, J.E., and Ananeh-Firempong, O. (2003) 'Defining cultural competence: a practical framework for addressing racial/ethnic disparities in health and healthcare,' *Public Health Reports*, 118: 293–302.

Blake, K.D., Flynt Wallington, S., and Viswanath, K. (2011) 'Health communication channel preferences by class, race, and place.' In G. Kreps (ed.) *Health Communication: Building the Evidence Base in Cancer Control*, Cresskill, NJ: Hampton Press.

Booth-Butterfield, S. and Reger, B. (2004) 'The message changes belief and the rest is theory: the "1% or less" milk campaign and reasoned action,' *Preventative Medicine,* 39: 581–588.

Bradley, P.K., Berry, A., Lang, C., and Myers, R.E. (2006) 'Getting ready: developing an educational intervention to prepare African American women for breast biopsy,' *ABNF Journal*, 17: 15–19.

Bronfenbrenner, U. (1977) 'Toward an experimental ecology of human development,' *American Psychologist*, 32(7): 513–531.

Calderón, J.L. and Beltran, R.A. (2005) 'Culture and linguistics: neglected variables in the health communication equation,' *American Journal of Medical Quality,* 20: 179–181.

Campbell, D.T. and Stanley, J.C. (1966) *Experimental and Quasi-experimental Designs for Research*, Chicago, IL: Rand McNally.

Campbell, S.M., Braspenning, J., Hutchinson, A., and Marshall, M.N. (2003) 'Research methods used in developing and applying quality indicators in primary care,' *British Medical Journal*, 326: 816–819.

Centers for Disease Control and Prevention. (2011a) 'Observances, September 15th–October 15th Hispanic/Latino Heritage Month: examples of important health disparities experienced by Hispanics/Latinos.' Retrieved June 25, 2012, from: http://www.cdc.gov/minorityhealth/observances/HL.html

——(2011b) 'Rationale for regular reporting on health disparities and inequalities. Morbidity and Mortality Weekly Report.' Retrieved August 9, 2012, http://www.cdc.gov/mmwr/pdf/other/su6001.pdf

——(2011c) 'Social ecological model.' Retrieved March 15, 2012, from: http://www.cdc.gov/cancer/crccp/sem.htm

Chou, W.Y., Hunt, Y., Folkers, A., and Augustson, E. (2011) 'Cancer survivorship in the age of YouTube and social media: a narrative analysis,' *Journal of Medical Internet Research,* 13: e7.

Collins, T.C., Clark, J.A., Petersen, L.A., and Kressin, N.R. (2002) 'Racial differences in how patients perceive physician communication regarding cardiac testing,' *Medical Care,* 40: 127–134.

Concato, J. (2004) 'Observational versus experimental studies: what's the evidence for a hierarchy?' *NeuroRx*, 1: 341–347.

Cook, T.D. and Campbell, D.T. (1979) *Quasi-experimentation: Design and Analysis for Field Settings*, Chicago, IL: Rand McNally.

Creswell, J.W., Fetters, M.D., and Ivankova, N.V. (2004) 'Designing a mixed methods study in primary care,' *Annals of Family Medicine*, 2: 7–12.

Da Pidgin Coup. (1999) 'Pidgin and education.' University of Hawaii. Retrieved May 2013 from: http://www.hawaii.edu/sls/pidgin.html

D'Alonzo, K.T. (2010) 'Getting started in CBPR: lessons in building community partnerships for new researchers,' *Nursing Inquiry*, 17: 282–288.

DiMaggio, P., Hargittai, E., Neuman, R.W., and Robinson, J.P. (2001) 'The Internet's implications for society,' *Annual Review of Sociology*, 27: 307–336.

Doak, C.C., Doak, L.G., and Root, J.H. (1996) *Teaching Patients with Low Literacy Skills*, 2nd edn, Philadelphia, PA: J.B. Lippincott.

Emmons, K.M. (2000) 'Behavioral and social science contributions to the health of adults in the United States.' In B. Smedley and S.L. Syme (eds) *Promoting Health: Intervention Strategies from Social and Behavioral Research* (pp. 254–321), Institute of Medicine, Washington, DC: National Academy Press.

Fanon, F. (1967) *Black Skin, White Masks*, New York: Grove Press.

Fishbein, M. and Ajzen, I. (1981) 'Acceptance, yielding, and impact: cognitive processes in persuasion.' In R.E. Petty, T.M. Ostrom, and T.C. Brock (eds) *Cognitive Responses in Persuasion* (pp. 339–359), Hillsdale, NJ: Erlbaum.

Ford, M.E., Hill, D.D., Blount, A., Morrison, J., Worsham, M., Havstad, S.L., and Johnson, C.C. (2002) 'Modifying a breast cancer risk factor survey for African American women,' *Oncology Nursing Forum*, 29: 827–834.

Frey, L.R., Botan, C.H., and Kreps, G.L. (2000) *Investigating Communication: An Introduction to Research Methods*, 2nd edn, Boston, MA: Allyn and Bacon.

Giuliano, A.R., Mokuau, N., Hughes, C., Tortolero-Luna, G., Risendal, B., Ho, R.C.S., et al. (2000)'Participation of minorities in cancer research: the influence of structural, cultural, and linguistic factors,' *Annals of Epidemiology*, 10 (8 suppl): S22–34.

Glanz, K., Rimer, B.K., and Viswanath, K.E. (2008) *Health Behavior and Health Education: Theory, Research and Practice*, 4th edn, San Francisco, CA: Jossey-Bass.

Glasgow, R.E., Klesges, L.M., Dzewaltowski, D.A., Bull, S.S., and Estabrooks, P. (2004) 'The future of health behavior change research: what is needed to improve translation of research into health promotion practice?' *Annals of Behavioral Medicine*, 27: 3–12.

Grol, R.P., Bosch, M.C., Hulscher, M.E., Eccles, M.P., and Wensing, M. (2007) 'Planning and studying improvement in patient care: the use of theoretical perspectives,' *Milbank Quarterly*, 85: 93–138.

Halliday, M.A.K. and Webster, J. (2006) *On Language and Linguistics*, New York: Continuum.

Hamilton, H.E. (2008) 'Language and dementia: sociolinguistic aspects.' In C.L.J. de Bot (ed.) *Language and the Brain, Vol. 28 of the Annual Review of Applied Linguistics (ARAL)*, pp. 91–110, Cambridge: Cambridge University Press.

Hawley, A.H. (1950) *Human Ecology: A Theory of Community Structure*, New York: Ronald Press.

Harvey, K., Churchill, D., Crawford, P., Brown, B., Mullany, L., Macfarlane, A., and McPherson, A. (2008) 'Health communication and adolescents: what do their emails tell us?' *Family Practice.*, 25: 304–311.

Hesson, A.M., Sarinopoulos, I., Frankel, R.M., and Smith, R.C. (2012) 'A linguistic study of patient-centered interviewing: emergent interactional effects,' *Patient Education and Counseling,* 88(3): 373–380.

Hibbard, J. and Lorig, K. (2012) 'The dos and don'ts of patient engagement in busy office practices,' *Journal of Ambulatory Care Management,* 35: 129–132.

Hill-Briggs, F. and Smith, A.S. (2008) 'Evaluation of diabetes and cardiovascular disease print patient education materials for use with low-health literate populations,' *Diabetes Care*, 31: 667–671.

Hodge, F.S., Fredericks, L., and Rodriguez, B.T. (1996) 'American Indian women's talking circle. A cervical cancer screening and prevention project,' *Cancer,* 78: 1592–1597.

Hornik, R C. (1988) *Development Communication*, New York: Longman.

Houts, P.S., Doak, C.C., Doak, L.G., and Loscalzo, M.J. (2006) 'The role of pictures in improving health communication: a review of research on attention, comprehension, recall, and adherence,' *Patient Education and Counseling,* 61: 173–190.

Hovland, C., Lumsdaine, A., and Sheffield, F. (1949) *Experiences on Mass Communication*, Princeton, NJ: Princeton University Press.

Huang, A.C.Y. (2010) 'East–West Montage: Reflections on Asian Bodies in Diaspora (review),' *Comparative Literature Studies*, 47: 96–98.

Institute of Medicine (IOM) (2002) 'Improving the health of diverse populations: speaking of health: assessing health communication strategies for diverse populations,' Washington, DC: National Academies Press.

——(2003) 'Unequal treatment: confronting racial and ethnic disparities in healthcare,' Washington, DC: National Academies Press.

Israel, B.A., Coombe, C.M., Cheezum, R.R., Schulz, A.J., McGranaghan, R.J., Lichtenstein, R., et al. (2010) 'Community-based participatory research: a capacity-building approach for policy advocacy aimed at eliminating health disparities,' *American Journal of Public Health,* 100: 2094–2102.

Jaspal, R. (2009) 'Language and social identity: a psychological approach,' *Psychtalk,* 64: 17–20.

Johnson, J.L., Lovato, C.Y., Maggi, S., Ratner, P.A., Shoveller, J., Baillie, L., and Kalaw, C. (2003) 'Smoking and adolescence: narratives of identity,' *Research in Nursing & Health,* 26: 387–397.

Johnstone, P.L. (2004) 'Mixed methods, mixed methodology health services research in practice,' *Qualitative Health Research,* 14: 259–271.

Kagawa-Singer, M., Dadia, A.V., Yu, M.C., and Surbone, A. (2010) 'Cancer, culture, and health disparities: time to chart a new course?' *CA: A Cancer Journal for Clinicians,* 60: 12–39.

Katz, D.L. (2004) 'Representing your community in community-based participatory research: differences made and measured,' *Preventing Chronic Disease,* 1: A12.

Kehl, K.A. and McCarty, K.N. (2012) 'Readability of hospice materials to prepare families for caregiving at the time of death,' *Research in Nursing & Health*, 35: 242–249.

Kim, K., Yu, E., Chen, E., Kim, J.K., and Brintnall, R. (1999) 'Breast cancer screening knowledge and practices among Korean American women,' *Asian American and Pacific Islander Journal of Health,* 6: 263–275.

Koelen, M.A., Vaandrager, L., and Colomer, C. (2001) 'Health promotion research: dilemmas and challenges,' *Journal of Epidemiology and Community Health,* 55: 257–262.

Kontos, E.Z., Bennett, G.G., and Viswanath, K. (2007) 'Barriers and facilitators to home computer and internet use among urban novice computer users of low socioeconomic position,' *Journal of Medical Internet Research*, 9: e31.

Korsch, B.M. and Negrete, V.F. (1972) 'Doctor–patient communication,' *Scientific American,* 227: 66–74.

Kotler, P. and Roberto, E.L. (1989) *Social Marketing: Strategies for Changing Public Behavior*, New York: Free Press.

Kreps, G.L. (2008) 'Qualitative inquiry and the future of health communication research,' *Qualitative Research Reports in Communication*, 9: 2–12.

——(2011) 'Methodological diversity and integration in health communication inquiry,' *Patient Education and Counseling*, 82: 285–291.

Kreps, G.L., Bonaguro, E.W., and Query, J.L. (1998) 'The history and development of the field of health communication.' In L.D. Jackson and B.K. Duffy (eds) *Health Communication Research: Guide to Developments and Directions*, Westport, CT: Greenwood Press.

Lazarsfeld, P., Berelson, B., and Gaudet, H. (1948) *The People's Choice,* New York: Columbia University Press.

Lee, S.K. (2003) 'Exploring the relationship between language, culture, and identity,' *GEMA Online Journal of Language Studies*, 3: 1–13.

Lim, J.W. (2010) 'Linguistic and ethnic disparities in breast and cervical cancer screening and health risk behaviors among Latina and Asian American women,' *Journal of Women's Health (Larchmont)*, 19: 1097–1107.

Lipsey, M.W. and Wilson, D.B. (2001) *Practical Meta-analysis*, Thousand Oaks, CA: Sage.

McAllister, M., Dunn, G., Payne, K., Davies, L., and Todd, C. (2012) 'Patient empowerment: the need to consider it as a measurable patient-reported outcome for chronic conditions,' *BMC Health Services Research,* 12: 157.

McLeroy, K.R., Bibeau, D., Steckler, A., and Glanz, K. (1988) 'An ecological perspective on health promotion programs,' *Health Education Quarterly,* 15: 351–377.

Meiring, D., Van de Vijver, F., Rothmann, S., and Barrick, M.R. (2005) 'Construct, item and method bias of cognitive and personality tests in South Africa,' *South African Journal of Industrial Psychology,* 31(1): 1–8.

Meyer, A.L., Allison, K.W., Reese, L.E., and Gay, F.N. (2004) 'Choosing to be violence free in middle school: the student component of the GREAT Schools and Families Universal Program,' *American Journal of Preventive Medicine,* 26: 20–28.

Minkler, M. and Wallerstein, N.E. (2003) *Community-based Participatory Research for Health*, San Francisco, CA: Jossey-Bass.

Muller, N. and Mok, Z. (2012) 'Applying systemic functional linguistics to conversations with dementia: the linguistic construction of relationships between participants,' *Seminars in Speech and Language*, 33: 5–15.

Mutchler, J.E. and Brallier, S. (1999) 'English language proficiency among older Hispanics in the United States,' *Gerontologist*, 39: 310–319.

National Institutes of Health (NIH) (2012) 'Using mixed methods to optimize dissemination and implementation of health interventions.' Retrieved August 14, 2012, from: http://obssr.od.nih.gov/scientific_areas/methodology/mixed_methods_research/index.aspx

Nelson, M. and Hamilton, H.E. (2007) 'Improving in-office discussion of chronic obstructive pulmonary disease: results and recommendations from an in-office linguistic study in chronic obstructive pulmonary disease,' *American Journal of Medicine*, 120: S28–32.

Nussbaum, J.F. (1989) 'Directions for research within health communication,' *Health Communication,* 9: 35–40.

Oakley, A. (1998) 'Experimentation and social interventions: a forgotten but important history,' *British Medical Journal*, 317: 1239–1242.

Paisley, W. (1989) 'Public communication campaigns: the American experience.' In R.E. Rice and C.K. Atkin (eds) *Public Communication Campaigns*, Newbury, CA: Sage.

Pasick, R., Burke, N.J., Barker, J.C., Galen, J., Bird, J., Otero-Sabogal, J.A., et al. (2009) 'Behaviorial theory in a diverse society: like a compass on Mars,' *Health Education and Behavior*, 36 (5 suppl): 11S–35S.

Prochaska, J.O. (1979) *Systems of Psychotherapy: A Transtheoretical Analysis*, Homewood, IL: Dorsey Press.

Prochaska, J.O., Redding, C.A., and Evers, K. (2002) 'The transtheoretical model and stages of change,' Chapter 5. In K. Glanz, B.K. Rimer, and F.M. Lewis (eds) *Health Behavior and Health Education: Theory, Research, and Practice,* 3rd edn (pp. 99–120), San Francisco, CA: Jossey-Bass.

Rawson, K.A., Gunstad, J., Hughes, J., Spitznagel, M.B., Potter, V., Waechter, D., and Rosneck, J. (2010) 'The METER: a brief, self-administered measure of health literacy,' *Journal of General Internal Medicine*, 25: 67–71.

Rodriguez, H., Saenz, R., and Menjivar, C. (eds) (2008) *Latinas/os in the United States: Changing the Face of America*, New York: Springer.

Rosenstock, I.M. (1974) 'Historical origins of the health belief model,' *Health Education Quarterly*, 2: 328–335.

Sallis, J.F., Owen, N., and Fisher, E.B. (2008) 'Ecological models of health behavior.' In K. Glanz, B.K. Rimer, and K. Viswanath (eds) *Health Behavior and Health Education: Theory, Research, and Practice,* 4th edn (pp. 465–486), San Francisco, CA: Jossey-Bass.

Savitz, L. and Umble, K. (2002) 'Social marketing: a vehicle for employer-driven health promotion and disease prevention.' Retrieved September 30, 2003, from: http://www.nhcpi.net/pdf/socialmarketing.pdf

Schulz, A.J., Israel, B.A., Coombe, C.M., Gaines, C., Reyes, A.G., Rowe, Z., et al. (2011) 'A community-based participatory planning process and multilevel intervention design: toward eliminating cardiovascular health inequities,' *Health Promotion Practice,* 12: 900–911.

Shadish, W., Campbell, T., and Cook, D. (2002) *Experimental and Quasiexperimental Designs for Generalized Causal Inference,* Boston, MA: Houghton Mifflin.

Smedley, B.D. and Syme, S.L.E. (2000) *Promoting Health: Intervention Strategies from Social and Behavioral Research*, Washington, DC: National Academy Press.

Storey, J.D., Saffitz, G.B., and Rimon, J.G. (2008) 'Social marketing.' In B. Glanz, B.K. Rimer, and K. Visawanath (eds) *Health Behavior and Health Education: Theory, Research, and Practice*, 4th edn (pp. 435–464), San Francisco, CA: Jossey-Bass.

Tanjasiri, S.P., Kagawa-Singer, M., Foo, M.A., Chao, M., Linayao-Putman, I., Nguyen, J., et al. (2007) 'Designing culturally and linguistically appropriate health interventions: the "Life Is Precious" Hmong breast cancer study,' *Health Education & Behavior,* 34: 140–153.

Thomas, R.K. (2006) *Health Communication*, New York: Springer.

Thompson, A.G.H. (2003) 'Questioning practices in healthcare research: the contribution of social surveys to the creation of knowledge,' *International Journal for Quality in Health Care*, 15: 187–188.

Thompson, T.L., Robinson, J.D., Anderson, D.J., and Federowicz, M. (2008) 'Health communication: where have we been and where can we go?' In K.B. Wright and S.D. Moore (eds) *Applied Health Communication* (pp. 3–34), Cresskill, NJ: Hampton Press.

Timberlake, J.M. and Williams, R.H. (2012) 'Stereotypes of US immigrants from four global regions,' *Social Science Quarterly,* 93: 867–890.

US Census Bureau (2002) 'US Summary: 2000, profile of general demographic characteristics: 2000.' Retrieved July 25, 2012, from: http://www.census.gov/prod/2002pubs/c2kprof00-us.pdf

——(2010) *The Next Four Decades, The Older Population in the United States: 2010 to 2050.* Retrieved July 26, 2012, from: http://www.census.gov/prod/2010pubs/p25-1138.pdf

US Department of Health and Human Services (HSS) (2000) 'Healthy people 2010: understanding and improving health,' Washington, DC: US Government Printing Office.

——(2008) 'A strategic framework for improving racial/ethnic minority health and eliminating racial/ethnic health disparities,' Washington, DC: US Government Printing Office.

——(2012) 'Healthy people 2020: improving the health of America.' Retrieved August 9, 2012, from: http://www.healthypeople.gov/2020/default.aspx

Viswanath, K. (2005) 'The communication revolution and cancer control,' *Nature Reviews Cancer*, 5: 828–835.

Viswanath, K., Breen, N., Meissner, H., Moser, R.P., Hesse, B., Steele, W.R., and Rakowski, W. (2006) 'Cancer knowledge and disparities in the information age,' *Journal of Health Communication,* 11(Suppl 1): 1–17.

Viswanath, K., Ramanadhan, S., and Kontos, E.Z. (2007) 'Mass media and population health: the macrosocial view.' In S. Galea (ed.) *Macrosocial Determinants of Population Health*, New York: Springer.

Weiss, J.B. and Lorenzi, N.M. (2008) 'Synthesizing community wisdom: a model for sharing cancer-related resources through social networking and collaborative partnerships,' *AMIA Annual Symposium Proceedings,* 793–797.

Witte, K. (1997) 'Preventing teen pregnancy through persuasive communications: realities, myths, and the hard-fact truths,' *Journal of Community Health,* 22: 137–154.

Wright, K., Sparks, L., and O'Hair, D. (2007) *Health Communication in the 21st Century*, Malden, MA: Blackwell.

12

Web 2.0 and the changing health communication environment

Abby Prestin and Wen-ying Sylvia Chou

Introduction

The emergence of Web 2.0 technologies sparked a digital revolution that has dramatically altered the ways in which we communicate: in less than a decade, the online landscape shifted from a static, read-only space to a dynamic, multidirectional ecology characterized by participation, collaboration, and network effects. In this new online environment, we are no longer a passive audience that simply receives information 'pushed' on us by publishers and experts – we are now active agents who both consume *and* produce web content.

This shift has had profound implications for health. The broad range of Web 2.0 applications – from health-oriented online social networks to patient portals to the mhealth explosion – has increased access to health information and opened channels of communication between individual users and health stakeholders. At their core, these platforms are tools to foster participation, collaboration, and involvement, ultimately facilitating a dialogue that can empower individuals to take a greater role in improving or maintaining their own health. And yet, with this promise come pitfalls, as health experts must learn to best leverage the power of Web 2.0 in the advocacy of health, and healthcare consumers must become comfortable in their place at the table.

The purpose of this chapter is to explore the ways in which Web 2.0 has influenced health communication. We begin with a background of Web 2.0, tracing its history and defining its foundational characteristics. Next, we examine vital threads of research that illuminate the impact of Web 2.0 on: (a) healthcare interactions, (b) peer-to-peer communication about health, and (c) public health communication and promotion efforts. We will provide approaches and exemplars from multiple disciplines to highlight key work in communication, linguistics, and health research to date. After discussion of the challenges and opportunities inherent in this work, this chapter concludes by setting a research agenda for the implementation of health communication efforts in our ever-evolving online environment.

Historical perspectives

What is Web 2.0?

The term Web 2.0 gained popularity when Tim O'Reilly used it to describe the turning point at which technology corporations began to utilize the Web, rather than the desktop, as a platform for software applications (O'Reilly 2005). It has since been adopted in reference to online applications and technologies built on the premise of participatory information sharing, collaboration, social connectedness, user-centered design, and user-generated content. The diverse array of Web 2.0 applications is unified by three key themes: participation, networks, and collaboration. In the Web 1.0 environment, experts and publishers controlled online content and, for the average user, the Web was primarily a repository of information. In contrast, in the Web 2.0 environment, the average user makes a much larger contribution to web content, as evidenced by the proliferation of wikis, blogs, and media sharing sites populated by user-generated content. Currently, users generate content at a rapid rate: millions of images are uploaded to photo sharing sites such as Flickr and Instagram every day, three days' worth of video content are uploaded to YouTube every minute, and there are more than 100 million blogs on tumblr and WordPress combined.

Second, Web 2.0 platforms (e.g., Facebook, LinkedIn) can model connections between individual users in a network of relations that engender sharing, collaboration, and exchange of social capital. Online social networks (OSN) recombine features of earlier technologies into a new context that supports the formation and maintenance of a wide network of social connections (Ellison et al. 2011). Although these platforms include a suite of features that facilitate the creation of new connections, individuals typically use OSN to articulate offline social relationships; for instance, most Facebook connections represent 'in person' relationships (Subrahmanyam et al. 2008). This usage distinguishes OSN from blogs, forums, and other online communities that bring people together based on shared interests.

Lastly, the interactivity of new media fosters collaboration. The terms 'collective intelligence' and 'crowdsourcing' are used to describe online processes by which groups and individuals synergistically create and organize information (Surowiecki 2005). This phenomenon is illustrated by online products such as Wikipedia, wherein the community provides quality control over user-authored content. The theory behind such efforts is the belief that, without central control, information will become naturally structured as critical mass is reached (Weiss 2005). As such, the product of collective intelligence is more than just the sum of its parts.

Use of Web 2.0 for health in the US

The percentage of US adults online has been increasing at a steady rate. According to the latest statistics from the Health Information National Trends Survey (HINTS), over 78 percent of American adults have accessed the Internet (Chou et al. 2013a). It is noteworthy that while a majority of US adults are online, inequalities in access to the Internet persist, whereby those of lower socio-economic status, minority race/ethnicity, older age, poorer health, and rural regions are afforded less access (Jackson et al. 2008; Jansen 2010). Furthermore, the main dividing lines for broadband access are along socio-economic dimensions such as income and education (Horrigan 2009), and research on health information technology adoption has found disparities in access and utilization patterns across socio-economic groups and health literacy levels (Sarkar et al. 2011).

There is some reason to believe that the digital divide picture is more nuanced than these figures indicate. Although Internet access is influenced by available infrastructure and cost of service, mobile technologies may be helping to bridge the access gap: in 2012, 88 percent of US adults owned a mobile phone and more than half of these cell owners (55 percent) used their phone to go online (Smith 2012). Latinos and African Americans are now more likely than Whites to use mobile phones to access health information (Fox and Duggan 2013). Further, race/ethnicity is no longer a predictor of social media use for US adults with Internet access, as once online, minorities are equally likely to use sites such as Twitter and Facebook (Chou et al. 2009).

Given overall high and growing Internet penetration, the next logical question is: How are people interacting with health information online? Of those US adults online, almost 70 percent reported that the Internet was the first source of health information (Chou et al. 2013a). Traffic to the top five health-related websites – Yahoo! Health, National Institutes of Health, WebMD, Medicine Net, and Mayo Clinic – averages almost 80 million unique visitors monthly. The popularity of these sites reflects the frequency with which individual users seek health information from credible or 'expert' online sources. Yet, findings from HINTS 2012 indicate that some individuals are also turning to social media to participate in health-related activities and contribute health-related content online: of the 78 percent of adults online, 16 percent used social networking sites for health, 5 percent participated in an online health support group, and only 3 percent wrote on health topics in blogs (Chou et al. 2013a).

Note that while greater numbers of US adults reportedly use the Web to access health information, they are *contributing* health information in relatively smaller numbers: 18 percent of adults had consulted online peer-generated reviews of drugs or medical treatments, but only 3 percent reported contributing reviews of their own. We see a consistent trend whereby online adults consume more health information than they themselves generate. Despite these low prevalence rates, the emphasis of new media applications on content creation and sharing has encouraged a rapidly expanding volume of online user-generated health content, as illustrated by numerous descriptive studies.

One key area of concern is the quality of user-generated health content. Of note, concerns have been raised about the quality and credibility of user-generated health information. For instance, the majority of tweets about smoking cessation are found to not adhere to recommended clinical guidelines (Prochaska et al. 2011) and information quality of YouTube videos about prostate cancer screening were rated by physicians as only fair to poor in almost 75 percent of cases (Steinberg et al. 2010). Clearly, there is a disconnect between what healthcare experts consider to be standardized, well-vetted health guidelines and the information present in user-generated content. These findings give health advocates a point of intervention – if false or incorrect health information is promulgated via content sharing sites, efforts to correct the public's understanding of these topics may be needed.

Critical issues and topics

Current multidisciplinary research on the intersection of Web 2.0 and health can be grouped into three intersecting domains: (1) clinical communication and care, (2) peer-to-peer interactions about health, and (3) public health communication efforts. In each area, quantitative and qualitative methods have been used to understand how individuals and communities use the participative Web to seek and exchange health information, make healthcare decisions, provide support, and benefit from health education. We will introduce key issues and research questions, followed by illustrative examples, focusing on the role of language and communication in each domain.

Clinical care and communication

With the growth of health information technologies and the adoption of electronic medical records, many aspects of clinical care are significantly affected. To review current evidence, a framing question may be helpful: How can social media improve clinical communication and facilitate health care?

Social media and electronic patient portals have afforded patients unprecedented access to health information and medical records. Many would argue that easy access to knowledge and information is empowering (Samoocha et al. 2010). Patients have reported that ehealth applications have improved their knowledge and self-efficacy; this empowerment has been found to strengthen relationships with providers (Åkesson et al. 2007). Specifically, patients have reported feeling empowered by online learning to make health decisions and having more confidence to ask questions during healthcare visits with respect to managing chronic conditions (Fleisher et al. 2002; Fox 2005). Indeed, Web 2.0 platforms, once integrated into the electronic health record systems (e.g., Personalized Health Records (PHR)), have the potential to improve care management, particularly in facilitating communication with providers, viewing and commenting on medical records, filling prescriptions, and receiving reminders (Finney Rutten et al. 2012).

Moreover, online health information, including user-generated health content, has had significant impact on patient–provider relationships and communication patterns. The Internet has become the first source of health information in the US (Hesse et al. 2005); more importantly, it is a documented common practice for patients to bring information found online into a clinical encounter (Bylund et al. 2010). Physicians' responses to the changing health information ecology have varied: some react defensively and exert 'expert' opinion; while others acknowledged the 'opened flood gate' and collaborate with patients to evaluate online information. Some have noted physicians' 'philosophical shift' towards patient empowerment (Anderson and Funnell 2010): not trying to persuade patients to do what doctor thinks is right, but helping them to identify and pursue health goals. Similarly, while some patients feel empowered with online information, others worry about challenging a physician's authority by bringing up information from web sources (Jacobson 2007). In fact, research has noted conflicting results in terms of patients' disclosure of information in light of increased health information availability: does the less socially rich medium of the patient portal lead patients to disclose symptoms or concerns they may be too embarrassed to reveal in face-to-face encounters with providers?

Web 2.0 can also potentially increase access to healthcare providers. A small group of allied health professionals have begun to make themselves available on Facebook and Twitter, in many ways challenging the traditional healthcare and payment model (Hawn 2009). Moreover, physicians could reach patients through Twitter to update them with therapeutic options, to answer disease-related questions, or simply to remind a large group to wear sunscreen (Vance et al. 2009).

Despite the potentials of improved clinical communication through Web 2.0 technology, privacy and confidentiality concerns remain. Does it break certain institutional boundaries? When doctors are 'friended', does it raise ethical red flags? In a recent survey of physicians and trainees, most participants expressed a belief that it was ethically unacceptable to interact with patients on OSN due to threats to patient confidentiality (Bosslet et al. 2011). In addition, lapses of professionalism in providers and trainees have been found to negatively impact care delivery. For example, 60 percent of US medical schools reported incidents of students posting unprofessional content online, and 38 percent of schools had developed disciplinary policies for handling inappropriate online content posted by students (Chretien et al. 2009).

In summary, Web 2.0 platforms present opportunities for improved patient–doctor communication and clinical care. Empirical evidence is only beginning to emerge to demonstrate actual benefits in patient empowerment, chronic disease self-management, and patient–provider interactions. Moreover, challenges and potential pitfalls concerning privacy, care utilization patterns, and incentive models continue to raise concerns for real-world implementation of these platforms.

Peer-to-peer interactions about health

Enthusiasm has been growing with regard to using social media for peer-to-peer health communication in order to improve information exchange, social support, and behavior change. Whether by reaching out to online communities for treatment information, sharing personal illness experiences on a blog, or using an mhealth app within a social network, users are producing and sharing health content online in a myriad of meaningful ways. We are just beginning to understand how the emergence of platforms such as blogs and social networking sites are facilitating online peer-to-peer discussions about health. Indeed, a number of open questions remain with regard to the ways in which users participate in health communication online, motivations for information or support exchange, and the impact of these behaviors on health outcomes. Below, we outline several important influences of the Web 2.0 environment on peer-to-peer health communication.

Existing online social networks

Online social networks such as Facebook have, in recent years, made networks of family, friends, colleagues, and acquaintances more visible and accessible. These social tools have implications for health communication, and might even confer unique benefits for physical and psychological wellness. Yet, it is important to distinguish general OSN engagement and health-specific activities on OSN. A national survey reveals that only 16 percent of Internet users reported visiting an OSN for health purposes (HINTS 2012 – Chou et al. 2013a). Additionally, only 11 percent of adults have followed a friend's health experience, 7 percent have received health information, and 4 percent have started or joined a health-related group on an OSN (Fox 2011). Motivations to consume or share information within OSNs are just beginning to be identified, but it could be the case that for those with chronic disease, posting about their health on OSNs could be seen as overloading or boring their connections with 'inappropriate' communications that conflict with impression management goals (Newman et al. 2011).

Although OSNs are not yet spaces for health-related dialogue, they do uniquely support sharing health activity and experience with social networks. A diverse array of apps allows users to share their progress toward a health goal, such as the map of a route they ran or the number of steps taken in a day. These apps can foster friendly competition among social network members that may increase physical activity (Young 2010).

Among health topics and populations, adolescent health represents an area most readily receptive to leveraging the existing Web 2.0 environment. Evidence suggests that adolescents and young adults are posting messages about depression or risky behaviors, such as sexual activity and drug or alcohol use (Moreno et al. 2009). The influence of these online disclosures within one's social networks and the exchanges they spark are not yet known. For instance, disclosure of risky behaviors could potentially normalize these behaviors, or they might provide a point at which family, friends, or other peers can intervene with messages that discourage these behaviors. As well, messages that reference depressive symptoms may indicate clinical depression, and social connections may respond with emotional or informational social support (Moreno et al. 2011). University counseling centers may take advantage of the targeted advertising feature (e.g., on Facebook) by linking messages about counseling services or online screening to keywords that indicate dysphoria (e.g., 'depressed').

Finally, there is speculation that participation in OSNs may directly affect health by enhancing salience of our social networks and, in turn, increasing perceptions of the availability of social support, or the belief that social relationships can provide emotional or informational resources. Recent studies have explored how Facebook and related platforms serve as opportunities for social support seeking and provision (Bender et al. 2011; Skeels et al. 2010). One study found that one's number of Facebook friends was positively associated with well-being despite that this relationship was not mediated by perceived social support (Kim and Lee 2011).

Online health communities

The online environment is an increasingly popular venue for the exchange of health information and experience as well as social support. Since the early 1990s, long before the terms 'Web 2.0' and 'social media' became popular, there were various digital spaces that facilitated peer interactions, including online bulletin boards, chat rooms, and email listservs. Virtual communication about health offers several advantages over face-to-face contexts, including access to heterogeneous peer groups with shared health concerns, time and space independency, anonymity or 'pseudonymity', invisibility, disinhibition, and status neutralization (Eysenbach et al. 2004). As well, individuals derive benefit as active participants, casual browsers, or passive recipients in online health communities. Evidence of a positive relationship between online peer-to-peer health communication and favorable health outcomes has emerged in areas of physical and psychosocial wellness. For instance, participation in online support groups has led to reduced depression and stress (Winzelberg et al. 2003) and support functions (e.g., web chats) were the best predictors of weight loss maintenance in an online intervention (Krukowski et al. 2008).

The Web 2.0 environment builds on these earlier models by offering a greater range of opportunities for the exchange of social support about health issues. This includes gathering users who share a common health condition. These platforms facilitate the exchange of information, encouragement and motivation toward goals, shared experiences, empathy, non-judgmental interactions, accountability, and a sense of belonging (Hwang et al. 2010). These communities are described as 'the glue that holds people together so that they can collectively solve each other's problems' (Preece et al. 2004: 202).

PatientsLikeMe is a well-known example. On this site, patients can connect with others who share their condition via forums, private messages, and profile comments. Here patients can network with others who can provide empathy, support, advice, and knowledge that may help them to better manage their own care. The site also provides customized disease-specific outcome and visualization tools to help patients understand and share information about their condition; these individual patient data are aggregated to produce information about specific diseases, treatments, and side effects (Frost and Massagli 2008). The data that users provide through interaction on this site allow researchers to become more informed about these illnesses and accelerates progress toward the development of more effective treatments (Wicks et al. 2010).

In addition to identifying the benefits of online health communities, researchers are interested in understanding the communicative processes by which these platforms help to deliver health benefits. Although traditional social science methods (e.g., ethnography, interviews, surveys, and content analysis) continue to be used, new and innovative approaches are brought to bear in analyzing online Web 2.0 interactions. As an illustration, in a large-scale analysis of the influence of participation in the American Cancer Society's Cancer Survivors Network, researchers employed a computational linguistic approach that utilized text mining and machine learning techniques to automatically estimate the sentiment of forum posts made by community members to explore patterns of sentiment change (Qiu et al. 2011). This analysis documented the sentiment of a member's original post and compared it to his or her final reply in the same thread, finding that the majority of participants shifted toward more positive sentiment over time. Sentiment was positively influenced by a greater number of thread responses, higher degree of involvement of the original poster, and more positive sentiment of responses. This Natural Language Processing (NLP)-based approach was able to distill a half-million posts across 10 years, concluding that online health interactions conferred important benefits for psychological well-being.

Members influence and benefit from online health communities in different ways. For example, 'leaders' affect the functioning and effectiveness of the community, whereas 'lurkers' consume but do not contribute content. Novel computational linguistic methods are employed to identify influential users in large-scale online communities using interactional matrices such as the amount, frequency, and content of posts, as well as their centrality and activity within social networks. This work has important implications for maintaining an active, supportive, and effective online health community, such as helping to identify influential users and leverage their influence to promote wider participation (Zhao et al. 2011). Encouragement from influential users or supportive moderators may help some lurkers to feel more comfortable contributing to these communities (Preece et al. 2004).

Communicating the illness experience

Another type of peer-to-peer health interaction occurs when individuals share narratives of personal health experience online, often through prose and video content. For instance, many cancer survivors post YouTube videos in which they describe their personal experience of a cancer diagnosis and how they make meaning out of the cancer diagnosis (Chou et al. 2011). In addition to authentic voices of 'everyday' survivors, personal narrative videos are also featured on the websites of organizations (e.g., Livestrong and the American Cancer Society) to educate and inspire viewers. Some of these narratives can be seen as having health advocacy messages. For instance, the story of a breast cancer survivor may recount a self-exam in which the narrator found a lump, serving as an implicit recommendation or reminder to female viewers to conduct self-exams or schedule a screening mammogram. In online breast cancer support forums, storytelling has been shown to empower women and help them cope (Høybye et al. 2004). As well, blogs offer several key utilities to those with chronic illness, allowing them to update others on their activities and experiences, seek opinions or advice, work out ideas through writing, and manage emotions. Some cancer patients use blogs to discuss issues of prevention and care, solve problems, manage their emotions, and share information (Chung and Kim 2007). In particular, hosting one's own blog (in comparison to commenting on or reading other blogs) has been linked to greater ability to manage emotions, which dovetails with the literature on the benefits of expressive writing (Pennebaker and Chung 2007).

Public health communication campaigns

Health campaigns have traditionally utilized broadcast media channels to reach audiences. Although campaigns vary in their effectiveness, a meta-analysis found that across 48 published evaluations, communication campaigns had, on average, a small effect on health behavior change (Snyder and Hamilton 2002). Several factors account for this limited impact, such as low exposure rates, 'one size fits all' messages that sacrifice individual-level specificity, and a potentially disempowering top-down approach 'pushing' information to consumers, which could lead to message rejection (Kreps and Neuhauser 2010).

Given these barriers to campaign effectiveness, Web 2.0 technologies and related social marketing approaches were met with enthusiasm by experts who recognize the advantages these channels offered for health communication. Widespread engagement with social media platforms means that Web 2.0 has opened channels of communication between health experts and the public, offering substantial improvement for the reach of health messages, particularly among traditionally 'difficult to reach' populations (e.g., adolescents and racial/ethnic minorities). Social media can also deliver highly specific messages to targeted groups. Moreover, platforms provide data that allow messages to be targeted not only on traditional demographic variables (i.e., age, location, and education), but also on relationship status, religious or political affiliations, and other personal characteristics such as favorite movies, music, sports teams, and television shows. Finally, given the low cost of social media use, organizations can offer multiple messages that can move people through stages of behavior change or build on their knowledge over time. In many ways, Web 2.0 represents a hybrid channel for message delivery that has the benefits of mass media (e.g., low cost, wide reach) and the immediacy and personalization of interpersonal communication.

The participatory nature of Web 2.0 also plays an important role: health communication is no longer a unidirectional effort, but a collaborative and dynamic conversation. In other words, the audience talks back and, of equal importance, they talk to each other. Owing to the central characteristics of Web 2.0, the typical sender–message–receiver health communication transaction is losing relevancy. In sum, Web 2.0 technology facilitates interactive health communication. Further, the more involved people are in the communication process, the more likely they are to make healthy changes (Neuhauser and Kreps 2003). The task now is to consider the ways to involve individuals (formerly the 'audience') as collaborators in health communication efforts. Below we offer key strategies.

User-generated content and user-designed interventions

In keeping with Web 2.0's hallmark characteristics of participation, collaboration, and connectedness, the audience or end-users of the health intervention can be incorporated into the design of the intervention or campaign. This idea takes formative research a step further and involves the user as co-designer. According to Lefebvre (2007: 37), 'the best way to improve programs, products, and services is to bring them to the marketplace and let the user/audience comment, hack, provide feedback, and even write copy'. As an illustration of the process of involving the user in the design process, researchers collaborated with breast cancer survivors to develop a social networking site using Facebook's 'Connect' app extension to correct the underutilization of social support in cancer care (Skeels et al. 2010). Through a series of participatory design activities, patients, survivors, and caregivers identified barriers to social support and ways in which technology could facilitate information dissemination, requests for help, and care coordination. The resulting prototype was designed for users by users to meet their specific needs. Although to date, few empirical tests of these user-designed social media health interventions are present in the literature (Chou et al. 2013b), evaluations of these projects are necessary to determine their impact.

Web 2.0 platforms also offer the ability to harness user-generated content to create more effective health messages. Health promotion efforts can motivate user participation by offering the intrinsic rewards of contributing their knowledge, experience, insight, and skill in the creation of a health-related product or message, or the extrinsic reward of a prize or special acknowledgment. For example, as part of the Youth Speaks Program, teenagers were invited to participate in a contest to create the best video around obesity and urban food deserts. Contestants produced videos wherein they rapped about environmental factors that contributed to obesity in their communities and dietary patterns that influenced their own weight struggles. These types of crowdsourcing 'interventions' offer new opportunities to foster participation and community engagement. Perhaps most exciting is the way in which content creators themselves step into the role of health advocates. Examples such as this highlight the value of evaluative research to better understand the role that content creation might have on participants' interest in and commitment to health issues. Health experts can construct messages that combine wisdom derived from user-generated content with expert advice – e.g., pairing clinical smoking cessation guidelines with advice from former smokers who made successful quit attempts.

Finally, online social networking sites can expand the reach of a campaign message, either through strategic campaign messaging, or via the spontaneous sharing and reposting of content. In successful cases, content goes 'viral', spreading rapidly and effortlessly through online communities. One recent example of a viral campaign was the Centers for Disease Control's 'Zombie Apocalypse' campaign, which tied disaster preparedness to a hot pop culture topic. The campaign began with a blog post on the CDC's site which instructed readers on how to get a kit and make a plan, and a push on social media channels to help the message reach a wider audience. The initial campaign tweet received more than 70,000 retweets, and both 'CDC' and 'Zombie Apocalypse' became worldwide trending topics on Twitter. Its popularity on social media attracted wide mainstream media coverage to the campaign, and drove record numbers of visitors to the CDC website (Silver 2012). The campaign continued even a year later, with increasing involvement from online participants, who engage in challenges such as creating their own 'zombie preparedness' videos to share with family and friends.

The rapid diffusion of viral content is the 'Holy Grail' that all marketers strive to attain, though the mechanisms behind how and why content goes viral are not yet understood. Health promotion efforts can take advantage of diffusion of information via social media platforms through a number of strategies. First, health messages can include an appeal to share the message with loved ones. Simply asking users to forward a message could expand its reach and to the extent that the message has been co-authored by these users, sharing behavior should be enhanced. Second, health advocates can identify opinion leaders and gatekeepers in social networks and target these individuals for involvement in message design and dissemination. Identifying and involving influential community members could provide a positive influence on the community's reception of the health message or intervention. Lastly, health communication experts must be mindful that health messages often generate conversation that could enhance – or detract from – effectiveness. Traditionally, mass-mediated health campaigns that generate interpersonal communication have enjoyed improved effectiveness. However, in this participatory online environment, comments on health messages also become a part of the message experience. A recent experimental study demonstrated the influence of viewer comments on other audience members' perceptions of health-related YouTube clips, demonstrating the power of the participatory nature of the Web to enhance or detract from the efficacy of health promotion efforts (Walther et al. 2010).

Innovative research methods in studies of Web 2.0 and health

Web 2.0 has provided a fertile ground to test innovative analytic research techniques. We highlight a few emerging health communication research methodologies. First, the Web 2.0 landscape offers access to unlimited amounts of online textual data. Data mining and cloud-based computing techniques are increasingly recognized and utilized to facilitate the acquisition and analysis of large volumes of user-generated social media content. Specialized platforms are used to monitor as well as quantitatively and qualitatively analyze social media content around particular key words or phrases (Wollan and Smith 2010). Computational linguistics – in particular, natural language processing (NLP) approaches – are useful in synthesizing the content, sentiment, and associated interactions surrounding a particular health topic. All in all, computational techniques are poised to bring in expertise for the analysis of online discourse. For example, validated machine learning models can be built to assess patterns of social media content (Wang et al. 2012). Sentiment analysis applied to Web 2.0 discussions can broadly describe overall attitudes and perceptions towards a specific topic. Coupled with network analysis, researchers can trace the diffusion of knowledge through social networks. This is particularly useful with data derived from Twitter and online social networks, such as online smoking cessation communities (Poirier and Cobb 2012). This methodology helps researchers to better understand information diffusion and complex interactions across users and platforms.

The data that individual users contribute to a platform, system, or application can be aggregated into meaningful patterns used for disease surveillance. For instance, geo-located tweets and Facebook posts containing references to the flu or flu-like symptoms have collected, classified, and correlated with the CDC's maps of actual flu incidence (Achrekar et al. 2011). Relatedly, researchers are using social media data (e.g., tweets) to identify and estimate health-oriented beliefs (i.e., *belief surveillance*). Belief surveillance can be approached by exploring the prevalence of a predetermined set of statements representing specific propositions, or 'probes', and measuring the extent of belief or disbelief for each, or by automatically mining probes to identify naturally occurring health beliefs in the online population (Bhattacharya et al. 2012). As these technologies become more sophisticated and methodologies are further refined, social media may be leveraged for their insight into health trends.

In addition to quantitative methods for descriptive and predictive research, qualitative approaches continue to be important. As illustrated in several chapters of this *Handbook*, discourse analysis, including conversation analysis, narrative analysis, and interactional sociolinguistics, helps ascertain the communication processes and motivations beyond the simple content of a conversation. For example, while a quantitative analysis may identify general content or accuracy of information shared in an online health community (such as a discussion on the pros and cons of the HPV vaccine), a qualitative study describes the types of framing and interactive positioning of participants and their ways of aligning or disaligning with one another. This knowledge cannot be obtained through surveys or content analyses, but is crucial in discerning the motivations behind joining the discussions and being outspoken about particular positions.

Beyond descriptive methods, a new array of innovative measurement tools for assessing dissemination, exposure, engagement, and effectiveness now exist, ranging from Facebook 'likes' to more sophisticated assessments of time spent watching a video or number of content downloads from a link included in a tweet. These metrics can illuminate the reach and impact of a particular message, as well as user-generated content in response to the message. The challenge is to define the meaning of these measures with regard to traditional campaign effectiveness outcomes, such as knowledge acquisition and attitude or behavior change. For instance, the CDC 'Zombie Apocalypse' campaign was by all accounts a success in terms of its exposure to a wide and diverse audience, but its impact on disaster preparation attitudes and behavior are not yet known. Research evaluating the impact of social media campaigns for public health is still in its infancy and researchers and health practitioners are still developing a set of best practices for its use in health communication work (Chou et al. 2013b).

Finally, in health interventions, rapidly evolving technologies require dynamic intervention design, as opposed to traditional designs such as a randomized controlled trial. For instance, systems science and engineering perspectives can potentially be maximized to offer more nimble and rapid experimental design and modeling opportunities.

Conclusion

This chapter has introduced a variety of ways in which Web 2.0/social media have intersected with health communication, from clinical care to peer-to-peer health exchange to public health efforts. We have also highlighted advances in multidisciplinary research as well as scientific gaps and research priorities going forward. Linguists, communication scientists, and researchers in health behavior and public health face unique and timely opportunities to 'move beyond buzzwords' and understand how Web 2.0 technology, including a variety of social media platforms, has shaped and can improve the way we communicate and make health decisions.

Related topics

Social media; mhealth; health promotion; patient–physician communication; patient empowerment; information seeking; health communication campaigns.

Further reading

Chou, W.-Y.S., Prestin, A., Lyons, C., and Wen, K.-Y. (2013) 'Web 2.0 for health promotion: reviewing the current evidence', *American Journal of Public Health*, 103: e9–e18.

Eysenbach, G. (2008) 'Medicine 2.0: social networking, collaboration, participation, apomediation, and openness', *Journal of Medical Internet Research*, 10: 5–6.

Hawn, C. (2009) 'Take two aspirin and tweet me in the morning: how Twitter, Facebook, and other social media are reshaping health care', *Health Affairs*, 28: 361–368.

Kreps, G.L. and Neuhauser, L. (2010) 'New directions in eHealth communication: opportunities and challenges,' *Patient Education and Counseling*, 78: 329–336.

References

Achrekar, H., Gandhe, A., Lazarus, R., Yu, S.H., and Liu, B. (2011) 'Predicting flu trends using twitter data', in *Computer Communications Workshops* (pp. 702–707), *2011 IEEE Conference*, IEEE.

Åkesson, K.M., Saveman, B.I., and Nilsson, G. (2007) 'Health care consumers' experiences of information communication technology – a summary of literature', *International Journal of Medical Informatics*, 76(9): 633–645.

Anderson, R.M. and Funnell, M.M. (2010) 'Patient empowerment: myths and misconceptions', *Patient Education and Counseling*, 79: 277–282.

Bender, J.L., Jiminez-Marroquin, M.C., and Jadad, A.R. (2011) 'Seeking support on Facebook: a content analysis of breast cancer groups', *Journal of Medical Internet Research*, 13(1): e16.

Bhattacharya, S., Tran, H., and Srinivasan, P. (2012) 'Discovering health beliefs in Twitter', Association for the Advancement of Artificial Intelligence Fall Symposium Series, North America, October. Online. Available HTTP: <http://www.aaai.org/ocs/index.php/FSS/FSS12/paper/view/5591> (accessed 1 December 2012).

Bosslet, G.T., Torke, A.M., Hickman, S.E., Terry, C.L., and Heflt, P.R. (2011) 'The patient–doctor relationship and online social networks: results of a national survey', *Journal of General Internal Medicine*, 26: 1168–1174.

Bylund, C.L., Gueguen, J.A., D'Agostino, T.A., Li, Y., and Sonet, E. (2010) 'Doctor–patient communication about cancer-related Internet information', *Journal of Psychosocial Oncology*, 28: 127–142.

Chou, W.-Y.S., Hunt, Y., Beckjord, E., Moser, R., and Hesse, B. (2009) 'Social media use in the United States: implications for health communication', *Journal of Medical Internet Research*, 11: e48.

Chou, W.-Y.S., Hunt, Y., Folkers, A., and Augustson, E. (2011) 'Cancer survivorship in the age of YouTube and social media: a narrative analysis', *Journal of Medical Internet Research*, 13(1): e7.

Chou, W.-Y.S., Prestin, A., and Naveed, S. (2013a) 'Inequalities in access to and use of the Internet for health information seeking online: findings from the 2011 Health Information National Trends Survey (HINTS)', Paper presented to the annual conference of the Society of Behavioral Medicine, March, San Francisco, CA.

Chou, W.-Y.S., Prestin, A., Lyons, C., and Wen, K.-Y. (2013b) 'Web 2.0 for health promotion: reviewing the current evidence', *American Journal of Public Health*, 103: e9–e18.

Chretien, K.C., Greysen, S.R., Chretien, J.-P., and Kind, T. (2009) 'Online posting of unprofessional content by medical students', *Journal of the American Medical Association*, 302: 1309–1315.

Chung, D.S. and Kim, S. (2007) 'Blogging activity among cancer patients and their companions: uses, gratifications, and predictors of outcomes', *Journal of the American Society for Information Science and Technology*, 59: 297–306.

Ellison, N.B., Steinfeld, C., and Lampe, C. (2011) 'Connection strategies: social capital implications of Facebook-enabled communication practices', *New Media and Society*, 13: 873–892.

Eysenbach, G., Powell, J., Englesakis, M., Rizo, C., and Stern, A. (2004) 'Health related virtual communities and electronic support groups: systematic review of the effects of online peer to peer interactions', *British Medical Journal*, 328: 1166.

Finney Rutten, L.J., Davis, T., Beckjord, E.B., Blake, K., Mose, R.P., and Hesse, B.W. (2012) 'Picking up the pace: changes in method and frame for the Health Information National Trends Survey (2011–2014)', *Journal of Health Communication*, 17: 979–989.

Fleisher, L., Bass, S., Ruzek, S.B., and McKeown-Conn, N. (2002) 'Relationships among Internet health information use, patient behavior and self efficacy in newly diagnosed cancer patients who contact the National Cancer Institute's NCI Atlantic Region Cancer Information Service (CIS)'. In *Proceedings of the AMIA Symposium* (p. 260), American Medical Informatics Association.

Fox, S. (2005) *Health information online*, Pew Internet and American Life Project. Washington, DC, http://pewinternet. org/pdfs/PIP_Healthtopics_May05. pdf

——(2011) *The social life of health information 2011*, Pew Internet and American Life Project, Washington, DC: Pew Research Center.

Fox, S. and Duggan, M. (2013) *Health online 2013*, Pew Internet and American Life Project, Washington, DC: Pew Research Center.

Frost, J.H. and Massagli, M.P. (2008) 'Social uses of personal health information within PatientsLikeMe, an online patient community: what can happen when patients have access to one another's data', *Journal of Medical Internet Research*, 10(3): e15.

Hawn, C. (2009) 'Take two aspirin and tweet me in the morning: how Twitter, Facebook, and other social media are reshaping health care', *Health Affairs*, 28: 361–368.

Hesse, B.W., Nelson, D.E., Kreps, G.L., Croyle, R.T., Arora, N.K., Rimer, B.K., and Viswanath, K. (2005) 'Trust and sources of health information: the impact of the Internet and its implications for health care providers: findings from the first Health Information National Trends Survey', *Archives of Internal Medicine*, 165: 2618.

Horrigan, J. (2009) 'Broadband adoption and use in America', *OBI Working Paper Series*, Washington, DC: Federal Communications Commission.

Høybye, M.T., Johansen, C., and Tjørnhøj-Thomsen, T. (2004) 'Online interaction: effects of storytelling in an Internet breast cancer support group,' *Psycho-Oncology*, 14: 211–220.

Hwang, K.O., Ottenbacher, A.J., Green, A.P., Cannon-Diehl, M.R., Richardson, O., Bernstam, E. V., and Thomas, E.J. (2010) 'Social support in an Internet weight loss community', *International Journal of Medical Informatics*, 79: 5–13.

Jackson, L.A., Zhao, Y., Kolenic III, A., Fitzgerald, H.E., Harold, R., and Von Eye, A. (2008) 'Race, gender, and information technology use: the new digital divide', *CyberPsychology and Behavior*, 11: 437–442.

Jacobson, P. (2007) 'Empowering the physician–patient relationship: the effect of the Internet', *Partnership: The Canadian Journal of Library and Information Practice and Research*, 2(1): 1–13.

Jansen, B.J. (2010) *Use of the internet in higher-income households*, Washington, DC: Pew Research Center.

Kim, J. and Lee, J.E.R. (2011) 'The Facebook paths to happiness: effects of the number of Facebook friends and self-presentation on subjective well-being', *CyberPsychology, Behavior, and Social Networking*, 14: 359–364.

Kreps, G.L. and Neuhauser, L. (2010) 'New directions in eHealth communication: opportunities and challenges', *Patient Education and Counseling*, 78: 329–236.

Krukowski, R.A., Harvey-Berino, J., Ashikaga, T., Thomas, C.S., and Micco, N. (2008) 'Internet-based weight control: the relationship between web features and weight loss', *Telemedicine and e-Health*, 14: 775–782.

Lefebvre, R.C. (2007) 'The new technology: the consumer as participant rather than target audience', *Social Marketing Quarterly*, 13: 31–42.

Moreno, M.A., Parks, M.R., Zimmerman, F.J., Brito, T.E., and Christakis, D.A. (2009) 'Display of health risk behaviors on MySpace by adolescents: prevalence and associations', *Archives of Pediatrics and Adolescent Medicine*, 163: 27.

Moreno, M.A., Jelenchick, L.A., Egan, K.G., Cox, E., Young, H., Gannon, K.E., and Becker, T. (2011) 'Feeling bad on Facebook: depression disclosures by college students on a social networking site', *Depression and Anxiety*, 28: 447–455.

Neuhauser, L. and Kreps, G.L. (2003) 'Rethinking communication in the e-health era', *Journal of Health Psychology*, 8: 7–23.

Newman, M.W., Lauterbach, D., Munson, S.A., Resnick, P., and Morris, M.E. (2011) 'It's not that I don't have problems, I'm just not putting them on Facebook: challenges and opportunities in using online social networks for health', in *Proceedings of the ACM Conference on Computer-supported Cooperative Work*, New York, NY: Association for Computing Machinery (ACM): 341–350.

O'Reilly, T. (2005) 'Web 2.0: compact definition,' Online. Available HTTP: <http://radar.oreilly. com/ archives/2005/10/web_20_compact_definition.html> (accessed 10 Novemer 2011).

Pennebaker, J.W. and Chung, C.K. (2007) 'Expressive writing, emotional upheavals, and health', in H.S. Friedman and R.C. Silver (eds) *Foundations of Health Psychology* (pp. 263–284), Oxford: Oxford University Press.

Poirier, J. and Cobb, N.K. (2012) 'Social influence as a driver of engagement in a web-based health intervention', *Journal of Medical Internet Research*, 14(1): e36.

Preece, J., Nonnecke, B., and Andrews, D. (2004) 'The top five reasons for lurking: improving community experiences for everyone', *Computers in Human Behavior*, 20: 201–223.

Prochaska, J.J., Pechman, C., Kim, R., and Leonhardt, J.M. (2011) 'Twitter = quitter? An analysis of Twitter quit smoking social networks', *Tobacco Control*, 21: 447–449.

Qiu, B., Zhao, K., Mitra, P., Wu, D., Caragea, C., Yen, J., Greer, G.E., and Portier, K. (2011) 'Get online support, feel better: sentiment analysis and dynamics in an online cancer survivor community', in *Privacy, Security, Risk and Trust*, Third international conference on social computing, IEEE: 274–281.

Samoocha, D., Bruinvels, D.J., Elbers, N.A., Anema, J.R., and Van Der Beek, A.J. (2010) 'Effectiveness of web-based interventions on patient empowerment: a systematic review and meta-analysis', *Journal of Medical Internet Research*, 12(2): e23.

Sarkar, U., Karter, A.J., Liu, J.Y., Adler, N.E., Nguyen, R., Lopez, A., and Schillinger, D. (2011) 'Social disparities in internet patient portal use in diabetes: evidence that the digital divide extends beyond access', *Journal of the American Medical Informatics Association*, 18: 318–321.

Silver, M. (2012) 'Going viral: CDC's Zombie Apocalypse', in National Conference on Health Communication, Marketing, and Media, August 7–9, 2012, Atlanta, GA: Centers for Disease Control.

Skeels, M.M., Unruh, K.T., Powell, C., and Pratt, W. (2010) 'Catalyzing social support for breast cancer patients', in *Proceedings of the 28th International Conference on Human Factors in Computing Systems*, Atlanta, GA: ACM: 173–182.

Smith, A. (2012) *17% of cell phone owners do most of their online browsing on their phone, rather than a computer or other device*, Washington, DC: Pew Research Center.

Snyder, L.B. and Hamilton, M.A. (2002) 'A meta-analysis of US health campaign effects on behavior: emphasize enforcement, exposure, and new information, and beware the secular trend', in Hornik, R.C. (ed.) *Public Health Communication: Evidence for Behavior Change*, 3rd edn, pp. 357–83, Mahwah, NJ: Lawrence Earlbaum.

Steinberg, P.L., Wason, S., Stern, J.M., Deters, L., Kowal, B., and Seigne, J. (2010) 'YouTube as source of prostate cancer information', *Urology*, 75: 619–622.

Subrahmanyam, K., Reich, S.M., Waechter, N., and Espinoza, G. (2008) 'Online and offline social networks: use of social networking sites by emerging adults', *Journal of Applied Developmental Psychology*, 29: 420–433.

Surowiecki, J. (2005) *The Wisdom of Crowds*, New York: Anchor.

Vance, K., Howe, W., and Dellavalle, R.P. (2009) 'Social internet sites as a source of public health information', *Dermatologic Clinics*, 27: 133–136.

Walther, J.B., DeAndrea, D., Kim, J., and Anthony, J.C. (2010) 'The influence of online comments on perceptions of antimarijuana public service announcements on YouTube', *Human Communication Research*, 36: 469–492.

Wang, Y.-C., Kraut, R., and Levine, J.M. (2012) 'To stay or leave? The relationship of emotional and informational support to commitment in online health support groups', in *Procceedings of the ACM Conference on Computer-supported Cooperative Work*, New York, NY: Association for Computing Machinery (ACM): 833–842.

Weiss, A. (2005) 'The power of collective intelligence', *netWorker*, 9: 16–23.

Wicks, P., Massagli, M., Frost, J., Brownstein, C., Okun, S., Vaughan, T., Bradley, R., and Heywood, J. (2010) 'Sharing health data for better outcomes on PatientsLikeMe', *Journal of Medical Internet Research*, 12(2): e19.

Winzelberg, A.J., Classen, C., Alpers, G.W., Roberts, H., Koopman, C., Adams, R.E., et al. (2003) 'Evaluation of an internet support group for women with primary breast cancer', *Cancer*, 97: 1164–1173.

Wollan, R. and Smith, N. (2010) *The Social Media Management Handbook : Everything You Need to Know to Get Social Media Working in Your Business*, New York: Wiley.

Young, M. (2010) 'Twitter me: using micro-blogging to motivate teenagers to exercise', in *Global Perspectives on Design Science Research: 5th International Conference, DESRIST 2010, St. Gallen, Switzerland, June 4–5, 2010. Proceedings*: 439–448.

Zhao, K., Qiu, B., Caragea, C., Wu, D., Mitra, P., Yen, J., Greer, G.E., and Portier, K. (2011) 'Identifying leaders in an online cancer survivor community', in *Proceedings of the 21st Annual Workshop on Information Technologies and Systems*, Shanghai, China: 115–120.

13

Interaction in online support groups

Advice and beyond

Wyke Stommel and Joyce Lamerichs

Introduction

Online Support Groups (OSGs) entered the health domain in the early 1990s. Although their technical setup and layout has changed considerably since then, even today they are important sites for people who wish to discuss illness-related issues and experiences. Researchers have been interested in these peer environments and have focused on issues such as therapeutic relevance (King 1994; Wright and Bell 2003), withdrawal from OSGs and barriers to their use (Sandaunet 2008), the role of diagnosis in OSG discussions (Giles and Newbold 2011) and the performance of emotions in such groups (Bar-Lev 2008).

Interaction analysts have looked more specifically at the interaction between members in OSGs and have examined issues including the factual status of (causal) claims about the illness (Lamerichs and Te Molder 2003; Guise et al. 2007), the co-construction of consensual views which functions as a backdrop against which to compare individual member's personal experiences (Stommel and Koole 2010; Vayreda and Antaki 2009), the construction of illness identities and community (Stommel 2009; Horne and Wiggins 2009; Stommel 2008) and the role of asking and providing advice (Kouper 2010; Vayreda and Antaki 2009; Morrow 2006).

In this chapter, we present relevant findings of previous studies of OSG interaction and an analysis that builds on these results. We begin with historical perspectives and address several methodological questions that have been considered within studies of OSG interaction. In the following section on current contributions and research, we outline the dimensions of advice in OSGs based on previous discourse analytic studies. We then provide an analysis that systematically examines the issue of requesting and giving advice in an OSG about eating disorders in order to gain more insight into how questions directed at the group make relevant particular illness-related concerns, as well as how these questions invite particular answers by other OSG users. Our analysis includes not only initial postings and responses, but also the subsequent message(s) from the initial poster.

Historical background

Since roughly the end of the 1990s, research from different disciplinary backgrounds has documented the unique communicative affordances that online support groups offer to their participants to talk about matters relevant to their condition or illness (see for an overview Wright and Bell 2003; Murero and Rice 2006). Benefits that are typically mentioned are 24-hour availability independent of geographical or temporal constraints (Mickelson 1997); greater access to a diverse set of illness narratives, experiences, and advice than are typically available in face-to-face settings (Rice and Katz 2001); anonymous access which poses fewer risks than usually experienced in face-to-face encounters (Walstrom 2000); and more heterogeneous supportive relationships due to the fact that social status cues are believed to operate in a diminished fashion when online (King and Moreggi 1998). Special benefits are ascribed to the characteristics of written communication in OSGs, such as the therapeutic value that can be attributed to formulating illness narratives, personal triumphs, or health self-disclosures in written form, as well as the possibility of careful editing of typed text (Miller and Gergen 1998; King 1994; Wright and Bell 2003).

In this chapter we focus on the central analytical concepts and thematic areas that are highlighted in those studies that have examined OSGs from an interactional perspective. Studies within this domain generally apply insights from conversation analysis (CA), category membership analysis, and discursive psychology to study the interactional work participants accomplish when they take part in an OSG. Two broad trends can be distinguished here. One trend focuses on the applicability of CA to the study of computer-mediated communication (CMC). In early years, attention was strongly focused on determining whether the conceptual apparatus of CA holds explanatory power when applied to computer-mediated communication. A second trend, which has been the focus of more recent studies, involves explorations of what people do with their contributions in an OSG in terms of accountability, identity/community, and advice. We will discuss this second trend in the upcoming section.

Discussions about the applicability of CA have focused on key concepts such as turn-taking, adjacency pairs, and sequential placement of messages, given that in a-synchronous communication there is a temporal delay between messages that has consequences for the sequential development of the interaction. In considering participants' local management of interaction in newsgroups, Reed (2001) has pointed out how turn-taking can be seen as a participants' concern: a practical achievement in the hands of participants when engaging in interaction in online newsgroups. He stresses that 'participants *actively construct* turn-taking units through particular practices and that these practices act to *construe textual interaction as conversation-like*' (2001: 2; emphasis in original). Reed's analysis highlights the practice of quoting as a way to achieve intersubjectivity (2001: 3).

In addressing aspects of sequentiality in online interaction Antaki et al. (2005) and Vayreda and Antaki (2009) have taken up the position that written contributions in online forums can be considered equal to synchronous turns in face-to-face interaction or in telephone talk. This means that, within computer-mediated communication, actions such as questions open up a space for corresponding actions such as answers (Sacks et al. 1974). However, in OSG interactions, such relationships are enacted through a-synchronically produced postings. As Vayreda and Antaki (2009) point out: 'One post shapes a space (makes a context for) the next, and the next occupies that space in its own way, and makes another space in its turn' (2009: 933). We propose a similar position in this chapter, arguing that participants convey social actions in their postings and orient to their sequential implicativeness (Schegloff and Sacks 1967).

Current contributions and research

With regard to the second trend we mentioned earlier, scholars have used the central concepts of CA as if they can be applied to CMC. Thus, they explored interactional features of OSGs and other online groups, such as accountability, identity/community, and advice within their sequential context in OSG interactions. We discuss these issues briefly.

Generally, participants attend to matters of accountability in interaction (Edwards and Potter 1992). Within OSGs, accountability may be attended to vis-à-vis the legitimacy of participants' claims or the factual status of their descriptions (Lamerichs 2003). It has been pointed out that the kinds of concerns participants in OSGs make relevant are not fundamentally different from those in face-to-face settings. This calls into question a number of assumptions of earlier research that considers CMC an impoverished medium that somehow fundamentally differs from face-to-face communication (see Lamerichs and Te Molder 2003; Guise et al. 2007).

At the same time, previous research has revealed *specific concerns* that may be attended to in OSGs (Stommel 2009; Stommel and Koole 2010; Vayreda and Antaki 2009). Upon joining an OSG, new users present themselves to the OSG population. It has been shown that identity is essentially constructed through diagnosis here, because diagnosis serves to legitimize the newcomer's membership of the group (Stommel and Meijman 2011; Stommel 2009). In these 'new here' interactions, members additionally construct the group as a community and articulate its affordances. This allows them to correct 'deviant' illness ideologies, such as pro-anorexia (Stommel and Koole 2010) or perspectives that do not adhere to the biomedical ideology of bipolar disease (Vayreda and Antaki 2009).

Advice is another important aspect of OSG interaction that interaction studies have illuminated. Since our analysis is focused on advice, we turn now to a more extensive discussion of previous work on requesting and giving advice in OSGs.

Requesting advice

Even though OSGs are lay environments (as opposed to institutional settings in the health domain), advice giving is still one of the core activities users engage in (Kouper 2010; Morrow 2006). Various studies on interaction in OSGs have focused on ways in which advice is asked for and given (Veen et al. 2010; Vayreda and Antaki 2009; Morrow 2006; Lamerichs and Te Molder 2003; Stommel and Koole 2010; Sneijder and Te Molder 2005). Most of the time, discussions in OSGs consist of a 'problem' message that receives one or more replies. Problem messages usually contain a request for advice, although there is variation in the realization of such a request (Morrow 2006). Among the variations, there are general requests for advice ('What can I do to help myself?' or 'Please help'), requests that ask for other members' experience with a certain treatment or medication, or requests asking for a confirmation of one's self-diagnosis.

There is reason to approach the issue of requesting advice with scrutiny. A study by Vayreda and Antaki (2009) revealed that frequently the first posting ends not with a specific request but with a rather general help question that is not cast as a request for advice. The authors have analyzed such questions as being 'low contingent' (cf. Curl and Drew 2008) to the possible advice provider and thus lowering the bar for responses to come. In addition to making responses more likely, there could be other reasons for requests to be formulated indirectly. Veen et al. (2010: 29) presented a case in which the request was formulated as a question designed to prefer descriptive experiences (e.g., 'what happened?') over evaluative options (e.g., 'do you think this is the right thing to do?'). As a response, this user did not receive direct advice, but second stories that only indirectly presented an evaluative stance towards the issue brought up in the initial posting. So, *in*directly requesting advice could be a way to make responses with unfavored advice less likely. Yet another study revealed that the requirement of a response to a request may be alleviated at the end of the posting (Stommel and Koole 2010). This study involved a case analysis of one thread that started with a lengthy initial posting. Although the beginning of the posting contained an indirect request for advice ('I don't know if this is right'), the call for advice giving as a corresponding action within the next turn was retracted by the original poster's suggestion that addressees need not respond since writing-up the posting had already helped.

In sum, previous research suggests that requests for advice in OSGs are frequently not presented straightforwardly. This could be explained by the need for participants to appear competent in managing their affairs, despite the fact that they need some help or advice (Heritage and Sefi 1992; Lamerichs 2003; Morrow 2006). It implies that all kinds of questions can be treated as requests for advice. We now discuss what previous studies have revealed about advice giving in OSGs.

Giving advice

When examining the delivery of advice in OSGs, observations in the literature relate to formats of advice and the role of personal experience (Lamerichs 2003; Morrow 2006; Sneijder and Te Molder 2005; Vayreda and Antaki 2009; Veen et al. 2010). Since advice givers are non-professionals, they need to establish that they are qualified to give advice. Reference to their own experience fulfills this need (Morrow 2006). In other words, personal experience is treated as a pre-condition for giving advice. However, it appears that the 'validity and scope of personal experience with [the illness] as a basis to provide advice is a negotiable matter' (Lamerichs 2003: 181).

Personal experience in the form of a second story can also work as advice without being articulated as such (Veen et al. 2010). The second story format enables respondents to formulate an answer in such a way that does not undermine the first poster's position. Veen et al. (2010: 43) point out: 'By providing their own reasons ..., they also offered advice without affecting the first poster's experiential territory.' In other words, advice can be implied by a second story in the sense that parallel experiences can show recipients how to deal with certain issues without stating this resemblance in a more explicit fashion.

Another format that has been shown to attribute responsibility for possible deficiencies and in this sense also works as advice is the if–then formulation with certain modal constructions, such as 'if you eat a varied diet, you shouldn't have problems' (Sneijder and Te Molder 2005 in reference to a vegan diet). However, more directive advice also occurs in OSGs. Vayreda and Antaki (2009) have found that directive advice, such as 'it's crucial to follow the psychiatrist's instructions', is given in response to a low-contingent question by the new user. In this case, the authors speak of 'unsolicited' advice. They argue that the low-contingent request of the initial posting can be treated as an occasion to direct the new user to the ideology of the OSG in cases where the initial posting presented a view that did not fit that ideology. In other words, it seems clear that in OSGs advice is presented in various formats.

This exploration of studies of advice in OSG suggests that asking and giving advice are sequentially related. That said, advice may occur in response to a question that is not clearly formatted as a request and may frequently not even be formatted as clear advice. Some requests for advice display features that mitigate the request character and, similarly, some instances of advice are not packaged as straightforward pieces of advice.

With an additional analysis of OSG interaction with newcomers, we wish to consider the relation between first postings containing questions that could be treated as requests, and responses being readable as advice or non-advice. This allows us to discuss issues of sequential organization of advice in OSGs and possible alternatives to advice giving. So even if a question could be treated as a request for advice, is it actually treated that way? If not, in what way does the respondent treat the question in the initial posting? And how does the initial poster react to this response in the third turn? We examine two threads that begin with very similar postings. In the first case, the response provides advice; in the second, the response contains further questions that project a continuation of the interaction with the new user.

Sample analysis

Data

The data consist of 27 threads from the largest German OSG on eating disorders, hosted by the association *Hungrig-Online* (HO). All threads are taken from the sub-forum for new users *New Here*. For reasons of space, we refer to Stommel (2009) for a detailed description of this OSG. We gained informed consent from the HO administrators to use the threads as research materials. We also used pseudonyms for nicknames[1] and modified person-related information in the excerpts such as age to ensure the privacy of the participants. Moreover, we show a fictitious date together with the original timestamp of when each posting appeared on the forum board.[2] The excerpts we show are translations; the German originals are in Appendix 13.1 at the end of this chapter.

Preliminary review of the data revealed that only in three of the 27 threads did the first response provide straightforward advice.[3] Advice was formulated either in the form of generalized information ('The best thing is really a therapy'), a suggestion ('In your case I would ... '), or an imperative ('just apply for ... ' or 'don't go there ... ').

Among the 27 threads were two threads that were initiated by a single new user: Laura. We are certain that it is the same user who initiated both threads, because nicknames can be registered only once. Table 13.1 shows how the two threads developed chronologically.

Table 13.1 Date and time of postings' placement in case 1 and 2

Date	*Time*	*Case 1*	*Case 2*
Febr. 3	18:56		Posting 1 – Laura
	19:20		Posting 2 – Mandy
Febr. 4	11:49		Posting 3 – Laura
Febr. 7	10:13	Posting 1 – Laura	
	10:30	Posting 2 – Angela	
	10:35	Posting 3 – Laura	
	10:48		Posting 4 – Mandy
	10:53		Posting 5 – Laura
	11:07		Posting 6 – Mandy
	11:13		Posting 7 – Laura

Although the structure of both initial postings is roughly similar (a greeting, a narrative, a question, and a closing), in one case the response appeared to provide advice, while in the other it did not. Moreover, in the first case, the interaction consisted of three postings, while in the second, it stretched to seven postings. We decided to use these two interactions for more detailed analysis because they offer an unusual opportunity to compare and contrast two naturalistic interactions that are structurally very similar (same initiator, similar initial posting). We now analyze the ways in which advice is observably provided and *not* provided, along with the interactional consequences of each. Although it was initiated later, we start the analysis with the thread that started on Feb. 7, because it appears to have the more common sequential structure of advice in OSGs: request – advice – thank you (Morrow 2006).

Analysis

Case 1

Excerpt 1 (#26)

07.02.2005 10:13 fear – Laura hi guys! somehow i[4] am afraid that bulimia could also hit me. i have binging addiction[5] you see and often think of hanging myself over the loo. but have never done it though. is that the beginning? love laura
07.02.2005 10:30 Re: fear – Angela Hello Laura, i can't tell you where bulimia begins. In my case it gradually developed from AN to B. before though i never thought about how it would be to vomit ... in my case in the beginning it went just like that. everything just came out again ... if i were you i wouldn't start thinking deeper along these lines, who knows what you will trigger with that. B is disgusting ... i know that ... it is extremely costly, smells disgusting and is just obnoxious ... don't go there ...
07.02.2005 10:35 Re: fear – Laura thanks for your response! you are certainly right. but it is really quite tough when the thought to do it is there and it doesn't go away anymore. because often i just eat and eat everything in, afterwards i feel nauseous and think, when you vomit, you will certainly feel better again.

In excerpt 1, the initial posting contains a report of Laura's problem followed by a question. The fear that bulimia could 'hit' her is presented as Laura's reason for posting (line 3). Note that this description treats the illness as the agent and Laura as the potential victim, which is a way to ward off personal responsibility for developing bulimia (Lamerichs 2003; Sneijder and Te Molder 2005). Through the use of 'also' (line 3) Laura displays an orientation to the recipients as 'also' having bulimia, and thus having experience with the start of bulimia.

The question 'is that the beginning?' (line 6) can be considered a difficult one. This is mainly related to its yes/no format. In spoken interaction, yes/no questions set the agenda of the interaction in the sense that they make the recipient accountable to respond in the question's terms (Heritage 2003). Here, the question presupposes that it is possible to determine the start of bulimia, more specifically on the basis of a brief description of Laura's situation (line 4–5). It is a way of asking others to judge a 'B-event' (Labov and Fanshel

1977); i.e., an event to which they do not have direct access. Such questions are not rare in OSGs and can receive advice as a response (Stommel 2009; Morrow 2006).

Approximately 15 minutes later, Laura receives a response from Angela. Angela first claims she is unable to determine the onset of bulimia (line 10) and thus objects to the presupposition embedded in Laura's question. By continuing to describe her own experience as very different from Laura's ('in my case', line 10, 'though', line 11), she stages her own experience to account for her inability to answer Laura's question in the terms in which it was framed. The fact that in her case bulimia developed gradually (line 10) and spontaneously ('everything just came out again', line 12) also implies that the beginning of bulimia may be impossible to determine. In other words, Angela's answer relates to various aspects of the question: its sequential implicativeness, its presupposition (the possibility to determine the start of bulimia), and personal experience as an insufficient epistemic basis for an answer.

Angela's alternative experience with the start of bulimia can also be read as an account for the advice she continues to provide (line 13–14). By emphasizing her own personal experience ('in my case', line 10 and 12), she wards off the assumption that her experience is necessarily applicable to Laura, but her advice to stop thinking about vomiting contributes to the implication that Laura has an active role in the development of bulimia ('who knows what you will trigger with that').[6] The hedging ('if i were you i wouldn't', line 13), however, discounts the imposition of the advice and offers room to resist it.

The last line of the posting provides advice in a very different form. It consists of an evaluation, an epistemic claim, an evaluative 'three-part list' (Atkinson 1984) and advice, all connected by a series of punctuation dots. Through the use of extreme case formulations (Pomerantz 1986) the claims Angela makes are legitimized. Another type of legitimization is added with the epistemic statement 'i know that' (line 15), staging Angela's own experience as the grounds for providing the advice. The three-part list suggests completeness, meaning that Angela's claims about bulimia are presented as definite and conclusive. The punctuation dots articulate the implications of the claims.[7] In their connecting function, they also accumulate to the directive advice following the claims: 'don't go there ...' (line 15–16). As the advice in line 13–14, this second piece again treats Laura as personally responsible for developing bulimia (further), but this time there is no orientation to a limitation of the advice due to personal experience. The directness and absence of hedging offer little room for objection. So, with this response, Angela has managed to (1) bypass the question that projected confirmation of a self-diagnosis, (2) deny that bulimia has an observable beginning, (3) treat Laura not as the victim but as responsible herself for developing bulimia, and (4) give advice.

How does Laura attend to the advice subsequently? In message 3, she begins with a 'thank you' and affirmation (line 18–19). This suits a 'request – advice – thank you' sequence that appears to be common in OSG interaction (Morrow 2006). Thus, Laura seems to accept the advice and initiates the closing of the interaction (cf. Stommel and Koole 2010). However, she continues with something that could be read as resistance to the advice ('but', 'really quite', line 20). The advice, implying that Laura should control her thoughts, is indirectly deflected with the explanation that she is unable to dismiss these thoughts. After a binging attack, she thinks of vomiting as something that would make her feel better (line 21–22). In other words, vomiting is presented as the solution to something, not as the problem itself, which stands in strong contrast to Angela's description of bulimia. So Laura treats the advice initially as appropriate but subsequently as inappropriate. This could be read as projecting the relevance of another message by Angela or another user to discuss Laura's problem more extensively. However, Laura's second message receives no response. Although this would be a highly accountable matter in face-to-face interaction, in online interaction it seems to be unproblematic (Veen et al. 2010; Antaki et al. 2005). It could, however, also imply that something about Laura's message was inappropriate. In a forum on suicide, a posting containing an explicit request was analyzed as the reason the posting received no replies, because such requests put the OSG members in a position with which they could not identify (Horne and Wiggins 2009). Similarly, we could argue that Laura's resistance is the reason she does not receive replies, because it implies resistance to the OSG's view on bulimia (that it is 'disgusting'). Such explanations, however, remain speculative.

Case 2

As we have already written, the thread in excerpt 2 is initiated by the *same* user as excerpt 1 (Laura) with a different posting.[8] Instead of providing an answer that can be heard as advice, Mandy invites Laura to tell more about herself (line 18).

Excerpt 2 (#27)

03.02.2005 18:56 I'm new – Laura Hi People! Came across this site by accident and I hope I can find help here. I am just 17 and have had eating disorders for as long as i can remember. I constantly have the desire to eat something. What I like most is to nibble at things. I've hardly finished eating something when i need something else. When shopping an extra bag of chips or chocolate always has to come along. Is that normal? Hope to get answers soon. Love laura
03.02.2005 19:20 Re: I'm new – Mandy Hello laura I am also 'just' 17. In my case the thing is that I often have the desire to eat something although I am totally not hungry. Do you also have real binging attacks or not? (sorry, if you don't want to answer that question that's fine too. I am always so curious) Would you like to tell a bit more about yourself? Love, Mandy
04.02.2005 11:49 Re: I'm new – Laura Hello Mandy! I'm pleased you have replied! Well binging attacks I don't really have. Or do I? I can't really make a judgment about that. Sometimes I eat constantly during the day, at times I don't eat anything for hours. In my case it all started when I was 6 or 7, when my father was ill and eventually passed away. I can remember that I always used to secretly nibble and also when I was younger I also always had what they call puppy fat. I would be pleased to receive another response from you. Love Laura
[omitted message 4–7]

As in excerpt 1, the initial posting develops towards a yes/no question concerning self-diagnosis ('is that normal?' line 9). Also in this case, the yes/no question sets the agenda of the interaction, making a response in the question's terms relevant (Heritage 2003) and again this concerns a B-event (Labov and Fanshel 1977). The description of the problem is focused on the constant desire to eat (line 5–8). In addition to a question, the posting contains two more explicit orientations to receiving responses: 'I hope I can find help here' (line 3) and 'Hope to get answers soon' (line 10).

In response, Mandy first articulates affiliation with Laura by producing a hug (line 13) and by pointing to the fact that they are the same age (line 14). She then offers a report of her own experience. Its construction puts emphasis on the particularity of the experience ('In my case the thing is', line 15), although it resembles Laura's description ('constantly have the desire to eat something' versus 'I often have the desire to eat something although I am totally not hungry').[9] This implies that Mandy treats Laura's question as a topic rather than as a question that makes relevant an answer in the specific terms it projected. This topic is used to describe a similar experience and thus Mandy enacts solidarity without providing advice.

Subsequently, Mandy poses two questions inviting Laura to tell more about her eating problem and about herself more generally. Both questions are oriented to as sensitive business (the apology, line 17–18 and 'Would you like' and 'a bit', line 19). Thereby, Mandy displays awareness of the fact that these questions require Laura to reveal more about herself and therefore might be taken as inappropriate. In terms of sequential implicativeness, posing questions projects a different type of continuation of the interaction with Laura than the advice by Angela in excerpt 1, making relevant answers rather than a 'thank you'.

In message 3, Laura attends to the questions by first displaying positive feedback (exclamation mark in the greeting and explicit appreciation, line 24). She then provides answers to both questions. Additionally, she refers to the fact that she would appreciate another response from Mandy (line 32), which again projects a continuation of the interaction. In other words, throughout the posting, Laura displays that she accepts the implicit invitation to continue 'talking' to Mandy. This is confirmed by the fact that in this thread four more messages are posted, in which, notably, the question that Laura posed in her first message is not referred to again. So, although the new user's initial question is not answered, the trajectory of 'continued talking' is gratefully accepted.

Conclusion

We have seen two similar initial postings that contained a very specific question containing a presupposition about the condition that may be contested. The response in both cases bypassed the agenda implied by the new user's question, although different strategies were used to do so. In case 1, the respondent indirectly denied the presupposition that the start of bulimia can be determined. She subsequently offered advice, thereby treating the initial posting as a request for advice. Personal experience was attended to in several ways. First, it was used to counter the presupposition embedded in the question that the start of bulimia could be determined. Second, it was used to orient to the potential inapplicability of the advice. Third, it was attended to as an epistemic foundation for markedly directive advice in such a way that it left little room for discussion. The new user's uptake of this advice treated it as sequentially matching, but additionally as inappropriate. We have suggested that this 'resistance' may have led to the end of the interaction.

In case 2, the response did not observably provide advice, but the respondent described herself in terms similar to the new user and posed further questions about the new user's situation. The question in the initial posting was thus treated as the initiation of a topic, not as requiring a specific answer. In the third turn of this thread, the new user treated the response as appropriate by explicitly referring to being pleased and wishing for another response, without referring back to the question from her first posting that still remained unanswered.

Thus, it appears that even when a new user's question may set the agenda for a reply, the respondents find ways to continue the interaction in various directions. It, therefore, seems that the sequential implications of a question in an initial posting are weak. This is in line with Vayreda and Antaki's (2009) analysis of what they call 'low bid' initial postings. In addition, our analysis has revealed that in the third turn, the new user treats two very different types of responses (advice or non-advice) both as sequentially congruent, thus confirming that the question in the initial posting did not set strict limitations to the type of responses. It appears then that any response in principle is welcome. That said, some responses do appear to be more welcome than others. The response that posed further questions was received much more positively by the new user than was the advice. The advice implied a demand on the new user to look more critically at her situation and to actively prevent the development of bulimia. So the advice seemed to impose a specific view on the illness that the new user treated as impossible to subscribe to within her subsequent posting.

These observations imply that advice giving in OSGs involves risks for all participants. The advice giver runs the risk of the advice being resisted and the new user may have to deal with impositions embedded in the advice. As the norm of presenting a diagnosis can work as a threshold to become active in an OSG (Stommel and Meijman 2011), it seems that advice can similarly work counterproductively. We have shown that posing further questions to a new user is an alternative to advice giving, while simultaneously still serving the aim of exchanging personal experiences that are relevant to the illness. There is no reason to assume that these findings are unique to OSGs on eating disorders. Our analysis suggests that OSG participants open up an interactional space for telling their troubles without necessarily seeking advice and that providing advice in those cases may actually implicate closure of the thread.

Future directions

The analysis presented in this chapter has provided an important first step in the more detailed examination of particular types of requests for advice within OSGs. We have shown not only that there are indirect requests for advice and explicit (directive) ways in which advice is given, but also that it is possible to describe similar experiences without providing advice. We have shown that personal experience may be oriented to as an insufficient epistemic basis for advice, or, instead, as the basis for the enactment of solidarity. Research is needed to further explore the variations in responses; such research could unpack the interactional work that participants accomplish in the context of advice giving in OSGs and illuminate the role of personal experience in that process. This would shed more light on the local production of expertise and experience in OSGs. The role of personal experience is particularly relevant given the increased use of OSGs and social media. Together they create social networks around particular illnesses that may shift the boundaries of what is considered 'authoritative knowledge' to include experiential knowledge. Empirical research is still scarce, but it has been shown how the online health resources provided by some OSGs allow for 'an interweaving of personal experiences, lay and scientific knowledges' (Schaffer et al. 2007: 146), turning patients and their caregivers into information managers and co-producers of knowledge, as well as providing access to perspectives that are overlooked in regular treatments. Rather than treating these types of knowledge as pre-existing and clearly defined categories, the ways they are oriented to in participants' contributions in OSGs should be the starting point for detailed empirical research (cf. Horton-Salway 2004).

From a sequential point of view, our analysis has illustrated that it is important to take seriously the fact that OSG threads consist of multiple turns. Whereas most of the studies we have discussed in this chapter present one (opening) posting and two or three replies as 'dyads' (cf. Sneijder and Te Molder 2005), it is important to consider that threads are often 'messier', with more users participating in the discussion, and in diverse ways. Users may respond to multiple previous posters at once or selectively to parts of a previous post. How initial postings can be met with various replies from various participants deserves more attention in future research.

Related topics

Computer-mediated communication – requesting – advice – support – conversation analysis – discursive psychology.

Notes

1 See Stommel (2007) for examples and an analysis of nicknames used in this particular OSG.
2 For a more elaborate ethical account of the way in which the data were obtained and treated, see Stommel (2009).
3 This seems exceptional in the sense that there are other forums in which advice is offered in the majority of the responses (Morrow 2006). However, a possible explanation is that the data come from the sub-forum New Here, in which advice could be less appropriate. For the analysis we present this is irrelevant because we are interested in cases in which advice *does* occur compared to cases in which it does not.
4 Because the German extract is written without capitals (contrary to the conventions for German) we have chosen to not use capitals in the English translation either.
5 'Binging addiction' is used as a translation of 'Essucht' because neither is an official diagnosis. Therefore they work as a distinction from the DSM IV-diagnosis Binge Eating Disorder.
6 Note also that in line 13–14 Laura ascribes an important role to the thoughts about hanging oneself over the toilet, implying that once you become too involved in them, they will control you. Indirectly, the thoughts are thus staged as autonomous.
7 It is hard to interpret the punctuation dots (Lamerichs and Stommel 2010), but we will give it a try. The dots after 'disgusting' and 'obnoxious' imply that it is a disgusting affliction and the dots after 'i know that' imply that Angela has some hard-won experiences with the illness. The repetition of these sets of dots here works cumulatively towards the advice. Thus, the advice is presented as the climax and on top of that the last set of dots may work to stress the urgency of the advice to NOT go down the lane of bulimia.
8 We do not want to speculate on the new user's reasons to initiate a second thread three days after the first. Since the participants do not orient to the fact that the new user has initiated two interactions, we do not pay attention to this aspect in our analysis.
9 Note that Mandy does not refer to actual eating/nibbling in her description, while Laura did (line 6–7). The question in line 17 however connects the desire to eat with binging (attacks).

Further reading

Antaki, C., Ardévol, E., Núñez, F., and Vayreda, A. (2005) '"For she who knows who she is": managing accountability in online forum messages', *Journal of Computer-Mediated Communication,* 11: art. 6.
Lamerichs, J. and Te Molder, H. (2003) 'Computer-mediated communication: from a cognitive to a discursive model', *New Media & Society,* 5: 451–473.

Stommel, W. and Koole, T. (2010) 'The online support group as a community: a micro-analysis of the interaction with a new member', *Discourse Studies,* 12: 357–378.

Vayreda, A. and Antaki, C. (2009) 'Social support and unsolicited advice in a bipolar disorder online forum', *Qualitative Health Research,* 19: 931–942.

Veen, M., Te Molder, H., Gremmen, B., and Van Woerkum, C. (2010) 'Quitting is not an option: an analysis of online diet talk between celiac disease patients', *Health,* 14: 23–40.

References

Antaki, C., Ardévol, E., Núñez, F., and Vayreda, A. (2005) '"For she who knows who she is": managing accountability in online forum messages', *Journal of Computer-Mediated Communication,* 11, art. 6: n.p.

Atkinson, J.M. (1984) 'Public speaking and audience responses: some techniques for inviting applause', in J.M. Atkinson and J. Heritage (eds) *Structures of Social Action: Studies in Conversation Analysis*, Cambridge: Cambridge University Press.

Bar-Lev, S. (2008) '"We are here to give you emotional support": performing emotions in an online HIV/AIDS support group', *Qualitative Health Research,* 18: 509–521.

Curl, T. and Drew, P. (2008) 'Contingency and action: a comparison of two forms of requesting', *Reseach on Language and Social Interaction,* 41: 1–25.

Edwards, D. and Potter, J. (1992) *Discursive Psychology,* London: Sage Publications.

Giles, D. and Newbold, J. (2011) 'Self- and other-diagnosis in user-led mental health online communities', *Qualitative Health Research,* 21: 419–428.

Guise, J., Widdicombe, S., and McKinlay, A. (2007) '"What is it like to have ME?" The discursive construction of ME in computer-mediated communication and face-to-face interaction', *Health,* 11: 87–108.

Heritage, J. (2003) 'Designing questions and setting agendas in the news interview', in P. Glenn, C. Lebaron, and J. Mandelbaum (eds) *Studies in Language and Social Interaction*, Mahwah, NJ: Lawrence Erlbaum.

Heritage, J. and Sefi, S. (1992) 'Dilemmas of advice: aspects of the delivery and reception of advice in interactions between health visitors and first-time mothers', in P. Drew and J. Heritage (eds) *Talk at Work: Interaction in Institutional Settings*, Cambridge: Cambridge University Press.

Horne, J. and Wiggins, S. (2009) 'Doing being "on the edge": managing the dilemma of being authentically suicidal in an online forum', *Sociology of Health and Illness,* 31: 170–184.

Horton-Salway, M. (2004) 'The local production of knowledge: disease labels, identities and category entitlements in ME support group talk', *Health,* 8: 351–371.

King, S. (1994) 'Analysis of electronic support groups for recovering addicts', *Interpersonal Computing and Technology: An Electronic Journal for the 21st Century,* 2: 47–56.

King, S. and Moreggi, D. (1998) 'Internet therapy and self-help groups – the pros and cons', in J. Gackenbach (ed.) *Psychology and the Internet: Intrapersonal, Interpersonal, and Transpersonal Implications*, San Diego, CA: Academic Press.

Kouper, I. (2010) 'The pragmatics of peer advice in a LiveJournal community', *Language@Internet,* 7: 1–19.

Labov, W. and Fanshel, D. (1977) *Therapeutic Discourse: Psychotherapy as Conversation,* New York: Academic Press.

Lamerichs, J. (2003) 'Discourse of support: exploring online discussions on depression'. Unpublished Thesis, Wageningen University, the Netherlands.

Lamerichs, J. and Te Molder, H. (2003) 'Computer-mediated communication: from a cognitive to a discursive model', *New Media & Society,* 5: 451–473.

Lamerichs, J. and Stommel, W. (2010) 'Exploring interactional functions of three dots (...) in CMD', paper presented at the AWIA symposium Interaction in Institutional Settings, June, Amsterdam.

Mickelson, K.D. (1997) 'Seeking social support: parents in electronic support groups', in S. Kiesler (ed.) *Culture of the Internet,* Mahwah, NJ: Lawrence Erlbaum.

Miller, J.K. and Gergen, K.J. (1998) 'Life on the line: the therapeutic potentials of computer-mediated conversation', *Journal of Marital & Family Therapy,* 24: 189–202.

Morrow, P. (2006) 'Telling about problems and giving advice in an Internet discussion forum: some discourse features', *Discourse Studies,* 8: 531–548.

Murero, M. and Rice, R.E. (eds) (2006) *The Internet and Health Care: Theory, Research and Practice*, Mahwah, NJ: Lawrence Erlbaum.
Pomerantz, A. (1986) 'Extreme case formulations', *Human Studies*, 9: 219–229.
Reed, D. (2001) 'Making conversation: sequential integrity and the local management of interaction on Internet newsgroups', paper presented at the 34th International Conference on System Sciences, Hawaii.
Rice, R.E. and Katz, J.E. (eds) (2001) *The Internet and Health Communication: Experiences and Expectations*, Thousand Oaks, CA: Sage Publications.
Sacks, H., Schegloff, E., and Jefferson, G. (1974) 'A simplest systematics for the organization of turn-taking in conversation', *Language*, 50: 696–735.
Sandaunet, A-G. (2008) 'The challenge of fitting in: non-participation and withdrawal from an online self-help group for breast cancer patients', *Sociology of Health and Illness*, 30: 131–144.
Schaffer, R., Kuczynski, K., and Skinner, D. (2007) 'Producing genetic knowledge and citizenship through the Internet: mothers, pediatric genetics, and cybermedicine', *Sociology of Health and Illness*, 30: 145–159.
Schegloff, E. and Sacks, H. (1967) 'Opening up closings', *Semiotica*, 7: 289–327.
Sneijder, P. and Te Molder, H. (2005) 'Moral logic and logical morality: attributions of responsibility and blame in online discourse on veganism', *Discourse and Society*, 16: 675–696.
Stommel, W. (2007) '"Mein Nick bin ich!" Nicknames in a German forum on eating disorders', *Journal of Computer-Mediated Communication*, 13, art. 8: n.p.
——(2008) 'Conversation analysis and community of practice; an approach to studying online community', in J. Androutsopoulos and M. Beißwenger (eds) *Data and Methods in Computer-mediated Discourse Analysis*. Special Issue: *Language@Internet*, 5, art. 5: n.p.
——(2009) *Entering an Online Support Group on Eating Disorders; A Discourse Analysis*, Amsterdam: Rodopi.
Stommel, W. and Koole, T. (2010) 'The online support group as a community: a micro-analysis of the interaction with a new member', *Discourse Studies*, 12: 357–378.
Stommel, W. and Meijman, F.J. (2011) 'The use of conversation analysis to study social accessibility of an online support group on eating disorders', *Global Health Promotion*, 18: 1–9.
Vayreda, A. and Antaki, C. (2009) 'Social support and unsolicited advice in a bipolar disorder online forum', *Qualitative Health Research*, 19: 931–942.
Veen, M., Te Molder, H., Gremmen, B., and Van Woerkum, C. (2010) 'Quitting is not an option: an analysis of online diet talk between celiac disease patients', *Health*, 14: 23–40.
Walstrom, M. (2000) '"You know who is the thinnest?": combating surveillance and creating safety in coping with eating disorders online', *CyberPsychology & Behavior*, 3: 761–783.
Wright, K.B. and Bell, S.B. (2003) 'Health-related support groups on the Internet: linking empirical findings to social support and computer-mediated communication theory', *Journal of Health Psychology*, 8: 39–54.

Appendix 13.1

Excerpt 1

1	07.02.2005 10:13 angst – Laura
2	he leute!
3	irgendwie habe ich angst, dass mich di bulimie auch treffen könnte.
4	Ich habe nämlich Essucht und denke oft daran, mich übers klo zu hängen.
5	habe es aber noch nie gemacht.
6	ist das der anfang?
7	lg laura

07.02.2005 10:30 Re: angst – Angela Hallo Laura, ich kann dir nicht sagen, wo der Anfang der Bulimie ist. Bei mir ging das recht fließend von MS in B über. ich habe aber davor nie darüber nachgedacht, wie es wohl wäre, mich jetzt zu übergeben ... bei mir ging das anfangs auch ganz von alleine. es kam einfach alles wieder raus ... ich würde an deiner Stelle mich aber jetzt nicht in den Gedanken hineinvertiefen, wer weiß, was du sonst damit auslöst. B ist eklig ... ich weiß das ... es ist scheißteuer, riecht eklig und ist einfach nur widerlich ... lass es ...
07.02.2005 10:35 Re: angst – Laura danke für deine antwort du hast sicher recht. aber es ist einfach schon schlimm, wenn man den gadenken dazu hat und nicht mehr weg bekommt. denn oftmals esse ich und esse ich alles in mich hinein, nachher ist mir schlecht und ich denke mir, wenn du dich übergibst, dann geht es dir sicher wieder besser.

Excerpt 2

03.02.2005 18:56 bin neu – Laura Hi Leute! Bin zufällig aud diese Seite gekommen und ich hoffe, ich finde hier hilfe. Ich bin erst 17 und habe schon so lange ich zurückdenken kann Essstörungen. Ich habe ständig das verlangen etwas zu essen. Am liebsten Nasche ich etwas. Kaum habe ich etwas fertig gegessen, brauche ich gleich noch etwas. Beim Einkaufen muss auch immer ne Extrapackung Chips oder Schokolade mitgehn. Ist das normal? Hoffe bald Antworten zu bekommen. Lg laura
03.02.2005 19:20 Re: bin neu – Mandy Hallo laura Ich bin auch ,,erst"17. Bei mir ist es so,dass ich oft das Verlangen habe etwas zu essen,obwohl ich gar nicht hungrig bin. Hast du auch richtige Essanfälle oder nicht? (sorry,wenn Du darauf nicht antworten möchtest ist es auch okay.Ich bin immer so neugierig) Magst Du noch ein bisschen über dich erzählen? Liebe Grüße, Mandy
04.02.2005 11:49 Re: bin neu – Laura Hallo Mandy! Freut mich, dass du mir geantwortet hast! Naja Essensanfälle habe ich eher nicht. Oder doch? Ich kann es nicht so richtig beurteilen. Ich esse mal den ganzen Tag hindurch, mal ess ich wieder stundenland nichts. Bei mir hat das ganze angefangen, als ich 6 oder 7 war, als mein Vater krank war und schließlich auch gestorben ist. Ich kann mich erinnern, dass ich schon immer heimlich genascht habe und einen sogennanten Babyspeck hab ich früher auch schon immer gehabt. Würde mich freuen, wenn du wieder Antwortest. Lg Laura
[omitted message 4–7]

14

Quality and usefulness of written communication for patients

Rosemary Clerehan

Introduction

The ill body finds its articulation in stories told by the patient to the doctor. Its spoken form is typically full of fits and starts, a grappling with what needs to be told and what can be identified. It is at once a conversation, a narrative, and a plea for understanding. For all of its dynamic complexity, it is a story that belongs to the ill person (Frank 2000). For the doctor's part, the disease is represented back to a patient in the form of a diagnosis (however tentative), and a proposed course of action: whether to some degree prescribed, or evolving from shared decision-making. For the patient then to be provided with written information of some kind testifies to the commonness of the disease experience, implying appropriation and 'generification' of their story by the doctor. The patient's willingness and capacity to engage with the material, both a re-contextualizing and transformation of their story, remains a complex and under-researched domain of linguistic healthcare research.

Spoken discourse is arguably the most salient, significant, and principal mode of healthcare communication and it is unsurprising that the research focus has been squarely on spoken interactions. Written provider–patient communication has been a comparatively neglected area of research into medical discourse, especially for linguistic research. However, the information needs of patients have come into greater focus for healthcare practitioners today, under such influences as the concept of patient-centered care and patient empowerment; longer-lived populations (but with an increase in a number of chronic diseases); and the rise of technologies which are Internet-driven.

Contemporary 'written' health professional communication can be categorized into three types: first, one-to-one, where a healthcare provider is responding to the needs of an individual who may or may not be previously known to them. In the second type, one-to-many, a provider is responding to a group of individuals who are participating in a common program (e.g., weight loss), or who have a disease in common. In the third, many-to-many communication takes place where a bank of practitioners provide advice or responses to a group (as in the second type), usually online.

In a comprehensive account of the general state of health communication, Kreps and Bonaguro (2009) provide ample evidence that there is increasing emphasis on strategies to enable healthcare consumers to take control of their health and health care. There are, therefore, correspondingly rich possibilities for the linguistics researcher interested in written communication. Moreover, the availability of written texts makes those data relatively less problematic to access than seeking subjects in healthcare settings for analysis of spoken communication. Difficulties remain, however, for researchers seeking to gain access to healthcare settings such as clinics and hospitals for research into written communication which aims to explore social and organizational contexts as well.

This chapter will mention in passing research into Internet and multimedia material, but those readers primarily interested in electronic communication should also read Chapters 12 and 13, in this volume. The discussion will exclude generic public health promotion materials and materials produced by other specific groups of practitioners such as nurses, physiotherapists, occupational therapists, chiropractors, and nutritionists. Pharmacy materials will be referred to from time to time where relevant, as the majority of the research literature has covered the subset of Patient Information Leaflets or PILs, also known as Patient Package Inserts (PPIs), which accompany all medications, as well as the supplementary leaflets commonly known as Consumer Medication Information (CMI).

Historical perspectives

Research into written health communication discourse has been a multidisciplinary field of scholarly activity since at least the 1970s, with two broad areas in particular being identifiable: healthcare-focused and health promotion-focused (Kreps and Bonaguro 2009). As in other areas of doctor–patient communication, mismatches have often been identified between healthcare providers' and healthcare consumers' views about the optimal extent and type of information required (Grime et al. 2007).

Provision of high quality healthcare-focused written information may result in better informed and satisfied patients, supporting them in tasks such as decision-making and/or taking medications. Studies of the effectiveness of such material have historically been limited by a biomedical approach which fails to take into account socio-cultural and linguistic issues. In 2001, Dixon-Woods surveyed the field and was able to distinguish two bodies of work. The first was based solely on the biomedical discourse model, in which attitudinal and behavioral change were valorized, and non-compliance represented as a consequence of patient incompetence. The second drew on a rather different set of assumptions including the 'Imagined Reader' (Coulthard 1994) and thus took into account patients' experience and context in a discourse which was fundamentally patient-centered and which sought to assist decision-making, but was rarely based on linguistic analysis. The division between these two approaches Dixon-Woods saw as possibly dissolving over time, but questions still lingered around the best approaches to safeguard patients and assist them to understand risk, while at the same time providing them with understandable information – enabling them, in certain circumstances, to exercise choice. She called for 'a rigorous theoretical framework within which to think about [printed] patient information' (2001: 1428).

Since that time, research into healthcare-focused materials has attracted researchers from such fields as medicine, informatics, sociology, psychology, education, and organizational behavior (Kreps and Bonaguro 2009). Methodologies have included quantitative approaches such as randomized controlled trials, case-controlled studies, observational studies, the quasi-experimental (questionnaires) and the purely qualitative, involving grounded analysis and ethnographies, using focus groups and interviews. Very little has involved linguistic analysis (Garner et al. 2012).

The majority of the published research has focused on patient information provided by pharmacies and drug companies and mandated by legislation, rather than the information produced or handed out by doctors and other healthcare practitioners, which is not subject to any government regulation. It is helpful to be clear about the different types of text that are covered by regulatory bodies (see also Askehave and Zethsen 2008). In Australia, the Therapeutic Goods Administration (TGA) mandates the types of documents, known as Consumer Medication Information (CMI), that accompany pharmaceuticals, using the approved product information written by the drug companies and available for healthcare professionals to use (Aslani 2007). This is distinct from the Patient Package Insert or PPI which is found in the medicine package itself. For the United States and the European Union, Connor et al. (2008) outline the differences between the respective regulatory bodies that mandate the Patient Information Leaflets (PILs). PILs is also a term used to denote any leaflets provided by health practitioners, with 'non-mandated [drug] information' (2008: 118). The term, even more confusingly, is widely used to cover any printed health-related patient information. This blurring of regulatory, authorial, and generic boundaries has beset analysis, with findings regarding one text type often simply transposed to another.

Traditionally, the literature on print materials in healthcare settings has focused on the patient and the difficulties experienced when patients attempt to understand and interpret health practitioners' printed information. Health literacy has long been a subject of interest because of assumptions that the problem lies with the patient (health literacy is the subject of Chapter 10). The measurement of health literacy as a construct, however, continues to be problematic, and thus the use of the various standardized tools available for testing health literacy for the population at large has been increasingly open to question (Elder et al. 2012).

Targeting health messages for particular sub-populations on, say, ethnic, religious, and cultural quadrants would appear, intuitively, an optimal way for information to be delivered to individuals by whatever technology. Communications can be designed for multiple lifestyle risk factors: say, older persons who are smokers and consume excessive alcohol. Abrams et al. (1999: 301) described the challenge as needing to develop a 'parsimonious but comprehensive theoretical model that outlines what is worth tailoring on and what is not'. Drawing on older behaviorist conceptions of 'the receiver' receiving the message 'as the sender sent it', they are nonetheless prepared to acknowledge that the format, language, and presentation may well prove in future to be the best targets of analysis for better communications. Kreuter and Wray (2003) make the distinction between tailoring and targeting, defining targeting as related to some population sub-group, and tailoring as directing material towards a specific individual, based on a previous assessment. They report that both can enhance message relevance, but caution that tailoring, while intuitively appealing, is not the only way to proceed and may, in some circumstances, actually be counterproductive. A useful research direction would be to broaden the terms of such investigations beyond behavior change, and herein lies one advantage of investigators with linguistic training.

Critical issues

This section will cover assumptions about readership and associated problems concerning previous approaches which have used readability formulas to gauge the fitness for purpose of written healthcare texts. The role of text types and genres and other qualitative research will be discussed, and an approach drawing on systemic functional linguistics is proposed.

The role of supplementary written communication in a patient-centered approach to health care has generally been accepted as an important adjunct to spoken information (Meade and Smith 1991; Hill and Bird 2003). An information leaflet provides a patient with a tangible record to which they can refer, check understanding, and use as a basis for asking further questions (Glenton and Polit 2002). There continues to be debate and uncertainty, however, about the quality and usefulness of the material, supplied variously by hospitals, individual practitioners, and professional organizations (Smith et al. 1998; Payne et al. 2000).

Patient information leaflets, particularly consumer medication information, play important roles in patients' health, safety, and relationship with their healthcare provider. As indicated above, many of the methodologies used to investigate written patient information to date have been non-linguistic. Possibly due to limitations of the databases typically searched by health practitioners and health researchers, linguistic research is rarely even cited. In spite of research suggesting that reluctance to take medication has alternative explanations (Pound et al. 2005), most methods to date have instead centered on patient comprehension, memory, and compliance. A further gap is that little published research of any kind on the topic has been carried out in patients whose first language is not English, or in non-Western settings.

Linked to the problems recognized in Dixon-Wood's (2001) biomedical model of communication for research into patient information materials has been an over-fondness in the literature for the use of one of many readability formulas. These have been used, principally by doctors, in their attempt to capture difficulties in the text for patients. As Dixon-Woods argues, 'the dominance of readability testing despite these known problems also appears to be related to the potency of the "incompetent patient" as a discursive resource' (2001: 1424). Much of this healthcare literature has focused on statistical estimates of readability of patient information leaflets (for example, Davis et al. 1990; Payne et al. 2000), and even of websites (Sabharwal et al. 2008). While their use still appears to be recommended to improve medical information, for example, by the Australian National Health and Medical Research Council (NHMRC), at the same time it is conceded that it is not possible from any formula to recommend the appropriate level at which to pitch 'most consumer documents' (NHMRC 1999).

A modified approach is offered by Garner et al. (2012) who support the idea of using a readability score of some kind – but in combination with other strategies. Their proposed framework also involves the identification of problematic lexical and structural elements in the text, followed by the assessment of response in relation to communicative aims, which would involve interviews with readers to check the appropriateness of their responses.

Readability scores presuppose readers (or 'users') as passive recipients, straining to catch 'the message' of the health professional. They also presuppose that the text by itself can yield information that tells us how well people are reading it, among numerous other well-canvassed problems (Schriver 2000). Contemporary reading theory, notwithstanding its many schools of thought, generally characterizes reading as pre-eminently a meaning-making activity, an engagement of reader and text. Readers do first need to come to grips with the fields of experience (or content) present in the text, but also to understand the positioning of themselves vis-à-vis the writer, and the purposes and the staging of the text; and be able to engage with the relative formality of the language used. Information design theory, as well as our own research (e.g., Hirsh et al. 2009), suggests that readers of functional texts read with their own particular purposes, and may, for example, approach the task by searching headings until they find the information they want (Pander Maat and Lentz 2010).

Interesting findings emerged from Gal and Prigat's (2005) study to probe the question of why poor quality leaflets continued to be produced (conducted in Israel where, tellingly, readability formulas cannot in any case be used for Hebrew). They interviewed ten informants (only two of whom were physicians) who had participated in development of a patient information leaflet in their organizations. How the resulting product was distributed, and to whom, was not under the developers' control, and the researchers concluded that these organizational pressures were often the root cause of a leaflet's lack of appropriateness. They urge a more 'ecological perspective' (2005: 491) when investigating and attempting to improve such leaflets.

Current contributions and research

Granted the field is a relatively under-researched and theorized one, as indicated earlier it is important to be clear about the text type being analyzed. Some examples of the range of identifiable text types which answer to the description 'Health Practitioner Written Communication' are listed in Table 14.1, but this is far from an exhaustive typology. Some references are given, though only one (Fage-Butler 2011) was wholly a linguistic study.

These texts range from brief handwritten notes to professionally produced booklets. Those in the right-hand column are produced according to a specific (and fairly invariable) format, with the primary reader either generically or specifically predefined (patient's work supervisor/a known specialist), and the sets of communicative purposes quite stable. The patient may view or read such texts incidentally. We may say that those in this column are thus readily identified as genres in their own right and, probably due to their relatively constrained nature, they have excited little research interest – even though patients may view

Table 14.1 Text types for healthcare practitioner written communications

Primarily designed for patient (not necessarily disease-specific)	*Primarily designed for patient (disease-specific)*	*Primarily designed for another healthcare provider/other*
Patient education brochures	Medication information (e.g., Grime and Ong 2007; Haw and Stubbs 2011)	Prescriptions for medications
Instructions to guide behaviors	Care plans	Sickness certificates
Injury prevention information	Information on risks/benefits/ alternatives (e.g., Berry 2004; Fage-Butler 2011)	Referral letters
Family information booklets	Information on managing lifelong chronic conditions (e.g., Payne et al. 2000)	Radiology reports
Information on use of equipment/technology	Discharge information (e.g., Johnson and Sandford 2005)	Bone densitometry reports
Medical questionnaires	Patient decision aids (e.g., Smith et al. 2008).	Imaging reports (radiology, nuclear medicine, bone densitometry)
Dietary information		Pathology reports
Consent forms (e.g., Mayberry and Mayberry 2002)		Procedural reports (coronary angiograms, endoscopies, etc.)
		Progress notes (in-patients or ambulatory care)
		Handover notes
		Organ donation lists

them. Those in the first and second column have been researched to a much greater degree, but linguistic accounts are still rare.

The scope of this chapter precludes a discussion of genre theory per se, but the brief review of genre theories by Moore and Tuckwell (2006), in their situating of Hasan's (1989) theory of generic structure potential (GSP), is of interest here. GSP has been used to account for the elements of a text that must be present for it to be considered to belong to a given genre and, at the same time, showing what variation can still occur within that identification (used in Clerehan at al. 2009). Moore and Tuckwell (2006: 206) refer to the Swales (1990) model whereupon genre identification is assigned according to similarity to a 'prototypical instance of the genre in question' or, in Martin's (1997) terms, how similar texts may be to 'agnate' genres. The role of 'context' poses a further problem. Swales in later work (e.g., Askehave and Swales 2001) points to the difficulty in choosing to follow a 'text-first' or a 'context-first' approach in genre analysis, and instead follows a highly provisional procedure aiming to be sensitive to the evolving and dynamic nature of many genres, such as those in the first and second column of communications in Table 14.1.

For the patient-centered text types listed above, it can be seen from our own work (see following section) that the disease-specific may leak into the non disease-specific, for example a leaflet on the drug Prednisolone may cover various diseases for which the drug is relevant (e.g., http://www.patient.co.uk/medicine/Prednisolone.htm). It may still be pragmatically useful, however, to consider such a leaflet as an instance of the genre of medication information leaflet (often subsumed, as explained above, under the broader genre of patient information leaflets). In Hallidayan (1985/1994) terms, we are allowing the registral variable of field (what is talked about) to be fairly elastic, as well as, to a lesser degree, the variable of tenor, construing the relationships between author and addressee.

Bypassing readability formulas, a growing body of work has undertaken more qualitative assessment of medical information for patients. This has included the development of a checklist of content and design characteristics for printed health education materials by means of a systematic review of the available literature (Paul et al. 1997). The authors commented, however, that 'there may be some aspects not accounted for, or not able to be accounted for, by the characteristics covered in the literature' (p. 158). Paul et al. (2003) reviewed the effectiveness of print material, with particular emphasis on effects on knowledge, attitudes, and behavior. They found that both the 'content' items identified as important from their systematic review and the design of the leaflets had little impact on the material's perceived effectiveness. Wright (1999) explored distinctive features of the way users read healthcare materials as functional documents, and stressed the importance of performance-based design, testing materials with members of the target audience. Related studies have been conducted into communication barriers in public health education, focusing on patient package inserts (Askehave and Zethsen 2003); and recent work in this area has opened up the issue of the potential problems arising when the package insert is translated from English into another language (Martínez Motos 2012; Nisbeth Jensen 2012; Nisbeth Jensen and Zethsen 2012).

Thematic discourse analysis has also been used to illuminate some of the disruptions in the writer–reader relationship. This approach was used by Grime and Ong (2007) in a study of six osteoarthritis (OA) leaflets which identified three themes: OA as joint pathology; causation of OA and implications for lifestyle and growing older; and the management of OA. They reported a range of interesting findings, allowing telling insights into the differences between the leaflets, but also the common feature that all were dominated by a 'disease discourse' (2007: 33), effectively creating a barrier between professional and patient.

Fage-Butler (2011) used Foucauldian analysis to chart the 'discursive landscape' of a corpus of six European pharmaceutical companies' PILs to examine how risk and trust were discursively constructed. Within the trust discourses, she identified different sub-discourses of science, care, and corporate responsibility and how they operated in these leaflets. As she argues, this suggests ways of locating textual problems and points the way to strategies for addressing them. Another approach is content analysis which was used by Haw and Stubbs (2011) to investigate 42 antidepressant PILs already mandated by European law. They found a range of significant weaknesses despite the supposed standardized nature of the texts. Dray and Papen (2004) drew on a promising combination of critical discourse analysis and ethnography. They presented a framework for studying the role of written language in materials provided by healthcare institutions, suggesting an alternative to narrow notions of health literacy and patient deficit.

Given the paucity of linguistic studies, tools of analysis from allied disciplines developed to assess and improve patient materials will be briefly mentioned. Among many, these include Rees et al. (2002) who examined DISCERN, a tool to assist patients to evaluate information on treatment choices. Moult et al. (2004) developed EQIP (Ensuring Quality Information for Patients) as a preferable tool for assessing quality of healthcare information in pediatric settings. Helitzer at al. (2009) combined two tools in a new venture, called SAM+CAM, to score patient education materials on content, literacy demands, numeric literacy, graphics, layout/typography, and learning stimulation variables. Document design principles were used by Pander Maat and Lentz in their work (e.g., Pander Maat and Lentz 2010) to improve text structure and visual signaling in patient package inserts previously approved by the Dutch Medicine Evaluation Board. They felt their freedom to innovate was constrained by the template, but document design, as outlined in their body of work, continues to offer considerable promise, allied with linguistic analysis.

An approach drawing on a systemic functional linguistics (SFL) framework has been offered as one that can provide insight and directions for the improvement of patient materials. While there has been a considerable body of SFL-influenced research into medical discourse, the majority has focused on oral discourse. One SFL study of written medical discourse investigated aspects of nurse–patient/patient's family discourse, both oral and written (Kealley et al. (2005); and one of the many studies of the patient package insert, Zethsen and Askehave (2010), used SFL concepts to identify that so-called best practice, as judged by regulatory agencies, may not be so when subjected to linguistic analysis.

Systemic functional linguistics is a theory of language which is primarily concerned with language function within a social context and provides analytical tools at the level of the discourse, as well as the lexicogrammar, to investigate the relations of text and context (Halliday 1985/1994). Its value is that it can provide a grounded theoretical basis to test our hypotheses about language and genre. It is also possible to adopt only those features of the theory that are relevant to conduct particular investigations. One impressively detailed study in this tradition (McManus 2009) employed SFL analysis to provide insights into historically different conceptions of the doctor–patient relationship and their world, comparing an early twentieth-century corpus of leaflets accompanying medications with a modern corpus.

Further work in the SFL tradition has resulted in the development of the Appraisal Framework (Martin and White 2005), an approach still being expanded for analyzing how evaluations are expressed linguistically and negotiated at the interpersonal level. Appraisal theory offers an intricate way of analyzing interpersonal meaning in a text at the discourse semantic level and at the lexicogrammatical level where it is realized in the writer's choice of modality and intensification, among other possibilities. Two sub-systems are of particular interest in the analysis of written patient information: that of 'engagement', which regulates the dialogic space made available for propositions made; and that of 'judgment' (a subcategory of the attitude sub-system) allowing normative assessments of behaviors. Adequately accounting for how this kind of approach works for specific genres of written patient information is a task that still awaits researchers.

Sample analysis

Since 2005, Clerehan and colleagues have worked on a subset of PILs – medication information leaflets. From a set of printed leaflets collected from rheumatologists throughout Australia (Buchbinder et al. 2001), we developed a framework drawing on systemic functional linguistics and genre theories, the Evaluative Linguistic Framework (or ELF), in Clerehan at al. (2005) and Clerehan and Buchbinder (2006). A total of 195 rheumatologists had been asked to send in copies of the written drug information they routinely provided to patients to supplement oral communication when commencing them on therapy. The leaflets were produced by individuals/hospitals (15); the Australian Arthritis Foundation; the periodical, *Current Therapeutics*; and a drug company (one each). We applied the framework to a subset of these (the largest single drug represented in the corpus, namely methotrexate). This set of 18 leaflets was analyzed at the levels of genre, discourse-semantics, and some aspects of the lexicogrammar, so as to identify their characteristics and possible shortcomings as comprehensible documents for patients (see Figure 14.1).

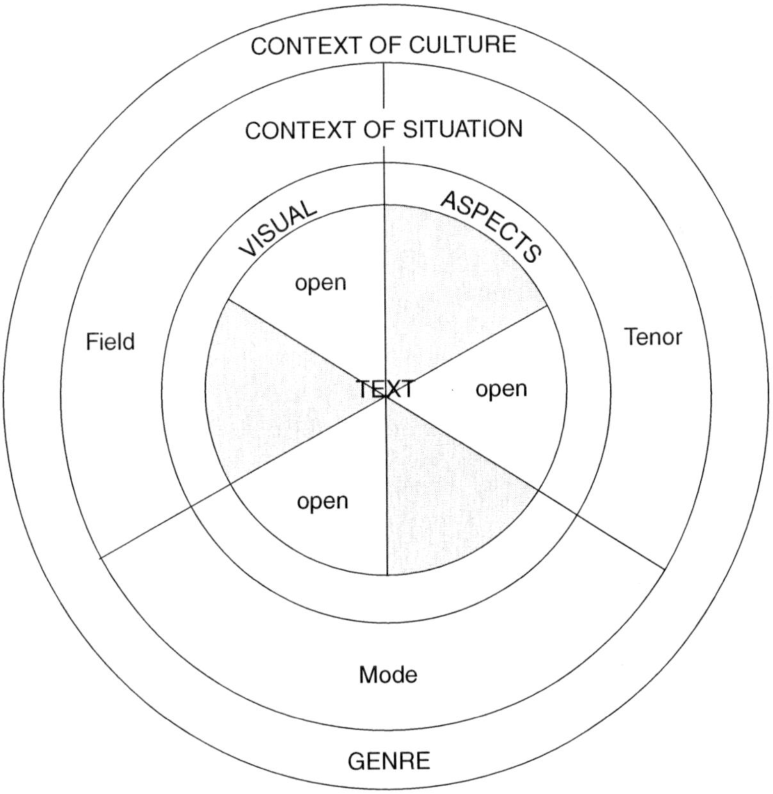

Figure 14.1 Model of text-focused evaluation

Source: Clerehan and Buchbinder (2006), after Lentz and Pander Maat (1992).

We found that the significant elements were: the overall structure, the technicality of the vocabulary used (terms such as 'mucocutaneous reactions'); the lexical density (number of content words per clause, Halliday 1985/1994); and the clarity of the role relationship between author and reader as inscribed in the interpersonal meanings in the text. While the drug information leaflet was identifiable as a genre with potentially up to nine structural moves where the writer initiates a particular activity, there was a high degree of variability in inclusion of moves, in rhetorical functions within moves, and in use of headings. The nine identifiable moves (only 3–8 of these present in any one leaflet) were found to be: Background on Drug, Summary of Use, Dosage Instructions, Outline of Benefits of Drug, Account of Side Effects, Information regarding Monitoring, Constraints on Patient Behavior, Storage Instructions, and Clinical Contact Availability.

Most leaflets contained a high number of content words per clause, and the identity of the author (their doctor/specialist/other) was clear in only three (17 percent), with implications for the writer–reader relationship, especially for their respective responsibilities. Headings were inconsistent so it was hard to discern the hierarchical structure of information. Within the moves, there were two main rhetorical elements employed in the leaflets – 'to inform', and 'to instruct'. Much of the information appeared to be provided 'to inform' the reader and was appropriately written as statements; however, the function of many moves appeared to be 'to instruct' the reader and the instruction was not clearly presented (e.g., 'special care must be taken'). This could be improved by explicitly considering who was responsible for each action, the importance and/or urgency of the action to be taken, and the strength of the reader's obligation to comply. We found further evidence for lack of congruity between rhetorical elements and the mood structure ('if serious problems occur, the treatment will be stopped'). It was concluded that the quality of patient information material could be improved by using an analysis which takes account of the suitability of generic structure and rhetorical functions, specialization of lexis, status relations, lexical density and modalization, together with critical assessment of factual and visual aspects (see Table 14.2).

We also concluded that a usability strategy with participants who were taking such medications should be employed to support the directions provided by the analysis.

Prior to this planned reader-focused evaluation of our framework, in the second stage of our research we established further the validity of the framework by applying it to sets of leaflets relating to two other drugs (Clerehan et al. 2009). Two of the moves previously identified, Dosage Instructions and Account of Side Effects, were present in all leaflets, and thus could safely be considered obligatory elements. None of the other moves occurred in all the leaflets and thus appeared to be optional elements. The new findings confirmed the applicability of the framework and were used to refine it. We identified a new stage or 'move' in the genre which caused us to re-evaluate our earlier generic structure analysis and raised the question of whether there were micro-moves operating within larger moves. The new move identified, Contra-indications, answered the question, 'When should the drug not be used?'

The leaflets still read more like academic text than spoken language because of the amount of nominalizations and, hence, the lexical density (for instance, '*Arising* out of its *use* in *cancer*, the *drug gained* a *reputation* for *causing damage* to the *liver* ...'). In the new set of leaflets, there was less inconsistency in the use of headings and in the use of medical or semi-technical language. On the whole, writer–reader relationships were clear, as was the responsibility for action; however, the factual content and the format of the leaflets varied considerably.

Table 14.2 Evaluative Linguistic Framework (ELF) for evaluating healthcare text based upon systemic functional linguistics

Item	*Description*	*Assessment*
Overall organizational or generic structure of the text	Series of moves in a text (e.g., background on drug, dosage instructions, account of side effects)	What identifiable moves are present? Are all essential moves included? What is the sequence of moves and is this appropriate?
Rhetorical elements	The function of each move in relation to the reader (e.g., to define, instruct, inform)	What are the rhetorical functions of each move in relation to the reader? Are these clearly defined and appropriate? Is there clear guidance about what to do with the presented information? Are instructions clear about what action needs to be taken?
Writer–reader relationship	Nature of the relationship between the writer and reader (e.g., medical expert to layperson; doctor to his/her patient)?	Is it clear who the writer and intended audience is? Is the relationship between writer and reader clear and consistent? Is the person who is expected to take responsibility for any actions clear? Is the importance and/or urgency of the action made clear?
Metadiscourse	Description of the purpose/structure of the text	Is there a clear description of the purpose of the text (if not already provided by the clinician)?
Headings	Signposts in the text for the reader	Are headings present? If present, are they appropriate?
Technicality of vocabulary	The technicality of the medical terminology/other vocabulary that is used	How technical is the vocabulary that is used in the text? Is this appropriate?
Lexical density	Density of the content words in the text	What is the average density of the text (content-bearing words per clause)? Is this appropriate (3 to 4 or below if possible)?
Factual content of text	Facts included in the text	Is the factual information correct, up to date, and dated? Is the source of information provided? Is the quality and strength of the evidence discussed?
Format	Visual aspects such as layout, font size, style, use of visual material etc.	What is the length, layout, font size and the visual aspect, and do these contribute to clarification of the meaning of the text?

Source: Clerehan et al. (2009).

To obtain patient feedback about the structure and quality of medication information leaflets and validate the usefulness of the ELF, we tested our findings by performing a reader-focused evaluation of the framework, using examples of what emerged from applying the framework as 'high' and 'low' quality leaflets, with a representative sample of 27 RA patients (Hirsh et al. 2009). Figure 14.2 illustrates our model of reader-focused evaluation.

Our data consisted of: (a) the reader's real-time response to the document in interview (process); (b) their written responses to the document after reading (product); and (c) their views about certain textual features, obtained in focus groups, which included a self-administered questionnaire (opinion) (Lentz and Pander Maat 1992). This triangulated feedback provided an in-depth reader-focused evaluation and our framework was revised, guided by the results of this and the findings from the second stage.

The principal elements of the framework were investigated: overall generic structure and functions of each stage, the interpersonal writer–reader relationship, technicality of language, and lexical density. Participant assessments of the leaflets aligned with the framework in terms of what constituted a 'good' leaflet. While the main purpose of the leaflets was identified as being information provision, participants also wanted clear instructions, benefits to be highlighted, and side effects to be comprehensively listed. For comprehensiveness and user-friendliness, leaflets developed with guidance of the ELF were consistently preferred.

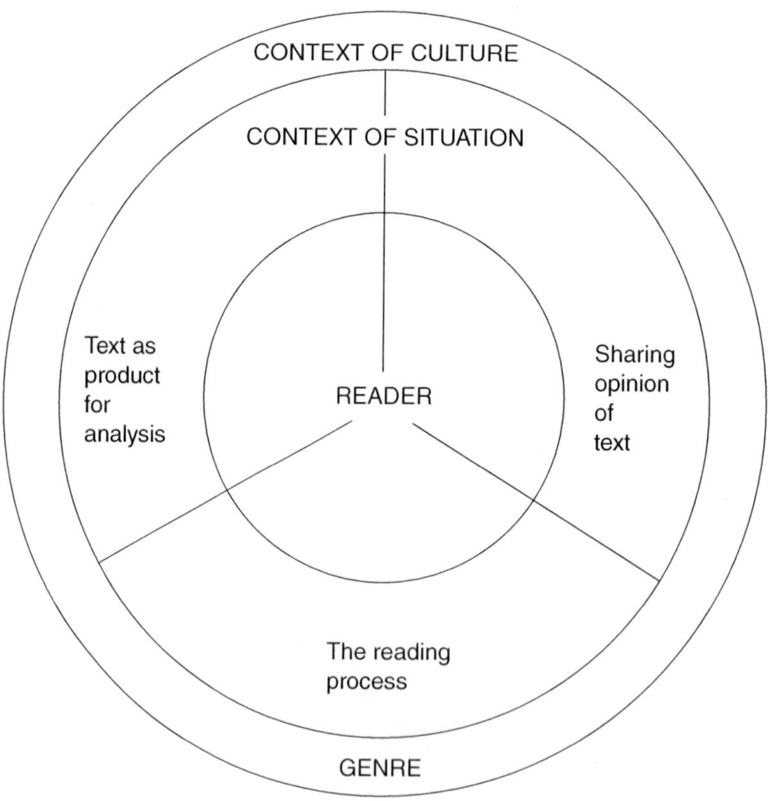

Figure 14.2 Model of reader-focused evaluation

Source: Clerehan and Buchbinder (2006), after Lentz and Pander Maat (1992).

Recommendations for practice

The strengths of the ELF are that it is a user-friendly, structured analytic framework that can assist with the development of effective high quality patient information materials, providing specific tools to produce and assess medication information leaflets to support readers in decision-making and taking medication. Future work could utilize the framework to evaluate information on other treatments and procedures, or on healthcare information more widely. To our knowledge, in addition to Connor et al. (2008), a comparison of medicine labeling in two countries, the ELF is currently being used to frame research in progress into decision aids, patient package inserts, and consent forms in Australia, Denmark, and Norway.

To assess the effects of multimedia 'educational interventions' on patients taking medications, the ELF was included as a potential instrument (Ciciriello et al. 2010), in a Protocol for a Cochrane Review. For use with multimedia texts, it will most likely be necessary to modify it to include further parameters such as navigation and the structure of given and new information; tailoring and interactivity; and how textual phases link together.

Future directions

Our own work could also usefully be extended by taking the context of initial planning and then the circumstances of patient reception and reading of the text into account, along the lines of Gal and Prigat's (2005) work. Approaches from other social sciences such as communication studies may also offer insights which can be potentially useful for future work. Papen's (2010) ethnography, for example, has offered an innovative approach to investigating reading and writing practices (including non-native speakers of English), exploring how patients 'read' the cultural practices of using written texts in health care. This involves not only the doctor's text, but the instrumental and emotional texts written by the patients themselves. Her claim that such texts need to be understood in relation to practices and policies highlights innovative directions for researchers.

It is hard to imagine the future for written doctor–patient communication research without taking into consideration the multiple roles played by electronic communications technology – and in forms we cannot yet even imagine. Today, patients are often attending their appointments with information gleaned from the Internet, notwithstanding significant issues with accuracy, completeness, readability, disclosures, and references on medical websites (Eysenbach et al. 2002). It seems certain that the printed patient information leaflet will continue to exist as an easy-access, concise, and potentially helpful aid to a community's health.

Summary

Patient information leaflets are an important adjunct to verbal exchange between healthcare practitioner and patient. Their value is dependent upon whether they contain useful information from the viewpoint of the patient, and are trusted and understood. While healthcare professionals may routinely use patient information leaflets, a poorly conceived leaflet has the potential to do harm and, despite a plethora of studies found in databases like MEDLINE, research into patient information of all kinds, which is sensitive to the uses of language, discourse and context, is still rare. Carefully planned research into the interactions between spoken and written communications – how healthcare practitioners develop or select, present, and deliver patient information – is the task awaiting applied linguistics researchers. The most promising research directions are likely to be taken by linguists in collaboration with healthcare professionals.

Acknowledgments

The author wishes to thank her co-authors on the various published papers, especially Professor Rachelle Buchbinder, and to express her gratitude to Arthritis Australia and the Cabrini Institute for their support.

Related topics

Doctor–patient written communication; healthcare provider texts; written patient information; written health communication; patient information leaflets.

Further reading

De Jong, M. and Schellens, P.J. (2001) 'Optimising public information brochures – formative evaluation in document design processes', in D. Janssen and R. Neutelings, *Reading and Writing Public Documents*, Amsterdam: John Benjamins. (One of many thoughtful and pragmatic papers from the Dutch school of document design.)

Raynor, D., Blenkinsopp, A., Knapp, P., Grime, J., Nicolson, D., Pollock, K., et al. (2007) 'A systematic review of quantitative and qualitative research on the role and effectiveness of written information available to patients about individual medicines', *Health Technology Assessment* 11(5). (Lengthy and interesting systematic review commissioned by the British National Institute for Health Research.)

Schriver, K.A. (1989) 'Evaluating text quality: the continuum from text-focused to reader-focused method', *IEEE Transactions on Professional Communication*, 3: 238–255. (An older text, but an excellent critical account of the advantages and disadvantages of the then existing quantitative and qualitative methods of assessing functional text quality.)

References

Abrams, D., Mills, S., and Bulger, D. (1999) 'Challenges and future directions for tailored communication research', *Annals of Behavioral Medicine*, 21(4): 299–306.

Askehave, I. and Swales, J. (2001) 'Genre identification and communicative purpose: a problem and a possible solution', *Applied Linguistics*, 22: 195–212.

Askehave, I. and Zethsen, K.K. (2003) 'Communication barriers in public discourse: the patient package insert', *Document Design*, 4: 22–41.

——(2008) 'Mandatory genres: the case of European Public Assessment Report (EPAR) summaries', *Text & Talk*, 28(2): 167–191.

Aslani, P. (2007) 'Consumer medicine information conundrums', *Australian Prescriber*, 30: 122–124.

Berry, D. (2004) *Risk, Communication and Health Psychology*, New York: Open University Press.

Buchbinder, R., Hall, S., Grant, G., Mylvaganam, A., and Patrick, M. (2001) 'Readability and content of supplementary written drug information for patients used by Australian rheumatologists', *Medical Journal of Australia*, 174: 575–578.

Ciciriello, S., Johnston, R., Osborne, R., Wicks, I., deKroo, T., Clerehan, R., and Buchbinder, R. (2010) 'Multimedia educational interventions for consumers about prescribed and over the counter medications', *Cochrane Library*, 3: 1–14.

Clerehan, R. and Buchbinder, R. (2006) 'Towards a more valid account of functional text quality: the case of the patient information leaflet', *Text & Talk*, 26(1): 39–68.

Clerehan, R., Buchbinder, R., and Moodie, J. (2005) 'A linguistic framework for assessing the quality of written patient information: its use in assessing methotrexate information for rheumatoid arthritis', *Health Education Research*, 20: 334–344.

Clerehan, R., Hirsh, D., and Buchbinder, R. (2009) 'Medication information leaflets for patients: the further validation of an analytic linguistic framework', *Communication and Medicine,* 6: 117–127.

Connor, U., Ruiz-Garrido, M.F., Rozycki, W., Goering, E., Kinney, E.D., and Koehler, J.M. (2008) 'Patient-directed medicine labeling: text differences between the United States and Spain', *Communication and Medicine,* 5: 117–132.

Coulthard, M. (1994) *Advances in Written Text Analysis,* London: Psychology Press.

Davis, T., Crouch, M., Wills, G., Miller, S., and Abdehou, D. (1990) 'The gap between patient reading comprehension and the readability of patient education materials', *Journal of Family Practice,* 31: 533–538.

Dixon-Woods, M. (2001) 'Writing wrongs? An analysis of published discourses about the use of patient information leaflets', *Social Science and Medicine,* 52: 1417–1432.

Dray, S. and Papen, U. (2004) 'Literacy and health: towards a methodology for investigating patients' participation in healthcare', *Journal of Applied Linguistics,* 1: 311–332.

Elder, C., Barber, M., Osborne, R., Clerehan, R., and Buchbinder, R. (2012) 'Assessing health literacy: a new domain for collaboration between language testers and health professionals', *Language Assessment Quarterly,* 9(3): 205–224.

Eysenbach, G., Powell, J., Kuss, O., and Sa, E.-R. (2002) 'Empirical studies assessing the quality of health information for consumers on the World Wide Web', *Journal of the American Medical Association,* 287: 2691–2700.

Fage-Butler, A.M. (2011) 'The discursive construction of risk and trust in patient information leaflets', *Hermes – Journal of Language and Communication Studies,* 46: 61–73.

Frank, A. (2000) 'The standpoint of storyteller', *Qualitative Health Research,* 10: 354–365.

Gal, I. and Prigat, A. (2005) 'Why organizations continue to create patient information leaflets with readability and usability problems: an exploratory study', *Health Education Research,* 20: 485–493.

Garner, M., Ning, Z., and Francis, J. (2012) 'A framework for the evaluation of patient information leaflets', *Health Expectations,* 15(3): 283–294.

Glenton, C. and Polit, C. (2002) 'Developing patient-centred information for back pain sufferers', *Health Expectations,* 5: 319–329.

Grime, J.C. and Ong, B.N. (2007) 'Constructing osteoarthritis through discourse – a qualitative analysis of six patient information leaflets on osteoarthritis', *BMC Musculoskeletal Disorders,* 8(34).

Grime, J., Blenkinsopp, A., Raynor, D., Pollock, K., and Knapp, P. (2007) 'The role and value of written information for patients about individual medicines: a systematic review', *Health Expectations,* 10(3): 286–298.

Halliday, M.A. (1985) *Spoken and Written Language,* Victoria: Waurn Ponds.

Halliday, M.A.K. (1985/1994) *An Introduction to Functional Grammar,* London: Edward Arnold.

Hasan, R. (1989) *Language, Linguistics and Verbal Art,* Oxford: Oxford University Press.

Haw, C. and Stubbs, J. (2011) 'Patient information leaflets for antidepressants: are patients getting the information they need?', *Journal of Affective Disorders,* 128: 165–170.

Helitzer, D., Hollis, C., Cotner, J., and Oestreicher, N. (2009) 'Health literacy demands of written health information materials: an assessment of cervical cancer prevention materials', *Cancer Control,* 16: 70–78.

Hill, J. and Bird, H. (2003) 'The development and evaluation of a drug information leaflet for patients with rheumatoid arthritis', *Rheumatology,* 42: 66–70.

Hirsh, D., Clerehan, R., Staples, M., Osborne, R., and Buchbinder, R. (2009) 'Patient assessment of medication information leaflets and validation of the Evaluative Linguistic Framework (ELF)', *Patient Education and Counseling,* 77: 248–254.

Johnson, A. and Sandford, J. (2005) 'Written and verbal information versus verbal information only for patients being discharged from acute hospital settings to home: systematic review', *Health Education Research,* 20(4): 423–429.

Kealley, J., Smith, C., and Winser, B. (2005) 'Information empowers but who is empowered?' *Communication and Medicine,* 1(2): 119–129.

Kreps, G. and Bonaguro, B. (2009) 'Health communication as applied communication inquiry', in L. Frey and N. Kissna (eds) *Routledge Handbook of Applied Communication Research,* New York: Routledge.

Kreuter, M. and Wray, R. (2003) 'Tailored and targeted health communication: strategies for enhancing information relevance', *American Journal of Health Behavior,* 27: S227–S232.

Lentz, L. and Pander Maat, H. (1992) 'Evaluating text quality: reader-focused or text-focused?', in H. Pander Maat and M. Steehouder (eds) *Studies of Functional Text Quality*, Amsterdam: Rodopi.
McManus (2009) 'The ideology of patient information leaflets: a diachronic study', *Discourse & Communication*, 3: 27–56.
Martin, J.R. (1997) 'Analysing genre: functional parameters', in F. Christie and J.R. Martin (eds) *Genre and Institutions: Social Processes in the Workplace and School*, London: Cassell.
Martin, J.R. and White, P.R.R. (2005) *The Language of Evaluation: Appraisal in English*, London: Palgrave Macmillan.
Martínez Motos, R. (2012) 'Models of quality assessment for patient package inserts in English and Spanish: a review from the translation perspective', in B. Fischer and M. Nisbeth Jensen (eds) *Translation and the Reconfiguration of Power Relations. Revisiting Role and Context of Translation and Interpreting*, Vienna: LIT.
Mayberry, M. and Mayberry, J. (2002) 'Consent with understanding: a movement towards informed decisions', *Clinical Medicine, Journal of the Royal College of Physicians*, 2: 523–526.
Meade, C. and Smith, C. (1991) 'Readability formulas: cautions and criteria', *Patient Education and Counseling*, 17: 153–158.
Moore, A. and Tuckwell, K. (2006) 'A tenorless genre? Forensic generic profiling of workers' compensation dispute resolution discourse', *Linguistics and the Human Sciences*, 2: 205–232.
Moult, B., Franck, L.S., and Brady, H. (2004) 'Ensuring quality information for patients: development and preliminary validation of a new instrument to improve the quality of written health care information', *Health Expectations*, 7: 165–175.
National Health and Medical Research Council (NHMRC) (1999) 'How to prepare and present evidence-based information for consumers of health services', Canberra: Commonwealth of Australia, Retrieved 2 November 2011, from: http://www.nhmrc.gov.au/guidelines/publications/cp72
Nisbeth Jensen, M. (2012) 'Patient information leaflet translators in the EU: mapping the hypothetical competences of professional translators and pharmacists-cum-translators', in B. Fischer and M. Nisbeth Jensen (eds) *Translation and the Reconfiguration of Power Relations. Revisiting Role and Context of Translation and Interpreting*, Vienna: LIT.
Nisbeth Jensen, M. and Zethsen, K.K. (2012) 'Translation of patient information leaflets: trained translators and pharmacists-cum-translators – a comparison', *Linguistica Antverpiensia NS – Themes in Translation Studies* 11: 31–50.
Pander Maat, H. and Lentz, L. (2010) 'Written patient information: improving the usability of patient information leaflets', *Patient Education and Counseling*, 80: 113–119.
Papen, U. (2010) 'Writing in healthcare contexts: patients, power and medical knowledge', in D. Barton and U. Papen (eds) *The Anthropology of Writing: Understanding Textually Mediated Worlds*, New York: Routledge.
Paul, C., Redman, S., and Sanson-Fisher, R. (1997) 'A review of the effectiveness of print material in changing health-related knowledge, attitudes and behaviour', *Health Promotion Journal of Australia*, 7: 91–99.
——(2003) 'Print material content and design: is it relevant to effectiveness?' *Health Education Research*, 18: 181.
Payne, S., Large, S., Jarrett, N., and Turner, P. (2000) 'Written information given to patients and families by palliative care units: a national survey', *The Lancet*, 355: 1792.
Pound, P., Britten, N., Morgan, M., Yardley, L., Pope, C., Daker-White, G., and Campbell, R. (2005) 'Resisting medicines: a synthesis of qualitative studies of medicine taking', *Social Science and Medicine*, 61: 133–155.
Rees, C., Ford, J., and Sheard, C. (2002) 'Evaluating the reliability of DISCERN: a tool for assessing the quality of written patient information on treatment choices', *Patient Education and Counseling*, 47: 273–275.
Sabharwal, S., Badarudeen, S., and Kunju, S.U. (2008) 'Readability of online patient education materials from the AAOS web site', *Clinical Orthopaedics and Related Research*, 466: 1245–1250.
Schriver, K.A. (2000) 'Readability formulas in the new millennium: what's the use?', *ACM Journal of Computer Documentation*, 24(3): 138–140.
Smith, H., Gooding, S., Brown, R., and Frew, A. (1998) 'Evaluation of readability and accuracy of information leaflets in general practice for patients with asthma', *British Medical Journal*, 317: 264–265.

Smith, S.K., Trevena, L., Nutbeam, D., Barratt, A., and McCaffery, K.J. (2008) 'Information needs and preferences of low and high literacy consumers for decisions about colorectal cancer screening: utilising a linguistic model', *Health Expectations*, 11(2): 123–136.

Swales, J. (1990) *Genre Analysis: English in Academic and Research Settings*, Cambridge: Cambridge University Press.

Wright, P. (1999) 'Writing and information design of healthcare materials', in C. Candlin and K. Hyland (eds) *Writing: Texts, Processes and Practices*, London: Longman.

Zethsen, K. and Askehave, I. (2010) 'PIL of the month – a study of best practice in patient information leaflets', *Journal of Applied Linguistics and Professional Practice*, 7: 97–120.

15

Persuasion vs. information in direct-to-consumer advertising of prescription drugs

Peter J. Schulz and Uwe Hartung

Introduction and definitons

Direct-to-consumer advertising (DTCA) of prescription drugs is a term that does not need a definition; it is self-explanatory. Pharmaceutical companies employ mostly magazines, television, and the Internet for the distribution of these ads, with television nowadays receiving the largest share of advertising expenditure (Donohue et al. 2007).

According to a classification of the United States Food and Drug Administration (FDA), three types of DTCA for prescription drugs can be distinguished: (1) product claim advertisements that make assertions about the product, its application, its effects and side effects, etc., (2) reminder advertisements that display the brand logo or the package, and (3) help-seeking advertisements that recommend individuals with certain conditions to seek treatment, but do not mention any particular medication (Gellad and Lyles 2007; Silver et al. 2009). There are also product claim and reminder ads explicitly or implicitly directed at physicians rather than patients; in this case ads are primarily distributed in medical journals. The object of debate are mostly product claim ads, for which FDA regulations apply, ruling for example that they must contain information of risks, side effects, and contraindications. This means that, in printed ads, for each page of advertising an equal amount of space is usually devoted to cautionary small print.

Advertising prescription medication directly to consumers is a controversial matter. To date, only two countries in the world allow it, the United States and New Zealand. The pharmaceutical industry wants it to be allowed in other countries, but many fear detrimental consequences. Before this background, DTCA has increasingly been critically studied, employing the conceptual apparatus of argumentation theory.

Argumentation theory, and more specifically the pragma-dialectical theory of argumentation (van Eemeren and Grootendorst 1992, 2004), provides a useful framework for the analysis of DTCA (and, by the way, other types of health discourse such as health brochures, e.g., van Poppel 2012, or doctor–patient interaction, e.g., Labrie 2012). The pragma-dialectical theory of argumentation views argumentation as a part of a critical exchange between two parties that is ideally aimed at resolving a difference of opinion. At the heart of the theory lies an ideal model of critical discussion which specifies the different stages that can be distinguished in a critical discussion as well as the corresponding verbal moves that are functional in resolving the issue at stake. The basic principles of a critical discussion are laid down in a set of ten commandments, which constitute a code of conduct for discussants engaging in an argumentative dialogue. Any violation of the code is seen as a hindrance of the resolution process and constitutes a *fallacious* move of argumentation (van Eemeren and Grootendorst 1992, 2004).

The pragma-dialectical ideal model not only provides a normative account of argumentative discourse but can also serve as a descriptive tool for analysts of argumentative discourse. Using the model as a 'blueprint' for constructive argumentative conduct, analysts can describe and assess the argumentation advanced by discussants in actual practice for its reasonableness and, thereby, determine its resolution-oriented character. Taking a pragma-dialectical approach, also the implicit dialogue between the pharmaceutical (the *protagonist*) and the consumer (the *antagonist*) in a DTCA, can be reconstructed as a critical discussion concerning the standpoint 'Buy drug X', or a variation of this claim. Pragma-dialectics allows assessing to what extent pharmaceutical companies advance sound argumentation in ads directed at the patients who consume their products.

History, issues, and topics around DTCA

Motives for advertising prescription drugs to the public

The very idea behind DTCA of prescription drugs appears absurd at first glance. That non-prescription drugs are advertised to consumers is a plausible idea. That prescription drugs are advertised to the persons who hand out the prescription (physicians) is equally plausible. But why advertise prescription drugs to consumers when they cannot go to a store and buy the commodity?

DTCA aims at the patient's involvement in medical decisions. This involvement has at least three relevant aspects. The first is the decision to seek medical help, which is made by the patient and whomever he decides to involve, but without any interference from healthcare providers. This decision is what help-seeking ads aim at.

The second aspect is a mutual power of veto in therapy decision. Employing all her knowledge and experience, the physician has to pick the most advisable therapy in a concrete situation, but she also has the right to object to therapies the patient might suggest if she considers them inadequate.[1] The patient has a similar right of veto in the sense that he can refuse any treatment suggested by the physician. The mutual power of veto to treatment suggestion requires some element of collaboration and consensus building in medical decision-making, and has done that long before concepts such as shared decision-making, patient empowerment, and patient autonomy became guiding principles for patient–physician interaction. It is this element that DTCA aims at addressing: to use the patient's involvement in therapy choice to influence the principal decision-maker, the physician. This is why DTCA poses a special challenge to physicians, who consequently are sceptical of the idea (Robinson et al. 2004; Weissman et al. 2004).

DTCA thus represents a shift in the attempts to influence physicians:

> from the emphasis on the more traditional 'push' strategy to a 'pull' strategy. The push strategy focused on pharmaceutical rep[resentative]s calling on medical providers to provide information and samples of medications which were then prescribed to patients. The pull strategy focuses on promoting the medications to the consumer who in turn will ask the medical provider about the product.
>
> *(Silver et al. 2009: 251)*

The advice to ask a physician about the advertised drug is indeed formulated in many ads in popular magazines (in almost 90 percent according to an unpublished study by the University of Lugano), while ads in medical journals do not formulate a corresponding advice to physicians. Research shows the advice is understood by student study subjects, who are also able to repeat arguments used in the ads (Rubinelli et al. 2008). Rubinelli and colleagues (2008) have rightly stressed that the wording used in many US ads for prescription drugs (variants of 'ask your physician about Drug A') is ambiguous. It can mean 'talk' in the sense of 'inquire with your physician whether Drug A is good for you', or it can mean 'demand', 'get your physician to prescribe Drug A', which puts pressure on the physician to justify his dissenting preference, which takes time and costs money, and which might even induce some physicians to give in to the demand against their better judgment. Thus the best treatment might be missed and unnecessary prescriptions might be handed out.

The patient has one more power of veto, and this is the third aspect of his involvement in medical decision-making. He can privately and without consultation with the physician decide not to comply with her recommendation. Avoiding or reducing non-compliance might also be a motive for DTCA. The ads might affect compliance in two ways: the encounter with advertising for the very same drugs one's physician has prescribed might bolster patients' readiness to do as the doctor said, and it can also be expected that patients are more inclined to comply when a drug was prescribed upon their own suggestion, initiative, or pressure.

Do advertisers have any advantage from compliance? One might argue that pharmaceutical companies should be satisfied if their products are sold; whether they are then also taken is of no concern to them. But this view is short-sighted. If a medication has the effects desired, this must be considered one of the best selling-arguments possible, but the patient can only experience this if she takes the drug. And if a medication does not help, this might only be noticed when the patient stops taking it. In case of chronic illnesses, low compliance moreover means the next refill is due later. Therefore pharmaceutical companies have an economic interest that patients take the medication they bought.

DTCA as an issue in public health policy

Generally DTCA has been allowed in the US since the mid-1980s. A decisive relaxation of rules for broadcast DTCA by the Food and Drug Administration in 1997 has considerably increased this type of advertising. Since 1997, broadcast DTCA has to name only the product's major risks and most frequent adverse effects and give a source where the complete information is available. This can be a toll-free phone number, print material (including ads that run at the time), asking recipients to turn to their healthcare provider for information or a website address (Gellad and Lyles 2007).

The pharmaceutical industry in other parts of the world, mainly in Europe, Australia, and Canada, lobbies lawmakers on many levels to lift the ban and allow DTCA. The European Union so far allows information-based disease awareness campaigns, which are usually conducted by pharmaceutical companies and patient associations together.

The arguments for and against DTCA[2] can be summarized as follows (Mastin et al. 2007; Auton 2004). Proponents argue that DTCA:

- by providing consumers with information and by creating awareness of health conditions improves consumers capabilities of caring for their own health;
- encourages consumers to seek more information elsewhere; and

- educates consumers with regard to, for example, better compliance with drug therapies and motivation to change behaviour.

Opponents argue that DTCA:

- like other advertising motivates consumers to choose overly expensive and overrated medications for needless consumption;
- redirects company funds away from research and other valuable fields and makes the product more expensive;
- instigates unnecessary consultations, tests, and unnecessary or inappropriate drug prescriptions;
- eases the erroneous definition of normal conditions as medical problems (medicalization);
- offers incomplete or misleading information, which leads to wrong decisions;
- offers too many and too strong emotional appeals;
- focuses too much on benefits and too little on risks; and
- changes the traditional physician–patient to a physician–consumer relationship or creates friction between physician and patient or increases physicians' workload.

Two articles, one arguing fervently for DTCA, the other equally engaged against it, published together in the *Journal of Public Policy & Marketing* in 2002, reviewed the evidence available then. The proponent argued that DTCA did not aim at consumer deception, provided information to consumers, instigated consumers to seek more information, did not create friction in consultations, was appreciated by consumers, and had beneficial spill-over effect for patients including better risk awareness, better compliance, and increased health behaviors (Calfee 2002). The critics argued that empirical evidence for many of these claims was painfully weak, that many ads failed to provide crucial information and did not comply with FDA standards, that a gain in accurate information due to exposure to DTCA had never been shown, that many physicians were sceptical about DTCA, that most advertising expenditure went to new medications while most new medications did not have any therapeutic advantage over existing ones, and that no evidence had ever been provided for a positive effect of DTCA on health outcomes (Lexchin and Mintzes 2002).

In as much as DTCA is a health policy issue, the public's thinking on it is relevant. Some studies have found the public to be sceptical of DTCA (e.g., Diehl et al. 2008).

Increasing role of DTCA

That DTCA is a reality only in the US and New Zealand has already been mentioned, as has the fact that it became more common in the US after changes in FDA rules in 1997. Recent developments, however, have augmented the possible functions and significance of DTCA, likely to increase the pressure to allow it in other countries. One development is technical, the advent of the Internet and the possibility of buying online. The other is normative, the ideal of the patient who participates actively in medical decision-making.

Online pharmacies have become an issue of concern (e.g., Orizio et al. 2009). As the Web is worldwide, you can easily buy prescription drugs from countries with more lenient rules on drug trade. There are also devices that circumvent true diagnosis and treatment decision processes, such as 'diagnosis' with ensuing prescription of medication by an anonymous 'physician' (who might or might not be real) after the patient filled in and sent a questionnaire.

Whatever the details in practice and regulation of online pharmacies, they do offer to some degree the possibility for acquisition of prescription drugs without having a prescription. The higher this potential, the more sense does DTCA make.

The traditional role of the physician is nowadays often referred to as paternalistic. Almost as in a caricature, physicians of past generations are conceived as figures of authority who, after anamnesis, examination, and tests, knew what the patient suffered from and accordingly chose the therapy that was best for her. A need to involve the patient, to explain the criteria for treatment decisions, to lay out alternatives – all that did not exist. This conception is contrasted by a more modern approach in which the physician involves the patient in decision-making, giving the patient the chance of participating more actively in the decision, to the benefit of both (Epstein et al. 1993). Concepts that advocate the new ideal include shared decision-making, the expert patient, health literacy, and patient empowerment. The more the ideal corresponds to reality, the more sense does it make to address consumers directly by advertising prescription drugs. Although notions of increasing patient participation and DTCA have very different origins – the former rooted in ideals of autonomy, self-determination, and maybe even democracy, the other in the commercial interests of the pharmaceutical industry – they get along rather well.

Current research

Effects of DTCA

Most of the arguments for and against allowing DTCA adduce consequences of these ads. Therefore research into the effects of DTCA is immediately relevant for the health policy issue. Three kinds of effects can be distinguished: (1) effects that coincide with the economic intention of the advertisers (increased sales, better product awareness, improved product evaluation, increased readiness to try the product, etc.); (2) unintended benefits (increased knowledge of diseases and their treatment, increased awareness of diseases, etc.); and (3) unintended damages (creating unnecessary demand for particular drugs, raising expectations addressed at pharmacological treatment to unreasonable levels, etc.). The existence of unintended benefits is likely to be controversial as proponents of DTCA may claim unintended were actually intended benefits, a claim hard to refute and hard to prove.

Methods for studying the effects of DTCA are as diverse as in advertising effects research in general. Every method has advantages and disadvantages. Controlled experiments are the best way to establish causality, but under the demands of controlling it is very difficult if not impossible to simulate exposure realistically, e.g., capturing the low salience of the ads in everyday life and the cumulative nature of their impact. Surveys have, in contrast, higher external validity but cannot equally well claim to be able to establish causality.

Frank Auton in 2004 summarized that opinions on DTCA were 'highly polarised and despite numerous studies and research there [was] as yet an absence of conclusive evidence about the real impact of DTCA' (Auton 2004: 5). Despite more studies conclusive evidence is still lacking.

The foremost effect is that on sales. One way to study this is to compare aggregate advertising spending with indicators of consumption or sales figures. Donohue et al. (2004), for instance, compared periods of high spending on DTCA with periods with low spending and found that there was a 32 percent higher probability of starting to take antidepressants during the former. Additionally, evidence suggested that DTCA for a particular drug increases the demand for the class of drugs, but not necessarily the market share of the advertised brand. Another study by the same group could make use of individual-level prescriptions of antidepressants for as many as 25,000 individuals, as well as of monthly industry spending on DTCA for six different brands of drugs, detailing to physicians (marketing by pharmaceutical representatives) for the very same medications and a number of patient variables and medication characteristics. In a nutshell, the study finds again that DTCA increases the market for antidepressants but detailing affects the choice of brand (Donohue and Berndt 2004).

Economic data indicate that, in the years after the liberalization of rules for DTCA in the US, the drug market grew. Drug expenditure, with annual growth rates between 17 and 19 percent, increased much more than other health expenditures. This was due to price increases, a shift to more expensive drugs and an increased number of prescriptions. Pharmaceutical promotion expenditure increased by approximately 16 percent annually, with DTCA expenditure slightly increasing its share. By far the largest part of industry promotion expenditure goes into promotion to healthcare providers. By far most DTCA expenditure (roughly 90 percent) goes into television (for details see Auton 2004: 14–20).

Increasing product awareness and medical knowledge are also among the effects claimed by DTCA proponents. In a survey study of 285 college students, An et al. (2009) found that high exposure to antidepressant TV spots improved respondents' ability to recognize depression cases, increased their awareness of antidepressants as a treatment option, and augmented their evaluation of this type of drug. The effect could be observed only in students who had never experienced depressive symptoms themselves. Note that the second and third effect are among the desired ones (as seen from the perspective of the advertiser), while the first will have to be counted as an unintended beneficial side effect. But note also that the effects may also constitute a social problem as some college students might be inclined to use antidepressants as recreational drugs to feel better, and the ads show them what they have to tell their physician to get a prescription. This is why DTCA for drugs prescribed against mood disorders are especially controversial.

Third, effects on social perception were studied. A recent study using a source-priming manipulation found that participants based their judgement of the prevalence of depression on antidepressant ads. Those who remembered seeing more antidepressant ads tended to believe that there were more people suffering from depression than those who remembered fewer ads (An et al. 2009).

Fourth, there are diverse aspects of possible effects of DTCA on the physician–patient relationship, and several methods to study this. Blose and Mack (2009), for instance, conducted an experiment using scenarios to investigate likely patient reactions to a physician denying a specific prescription demand. Denial led to many negative patient outcomes, but only for males in life-threatening scenarios. Irrespective of the situation, females tended to be dissatisfied with the consultation when denied a prescription request.

As was stated, a definitive picture is hard to draw. Auton (2004), in summary of his review of effect studies, considers two effects likely: more knowledgeable patients (entailing knowledge when to seek treatment as well as willingness to change behaviour in aspects relevant to health) and increased demand for unnecessary and inappropriate treatment, including lifestyle drugs against, e.g., being overweight and baldness. He also calls for evidence on cost/benefit relations in the short as well as the long run, from the patient and the social perspective, before DTCA can be allowed.

Argumentative contents of prescription drug ads

The contents of DTCA have been subject to investigation. A major concern was the informative value of DTCA. Bell et al. (2000) studied 320 ads from 18 popular magazines, mostly pre-1997. They found that most ads named the condition treated by the promoted drug and described the symptoms. Shortcomings existed with regard to precursors, prevalence, attempts to clarify misconceptions, mechanism of action, success rate, treatment details, and health behaviour changes capable of supporting therapy or reducing its necessity (see also Frosch et al. (2007) for comparable results on television spots). A more recent review concluded that the evidence supports the purported benefits of DTCA such as providing information, which can contribute to consumers' level of information and improve their communication with healthcare providers (Taylor et al. 2007).

A second concern of content analysis research is compliance with FDA standards. In a study of 39 ads on medication prescribed for bleeding disorders, Abel et al. (2008) concluded about one-third of the claims in these ads were not based on sufficient evidence and that information on risk and adverse effects was shorter and more difficult to read than information on benefits. This fails to meet FDA standards, which demand a balanced treatment of both.

Another concern has been the subtle cultural messages DTCA may convey about health and illness and the treatability of conditions, all with the potential to foster health beliefs in the population, some of which can easily become dysfunctional. A special concern in this regard is with the socio-demographic structure of the persons depicted in these ads (e.g., Mastin et al. 2007; Ball et al. 2009), which is relevant for the claim that DTCA might help to remove health disparities between gender, race, and other groups.

Only little attention was paid until recently to the arguments that are used in these ads to support the ad's central claim that patients with a particular medical condition are well advised to ask their physician to prescribe a particular medication. The study of such 'selling arguments' is based on argumentation theory (van Eemeren and Grootendorst 2004) and thus links the study of language with the field of public health. One of the rare studies looking at the selling arguments finds incomplete syllogisms in ads that aim at the medicalization of mood disorders (Arney and Rafalovich 2007). Bell et al. (2000) found the effectiveness of the advertised drug to be the most frequently used argument. Another study found that emotional appeals were far more prevalent than rational appeals in the promotional portion of DTCA. Slightly more than one-third of the ads made a rational appeal, while nearly 89 percent made an emotional appeal. The study covers the promotional section of ads and both verbal and pictorial messages (Main et al. 2004). Studies such as these support the claim that DTCA are texts primarily intended to persuade, not primarily to inform (which they also do, as stated).

There are primarily two types of studies addressing the arguments in the ads: (1) studies that qualitatively analyse a small number of arguments in depth, and (2) studies that quantitatively classify a large number of arguments according to selected criteria.

In-depth analysis of arguments and fallacies

Research of this type is concerned with the possibility that the economic motivations behind the ads might induce advertisers to use arguments in a fallacious way, which comes down to misinforming recipients and thus compromises the informative function claimed by proponents of DTCA. The problem can be illustrated by an analysis by Rubinelli et al. (2008), which focuses on just two ads and combines the scrutiny of the ads with a reception study conducted with students. The authors found that an ad for the anti-allergy prescription drug

Allegra 180 mg used subtle means to present itself as more unique than it actually was. The major premise adduced in the ad was, 'One dose of *Allegra 180mg* lasts up to 4x longer than one dose of most OTC [over the counter] allergy medicines', providing relief from allergies for 24 hours. It was illustrated by a heap of packages for three over-the-counter anti-allergy medicines, said to last for only six hours, on the top of which Allegra180mg was presented. This presentation is misleading in two respects. First, the depicted medication brands are also available in dosages that last longer than the six hours mentioned, and second, there are other brands that also last 24 hours, which are not mentioned or depicted in the ad at all. The premise, in other words, is technically correct, but the ad suggests Allegra 180 mg is more unique than it really is. The suggestion is primarily created by omission. A second critique of the same ad also refers to omission: Counterindications to the high-dosage Allegra were banned to the small print section, and not noticed by student readers in an experiment. Using design as a means to stress benefits and downplay risks is seen by the authors as an example of the fallacy of relevance.

A third critique was directed at an ad for the anti-depressant Zoloft. Respondents in the reception study were asked which premises from the ad they recognized and offered some premises in fact adduced in the ad, but also some which were not, although they were in line with what the ad claimed. A majority of respondents, for instance, said the ad claimed that 'taking Zoloft will make you happy'. In fact, the ad did not say anything to this effect, but it claimed that life with depression was hard and that Zoloft helps against depression. One can rightfully conclude from the two claims that Zoloft makes your life less hard, but if this is happiness, it is happiness as a measurable quantity, not happiness in the metaphysical sense of the word. The claim that student respondents recognized was thus more grandiose than the actual claims contained in the ad. This can be considered an example of invited inference (Rubinelli et al. 2006). A fourth critique is raised against the same ad, and it also addresses omission. The ad does not really reveal that all claims of a causal link between taking Zoloft and getting better are based on probability only, and may not work in individual cases.

Further experiments with manipulated ads from which the problematic parts were removed showed that subjects who read the modified ads were clearly less certain about their recall of reasons not mentioned in the ads, compared to subjects who saw the original ads. This suggests that the modified ad was less likely to cue inaccurate inferences. That respondents found these ads less persuasive also suggests that the strategic use of the faulty argument structure by the advertiser can have a persuasive impact, implying that the intended persuasive effect of the ads indeed rests to some degree on misinformation.

Further criticism of the same two ads points out more examples of fallacies. There is a fallacy of ambiguity in the Zoloft ad statement, 'You get one performance. Why do it with depression?' This statement has an indeterminate meaning caused by the loose way in which its words are used and combined. The sentence does not explicitly say that Zoloft stops depression, but it suggests this, and readers understand it. There is a suggestive element in the assertion that after taking Zoloft a cartoon character realized that the medicine was helping him at work and at home, suggesting a positive resolution of the problematic aspects of one's entire life. Again in the Zoloft ad, we find the fallacy of hasty generalization when it is claimed that Zoloft has treated more people than any other brand. This is misleading because the fact does not assure that the medicine will work well for the reader as an individual, although the claim may make people think that Zoloft will be good for them as it has been good for many others. We can also observe the fallacy of relevance when it is claimed that Zoloft is the most prescribed anti-depressant. There is no causal link between this fact and the drug's quality (Rubinelli et al. 2006).

Research such as this reveals examples of the use of fallacious argumentation in DTCA, which shows clear elements of misinformation and casts doubt on the proponents' claim that these ads serve to inform patients.

Classification of a large number of arguments

A comprehensive study of selling arguments was done at the Institute of Communication and Health (ICH) of the Università della Svizzera italiana, Lugano, in cooperation with the Department of Marketing of the Virginia Polytechnic Institute and State University, Blacksburg. The content analysis covered all advertisements for medical prescription drugs in the *Journal of the American Medical Association, New England Journal of Medicine, Time, Good Housekeeping* in the period 2002–2007. The journals and magazines were chosen to allow comparison of ads directed to a medical audience (the readers of the two scientific journals) with ads directed to consumers (the readers of the two magazines).

The analysis is based on 756 unique ads containing 3,837 selling arguments. Several ads were published repeatedly. If publications are counted, the number of ads is 1,686, containing 8,592 selling arguments. Approximately 71 percent of the ads appeared in the two medical journals; the remaining 29 percent were published in the two popular magazines. If the addressee is coded independent of the medium, the expected relationships emerge: 99 percent of the ads that appeared in popular magazines were directed at patients, while 66 percent of ads in medical journals aimed at physicians (5 percent at patients, 10 percent at both, and 19 percent could not be decided).

Every ad is understood to make the claim 'use this drug', or 'consider using this drug', or 'ask your physician about this drug', or 'prescribe this drug', depending on the addressee. A majority of ads in magazines formulates the claim, while a majority of ads in medical journals does not explicitly formulate anything that comes close to this claim, as Table 15.1 shows.

Table 15.1 Formulation of major claim in prescription drug advertisements (unique ads)

	Medical journals (n = 460) %	*Popular magazines (n = 296)* %	*Total (n = 756)* %
Claim is strongly formulated	10.0	1.4	6.6
Claim is weakly formulated	4.3	80.4	34.1
Claim is very weakly formulated	0.9	5.7	2.8
Relevant claim is not formulated at all	80.0	5.7	50.9
Claim is not directed to a medicament but to a disease the medicament is prescribed for	1.7	3.4	2.4
Claim is not addressed at prescription but at a previous step (e.g., 'ask for free samples', 'ask sales representative')	3.0	3.4	3.2
Total	100.0	100.0	100.0

Source: Content analysis of all advertisements for medical prescription drugs in the *Journal of the American Medical Association, New England Journal of Medicine, Time, Good Housekeeping*, 2002–2007.

Note: Every ad is understood to make the claim 'use this drug' or 'consider using this drug', or 'ask your physician about this drug', or 'prescribe this drug', depending on the addressee.

The medical conditions against which the advertised drugs are used show a great variety, as Table 15.2 illustrates. Interestingly, medication against some conditions are advertised more in medical journals and/or in ads directed at physicians. These conditions include cardiovascular diseases, depression and anxiety, and diabetes. On the other hand, drugs against allergies, asthma, and attention-deficit hyperactivity disorder (ADHD) are almost exclusively advertised to medical laity.

Table 15.2 Types of drugs advertised in different media and to different addressees in ads as published

	Medium of publication		*Addressee of ada*		*Total*
	Medical journal %	*Popular magazine* %	*Physician* %	*Patient* %	%
Cardiovascular diseases	20	17	24	15	19
Depression, anxieties	17	8	19	9	14
Diabetes, high blood sugar	11	3	9	6	9
Arthritis, rheumatism, etc.	6	6	7	6	6
Heartburn, stomach problems	5	7	4	7	6
Sleeping pills, insomnia	6	4	8	3	6
Erectile dysfunction, impotence	5	5	4	6	5
Alzheimer	5	3	8	2	5
Allergies of any kind, hay fever	x	11	x	10	3
Antibiotics	4	–	3	–	3
Migraine	2	4	2	4	3
Asthma	–	7	–	7	2
Osteoporosis	1	5	1	5	2
Attention-deficit hyperactivity disorder (ADHD)	–	6	–	6	2
Cancer	1	5	1	4	2
Pain relievers	2	x	2	1	1
Overactive bladder	x	3	x	3	1
Parkinson, Restless legs syndrome	1	1	1	1	1
Fungal infection	–	2	–	2	1
Common cold, sinusitis, rhinosinusitis	–	x	–	x	x
Other	5	4	6	3	5
Type of drug cannot be identified	9	–	3	2	7
Total	100	101	102	102	101
(N)	(1,197)	(489)	(541)	(798)	(1,686)

Source: Content analysis of all advertisements for medical prescription drugs in the *Journal of the American Medical Association*, *New England Journal of Medicine*, *Time*, *Good Housekeeping*, 2002–2007.

Notes

x = less than 0.5 %.

[a] Not shown: Addressed to both and Cannot be decided

The majority of selling arguments in DTCA are variations of the contention that the advertised drug is efficacious. More than two-thirds of all selling arguments in medical journals and/or in those directed at physicians state, in various ways, that the advertised drug helps. This argument is used less frequently in ads in popular magazines and those directed at patients, but it still makes up half of all arguments used. These arguments include statements that the drug helps, that their effect endures over a long period, that it helps comprehensively, that it helps fast. The only other notable difference is the arguments that deal with the disease rather than the medication. These include statements that the condition is bad and causes a lot of suffering, that it is incapacitating, painful, makes life difficult, that it means high risk for other and worse diseases, that it is embarrassing, and that it is widespread, occurs often, that many people have it. These arguments do not support, in terms of formal logic, the claim that it is good to use drug A against condition B. They rather imply that something can be done against unnecessary suffering and embarrassment. They pursue a similar aim as the help-seeking advertisements mentioned at the beginning of this chapter. In contrast to help-seeking ads, which by definition did and do not name any particular product, the arguments directed at the disease are usually juxtaposed to others that aim at (and name) a specific medication, and because they appear in the context of a product ad, one can expect recipients to make the connection. These arguments are, as are the help-seeking ads, an aspect of what is sometimes called disease marketing, a phenomenon discussed in connection with the tendency towards medicalization. Using these arguments (more often in ads in magazines and those directed at customers, as Table 15.3 shows), DTCA might contribute to medicalization.

Table 15.3 Selling arguments in ads as published in different media and to different addressees

	Medium of publication		*Addressee of ad*[a]		
	Medical journal (n = 5395) %	*Popular magazine (n = 3197) %*	*Physician (n = 4089) %*	*Patient (n = 3436) %*	*Total (n = 8592) %*
Variations of: Medicament helps	71	50	71	52	63
Arguments directed at the disease drug is prescribed for	4	18	4	17	9
Variations of: no/low side effects	7	11	8	10	9
Arguments directed at research and development	7	9	8	9	8
Arguments directed at use	6	5	6	4	6
Variations of: widely used	3	4	3	4	4
Fringe benefits	x	3	x	3	1
Medicament is cheap, good cost–benefit relation	x	x	x	x	x
Other	1	x	1	x	1
Total	99	100	101	99	101

Source: Content analysis of all advertisements for medical prescription drugs in the *Journal of the American Medical Association*, *New England Journal of Medicine*, *Time*, *Good Housekeeping*, 2002–2007.

Notes

x = less than 0.5 %.

[a] Not shown: Addressed to both and Cannot be decided

This analysis suggests that in patient-oriented ads the fallacy of omission, which is associated with the disease-oriented arguments, might be a more widespread problem than the fallacy of hasty generalization associated with the argument of a drug being widely used.

Future directions

Analyses of the first type clearly have a potential to detect and explain dubious or fallacious argumentative elements, but have in practice been applied to a few examples only. Even if such work is continued, the database will necessarily remain small, and the question of how typical such malpractice is of the ads in general cannot really be answered. Analyses of the second type have identified structural features of the arguments used in DTCA and tell what types of medications are advertised and which arguments are used, etc. They can be conducted, at acceptable cost, for as large a sample as one wishes, but they remain descriptive. That is to say: content analysis studies have so far not helped much in detecting problems in the pharmaceutical industry's reasoning in DTCA. As mentioned, the analysis tells us that the ad populo argument that a particular medicine is widely used does not occur very often. Argumentation theory frowns upon this type of argument, but it is not always fallacious in the context of DTCA. So neither method alone can tell us the extent of the problem in using this argument.

Clearly a combination of the two methods has to be found which combines the advantages of both in data collection. A method has to be developed that allows the identification of fallacies on a wider scope than just in a few ads. That could be done either by enabling coders to identify fallacies or by having them code features that allow the identification of fallacies in data analysis. As the evidence for pronouncing an argument fallacious often lies in subtle details and displays high variety, and as it sometimes can be won only by researching external conditions, the first method appears to be the more promising choice. The challenge is to keep the codebook so simple that it can be used, after an acceptable time of training, by coders who have not majored in argumentation.

Related topics

Requests and refusals in primary care visits for pain management; language and discourse in the exchange of actionable health information; direct-to-consumer advertising; argumentation theory.

Notes

1 This is not meant to describe the legal situation in its full complexity, which binds the physician to complex rules and regulations. The veto is applicable only within this legal framework.
2 The arguments in a conflict over a public issue such as DTCA also provide a field of application for argumentation theory, but that is of no concern here.

Further reading

Auton, F. (2004) 'The advertising of pharmaceuticals direct to consumers: a critical review of the literature and debate', *International Journal of Advertising*, 23(1): 5–52. (Rich background information on many different aspects of the controversy.)

Calfee, J.E. (2002) 'Public policy issues in direct-to-consumer advertising of prescription drugs', *Journal of Public Policy & Marketing,* 21: 174–193. (A good summary of the arguments for DTCA, supported by scientific evidence.)

Lexchin, J. and Mintzes, B. (2002) 'Direct-to-consumer advertising of prescription drugs: the evidence says no', *Journal of Public Policy & Marketing,* 21: 194–201. (A good summary of the arguments against DTCA, supported by scientific evidence.)

Lyles, A. (2002) 'Direct marketing of pharmaceuticals to consumers', *Annual Review of Public Health,* 23: 73–91. (Overview of the controversy around DTCA with much background on US regulation history.)

References

Abel, G.A., Neufeld, E.J., Sorel, M., and Weeks, J.C. (2008) 'Direct-to-consumer advertising for bleeding disorders: a content analysis and expert evaluation of advertising claims', *Journal of Thrombosis and Haemostasis,* 6: 1680–1684.

An, S., Jin, H.S., and Brown, J.D. (2009) 'Direct-to-consumer antidepressant ads and young adults' beliefs about depression', *Health Marketing Quarterly,* 26: 259–278.

Arney, J. and Rafalovich, A. (2007) 'Incomplete syllogisms as techniques of medicalisation: the case of direct-to-consumer advertising in popular magazines, 1997 to 2003', *Qualitative Health Research,* 17(1): 49–60.

Auton, F. (2004) 'The advertising of pharmaceuticals direct to consumers: a critical review of the literature and debate', *International Journal of Advertising,* 23(1): 5–52.

Ball, J.G., Liang, A., and Lee, W.-N. (2009) 'Representation of African Americans in direct-to-consumer pharmaceutical commercials: a content analysis with implications for health disparities', *Health Marketing Quarterly,* 26: 372–390

Bell, R.A., Wilkes, M.S., and Kravitz, R.L. (2000) 'The educational value of consumer-targeted prescription drug print advertising', *Journal of Family Practice,* 49: 1092–1098.

Blose, J.E. and Mack, R.W. (2009) 'The impact of denying a direct-to-consumer advertised drug request on the patient/physician relationship', *Health Marketing Quarterly,* 26: 315–332.

Calfee, J.E. (2002) 'Public policy issues in direct-to-consumer advertising of prescription drugs', *Journal of Public Policy & Marketing,* 21: 174–193.

Diehl, S., Mueller, B., and Terlutter, R. (2008) 'Consumer responses towards non-prescription and prescription drug advertising in the US and Germany', *International Journal of Advertising,* 27(1): 99–131.

Donohue, J.M. and Berndt, E.R. (2004) 'Effects of direct-to-consumer advertising on medication choice: the case of antidepressants', *Journal of Public Policy and Marketing,* 23: 115–127.

Donohue, J.M., Berndt, E.R., Rosenthal, M., Epstein, A.M., and Frank, R.G. (2004) 'Effects of pharmaceutical promotion on adherence to the treatment guidelines for depression', *Medical Care,* 42: 1176–1185.

Donohue, J.M., Cevasco, M., and Rosenthal M.B. (2007) 'A decade of direct-to-consumer advertising of prescription drugs', *New England Journal of Medicine,* 357: 673–681.

Eemeren, F.H. van and Grootendorst, R. (1992) *Argumentation, Communication, and Fallacies,* Hillsdale, NJ: Lawrence Erlbaum.

——(2004) *A Systematic Theory of Argumentation: The Pragma-dialectical Approach,* Cambridge: Cambridge University Press.

Epstein, R.M., Campbell, T.L., Cohen-Cole, S.A., McWhinney, I.R., and Smilkstein, G. (1993) 'Perspectives on patient–doctor communication', *Journal of Family Practice,* 37: 377–388.

Frosch, D., Krueger, P.M., Hornik, R.C., Cronholm, P.F., and Barg, F.K. (2007) 'Creating demand for prescription drugs: a content analysis of television direct-to-consumer advertising', *Annals of Family Medicine,* 5(1): 6–13.

Gellad, Z.F. and Lyles, K.W. (2007) 'Direct-to-consumer advertising of pharmaceuticals', *American Journal of Medicine,* 120: 475–480.

Labrie, N.H.M. (2012) 'Strategic maneuvering in treatment decision-making discussions: two cases in point', *Argumentation,* 26(2): 171–199.

Lexchin, J. and Mintzes, B. (2002) 'Direct-to-consumer advertising of prescription drugs: the evidence says no', *Journal of Public Policy & Marketing,* 21: 194–201.

Main, K.J., Argo, J.J., and Huhmann, B.A. (2004) 'Pharmaceutical advertising in the USA: information or influence?', *International Journal of Advertising*, 23(1): 119–142.

Mastin, T, Andsager, J.L., Choi, J., and Lee, K. (2007) 'Health disparities and direct-to-consumer prescription drug advertising: a content analysis of targeted magazine genres, 1992–2002', *Health Communication*, 22(1): 49–58.

Orizio, G., Schulz, P., Domenighini, S., Bressanelli, M., Rubinelli, S., Caimi, L., and Gelatti, U. (2009) 'Online consultations in cyberpharmacies: completeness and patient safety', *Telemedicine Journal and e-Health*, 15: 1022–1025.

Poppel, L. van (2012) 'The strategic function of variants of pragmatic argumentation in health brochures', *Journal of Argumentation in Context,* 1(1): 97–112.

Robinson, A.R., Hohmann, K.B., Rifkin, J.I. et al. (2004) 'Direct-to-consumer pharmaceutical advertising: physician and public opinion and potential effects on the physician–patient relationship', *Archive of Internal Medicine*, 164: 427–432.

Rubinelli, S., Nakamoto, K., Schulz, P., and De Saussure, L. (2006) 'What are we to think about consumer advertising? A case-study in the field of misinterpreted argumentation', *Studies in Communication Sciences,* 6: 337–348.

Rubinelli, S., Nakamoto, K., and Schulz, P.J. (2008) 'The rabbit in the hat: dubious argumentation and the persuasive effects of prescription drug advertising (DTCA)', *Communication & Medicine,* 5: 49–58.

Silver, L.S., Stevens, R.E., and Loudon, D. (2009) 'Direct-to-consumer advertising of pharmaceuticals: concepts, issues, and research', *Health Marketing Quarterly*, 26: 251–258.

Taylor, C.R., Capella, M.L., and Kozup, J.C. (2007) 'Does DTC advertising provide information or create market power? Evidence from the U.S. and New Zealand', *Cross-Cultural Buyer Behavior,* 18: 9–30.

Weissman, J.S., Blumenthal, D., Silk A.J. et al. (2004) 'Physicians report on patient encounters involving direct-to-consumer advertising', *Health Affairs,* 4: 219–233.

Part II

Health professionals' communicative practices

16

Why read and write in the clinic?

The contributions of narrative medicine to health care

Rita Charon

At a medical conference on evidence-based medicine, that branch of clinical practice which strives to restrict its actions to those that have demonstrated efficacy, I was invited to run a workshop on narrative medicine. A small group that included pediatricians, geriatricians, an intensive care specialist, a pulmonary specialist, and emergency medicine doctors read a poem with me, talked about it, and then wrote in its shadow. My aim with this group of physicians committed to improving the scientific accuracy of their clinical decision-making was to enlist them in recognizing the evidence contained in language and to motivate them to learn how to capture evidence from what people say or write (Goyal et al. 2008). First, we read together Lucille Clifton's poem 'the death of fred clifton' (Clifton 2000):

the death of fred clifton
11/10/84, age 49

i seemed to be drawn
to the center of myself
leaving the edges of me
in the hands of my wife
and i saw with the most amazing
clarity
so that i had not eyes but
sight,
and, rising and turning,
through my skin,
there was all around not the
shapes of things
but oh, at last, the things
themselves.

(Clifton 2000: 51)

The doctors in the group grasped the image of centers and edges of persons. They understood the poem perhaps to be a poet-wife's wish that her husband had had a peaceful, even serene death. They appreciated the gravity and beauty of the phrase 'rising and turning, through my skin' as an image of the dying act, and they compared that image to the actual deaths they had witnessed. They wondered aloud what their own centers and edges might be, and to whom they could entrust parts of themselves. The writing prompt I provided, with four minutes in which to write in response to it, was: 'Write about the things themselves.'

The intensive care specialist, who had initially read the poem rather concretely ('rising and turning, through my skin' sounded to him like what the nurses do to patients to prevent bedsores), took a long time to get started. He ended with four words on his paper. He was the first to offer to read aloud what he had written. Here is what he had written in the shadow of Clifton's poem:

> Love
> Family
> Work
> Joy

When I asked the group to consider the genre of what he had written, we together recognized that he seemed to have written the motto for his own personal crest. He 'saw with the most amazing clarity' that these four words, emerging from deep inside him, uttered something true about his hopes for his own life. From then on, he was deeply and seemingly joyously engaged in the proceedings of my workshop.

I feel oddly sure that our work on this poem will at least invite this physician to *see deaths differently* in his own intensive care unit. Were he engaged in ongoing narrative training in his hospital, he would have the chance once a week or once a month to read and write so as to express and therefore to *see* the evidence of what he witnesses and undergoes.

Introduction

I want to invite health communication scholars and linguists and rhetoricians who study healthcare discourse to consider the narrative dimensions of health, illness, and health care. Not only the conversations between doctor and patient or the materials of so-called patient education can be fruitfully studied linguistically. So can the disease processes themselves, the responses of the person to shifts in the workings of his or her body, the positions of those listening to accounts of illness, and the cultures of health care. In describing health, illness, and health care as narrative events requiring narrative skill, I am widening the purview of the health communication practitioner to encompass the very foundations of what it means to have a body.

Narrative medicine proposes that narrative acts – having a sense of story, telling, listening, reading, writing, witnessing, imagining, remembering – are at the center of clinical care. The sick person must, before anything, give an account of his or her illness. Giving an account of one's illness entails giving an account of oneself. Those charged with the care of the sick must know how to receive these accounts. The neonatologist caring for a baby too young and ill to live, the chemotherapy nurse administering toxic medicines known by just about everyone involved to be futile, the social worker seeking organ donation from the grieving parents of a kid killed in a motorcycle accident, the physical therapist introducing the spinal-cord-injured patient to his new life as a paraplegic, the chaplain called to the Emergency

Room to break the news of death to the fireman's wife, the autism spectrum clinic receptionist who cannot comprehend the repetitive motor actions of the children in the waiting room – all are placed in challengingly close quarters to explosive or implosive events of illness as they unfold in strangers' lives. To give respectful and effective health care in all these such settings, the professional, whether a clinician or administrator or clerical staff person, has to know why he or she is there, has to accept the responsibility of witnessing someone else's suffering, and has to comprehend both logically and emotionally what is the matter and what is at stake.

The skills that might enable one to do these complex tasks in the face of illness are, I suggest, narrative skills – the capacities to cohere fragmented facts and findings into meaning, to recognize and convey what is being heard in another's account of illness, and to offer oneself as a witness to suffering. Narrative medicine is a clinical practice fortified by exactly these skills – the skills of hearing and recognizing stories, absorbing them, telling them, writing them, letting one's practice be amplified by the knowledge one obtains by attentive listening to what patients say and what one, as a clinician, might perceive about that patient. Since 2000, narrative medicine has grown exponentially, from a circle of clinicians and scholars at Columbia University in New York to an international network of narrativists and clinicians who are discovering the power of developing narrative skills for the care of the sick. Through training programs including intensive weekend workshops, a required curriculum for medical students at Columbia, a graduate program conferring a Master of Science in Narrative Medicine degree, and extensive international visits and training workshops, the Program in Narrative Medicine at Columbia has researched, refined, and developed the emerging conceptions and practices of this field.

The self-telling body

A person suffers a large stroke. He loses the power of speech and can only say 'mem-mem-mem' over and over. He is brought by ambulance to the hospital, emergently given an MRI of his brain, found to have had a devastatingly large stroke encompassing the language processing centers of the brain, established in a neurological intensive care unit berth, given medication to thin his blood and slow his heart rate and drop his blood pressure. His wife rushes intensively to his side to find him able to say only 'mem-mem-mem'. The person undergoing this stroke is poet and novelist Paul West and his wife is writer Diane Ackerman. Captured in Ackerman's brilliant memoir *A Hundred Names for Love*, the sequelae of West's massive stroke unfold over years and years of his physical therapy, speech therapy, writing again, reading again, always loving, always able to reach, deeply and movingly, the continent of his wife's love (Ackerman 2011). As I read this memoir, I realize what this marriage needs to 'recover' from this stroke – way beyond the anti-coagulation medicine and MRIs and braces for the dropping foot. The stroke ushers in a 'whole new life', to use the title of novelist Reynolds Price's memoir of living with his spinal cord tumor, that contrasts with and conflicts with and dazzles and illuminates the life that came before it (Price 1994).

Living as human beings do in or with or by virtue of bodies, and accepting as the conditions of living both corporeality and finality, the 'situation' of the self is always and ever tied to the situation of the body. The accounts of self are, in health care, amplified by the self-telling body. Bodies tell of selves in myriad ways. Not only can the spinal-cord-injured survivor of a gunshot wound tell of his attack in words, but the flaccid tone of his muscles, the upward-going flexion of his great toe, the demarcation along his upper thorax between skin that senses pinprick and skin that does not add to the account. These physical 'tellings' tell things that he, 'himself', does not know. The rehabilitation medicine doctor and the physical therapist interpret for him that which can only be told in the language of the body (Mattingly 1998). They translate what his body tells them into words that his 'self' might understand – you will never walk, you will never breathe, you will yet live.

Being sick, facing death, and dying are among the most challenging and honorable things humans do. Whether a patient is afflicted with an acute reversible sickness, a chronic illness, or a terminal disease, the very act of seeking health care 'admits' the fact that one's body can break its silence of health. Even the healthy person seeking preventive care or health-promoting care is aware of the potential for health to slow down. Sometimes the former state of health cannot be regained and the patient has to accept an altered state. Such events sometimes challenge a patient's very notion of who he or she is – now he or she is the person who cannot speak, now the person who cannot remember, now the person who cannot see, now the person whose cancer has come back for the final time. Those healthcare professionals who are relatively healthy can appreciate the *work* being done by the ill – the wherewithal to soldier on despite pain, despite uncertainly, despite all the losses. Those who are relatively healthy can stand in awe of the vision and ballast that must be required for a person to endure such reversals.

Because human beings are mortal, they 'carry' with them or are carried by bodies that operate systems of life – systems that take in nourishment, systems that extract needed gases from the universe and exhaust unwanted gases into it, systems that bring needed molecules – sugars, proteins, oxygen, fats, elements – to all tissues of the body, systems that recognize the difference between self and not-self, systems that permit sensation, perception, locomotion, and thought. Because these are physical systems that rely on chemical and biological *matter* and because the events governed by these systems are, on the whole, observable and even measureable, it is commonly thought that those who oversee or shepherd these systems need to know about chemical and biological matter. And yet we all know, from the time we are children, that our selves and our bodies exceed the realms of matter and enter the realms of dream, laughter, beauty, love, fear, fantasy, play, sadness, pain, and worry. In short, we have mental lives, metaphorical lives, aesthetic lives, emotional lives, lives of relation and attachment, and concepts of being selves. Narrative medicine admits all these dimensions into the care of the sick, not as 'humanistic' add-ons but as, well, the things themselves.

The sense of story

The capacities to imagine, perceive, and pay attention to that which a marriage needs in order to recover from a stroke or that which a person undergoes in living into the whole new life that a spinal cord tumor dictates are required for effective health care. That neurologist in the intensive care unit, that technician in the brace shop molding the plastic support for the patient's dropping foot, that chemotherapy nurse administering the anti-neoplastic drugs in the effort to slow the growth of the spinal cord tumor are each embroiled in an ongoing story. By virtue of their work, they are so embroiled. They cannot choose *not* to participate in an unfolding story of peril and consequence. Quite beyond the technical or biological significance of the cell counts or brain damage from the stroke, the unfolding stories *belong* to the sickness. The sickness cannot be effectively treated in absence of a rigorous sense of story that enables that neurologist, physical therapist, or chemotherapy nurse to imagine, perceive, and pay attention to the lived experiences dictated by these sicknesses.

The sense of story is built on language skills, cognitive depth, imaginative powers, and interpersonal sensibilities. Although the sense of story seems part of the natural equipment of the human being, there are many among healthcare professionals ungraced with it. It is a capacity present in humans in varying levels of intensity and acuity, although not, as some assume, distributed according to profession or specialty or 'college major'. To assume that psychiatrists have it and surgeons don't, or that English majors have it and molecular biology majors don't is to be terribly misled. I am convinced by all the work my team has done that one can strengthen one's sense of story, no matter at what level one starts, through purposeful narrative training.

Developing one's sense of story through training in narrative competence transforms the healthcare professional's enterprise. When met with narratively astute care, health problems are defined differently and by different persons – by the patient, by the family members, by their cultures or communities as well as by the individual professionals who take care of them. The narrative methods they use complement or even *become* the treatment, that is, the narrative methods themselves help to recognize, honor, and give voice to patients and family members. We see, and are in the process of demonstrating, that these things alter treatment and influence outcomes of care.

As health is increasingly considered to be the dynamic integral of all these forces – the physical, chemical, mental, metaphorical, aesthetic, emotional, relational, and self-conceptual – one's state of health takes in all these elements of self. To care for a sick person exceeds the fact-using sphere of disease recognition, diagnosis, and management to simultaneously require that the events befalling the patient be seen within the meaning-making sphere. Perhaps many persons who choose careers and professions in health care don't know, at the time of their choice, that they will have to operate within both these spheres. Narrative medicine arose in the effort to equip those who work with the sick with the wherewithal to travel constantly and skillfully between these spheres, and it is their sense of story that powers this travel.

Current contributions and research

Conceptual frameworks of narrative medicine

Events become appreciable when they are narrativized. Although the word 'story' has been overused of late, certainly and not only in health care, there is a fundamental and irreversible relationship between the befalling of something and its representation in either language or visual modes. I will in the remainder of this chapter, written for health communications scholars and linguists, restrict my attention to representation in words and language. This focusing choice is not meant to exclude visual, performative, or dramatic representation from consideration as narratives.

I need not rehearse centuries of narrative theory here to establish the necessity of representation for the occurrence of an event. What emerges as foundational for narrative medicine is the current of thought that seeks to see clearly the relationship among an event, the conferring of form on it, and the experiencing of it. The line runs straight from Aristotle's *Rhetoric* (Aristotle 1960) through the Romantic poets (Wordsworth and Coleridge 1940), the James brothers (Henry more than William) (Henry James 1948; William James 1968), Woolf's and Joyce's modernism (Woolf 1950), Barthean structuralism (Barthes 1977), Merleau-Ponty's phenomenology of the body (Merleau-Ponty 2002), the formalism of close reading (Lentricchia and DuBois 2003), reader-response criticism (Tompkins 1980), post-Structuralist transformations (Derrida 2001), psychoanalytic formulations of telling (Loewald 1988), trauma and memory studies (Hermann 1992) and the mournful post-apocalyptic contemporary self-telling fictions of W.G. Sebald (2001), Michael Ondaatje (1992), Anne Michaels (1996), or John Banville (2006) today. The line suggests that one does not perceive without composing; that writing grants to writers access to that which they do not know they know; that the form of an utterance or written text is as contributory to its meaning as is its content; and that experience, to be experienced, must be mediated by representation.

Barbara Herrnstein Smith wrote a pithy definition of narrative as 'someone telling someone else that something happened' (Smith 1981: 228). By bringing attention to the presence of the teller, the listener, and the thing that happened, Smith insists on the narrative contract's sociality and reality. However interior the telling or far-fetched the happening, narrative acts draw selves into contact. As readers and writers bend their heads over a mutually gazed-upon thing that exists or that happened, their heads touch (Berger and Mohr 1967). The line I seek to draw brings ever closer attention to the narrative contract itself – established between writer and reader, between teller and listener, between artist and production, between the giving and the receiving of an account, ultimately, of self. Those heads bent over the somethings that happened are, by virtue of the mutual bending of the head, in relation as they, together now, consider the thing beheld. This is the foundation of both relation and self-knowledge, that ground upon which narrativity and identity meet (Brockmeier and Carbaugh 2001).

Even those healthcare professionals who do not explicitly recognize their narrative duties are influenced by the gravity of accounts of illness. Narrative medicine brings attention to the presence and the power of these events of illness whose traces can only be found in the accounts given of them.

The movements of narrative medicine: attention, representation, affiliation

Narrative medicine has been described to have three movements (Charon 2006). In trying to appreciate why reading and writing in clinical settings seem to benefit students and colleagues, those scholars and clinicians who helped to develop this field realized the simultaneous efforts of *attention* and *representation* as clinicians considered and dwelt on things that happened in their practices. We observed that when attention was given in health care and when what was seen by the attentive witness was represented in language, there arose an *affiliation* between the ones engaged in these actions, whether doctor and patient, colleague and colleague, or clinician and more widely considered public. We even saw that this framework obtained between clinician and his or her self.

The formulation of the three movements of attention, representation, and affiliation remains a touchstone that approximates conceptual formulations of literary/narrative theory with clinical realities impinging on the clinician and the sick person seeking care. Although I will now discuss these as if separable, it must be clear to the reader that these are not consecutive 'steps' but rather simultaneous conditions that 'add up to' a narratively competent health care.

Attention

Attention is the position of the dutiful witness. Any act within health care requires the attentive presence of the person hoping to provide care. For the cover for my book *Narrative Medicine: Honoring the Stories of Illness* (2006), I found, in a small pastel by Mary Cassatt, a depiction of attention. Two women sit, one talking and the other listening. The painting focuses on the face of the one listening, head propped by bent arm, and body leaning forward.

Yet, the listener is in the drawing's shadow while the light of the work rests on the quarter-profile of the one being listened to. This pastel seemed to me to represent a keenness of listening, an acuity of presence. Not sympathy or pity; what it portrayed, to my eyes, was a listener who recruited her intelligence and her intention to absorb what the teller told her.

Attention is a state studied by such philosophers as Simone Weil and Iris Murdoch, by contemplative practitioners of Eastern traditions, by those engaged in consciousness studies from neurosciences and psychology, and by artists and aesthetic theorists who examine creative acts that culminate in or take up representations (Berger and Mohr 1967; Chalmers 1996; Dewey 2005; Gadamer 2004; Murdoch 2001; Weil 1973). To achieve a state of attention within a clinical setting, the doctor or nurse or social worker or X-ray technician has to lay aside distractions, focus sharply on the patient's matters, bring concentration of thought and perception to the present (Connelly 1999; Epstein 1999). The attentive clinician chooses to lay aside competing concerns for the period of time he or she spends with the patient, trying to donate his or her full presence to the tasks of absorbing whatever the patient emits.

Once attention has been achieved – and it generally requires training, practice, and constant intention – the patient can be seen *as* himself or herself. Attention recruits a radical unknowingness, a state in which presuppositions are not allowed to cloud perception or judgment (Bourdieu 1977). Such attention requires perceptive powers, psychological sensibility so as to register mood and affect, kinesthetic awareness to understand what the body tells by its posture and movements, and plain old curiosity so as not to squander any 'telling' aspect of the person with whom one sits (Noland 2009). It demands that the imagination be recruited into the process, for the doors of perception can only be opened by the one who is already guessing what might be inside. It is in the very act of imagining someone else's situation that the witness becomes invested in whatever will turn out to be the truth of the matter. I am beginning to think that this very act of curiosity or willingness to imagine the situation of the other is what constitutes empathy.

With attention, the clinician beholds that which the patient emits, in language and in all the other channels through which signals might show themselves. It is not so much 'getting the patient's history' as it is a placing oneself within the patient's force-field. The attentive one places himself or herself at risk for being changed by the process, for a force-field will influence that which comes into its presence. Contemporary clinicians prove their awareness of these forces, if only in the reverse, by trying so hard to resist them. To have valorized 'detached concern' as a necessary step in preserving one's clinical judgment may signal not the results of careful research but instead a way to get off the hook of being reached by and changed by one's patients.

Representation

In narrative medicine, we ask our learners to write down what they see and undergo in their practices. We find that beginning students and seasoned clinicians often stop before taking in all that is exposed to them in the complex situations encountered in health care. In the effort to encourage clinicians to more fully perceive the events of their practice, we ask our doctors, nurses, or social workers to describe, in writing, situations of care. Write about a patient whose suffering has moved you. Write about a patient you can't forget. Write about the last patient you saw today in clinic. Write about a time when you knew something about a patient without being told it. Write about a patient you love. Write about a patient you loathe. Write about a patient who breaks your heart.

Often times, the writing is preceded by close reading of a well-written text. Usually, this step can unlock powers that lay dormant unless writers absorb themselves in the representation given by an artist. For example, I've often brought the first page-and-a-half of Michael Ondaatje's (1992) magisterial novel *The English Patient* as my reading text. These first paragraphs set the stage of the immediately post-World-War-II field hospital set in a crumbling Italian villa. Only one patient is left in this place, an English pilot badly burned in an airplane crash in the North African desert. Only one clinician remains, a young Canadian nurse herself badly burned by losses of life. As she bathes the pilot's damaged body and feeds him gently as if he were an injured bird in her nest, the reader understands the wordless dimensions of care.

> She pours calamine in stripes across his chest where he is less burned, where she can touch him. She loves the hollow below the lowest rib, its cliff of skin. Reaching his shoulders she blows cool air onto his neck, and he mutters.
>
> What? she asks, coming out of her concentration.
>
> He turns his dark face with its grey eyes toward her. She puts her hand into her pocket. She unskins the plum with her teeth, withdraws the stone and passes the flesh of the fruit into his mouth.
>
> He whispers again, dragging the listening heart of the young nurse beside him to wherever his mind is, into that well of memory he kept plunging into during those months before he died.
>
> *(Ondaatje 1992: 4)*

One of the first times I used this excerpt of prose in a narrative medicine writing seminar, Annie Lawlor, the social worker in charge of the live organ donation program at Columbia, said through her tears as we read this short text together, 'All day, we walk in and out of these rooms of care.' Since then, the writing prompt I offer after a close reading of this short text is, 'Write about a room of care.'

Over the years, a social worker has written about a family in the Surgical Intensive Care Unit, unsure of what to do in the face of their mother's plunge toward death. An internist has written about her own deeply demented mother, now so far away, who believes her own daughter is the cab driver. One family doctor writes about his memory of being read to sleep by his mother when he was a little boy, the exquisite intimacy of it, the great good privilege, the safety. A 55-year-old internist is suddenly gripped by the never-consciously-thought-about first patient's death way back in her third year of medical school. The writers never know where they will be summoned by the careful reading of this scene of care and the invitation to write in its shadow about one of their own scenes of care. Writing exercises like this exemplify the deep methods narrative medicine has developed to open clinicians to their own experiences of caring for others.

These writers – however skilled or unskilled they may be in composition – find ways to confer form on whatever scene of care comes to mind. They reach for prose, poetry, or drama. One might describe a silent tableau, another a still life. Another might write an obituary of a patient. Sometimes, what is written seems more like a dream than anything else. Sometimes one can barely distinguish what is written from a clinical note that might have been written in a chart. However the representation unfolds, the writer and the readers are able to grasp a situation and what it might mean to the protagonists and to the writer by virtue of its form. Here is a paragraph written long ago by a participant in a far-away writing workshop:

> When I last saw you, Mom, it was two hours before you died. You stared at me with frightened eyes. Your mouth was open under the oxygen mask and you seemed to be gasping for breath. I'm not sure what you saw and understood. The nurses had told me that 'things weren't going well,' so I tried to say goodbye. I didn't want to frighten you more, so I waffled. I said, 'I'll see you soon,' but I didn't believe it. At least I had the presence of mind to say, several times, 'I love you.' I hope it was enough.

This older man was visibly moved by having written this paragraph. As we workshop participants listened to him read to us, we could appreciate the depth of the fear, the gasping, and the love. We recognized the immediacy of this representation through its sensory detail – the stare, the open mouth, the sound of breath, the words remembered, the words said. His own intention forms the interior monologue of the scene as he articulates what he 'tried' for – to say good-bye, to not frighten, to have the presence of mind that produced presence of love. All of this is telegraphed in one hundred and one words of care. We told the author that he had written a love letter to his mother. It *was* his good-bye to her, the one he felt he had not said. Until we readers told him, he did not recognize that he *had* written a love letter. Knowing that, now, was a source of comfort in his grief – simply that it could be said and had been said.

Writing gives form to the inchoate experiences lived through, including those undergone amid illness and death. By conferring form on the radically unformed, writing makes these events visible, potentially comprehensible, and communicable to others. Sharing these pieces of writing in the group can initiate genuine contact among the participants as they become, in effect, one another's readers. We have come to understand that this form of writing – the effort to represent complex events or states of affairs in whatever language will contain them – can gain a writer access to thoughts which have been, until they are written, out of awareness. Vast are the dividends of this method for self-awareness and accurate patient care.

Affiliation

Narrative medicine is a very practical undertaking. In addition to the intellectual discoveries we have made, our work leads to practical and demonstrable clinical outcomes. As methods of establishing and maintaining contact with patients, these narrative routines grant us entrance to dimensions of patients' lived and imagined experience that matter in the care of their illnesses. Whether the careful listening is done over decades in a generalist's practice or over the twenty-four hours of the day of the emergency medicine doctor and whether this is a patient one has written about or not, the proximity afforded by narrative methods transforms the clinical relationship. I remember caring for an ill young man – diabetes, high cholesterol, terrible psoriasis, depression, trouble at home – whose care became somehow illuminated and almost transfigured when I learned that he had about a hundred parakeets of all colors of the rainbow in his little apartment in the Bronx. That narrative feature, altogether unimaginable, transported our work into some midsummer night's fairy land. It didn't alter his diabetes but my knowing about the birds let us feel that we were on to one another's secrets. It gave us a new intimacy that has fueled a muscular clinical commitment of over 30 years.

Although still in the infancy of theorizing about the pathways of consequences of this kind of practice, we think that narrative methods alter the permeability of clinician to patient. I have written elsewhere about the 'membranes' of the doctor and patient as they sit together, and how stories might be the active agent that alters one's permeability to the other (Charon

2012). Stories fully told and heard seem as if they open something up in both teller and listener, letting them lean forward toward one another, activating the resources within each that will help them work productively together. The doctor's fund of scientific knowledge and determination to get needed things done for the patient need to be made available to the patient. The patient's trust and determination to do whatever it takes to get better needs to be activated by contact with this doctor or nurse. Through some intersubjective mechanism, stories told and heard somehow bring about shifts in availability, activation, and commitment. Maybe it is storytelling's leveling actions – there are no hierarchies as we sit around the campfire – that account for the profound shifts in comfort, openness, even power within these typically power-governed relationships.

The leveling actions of narrative medicine seen between clinician and patient are seen as well between members of the healthcare team. When clinicians gather for narrative training, reading and writing and reading aloud to one another what they have written, they quickly form sturdy and trusting bonds among one another. An unexpected dividend in our early work was the improvement in the effectiveness of the healthcare team that occurred as a result of narrative work (Charon 2012; Sands et al. 2008).

Improvement of the functioning of the healthcare team has become an urgent goal for all of health care. Narrative medicine methods are used to 'reset' the communication on a healthcare team. By focusing our learners squarely on the patient's suffering instead of conflictual aspects of management, we enable the doctor, nurse, social worker, and physical therapist to get 'under' the distinctions that typically divide them into separate siloes. They learn forcefully and emotionally that they are all engaged in trying to comprehend the plight of the patient and to improve his or her situation.

The movements spiral together

These three movements spiral on one another to bring about changes in the conventional clinician–patient transaction and in many, many clinical routines of interviewing, writing in charts, and inviting patients to write about their situations. The relation, the agenda, the decisions, the commitments, the goals of health care are all lifted from their reductivism toward becoming a buoyant living thing. These narratively inflected clinical relationships can do more than could their predecessors, both for the sick persons and for those who care for the sick. It is now narrative medicine's duty to clarify the consequences of these shifts in theory, training, and scope so as to continually improve the effectiveness of health care.

Future directions

My team in the Program in Narrative Medicine recently mounted an intensive training workshop for clinicians from Veterans' Administration Hospitals throughout the country. With members of the Veterans' Administration clinical faculty, we taught a weekend training workshop to doctors, nurses, social workers, and chaplains who work at a number of VA hospitals throughout the country. Of course, the issues of veterans' health is quite foregrounded in the news these days, with so many traumatized and injured veterans finding their way home from the vexed fronts at which they have been toiling and the history of untreated physical and psychical injury suffered by our men and women in the armed services.

My team did not know, though, to expect the power of response that we experienced. These clinicians were hungry for the narrative coherence that we were able to extend to their clinical practices caring for traumatized war veterans, demonstrating how urgent is narrative work for both the terribly injured veterans and for the swamped clinicians expected to care for them. The care of those injured in war is near its center an obligatory telling, that is, the recovery cannot proceed without some means of articulating or representing what has befallen the patient. Narrative medicine training equips clinicians exactly with the skills to beckon the telling of trauma, to permit it to be freed from its cage of the 'disremembered' (Morrison 1987), to witness whatever form of telling is possible, and to know what to do in the face of the admission of extreme trauma either suffered or inflicted.

Like narrative medicine training extended to other groups of clinicians and scholars, our work with VA clinicians opens new doors within our practice. Now we can see how the care of trauma survivors can be improved and intensified with the methods that have been developed in our field. We predict that we will continue to identify additional clinical areas – the care of cognitively impaired children, autism spectrum disorders, dementia, aphasias – that can be improved with narrative medicine methods.

Narrative medicine has helped to spearhead the use of reflective writing in health professionals' training and to conceptualize with rigor what is thought to occur as a consequence of such writing (Charon and Hermann 2012; Amiel et al. in press). More and more medical and nursing schools are adopting reflective writing as ways for students to be encouraged to think about their experiences with the ill. Typically, students are invited to write two or three short essays per year on such topics as their experience of dissecting the cadaver in anatomy lab, their meeting with their first patient, or their emotions on first being placed in the role of doctor or nurse. We have joined several other narrativists in recognizing the power of such writing, not as a means of 'reporting' sentinel events in professional development but as a means by which the trainee can experience these events to begin with. If writing is treated not as report but as discovery, then students can harvest tremendously powerful insights from their own writings done in response to well-crafted writing prompts (Wear et al. 2012). Building such programs requires that faculty be trained to read skillfully and perceptively what their students write, within trusting climates where a writer receives multiple interpretations to help the writer to envision what he or she has created in text and to begin to recognize what it might tell.

Ultimately, the task of narrative medicine is to demonstrate that clinical outcomes can improve with the use of narrative methods. Once there are enough clinicians well trained in narrative medicine methods, large-scale studies can be done to compare narrative medicine practices with standard practices assessing actual clinical endpoints. Some outcomes of interest will be process outcomes – patients' willingness to follow medical advice, patients' access to their physicians or nurses, rates of acceptance of health promotion recommendations like mammograms or flu shots, levels of knowledge and trust within clinical relationships, and patient and provider satisfaction with the care. I wonder if we can demonstrate that narratively skilled doctors and nurses keep learning new things about long-time patients. I wonder if we can demonstrate that patients of narratively trained doctors end up knowing more about their diseases or learn better how to control their physical symptoms. Other outcomes that may well change with narrative practices are actual disease management parameters – blood sugar control in diabetics, blood pressure control, smoking cessation success rates, pounds lost in overweight patients, or viral load in hepatitis C.

Health communication scholars and linguists bring particularly powerful knowledge and skill to this future work. I close this chapter with a précis of specific collaborative projects that are necessary to advance the work of narrative medicine and that are waiting for colleagues from health communication and linguistics.

1 *Linguistic analysis of narrative medicine training sessions.* Although we know, roughly speaking, what happens in narrative medicine seminars and we have standardized our approaches, our teaching texts, our writing prompts, and our style of responding to learners' writing, we have not undertaken close study of the transactions themselves of these seminars. I believe that much will be learned by close narrative analysis of transcribed speech of small narrative medicine seminars.
2 *Ethnographic study of receivers of training.* We have undertaken several qualitative outcomes studies of intensive narrative medicine teaching. No one has undertaken careful analysis of outcomes of clinician group training, for example, at the Narrative Medicine Workshops we hold in New York that attract participants worldwide. Immediate and longer-term follow-up interviews may unearth some unexpected outcomes of this work.
3 *Study of writing patterns before and after narrative training.* We hypothesize that narrative medicine training may alter the ways in which clinicians represent patients in medical charts or referral notes. We have not undertaken linguistic analysis of clinicians' patient-specific task-oriented writing as their narrative training proceeds. This would be the place to begin to query the clinical outcomes of narrative training. As importantly, it might illuminate the consequences of the conventional forms of writing about patients, either on the clinical impressions of doctors or nurses or on patients' assessment of their clinicians' capacity to comprehend their situations.
4 *Patients write too.* One sequel of narrative medicine clinical routines is that patients themselves are encouraged to write about their illness experiences. The narratively trained clinician who has invited such writing is then in a position to read it and to respond to what the patient has written. This sequence of narrative events contains nodal moments of importance, ultimately, for individual patients' outcomes and should be studied.
5 *Conceptual work in health communication.* Finally, the theoretical questions to be posed in the shadow of this work are protean – about the means and consequences of representing illness, about the power divides present in health care and language's responsibilities in bridging them, about the interior resources in the healthcare professional currently squandered for lack of capacity to articulate thought, and about the squandering of linguistic clinical evidence in routine health care for lack of the capacity of clinicians to decode it. In addition to these clinical questions, more global ones about language propose themselves – about the power of written language to expose thought, about the relations that develop between writer and reader or among readers of texts, and about the ways in which language nourishes the self.

Summary

Narrative medicine arose in response to the impoverishment of contemporary medicine in the dimensions of meaning-making and having a sense of story. By fortifying clinicians' practice with the capacity to recognize stories, to absorb them, to interpret them, to metabolize them, and to let them become part of self, narrative methods deepen the contact with patients and support deep care. As narrative medicine enters its second decade, it faces new and complex tasks. Not only will the field be expected to generate fresh pedagogical methods and to identify salient texts and composition teaching methods. It will also generate views on the underlying theoretical frameworks of creative composition work in general, of the consequences of interpretive communities on their members, and on the relations of matters of health to matters of telling and listening.

Narrative medicine's future certainly includes a growing collaboration between narrative medicine professionals and health communication scholars. Since our primary texts and primary data are the stories we hear in practice and retell in the efforts to help patients, we require sophisticated methods of probing the language, examining its structures, its means of production, its means of performance, its consequences on the narrating contexts. What we hope is that, as illness's stories expand in significance, our capacities enlarge ever more rigorously and generously to receive them, to comprehend them, and to be moved by them into action on behalf of our patients.

Related topics

Patient-centered care; relationship-centered care; patient–clinician communication; literature and medicine; disability studies; reflective practice; mindful practice.

Further reading

Berger, J. and Mohr, J. (1967) *A Fortunate Man*, New York: Pantheon Books.
Dewey, J. (2005) *Art as Experience*, New York: Penguin.
Jurecic, A. (2012) *Illness as Narrative*, Pittsburgh, PA: University of Pittsburgh Press.
Mattingly, C. (1998) *Healing Dramas and Clinical Plots*, Cambridge: Cambridge University Press.
Mishler, E. (1984) *The Discourse of Medicine: Dialectics of Medical Interviews*, Norwood, NJ: Ablex.

References

Ackerman, D. (2011) *One Hundred Names for Love: A Stroke, a Marriage, and the Language of Healing*, New York: W.W. Norton.
Amiel, Y., Armstrong-Coben, A., Bernitz, M., Glickstein, J., Graham, G., Hermann, N., Park, C., Taylor, D. and Charon, R. (in press) 'Narrative medicine in education and practice', in M. Feldman, J. Christensen, and J. Satterfield (eds) *Behavioral Medicine in Primary Care*, 4th edn, Columbus, OH: McGraw-Hill.
Aristotle. (1960) *The Rhetoric of Aristotle*, trans. L. Cooper, Upper Saddle River, NJ: Prentice-Hall.
Banville, J. (2006) *The Sea*, New York: Alfred A. Knopf.
Barthes, R. (1977) *Image Music Text*, trans. S. Heath, New York: Hill and Wang.
Berger, J. and Mohr, J. (1967) *A Fortunate Man*, New York: Pantheon Books.
Bourdieu, P. (1977) *Outline of a Theory of Practice*, trans. R. Nice, Cambridge: Cambridge University Press.
Brockmeier, J. and Carbaugh, D. (eds) (2001) *Narrative and Identity: Studies in Autobiography, Self and Culture*, Amsterdam: John Benjamins.
Chalmers, D. (1996) *The Conscious Mind: In Search of a Fundamental Theory*, New York: Oxford University Press.
Charon, R. (2006) *Narrative Medicine: Honoring the Stories of Illness*, New York: Oxford University Press.
——(2012) 'At the membranes of care: stories in narrative medicine', *Academic Medicine*, 87: 342–347.
Charon, R. and Hermann, N. (2012) 'A sense of story, or why teach reflective writing?', *Academic Medicine*, 87: 5–7.
Clifton, L. (2000) *Blessing the Boats: New and Selected Poems 1988–2000*, Rochester, NY: Boa Editions.
Connelly, J. (1999) 'Being in the present moment: developing the capacity for mindfulness in medicine', *Academic Medicine*, 74: 420–424.
Derrida, J. (2001) *The Work of Mourning*, ed. P-A. Brault and M. Naas, Chicago, IL: University of Chicago Press.
Dewey, J. (2005) *Art as Experience*, New York: Penguin.

Epstein, R. (1999) 'Mindful practice', *Journal of the American Medical Association,* 282: 833–839.
Gadamer, H-G. (2004) *Truth and Method,* London: Continuum.
Goyal, R., Charon, R., Lekas, H-M., Fullilove, M., Devlin, M., Falzon, L. and Wyer, P. (2008) '"A local habitation and a name": how narrative evidence based medicine transforms the translational research paradigm', *Journal of Evaluation in Clinical Practice,* 14: 732–741.
Hermann, J. (1992) *Trauma and Recovery*, New York: Basic Books.
James, H. (1948) *The Art of the Novel: Critical Prefaces*, New York: Charles Scribner's Sons.
James, W. (1968) *The Meaning of Truth*, New York: Greenwood Press.
Lentricchia, F and DuBois, A. (eds) (2003) *Close Reading: The Reader*, Durham, NC: Duke University Press.
Loewald, H. (1988) *Sublimation: Inquiries into Theoretical Psychoanalysis*, New Haven, CT: Yale University Press.
Mattingly, C. (1998) *Healing Dramas and Clinical Plots: The Narrative Structure of Experience*, Cambridge: Cambridge University Press.
Merleau-Ponty, M. (2002) *Phenomenology of Perception*, trans. C. Smith, London: Routledge.
Michaels, A. (1996) *Fugitive Pieces*, New York: Vintage/Random House.
Morrison, T. (1987) *Beloved*, New York: Penguin Books.
Murdoch, I. (2001) *The Sovereignty of Good*, London: Routledge.
Noland, C. (2009) *Agency and Embodiment: Performing Gestures/Producing Culture*, Cambridge, MA: Harvard University Press.
Ondaatje, M. (1992) *The English Patient*, New York: Random House/Vintage.
Price, R. (1994) *A Whole New Life: An Illness and a Healing*, New York: Atheneum.
Sands, S., Stanley, P., and Charon, R. (2008) 'Pediatric narrative oncology: interprofessional training to promote empathy, build teams, and prevent burnout', *Journal of Supportive Oncology*, 6: 307–312.
Sebald, W.G. (2001) *Austerlitz*, New York: Random House.
Smith, B. H. (1981) 'Narrative versions, narrative theories', in W.J.T. Mitchell (ed.) *On Narrative*, Chicago, IL: University of Chicago Press.
Tompkins, J. (ed.) (1980) *Reader-Response Criticism: From Formalism to Post-Structuralism*, Baltimore, MD: Johns Hopkins University Press.
Wear, D., Zarconi, J., Garden, R., and Jones, T. (2012) 'Reflection in/and writing: pedagogy and practice in medical education', *Academic Medicine*, 87: 603–609.
Weil, S. (1973) *Waiting for God*, trans. E. Craufurd, New York: Harper & Row.
Woolf, V. (1950) 'Reading', in V. Woolf *The Captain's Death Bed and Other Essays*, San Diego, CA: Harcourt Brace Jovanovich.
Wordsworth, W. and Coleridge, S. (1940) *The Lyrical Ballads, 1798–1805*, ed. G. Sampson, London: Methuen.

17

Presencing in the context of enhancing patient well-being in nursing care

Sally Candlin and Christopher N. Candlin

Preamble

In the discussion in this chapter, we draw particularly on two related constructs central to an understanding of the discourses of professional practice: that of *crucial sites of engagement* and their *critical moments* (see Candlin 2002; Scollon 2001; Scollon and Scollon 2004) as keys to the defining and understanding of professional practice. Following Cicourel (1992, 1996, 2007), such sites can be best seen as an ecology: involving their settings, their participants with their mediated actions and roles, focal themes and purposes, states of being, and where professional expertise is open to scrutiny and evaluation. In such sites, significant critical moments (Candlin 1987a, 1987b) are those where participants' actions, beliefs, and competencies are challenged, where their subjective realities are questioned and put on line (Candlin and Lucas 1986), where interactions may develop in unexpected ways, and where meaning-making is evidenced as an interactive process. The managing of such critical moments in such crucial sites may call upon and reveal particular communicative strategies of all kinds and modalities, both in terms of performance and of interpretation, by participants in the interaction who seek clarification and, where necessary, the re-attaining of equilibrium in the relationships in focus.

We locate these constructs in the domain of healthcare delivery, focusing on patient well-being in the context of a holistic perspective on nursing care, and informed by a view of health as:

> a relative state in which one is able to function well physically, mentally, socially and spiritually in order to express the full range of one's unique potentialities within the environment in which one is living. In the words of René Dubois: 'health is primarily a measure of each person's ability to do and become what he is capable of becoming … '.
>
> *(Encyclopaedia and Dictionary of Medicine, Nursing and Allied Health 1987)*

Within this multidimensional view of health we focus on the mutuality of contribution by nurse *and* patient to the healthcare encounter. As such, it is the exploration of professional practice in the context of providing nursing care that is central to this chapter. As part of the preamble to this chapter (and perhaps as a means of indicating to other professionals the relationships between a nurse's professional roles and functions and her discourse roles) Figure 17.1 from S. Candlin (2008) may be helpful.

Nurses, when asked to describe their work, typically analyze their roles in terms of the functions or, we might say, practices, that they perform, as in Figure 17.1. Notable here, however, is the overlapping and often concurrent exercise of different roles, engendering a polyphonic discourse marked by intertextuality and interdiscursivity. No function or role is closed off from any other, nor are such functions and roles a finite set. Such hybridity speaks to the holistic nature of nursing practice, incorporating not only healing and caring but also counseling, advocacy, management *inter alia.* As one concrete example, a nurse may draw on her technological knowledge in an educational role vis-à-vis the patient but enacts that role with the overarching caring and healing purpose of lowering patient anxiety and gaining the patient's cooperation and understanding. What is central in our view, however, is that in caring for persons across the lifespan and from all cultural backgrounds – whether sick or healthy – appropriate and ethical care is based on individual need: physical, emotional/psychological, social and spiritual, where all such needs are ineluctably interconnected in sites of nursing engagement. It is this that we characterize as holistic nursing. As McFarlane argues, and here with a focus on spirituality, the essence of nursing care is 'the entire person of the nurse interacting with the entire person of the patient in a caring relationship' (1981: 14–16).

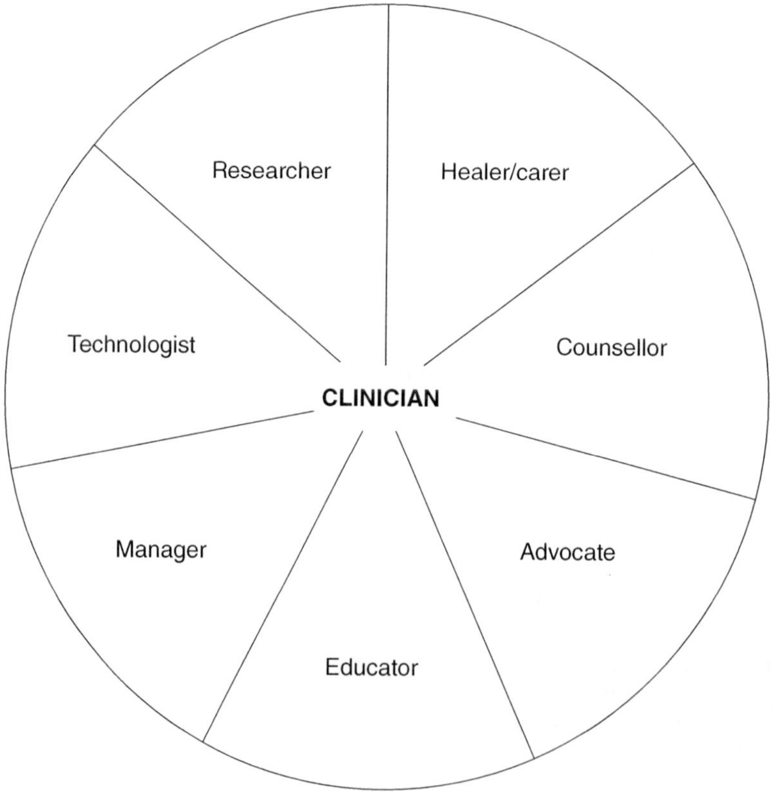

Figure 17.1 The role and function of the nurse

Source: S. Candlin (2008).

Accordingly, and against a background of professional practice seen from the perspective of socio-cultural mediation (Scollon 1998, 2001; Fairclough 1992), this chapter takes as its focus an emphasis on the holistic understanding of the interactional context by both nurse and patient, mediated through the practices of the researcher as analyst and as participant (Sarangi and Candlin 2003). We ground this approach to holistic understanding by means of an exploration of the construct of '*presencing*' (Fredricksson 1999; S. Candlin 2008; Walsh 2009) as a way of capturing and responding to the patient's physical, social, spiritual, and emotional condition. Presencing, as we shall argue, invokes Cicourel's (1973) concept of *reciprocity of perspective* (following Schutz 1962): the degree to which participants come to share what is needed to achieve, albeit temporarily, moments of understanding. In interpreting such mutuality as the sharing of the perspectives of the participants in the interaction and of the participants as analysts, researchers, and interactants, we establish two audiences and two types of mutuality. First, we can talk about mutuality in terms of the participants *within* an interaction, in this case the nurse and the patient, but, second, as the sharing of perspectives between the participants in the interaction themselves taken together, and the researcher as analyst seeking to make sense of the encounter.

Presencing as discursive practice in patient care

Here we discuss our understanding of the concept of *presencing*: its importance in nursing practice, and of particular elements such as listening only to that person and his/her agenda, so that the relationship is patient-centered as opposed to one that is nurse or institution-centered. We discuss how this may be achieved, and, importantly, how the philosophical literature (e.g., that of Heidegger 1927; Buber 1947) and that of nursing (e.g., Benner and Wrubel 1989) contribute to the development of a deeper understanding of the concept. This understanding relates to how the nurse's identity is revealed through its enactment in discourse (both verbal and non-verbal). We discuss this enactment below and later in the chapter as we present an analysis of the account of a nurse as she reminisces about an interaction with a patient in clinical practice.

Presencing as holistic understanding

The phrase 'to presence oneself' derives from the philosopher Martin Heidegger's seminal book on *Being and Time (Sein und Zeit)* (Heidegger 1927) where he suggests two related perspectives on 'presence': what he terms *Anwesenheit (*presence in the sense of being present with another*)* and *Zugegensein (*presence in the sense of attendance on or with another). Both terms taken together may incorporate what in English we might render as 'to enjoin' another, or even, 'to be accessible' to another. To presence oneself with another means that one is available to understand and be with someone, where each person can at times share in the 'being' of the other. Buber (1923) articulates this when he writes:

> when two individuals 'happen' to each other, there is an essential remainder which is common to them ... this is the 'sphere of between' ... that which happens within the souls of each, is only the secret accompaniment to the dialogue. The meaning of the dialogue is found neither in one nor the other of the partners, nor in both taken together, but in their interchange.
>
> *(Buber 1923: 62)*

and again (and more directly now in discourse terms):

> Dialogue, especially where people who are open to an I–You relation, is likely to involve both silence (stillness) and speech. In stillness there is communion. Where a person is able to release themselves to silence, unreserved communication streams from him and the silence bears it to his neighbor.
>
> *(Buber 1947: 4)*

Neither loses him/herself in the relationship but remains their unique self in relation to the other. We might infer from this that our individual identity is always in apposition to another, just as in dialogue our contribution is determined by our relationship with the other at a particular moment. Presencing oneself contrasts with standing aloof and outside the situation, or being preoccupied with other thoughts while being physically present with the person (Benner and Wrubel 1989: 13). Presencing is communicating to the patient a feeling of the patient's centrality within the situation. It need not be verbal communication, but just being there, sometimes in the silence of the moment, where the nurse can exude an aura of competence, caring, and dependability that may instill in the silence a knowledge in the patient that says: 'I am here for you, and only for you'. To instill a feeling in the patient to 'talk as you wish or just rest in the silence' demonstrates a sublimity in the human experience that at its most profound defies description, analysis, and explanation. This sense of ineffability is in our view characteristic of the responses of many healthcare professionals about their practice. The questions that so often remain unanswered include 'So how and why does this happen?', and the 'So what ... ?' question remains: 'So what does it add to our understanding of the human experience, to the ability to change ourselves and others – in the situation?' Does the ineffability of the human experience – and the data it produces – cause us to give up, or are we challenged to take the next step forward toward the completion of the jigsaw of human life?

Very much in the spirit of Heidegger, Fredricksson (1999) also identifies what he refers to as two modes of presence: *being there* (physical co-presence) involving interpersonality and intersubjectivity, grounded in the attention of the nurse (a matter of question and answer) and *being with,* encompassing communication and understanding (a matter of 'gift' of self) in response to what Pederson (1993) refers to as 'invitation', attaining a higher sense of intersubjectivity. Although not a discourse analyst, Fredricksson provides a useful basis for a discursive approach to presencing in that he highlights some quite specific features: being close to the patient, using a quiet tone of voice, making an appropriate choice of words, engaging eye contact, touch, all in the service of establishing rapport and communicating empathy. Such mediated actions (Wertsch 1991, 1994; Scollon 1998, 1999) have for Fredricksson clear professional purposes: to assist coping, to diminish intensity of feelings such as fear, powerlessness, anxiety, isolation, and distress, and to sustain encouragement and a sense of security and reassurance.

As a further example of the mediated actions of presencing, and drawing on a study of nurse–patient relationships in the Emergency Department, Walsh (2009) argues that:

> Strong characteristics for presencing included steadfast-in-being, being committed, having courage, instilling hope and being grateful. Nurses valued their interactions with patients and enjoyed caring for them giving the sense that 'we're in this together'. An important finding revealed the invisibility of the nurse presence.
>
> *(Walsh 2009: 1)*

Walsh's formulation adds another dimension to our understanding of presencing: how can one be present and yet invisible? Perhaps the answer lies in the perception of the actor and the skill of the agent, where, at a very profound level, the actor (the patient) perceives his or her centrality at that moment, and the nurse (as the agent) is part of the periphery, but is sensitive to the patient's centrality, who has been the architect of the perception. Here we refer to the actor not as one who is agentive but one who receives from the agent attention such that her being is transformed in that she is able to be an active participant. In the same way, the agent is one who has the skills to effect this transformation in the other. The nurse is just 'being', where verbal language is superfluous and indeed can be a distraction. Following Zerwekh (1997) and Owen-Mills (1998), we can suggest that presencing demands of the nurse that she consciously and deliberately focuses her attention on the patient, being open to the other and being aware of their shared humanity. Again, as with Fredricksson, Zerwekh identifies elements of presencing as the communication of empathy, providing of affirmation, and being without words. It would seem, then, that listening with sensitivity is also one hallmark of presencing. Cassidy (1988) talks about the doctor's perspective and the difficulties faced when cure is not possible, and the need to recognize the importance of sharing this powerlessness with the patient, staying with them and not deserting them. This sharing of powerlessness with the patient and not deserting them is as important for nurses as it is for the doctor, if not more so, since nurses are in a continual process of care for the person 'around the clock' (S. Candlin 1997).

Presencing and revelations of identity

How are these identities of '*agent*' and '*actor*' to be constructed and construed in the context of presencing? As Zimmerman and Wieder (1970) argue, rather than viewing identity as property of self alone, as it were as of some entity, or as the outcome of some process, we locate identity as closely connected to professional practices and professional roles and to the doing of professional work. This position is taken up below in the following section: 'Delivering holistic nursing care: supporting the concept of presencing' and in particular in the sub-section entitled: 'The identities, roles, and functions of the nurse' where we explore a narrative account of a nurse caring for a patient who is terminally ill.

Accordingly, we may expect that nursing as presencing will be complex, hybrid, and interdiscursive, and able only to be revealed through nurses' professional behaviors in practices linked to specific sites of engagement. Following Scollon (1998), but also Bamberg (1997), and Antaki and Widdicombe (1998), what is characteristic of mediated actions in such sites is that they are negotiable, subject to fragmentation, flows and disunity. They are typically relational, emergent from the interaction order (Goffman 1967, 1983) and always subject to the conventions of the institutional order of nursing as a set of professional beliefs, principles, and practices. At the same time, we acknowledge the professional capacity of the nurse to move across the boundaries of such practices, to extend them in particular moments of interaction, especially perhaps at those critical moments we alluded to earlier.

What do such accounts of communicative processes entail? We may explore these from two connectable perspectives: first, biographically, following Riessman's (1990, 2001, 2002, 2003) work in drawing on narratives of experience (as in this chapter in the nurse's (N) story) and resonating with Garfinkel's (1956, 1967) discussions of *accounts* – although here in terms of spoken not written texts – where such narratives do not just 'tell a story' but are indexically relevant of a professional practice (as here *presencing*) and of professional role. Here however we need to be conscious, as Garfinkel insists, that such narratives are not reproductions of 'fact', they are always likely to imbricate post hoc assumptions of order and coherence, influenced by the interaction order of the telling. Second, we may adopt a more interactionist position, in which such tellings are always, as Bamberg (1997) points out, products of an internal dialogue between the self and the other, or even of actual dialogues between, say, researcher and principal participant (as here between the nurse (N) and the researcher (R)), but where one consequence may well be some inconsistencies, gaps, or variabilities in the accounts provided, as it were, through the interaction.

So, how may we reconcile these approaches? Current research into narrative and identity from both perspectives (for example that of Riessman 1990, 2001, 2002; Schiffrin 1996; De Fina 2009; De Fina et al. 2006; Bamberg et al (2007); Georgakopoulou 2006; and De Fina and Georgakopoulou 2008) offers a set of practical research actions. It does so by anchoring such narratives of participants, both researchers and professional actors, in an exploration of identities; principally by offering accounts of how communicative strategies are deployed by participants; by combining local ethnographies with discourse analyses of interactions (see here Rampton et al. 2004; Rampton 2007), and by seeking to identify where possible, and, following Bamberg (1997), to harmonize distinctive positionings of participants. This notwithstanding, the issue for this chapter is more whether such studies also serve to connect their narrative analyses to the professional practices of members of communities of practice in their professional roles (see Candlin and Candlin 2007). Here we may discern two positions. First, that of Riessman (1990, 2001, 2002, 2003) where, especially in the discourse world of healthcare and against the background of institutional and professional philosophies and practices, her analyses are clearly so located, as is also the work of Greenhalgh and her colleagues (2005) with their focus on narrative method as a means towards quality improvement, again in the domain of healthcare. Second, we may identify the more generally and non-professionally and institutionally positioned studies of De Fina and Georgakopoulou (2008) inter alia. Here, although the contextualized 'small stories' with their discussion of emerging structures as set out in the studies of Georgakopoulou (2006) and Bamberg and Georgakopoulou (2008) do have considerable potential relevance to our work, they are not embedded in professional practice (although they might well be). In the world of discourse and professional practice in the domain of healthcare, it is central to keep firmly in mind that the analysis of narrative, interaction, and indeed communication generally, is not to be equated with the analysis and evaluation of therapeutic communication as a specific professional practice (S. Candlin 2008). Further, in evaluating the usefulness for our theme of such studies as those listed above, it is salutary to note the injunction by Sarangi and Candlin (2003), a matter to which we return in the final section of this chapter:

> So far, then, discourse analysis, whether primarily descriptive or seeking also interpretation, confines itself to the classification of pattern. The question remains, is pattern-seeking enough? Clearly, to meet the third challenge, that of explanation, much more work remains to be done; not just a matter of some internally generated warrant, from the data and the participants, but an external warrant in terms of what the analysis can offer to our understandings of (as here) professional or personal practice.
>
> *(Sarangi and Candlin 2003: 123)*

Delivering holistic nursing: supporting the concept of presencing

To locate our argument in nursing practice, and with ethical permission from Macquarie University's Ethics Committee, we approached nursing colleagues inviting them to reminisce on their nursing practice experiences and to give accounts of significant events which had impacted on their practice, specifically identifying any markers in the event which, in their view, had changed the direction of their care, that is, to indicate particular critical moments. We discussed the concepts of critical moments and crucial sites so that we could later discuss our analysis and align our interpretations of their data. Accordingly, in this section, and as one example of nursing care, we analyze and explain the account of one nurse (N) as given to the researcher (R) where critical moments were identified. It became clear from the outset that the concept of *presencing* was a significant strategy in her care, helped to identify the functions of her caring and, in so doing, gave indications of her own identity (see Figure 17.1 above).

We begin with what is an edited account of N's story – edited, because in the spirit of reflection and cooperation where the informant (N) is seen as a co-worker in the research – the researcher asked N to examine the transcript of the audio recorded data to verify it for accuracy. N chose to email her revised account to R. As this account displayed only few changes (but nonetheless important changes for N), R was able to use it in conjunction with the original audio recording so that pragmatic features such as pauses and placement of emphasis could be retained in the transcript. R and N then discussed R's analysis of the discourse and, as a result, N was able to articulate the impact that the event had had on her, and R was able to formulate her own account as the researcher. These perceptions are also addressed in this section of the chapter, but first we introduce the setting (the crucial site) which then leads to N's narrative of her interaction and nursing actions with the patient (P). Following later discussion between R and N, R was able to clarify the issues that had been raised, so that R was able to discuss with N and then provide her with a researcher's account of the event. We see this process as exemplifying joint participation in the research process (Sarangi and Candlin 2001) and collaboration in the provision of an account (Garfinkel 1967).

N's story

N is a recently retired registered nurse who has worked across a number of specialty areas of nursing practice. She is a single woman in her early sixties who spends her time performing community aid to those in need. We agreed, at her request, to sit in the garden and audio record our conversation. After clarifying with N the meaning of what is meant by critical moments, and crucial sites of engagement, she then talked about her experience of some years ago. The *crucial site* was the 'medicine round' in a palliative care ward in a healthcare facility and, within that, a situation which developed into a counseling session between nurse and patient in a single room.

Transcript conventions used in this extract of discourse

Bold typeface:	indicates a lexical item that is emphasized in the discourse
(*):	indicates pauses that are considered to be longer than that represented by a comma
(***):	indicates silence of approximately three seconds
plain font:	indicates a significant non-verbal gesture

Excerpt 1

1 N: The ***one*** *experience that hits home was about nine years ago.(*)*
2 I did a day's ***relief*** *as an RN in a Palliative Care Hospice which was a nice*

3 *change given my main area of practice being Adolescent Health.*
4 *It was a **busy** morning so after taking **report** I then proceeded to meet the*
5 *patients, of whom there were about 19, and to begin the **medications** round.*
6 *The layout of the unit consisted of three four bedded wards and seven or so*
7 *single rooms located in another corridor.*
8 *Arriving at the end single room I stepped into a dark sombre space (*)*
9 *curtains drawn with barely any light penetration.*
10 *Lying on the bed was an emaciated young woman (P) in her 20s (*) dying. (*)*
11 *I **returned** to the nurses' station at that point to collect additional medications*
12 *and check her notes then returned to her room.*
13 *The tea lady appeared so I enquired as to whether P would like a cup.*
14 *She de**clined** and seemed to want to just be left **alone**.*
15 *I quietly motioned to the lady to leave a cuppa*
(N waved her arm behind her – indicating that she said nothing to the tea lady but relied on non-verbal gesture, presumably so that conversation with P was uninterrupted)
16 *while saying to P, 'Is there anything **wrong** or that you would like to talk about*
17 *because I can have a cup of **tea with** you?' (*)*
18 *Her response went from someone limp and disinterested to one where her eyes*
19 *opened **wide** and her face became **animated**. (*)She turned her gaze toward me*
20 *and then blurted out poignantly (*) 'I've got 2 children and I'm dying of AIDS and I*
21 *am so **alone**'.(*)*
22 *In the next 10 to 15 minutes she shared **much** about her inner turmoil and*
23 ***sad**ness. I stood close **by** just listening holding the cup of **tea** not touched since*
24 *that first little sip she **took**.(*)*
25 *When I was leaving the room I asked if she wanted the curtains drawn **back**.*
26 *She said 'yes' and the room became **bathed** in the light that **streamed** through*
27 *the large windows. (*)*
28 *I don't know **what** happened to P as I only did **one** shift there*
29 *however I have **never** forgotten her*
(***)
30 *R: You were **pres**encing **wer**en't you?*

Discussion of the discourse

Identifying critical moments

The first *critical moment* in the encounter, i.e., the moment that determined its trajectory, was the initial perception of the ambience '*a dark sombre space*' (lines 8–10), alerting N to the possibility of a situation that was 'out of the ordinary' and might need to be approached with sensitivity. N's response was to gather further information (lines 11–12) so that she was able to plan appropriate nursing interventions. A further *critical moment* was the appearance of the tea lady (line 13) providing N with the opportunity to offer to have a cup of tea and talk with P (lines 16–17). This was the moment when P's demeanor changed (lines 18–19) and when she was able to take the opportunity to make painful self-disclosures (lines 20–22) (Coupland et al. 1991). P was able to share 'her inner turmoil and sadness' with N who 'stood close by just listening holding the cup of tea'. Here we might suggest that P recognized that she was in a 'safe place', one that had been provided by N.

Interestingly, neither of the critical moments (lines 8 and 13) were indicated by any verbal communication, but each provided an opportunity for N to demonstrate strategic presencing (line 30) with the consequence that the interaction took on a therapeutic character.

The context of presencing in a crucial site of engagement

Taking up our earlier discussion concerning presencing in the context of providing holistic nursing care, we argue that such care involves considering the *physical*, *psychosocial/emotional,* and *spiritual* needs of the patient. These constitute the parameters within which the individual patient is to be considered as a person. As such, any assessment and any consequent intervention, and any determination more generally of the evaluation and efficacy of care outcomes, involves considering *care* of the individual within each of these parameters of need. At the same time, such provision of care needs to acknowledge the *spatial dimensions of the encounter* and the particular use of *artifacts* in the particular site of engagement. Discourse in such a perspective is a matter not just of talk and its wording but one of mediated action involving a range of tools (Wertsch 1991).

What are these tools? Wertsch argues that they encompass a whole range of objects, technologies, practices, identities, even social institutions and communities, including, as we are emphasizing here, those of *presencing.* These tools are associated with a range of what Wertsch, following Gibson (1977), refers to as *affordances* and *constraints*. In sum, affordances afford, that is they enable purchase, contact, usability, while constraints have the reverse and inhibiting effect. It is this dynamic between affordances and constraints that characterizes much if not all of nursing practice, of which presencing is a key example.

Accordingly, rather than employing the term 'tools' in our analysis of presencing, we prefer here to use the term *affordances*, since for us such a term reminds us that we must consider all aspects of mediated interaction, just as nurses consider and take account of all aspects of health when engaging in healthcare situations (see S. Candlin 2008; and S. Candlin and Roger 2013). Thus, those affordances that we consider in this practice of presencing follow closely Wertsch's concept of mediated action, where the environment of the action is part of the total situation, much in the manner emphasized also by Benner (1984). We may indeed say that the utilization of the potential afforded by the total environment in the delivery of nursing care is an extension of the holistic care of the person we discussed earlier in this chapter, and which is at the heart of the concept of *total situation focused nursing care* (S. Candlin 2008; S. Candlin and Roger 2013) where *all* aspects of a situation must be considered if care is to be appropriate and effective, and desired outcomes achieved. Among such affordances are those of the ambience, the spatial dimensions, and the entirety of the physical characteristics of the site of engagement identified by R – in no small part as a result of her own clinical experiences – upon which the concept of *total situation focused nursing care* is built.

Analysis

Here we examine an extract from N's account of her interaction with P where she provides a background to the situation before she then engages with the situation of P, a terminally ill young woman.

Affordances to be considered when presencing is the mediated action

Affordance	*Discourse evidence from N's story*	*Line*
ambience	– *a busy morning*	4
patients	– *of whom there were about 19*	5
space	– *ward layout* – *end single room* – *a dark sombre space* – *curtains drawn* – *barely any light penetration*	6–7 8 8 9 9
physical	– *lying on the bed* – *an emaciated young woman in her 20s*	10 10
psychosocial aspects of P's health	– *is there anything wrong...* – *someone limp and disinterested* – *and then blurted out poignantly* – *I've got 2 children and I'm dying* – *I am so alone*	16 18 20 20 21
nursing actions	– *returned to nurses' station* – *collect additional medications* – *check her notes* – then *returned to her room*	11 11 12 12

In this analysis, we set out the situated interaction and identify in its discourse (columns 2 and 3) evidence of some of the affordances (column 1) of a total health situation to be considered in the context of presencing in nursing. However, if the process and practice of presencing, and the impact of presencing on the individual is to be explored and understood, what is now needed is to consider the responses by the participants to the mediated action. This can in part be achieved from the discourse data above, but to illuminate the outcomes of the interaction we need to augment our account with an analysis of the interaction between N and R as they engaged in discussion of the particular situation: a situation which had such an impact on N that she was prompted to say: '*I have **never** forgotten her*' (line 29), to which R replied: '*You were **pres**encing **wer**en't you?*' (line 30).

Responses and outcomes of mediated action

The nursing response as identified by R when talking with N

N continued as she reminisced further (see Excerpt 2), and from that discourse we can identify N's response to P's situation even though they had not engaged in any verbal interaction. N's description of the situation (lines 8–10) suggested that she needed further information, and she responded by returning to the nurses' station to collect additional medications and check P's notes (lines 11–12). In addition, N offered to talk and have a cup of tea with P (lines 16–17). This might suggest that without verbalizing the message, N was saying: 'I am here only for you – oblivious of all else.' This was the message which P understood, as can be seen in her positive response, having initially rejected the offer of a cup of tea. This was affirmed later in the conversation which continued between N and R, when N said: 'Yes I'm here for you – and oblivious to all else' (line 36) and line 37: 'She knew there was someone there for her.' N's response seemed to be considering the psychosocial needs of P (line 33): 'We talked about so many things … she seemed relieved, lightened up.'

But for N there was a spiritual aspect to the response as can be seen in line 32: 'It was the sacrament of the moment.' This was not part of the conversation with P but demonstrated in N a spiritual strength which she drew upon as appropriate in her work and her life.

Excerpt 2

31 N: She knew there was someone there for her.
32 It was the sacrament of the moment.
33 We talked about so many things … she seemed relieved, lightened up(')
34 R: This presencing was obvious in your demeanor when you must have given out
35 'I'm here only for you' It's something spiritual isn't it?
36 N: Yes I'm here for you – and oblivious to all else …
37 She knew there was someone there for her.

However, for P her concern was for her two children.

P's response as indicated in the discourse

Affordance	*Discourse evidence*	*Line*
Psychosocial	*– I've got 2 children*	20
	– and I'm dying	*20*
	– and I am so alone	*21*

N's perception of P's response

	– she shared so much about	22
	– her inner turmoil and sadness	22–23

In one sense, N's response to P's situation can be interpreted as a reflection of N's nursing values and their professional affordances.

- 'she shared' (an indication that she needed the support of another human being)
- 'her inner turmoil' (an indication of distress)
- 'and sadness' (an indication of regret for deprivation – of her children's lives and her (assumed) resulting loss of progeny ('I've got two children'))

At the same time, however, such psychosocial affordances, as identified above in the bracketed points, are driven by that deep and innate maternal longing that is part of the universal human condition, one that surpasses socio-cultural and professional boundaries. In such a situation of impending death the human response of N is to acknowledge and utilize available physical affordances, among which artifacts must be included.

Physical affordances	*Situation*	*Line*	*Response line*
artifacts	*– tea lady,*	*13*	
	– cup (of tea)	*13, 15*	*23*
	– curtains	*9,*	*25*

We note also that P's responses and the outcomes of the mediated action initiated by N are displayed not through any verbal discourse but through more powerful non-verbal displays of emotion, as when N said: '*her eyes opened **wide** and her face became **animated***'. (line 18/19) which N interpreted as indicators of patient health outcomes.

Physical signs of a change in emotional state		
	– Her response went from someone limp and disinterested	*18*
	to one where her eyes opened wide	*19*
	and her face became animated	*19*
	She turned her gaze towards me ...	*19*
	She shared so much ...	*22*

It is important to recognize that not only are affordances physical and psychosocial in nature but also involve a spatial dimension, itself also a powerful indicator of health outcomes.

Spatial artifacts as indicative of health outcomes – signs of change in emotional state

Spatial affordances	*Situation*	*Response*
	– a dark sombre space	*8*
	– curtains drawn with barely any light penetration	*9*
	– I asked if she wanted the curtains drawn back	*25*
	– room became bathed in light ... windows	26, 27

Significantly, the outcomes of the situation evidence the multidimensional nature of the responses of N and P, affordances that are physical and psychosocial as well as spatial. N did not just open the curtains but sought the opinion of P. In the same way, N did not simply accept the cup of tea from the tea lady but first asked P, and then offered to spend time and talk with P. Such micro examples of interaction display how in a situation of patient need, apparent weakness, and physical and psychosocial deficit, caring is co-constructed between, as here, N and P, evidenced both in talk and non-verbal action. Multidimensionality in interaction is thus aligned with multidimensionality in healthcare.

Presencing as a process and a practice

While presencing is an essential component of empathic behavior, it is not one that suddenly appears in the discourse. It is rather a strategy presupposing the development of a trusting relationship involving both participants. The onus is on N to demonstrate that she is a person who can be trusted, and to make clear to P that she is available for P to disclose her deep-seated needs. Trust and disclosure involve a developing and gradual process, not matters simply invoked by displays of professional identity. Indeed, the identity itself is one that is earned and develops with experience (and education) and this is not immediately and transparently obvious to one's interlocutor. But presencing as a process – and particularly in nursing situations – implies time – a factor that is not always available. This suggests that there must be an acceleration of the process and this demands expertise of the nurse – a factor that again comes only with education and experience (see Benner 1984; S. Candlin 1997) – if the patient's needs are to be met. The communicative expertise of the nurse is 'on the line' if she is to facilitate a positive outcome in P's health state. The process is indicated in the following extract of discourse when N and R are discussing the event.

Excerpt 2 (repeated partially here for ease of the reader)
31 *N:* *She knew there was someone there for her.*
32 *It was the sacrament of the moment.*
33 *We talked about so many things ... she seemed relieved, lightened up*
34 *R:* *This presencing was obvious in your demeanor when you must have given out*
35 *'I'm here only for you' It's something spiritual, isn't it?*
36 *N:* *Yes I'm here for you ...*

For N, her interaction with P was a spiritual experience (line 32) possibly even to be considered as a ministry.

N gave of her time (line 33) and P demonstrated an openness as indicated by her response – an obvious relief that she had unburdened herself. In the telling she had found what she wanted. We may note here the professionalism of N. She talked about her perceptions of P's situation, giving however no indication of P's deeper thoughts (line 33). N maintained the ethical code of confidentiality in respect of patient information. N was however prepared to discuss her own behavior (line 33) and her impressions of a changing situation (line 33).

The effects of presencing on N

Such intense interactions are not without their immediate effects on nurses. For N, this encounter with the young mother was a spiritual experience, as we see in her reference to the 'sacrament of the moment'. There are longer term effects as well. Such effects are not necessarily negative. We may say that the longer term effects of this brief episode in the care of P have remained as positive affordances with N as when she said (lines 28–29 in Excerpt 1):

... I don't know what happened to P as I only did one shift there
However I have never forgotten her.

This telling was repeated later (as in the following section of the conversation between N and R). While to some this might be interpreted as an indication of regret, N's professionalism allowed her to draw a line under the experience. She did not appear to be grieving for P but was able to share her experience with another nurse (R), something which may have effected her own healing process.

Researcher's (R) account

In her story, N demonstrates the deliberate focused attention discussed by Zerwekh (1997) as a prerequisite of presencing. But N also recognized that she (N) needed to initiate the interaction ('Is there anything wrong or that you would like to talk about because I can have a cup of tea with you?' – lines 16–17 Excerpt 1). Not only did she give the patient the opportunity to talk but re-enforced the sincerity of her offer by saying that she would have a cup of tea with her. She was not going to leave her. N, by gently asserting that she would stay with her, deliberately focused her attention on P. N would stay with her and listen. She gestured to the tea lady to go, both of them recognizing that P needed to talk with N. This focused attention supports Walsh's (2009) argument where, as we see from earlier discussion in this chapter, she talks about the nurse just 'being'; where verbal discourse is unnecessary and indeed can be a distraction. Nurses valued their interactions with patients and enjoyed caring for them, giving a sense of a cooperative action that 'we're in this together'. In our context, when discussing N's experience with her, R said that she thought that presencing was obvious in N's demeanor. This transcends words. R suggested that it had a spiritual element. To which N replied: 'Yes I'm here for you – and oblivious to all else'.

N and R were able to discuss nursing practices thereby providing some explanatory value to the situation.

Excerpt 3
Conversation between N and R

ix	R:	The spiritual experience affects all other dimensions of communication:
x		the non-verbal signs when P became animated, the physical
xi		when P lifted up her head,
xii		the spatial – the darkened room
xiii		and the artifacts – the cup of tea.
xiv	N:	Yes, and when I left, we had opened the curtains and
xv		the room was bathed in light.
xvi		I don't know what happened to that woman,
xvii		I never went back to the hospital so I don't know how long she lived.
xviii		I reported to the nurses what had happened and then I had to leave but I
xix		have never forgotten that experience. It's stayed with me all these years.

The conversation continued after a pause – again with repetitions of her first narrative – when R talked with N about N's conversation:

Excerpt 4

xx	N:	She knew there was someone there for her.
xxi		It was the sacrament of the moment. We talked about so many things.
xxii		She seemed relieved, lightened up.
xxiii		Yes I held the cup of tea and **then** there was the discourse.
xxiv	R:	This presencing was obvious in your demeanour when you must have
xxv		given out 'I'm here only for you'. It's something spiritual.
xxvi	N:	Yes I'm here for you – and oblivious to all else.
xxvii	R:	This was an opportunity for her to give meaning to the moment.
xxviii	N:	She knew there was someone there for her.

Perhaps N was placing herself here in a risky position (Candlin and Candlin 2002; S. Candlin 2002) by inviting the patient to talk, having little idea of what P was going to disclose, or request. But by deliberately focusing her attention on P, N recognized the patient's need and was able to move into a counseling role. That P was able to talk freely indicates how N was engaging in active and empathic listening. She was displaying empathy with P by being there at the point of P's need, and at that moment sharing in her humanity.

There were critical moments in this interaction that seemed to us to be evidenced not in the talk-in-interaction itself, but in relation to surrounding spatial factors. For example, N, who we recall was orienting herself to a new environment, was confronted by a darkened room and a young woman who appeared to be distressed. This was a critical moment that suggested to N she was entering into a situation requiring more explanatory information about P if she was to attempt to meet P's needs. Indeed, this determined N's next move 'I **returned** to the nurses' station at that point to collect additional medications and check her notes' (lines 11–12). Other factors included the presence of the artifacts, for example in the form of a cup of tea, which allowed N to say 'I can have a cup of tea with you' (line 17). A consequent critical moment, displayed in the discourse (both verbal and non-verbal), was when N was confronted with a change in P's non-verbal behavior when P looked up and established eye contact (line 19) where she made painful self-disclosures (PSDs) (lines 20–21) (Coupland et al. 1991). Such actions by P placed a responsibility on N to respond. It is through this taking on of this counseling role that N was able to demonstrate her presencing, compassion, and empathy. The meaning of the encounter was not lost on N and she was thus able to say, 'It was the sacrament of the moment' (line 32).

The identities, roles, and functions of the nurse

If we return now to our earlier discussion in the Preamble to this chapter concerning nurses' roles and functions, and in a later section to how identities may be revealed through narrative and interactional accounts, we can discern how N in the enactment of various professional nursing roles embraces a number of identities within this brief interaction.

She is seeable

- as a nurse in palliative care, evidenced by her taking report, doing the medication round, returning to the nurses' station to collect additional medications and check the notes;
- as a counselor, evidenced when she engages in her active listening role;
- as an informant and as a collaborative and joint participant in the research; and, above all
- as a person who shared in the humanity of another.

In sum, we may say that by adopting an overarching *presencing role,* N is seeable as a deeply caring human being. Nurses who allow their silent presence to communicate their caring can eliminate the loneliness that people may experience at the end of life. This for us constitutes *presencing,* being there only for the other person, regardless of one's own needs and desires. *Presencing* is thus unconditional love and service in action. It is an offering of self that makes no demands. It can be costly in terms of emotion and as such ought not be performed as an isolated activity. It requires the practical and emotional support of team members, as when, for example, colleagues seek to ensure that a nurse who is upset at the death of 'his/her' patient does not remain alone (if s/he doesn't want to be) at, say, morning tea or lunch. The nursing response to the patient is both complex and participatory since to practice her caring role the nurse necessarily draws support and strength from others. Such activity makes for a strong and caring team, demonstrated many times in the caring environment and not only in palliative care settings. Perhaps, then, the art of *presencing* is the hallmark of the expert nurse, demonstrating the highest level of communication skills and strategies (S. Candlin 2008: 246).

Preparing for presencing: Going beyond skills training in professional development

The above mini case study, not at all unusual in clinical nursing practice, can serve to demonstrate the manner in which critical moments may be handled by experienced nurses. We note how N was able to adapt her discourse and her mediated actions so that new trajectories were established that fitted a changing reality. New nursing goals had to be recognized and worked towards, and nursing functions had to be successfully employed to meet those goals. This change in functions with its accompanying change in mediated action is, in our view, entirely commensurate with the display of nursing experience and expertise. Characteristically it is evidenced by a resourcefulness in communicative action, frequently realized by polyphonic discourse.

However, such capacity and resourcefulness is not some simple matter of skill, although it is all too frequently labeled as such. It demands considerable knowledge and experience – institutional, professional, and interpersonal (see Sarangi and Roberts 1999), together with an awareness of the practices demanded in and appropriate to particular crucial sites of engagement. The testing of such practices and such capacity arises at critical moments in such sites, as with the interaction between N and P. Such expertise is not the outcome merely of some natural gift. It is fostered by that continuing reflection *in* and *on* practice called for by Schön (1983) and which is rightly the property of tailored professional development programs. These programs, in turn, to achieve such a goal, need to be data-driven and situation-focused, resourced from recognizable and authenticable sites of engagement.

One such approach is through those data-driven programs that follow a pedagogic and exploratory cycle of teaching and learning phases of *Awareness, Knowledge, Critique,* and *Action*, culminating in potential modifications to professional practice. An example, originally drawing on work in intercultural English as a Second Language (ESL) contexts in the US by Auerbach and Wallerstein (1997, 2004), was adapted by Candlin et al. (1995) for use in legal communication training, and subsequently by S. Candlin (1997) for use in nurse education, and by O'Grady (2011) in the communications training of registrars and novice doctors. In the context of nursing, S. Candlin (1997) sets out in some detail the content and process of such a curriculum. Beginning with the *Awareness* phase, and addressing the question: 'What do we know?' participants engage with consciousness-raising tasks, invoking personal experiential commentary, and directly drawing on authentic data (audio/video recorded and transcribed) relevant to the theme of the program. One such theme, and perhaps making use of similar data to that presented in this chapter, would be that of *Presencing* in nursing care. In the *Knowledge* phase, addressing the question: 'What do we need to learn?' new knowledge is accessed from multiple sources to enable fuller and more focused discussion of what appears to the participants, as in Goffman's (1983) sense, to be 'going on' in the data extracts in question, and much in the manner of the commentary on N's story provided earlier in this chapter. In this phase, too, participants come to determine and adopt a common analytical language in terms of which the data in question can be described, interpreted, and explained. In the *Critique* phase, and now addressing the question: 'Why are matters as they are?' there are two main foci. First, to inquire about the structural and organizational circumstances in the institutional order (Cicourel 1992; Sarangi and Roberts 1999) which give rise to the particular examples of the interaction order in question, and second, now more participant-focused, to engage with the reasons behind the particular performances in question, how these may or may not relate to broader professional concerns of degrees of expertise, or the appropriateness of situation-specific practices. Here the matters surrounding the identification and management of crucial sites and critical moments (again, see the discussion earlier in this chapter) would usefully be explored. In the final phase, that of *Action*, participants now draw on, and engage with their *own* recorded and transcribed data from their *own* professional practice, addressing the question: 'What can be done?'. Here the emphasis is on potential modifications to professional practices and behaviors which now become salient and possible as a consequence of the phased work undertaken to that point in the program. Such personally relevant data can then, suitably anonymized and with the ethical permissions of all involved, be recycled as input to the initial phases of any subsequent program, in this way completing what is a continuing and practice-generating cycle of description, interpretation, and explanation aimed at enhancing professional judgment in performance. In short, the achievement of *praxis*.

In our view, and in the light of our experience, such practices as these have considerable traction in clinical settings, raising awareness in program participants of discourse in use, but also enabling the translating of such awareness into practical action. Teacher/facilitator support with planned resources can increase knowledge, while experiential learning (in the form of Total Situation Focused Learning – see S. Candlin 2008; S. Candlin and Roger 2013) can be highly valuable in the development of professional competence in critical analysis. As we argue throughout this chapter, such a process goes far beyond mere skills training and modeling. It can have profound effects on the improvement of professional practice, impacting positively on patient care, and on healthcare more generally.

Related topics

Presencing; nursing; healthcare; healing; holistic.

Further reading

Bradshaw, A. (1994) 'Lighting the lamp', in *The spiritual dimension of nursing care*, London: Scutari Press.

Donohue, M.P. (1985) 'Nursing', in *The finest art: an illustrated history*, St Louis: The C.V. Mosby Company.

Iedema, R. (ed.) (2007) *The discourse of hospital communication: tracing complexities in contemporary health care organizations*, Basingstoke: Palgrave Macmillan.

Kember, D. et al. (2001) *Reflective teaching and learning in the health professions*, Oxford: Blackwell Science.

Women's Cancer Group (1997) *Songs of strength*, Sydney: Macmillan.

References

Antaki, C. and Widdicombe, S. (1998) *Identities in talk*, London: Sage.

Auerbach, E. and Wallerstein, N. (1997) *ESL for action: problem posing at work*, Menlo Park, CA: Addison Wesley.

——(2004) *Problem posing at work: ESL for action*, 2nd edn, Edmonton, Alberta: Grass Roots Press.

Bamberg, M. (1997) 'Positioning between structure and performance', *Journal of Narrative and Life History*, 7: 335–342.

Bamberg, M. and Georgakopoulou, A. (2008) 'Small stories as a new perspective in narrative and identity analysis', *Text & Talk*, 28: 377–396.
Bamberg, M., De Fina, A., and Schiffrin, D. (2007) *Selves and identities in narrative and discourse*, Philadelphia, PA: John Benjamins.
Benner, P. (1984) *From novice to expert. Excellence and power in clinical nursing practice*, Menlo Park, CA: Addison Wesley.
——(2004) 'Relational ethics of comfort, touch and solace – endangered arts?', *American Journal of Critical Care*, 13(4): 346–349.
Benner, P. and Wrubel, J. (1989) *The primacy of caring: stress and coping in health and illness*, Menlo Park, CA: Addison Wesley.
Buber, M. (1923/1967) *Ich und Du (I and thou)*, trans. W. Kaufmann, New York: Charles Scribners's.
——(1947/1979) *Between man and man*, trans. R.G. Smith, London: Kegan Paul.
Candlin, C.N. (1987a) 'Explaining moments of conflict in discourse', in R. Steele and T. Threadgold (eds) *Learning, keeping and using language: Language Topics Vol. 2 Proceedings of the 1987 AILA Congress, Sydney*, Amsterdam: John Benjamins.
——(1987b) 'What happens when applied linguistics goes critical?', in R. Steele and T. Threadgold (eds) *Learning, keeping and using language: Language Topics Vol. 2 Proceedings of the 1987 AILA Congress, Sydney*, Amsterdam: John Benjamins.
——(2002) 'Introduction: research & practice in professional discourse', in C.N. Candlin (ed.) *Research and practice in professional discourse*, Hong Kong: City University of Hong Kong Press.
Candlin, C.N. and Candlin, S. (2002) 'Introduction: discourse, expertise and the management of risk in health care settings', in C.N. Candlin and S. Candlin (eds) Special Issue of the *Journal of Research on Language and Social Interaction*, 35(2):115–137.
Candlin, C.N. and Lucas, J. (1986) 'Interpretations and explanations in discourse: modes of "advising" in family planning', in T. Ensink, A. van Essen, and T. van der Geest (eds) *Discourse analysis and public life*, Dordrecht: Foris
Candlin, C.N., Maley, Y., Koster, P., and Crichton, J. (1995) *Lawyer–client conferencing: a report to the Law Foundation of NSW*, Sydney: Law Foundation of NSW.
Candlin, S. (1997) 'Towards excellence in nursing: an analysis of the discourses of nurses and patients in the context of health assessments', PhD thesis, University of Lancaster.
——(2002) 'Taking risks: an indicator of expertise?', *Research on Language and Social Interaction*, 35(2): 173–194.
——(2008) *Therapeutic communication: a lifespan approach*, French's Forest, NSW: Pearson Education.
Candlin, S. and Candlin, C.N. (2007) 'Nursing over time and space: some issues for the construct "community of practice"', in R. Iedema (ed.) *The discourse of hospital communication: tracing complexities in contemporary health care organizations*, London: Palgrave Macmillan: 244–267.
Candlin, S. and Roger, P. (2013) *Communication and professional relationships in healthcare practice*, Sheffield: Equinox.
Cassidy, S. (1988) *Sharing the darkness: the spirituality of caring*, London: Darton, Longman, and Todd.
Cicourel, A. (1973) *Cognitive sociology*, Harmondsworth: Penguin.
——(1992) 'The interpenetration of communicative contexts: examples from medical encounters', in A. Duranti and C. Goodwin (eds) *Rethinking context: language as an interactive phenomenon*, Cambridge: Cambridge University Press.
——(1996) 'Ecological validity and "white room effects": the interaction of cognitive and cultural models in the pragmatic analysis of elicited narratives from children', *Pragmatics and Cognition*, 4(2): 221–264.
——(2007) 'A personal, retrospective view of ecological validity', *Text & Talk*, 27: 735–752.
Coupland, N., Coupland, J., and Giles, H. (1991) *Language, society and the elderly*, Oxford: Blackwell.
De Fina, A. (2009) 'Narratives in interview – the case of accounts: for an interactional approach to narrative genres', *Narrative Inquiry*, 19(2): 233–258.
De Fina, A. and Georgakopoulou A. (2008) 'Analysing narratives as practices', *Qualitative Research*, 8(3): 379–387.
De Fina, A., Schiffrin, D., and Bamberg, M. (2006) *Discourse and identity*, Cambridge: Cambridge University Press.

Encyclopaedia and dictionary of medicine, nursing and allied health (1987) B.F. Miller and C. B. Keane (eds) 4th edn, Philadelphia, PA: W.B. Saunders.
Fairclough, N.L. (1992) *Discourse and social change*, Cambridge: Polity Press.
Fredricksson, L. (1999) 'Modes of relating in a caring conversation: a research synthesis on presence, touch and listening', *Journal of Advanced Nursing,* 30(5): 1167–1176.
Garfinkel, H. (1956) 'Conditions of successful degradation ceremonies', *American Journal of Sociology,* 61: 420–424.
——(1967) 'Good organizational reasons for "bad" clinical records', in H. Garfinkel (ed.) *Studies in Ethnomethodology*, Englewood Cliffs, NJ: Prentice-Hall.
Georgakopoulou, A. (2006) 'Thinking big with small stories in narrative and identity analysis', *Narrative Inquiry,* 16:122–130.
Gibson, J.J. (1977) 'The theory of affordances', in R. Shaw and J. Bransford (eds) *Perceiving, acting, and knowing: toward an ecological psychology*, Hillsdale, NJ: Lawrence Erlbaum.
Goffman, E. (1967) *Interaction ritual: essays on face-to-face behavior*, New York: Doubleday Anchor.
——(1983) 'The interaction order', *American Sociological Review,* 48: 1–17.
Greenhalgh, T., Russell, J., and Swinglehurst, D. (2005) 'Narrative methods in quality improvement research', *Quality & Safety in Health Care,* 14: 443–449.
Heidegger, M. (1927/1962/1977) *Sein und Zeit (Being and Time)*, in F.W. von Hermann (ed.) *M. Heidegger Gesamtausgabe Vol. 2 XIV*, trans. J. Macquarrie and E. Robinson, London: SCM Press.
McFarlane, J. (1981) 'Spiritual care', *Contact,* 73(4): 14–16.
O'Grady, C. (2011) 'Teaching the communication of empathy in patient-centred medicine', in B. Hoekje and S. Tipton (eds) *English language and the medical profession: instructing and assessing the communication skills of international physicians*, Bingley, UK: Emerald: 43–72.
Owen-Mills, V. (1998) 'Presencing in practice: utilising the core of the caring process', *Australian Journal of Holistic Nursing,* 5(1): 4–9.
Pederson, C. (1993) 'Presence as a nursing intervention with hospitalized children', *Maternal-Child Journal,* 3: 75–81.
Rampton, B. (ed.) (2007) *Linguistic ethnography:* Special Issue of *Journal of Sociolinguistics*, 11(5).
Rampton, B., Tusting, K., Maybin, J., Barwell, R., Creese, A., and Lytra, V. (2004) 'UK linguistic ethnography: a discussion paper', Coordinating Committee UK Linguistic Ethnography Forum.
Riessman, C.K. (1990) 'Strategic uses of narrative in the presentation of self and illness: a research note', *Social Sciences and Medicine,* 30(11): 1193–1200.
——(2001) 'Analysis of personal narratives', in J.F. Gubrium and J.A. Holstein (eds) *Handbook of interviewing*, London: Sage.
——(2002) 'Illness narratives: positioned identities', annual lecture to the Health Communication Research Centre, Cardiff University, Wales, May.
——(2003) 'Performing identities in illness narrative: masculinity and multiple sclerosis', *Qualitative Research,* 3(5): 5–33.
Sarangi, S. and Candlin, C.N. (2001) '"Motivational relevancies": some methodological reflections on social theoretical and sociolinguistic practice', in N. Coupland, S. Sarangi, and C.N. Candlin (eds) *Sociolinguistics and social theory*, London: Pearson.
——(2003) 'Editorial: categorization and explanation of risk: a discourse analytical perspective', *Health, Risk & Society,* 5: 115–124.
Sarangi, S. and Roberts, C. (eds) (1999) *Talk, work and the institutional order: discourse in medical, mediation and management settings*, Berlin: Mouton de Gruyter, Language, Power and Social Process series.
Schiffrin, D. (1996) 'Narrative as self-portrait: sociolinguistic constructions of identity', *Language and Society,* 25: 167–203.
Schön, D. (1983) *The reflective practitioner: how professionals think in action*, New York: Basic Books.
Schutz, A. (1962) *Collected papers I: the problem of social reality,* M. Natanson (ed.) The Hague: Martinus Nijhoff.
Scollon, R. (1998) *Mediated discourse as social interaction*, London: Longman.
——(1999) 'Mediated discourse and social interaction', *Research on Language & Social Interaction,* 32: 149–154.
——(2001) 'Action and text: towards an integrated understanding of the place of text in social (inter) action, mediated discourse analysis and the problem of social action', in R. Wodak and M. Meyer (eds) *Methods of critical discourse analysis*, London: Sage.

Scollon, R. and Scollon, S.W. (2004) *Nexus analysis: discourse and the emergent internet*, London: Routledge.
Walsh, K.M. (2009) 'Disciplined silence: a focused ethnography of exemplary emergency nursing practice', PhD thesis, University of Connecticut.
Wertsch, J.V. (1991) *Voices of the mind: a sociocultural approach to mediated action*, Cambridge, MA: Harvard University Press.
——(1994) 'The primacy of mediated action in sociocultural studies', *Mind, Culture & Activity*, 1: 202–208.
Zerwekh, J.V. (1997) 'The practice of presencing', *Seminars in Oncology Nursing*, 13(4): 260–262.
Zimmerman, D.H. and Wieder, D.L. (1970) 'Ethnomethodology and the problem of order: comment on Denzin', in J.D. Douglas (ed.) *Understanding everyday life*, Chicago, IL: Aldine.

18

Transforming medical school culture

A case of changing conversations

Richard M. Frankel and Elaina Chen

Introduction

As a discipline, linguistics has traditionally been concerned with studying the nature, structure, and variation of language within the boundaries of single sentences. In sociolinguistics and in some areas of pragmatics, analysts take the study of speech production a step further by looking at the influence of social context on the choice of a speaker's words, and the impact of those words on a co-conversationalist. Yet one step further into the world of language-in-use, conversation analysis focuses on the sequential organization of talk as it emerges in real time. The goal of conversation analysis is to understand the organizing principles that account for the coordinated use of language by speakers and hearers, whether they are strangers or intimates, having a casual chat or seeking medical care in a large group practice. Given its focus on how speakers and hearers coordinate their interactions, the smallest unit of measure in conversation analysis is a sequence in which turns at talk are exchanged.

In this chapter we build on the goals of sociolinguistics and conversation analysis to understand language in context. Our point of departure is in moving from sentences and sequences to whole conversations that occur in complex bureaucratic organizations like medical schools. Our overriding question is whether it is possible to transform the nature of these conversations and in so doing change the patterns of social relationships that create and sustain organizational culture. Two developments in medical education and the positive social sciences inform our approach: the first is a growing recognition among medical educators that a substantial gap exists between the language of pre-clinical classroom instruction and what is experienced in the hospital during clinical rotations; the second is an area of scholarship known as Appreciative Inquiry (AI), an organizational change framework that focuses on the positive potential for storytelling in conversation to change organizational culture. We briefly describe both below.

Linking language in the classroom with actual care contexts

Perhaps the most important need in medical education today is to reconcile what is being taught in the 'classroom' in the first two years, with what is observed and experienced by students in their third and fourth year clinical rotations, when they are immersed in the types of work settings in which they will one day practice. At root is what Hafferty and others have labeled an informal or 'hidden curriculum' problem (Hafferty and Franks 1994) in which the formal language of classroom instruction and the day-to-day or moment-to-moment lived experience of trainees in the hospital or clinic don't match. Although it is not a causal relationship, the gap has been associated with declines in medical student empathy from first to fourth year (Hojat et al. 2009) an increase in cynicism over time (Wear et al. 2006), increased amounts of burnout (Santen et al. 2010) and a degradation in standards of ethical behavior (Dyrbye et al. 2010). In addition, recent studies of student narratives document a range of unprofessional behaviors observed by students during clinical rotations (Karnieli-Miller, Vu et al. 2010; Karnieli-Miller, Taylor et al. 2010; Karnieli-Miller et al. 2011). It is clear from these studies that there is a language gap in medical education, one that is associated with a number of negative outcomes, including disavowal of the formal curriculum (Ginsburg et al. 2003).

Appreciative Inquiry was developed in the 1980s by David Cooperrider (2001), a professor in the Business School at Case Western University. Cooperrider was studying automobile manufacturing processes at a time when the quality of American cars was waning and Japanese car quality had increased substantially. Interested to know what accounted for the differences, he observed how Japanese automobile workers at a Toyota plant went about their work and dealt with quality issues. While policing and inspection were used to 'control' quality in American plants by weeding out 'bad apples' and punishing poor performance, Cooperrider discovered that the Japanese had an entirely different approach to problems of quality. In the Japanese context mistakes were seen as a 'gift' to the community that everyone could learn and benefit from. The difference in approach led Cooperrider to conclude that in every organization something is going well and that if one can shift the conversational frame from what's wrong and how to fix it to what's right and how to get more of it one can essentially change the nature of the organization. Appreciative Inquiry has been used worldwide in many different organizational contexts with positive results (Bushe and Kassam 2005). It has also been used in some areas of medicine and nursing (Carter et al. 2007; Shendell-Falik et al. 2007; Helms et al. 2012).

A related concept to AI is the concept of Relational Coordination, a term coined by Jody Gittell, a professor in the Business School at Brandeis University, to describe findings from her research on the success of Southwest Airlines (Gittell 2002). Relational Coordination refers to, 'a mutually reinforcing process of interaction between communication and relationships carried out for the purpose of task integration' (Gittell 2009). Gittell found that the company's success lay primarily in its ability to encourage and support high levels of communication across multiple job classifications and management. Applying her approach to health care, Gittell has shown that organizations with high levels of Relational Coordination have better care outcomes and lower overall costs (Gittell 2009). In short, language that focuses on creating and sustaining positive potential and relationships relates to individual and organizational success.

Neither Cooperrider nor Gittell draw explicitly on work in sociolinguistics or conversation analysis. Nonetheless, both of their approaches depend on an understanding of how language shapes context and vice versa. For example, Cooperrider et al. assert,

> AI seeks, fundamentally, to build a constructive union between a whole people and the massive entirety of what people talk about as past and present capacities: achievements, assets, unexplored potentials, innovations, strengths, elevated thoughts, opportunities, benchmarks, high point moments, lived values, traditions, strategic competencies, stories, expressions of wisdom, insights into the deeper corporate spirit or soul – and visions of valued and possible futures.
>
> *(Cooperrider et al. 2005)*

Here, as in many other aspects of his writing, there is a deep, but unstated, connection to linguists such as Sapir and Whorf (Whorf 1940) and the idea that language has an effect (strong or weak) in determining perception (Rossi-Landi 1983).

Likewise, Gittell's work on Relational Coordination shares much in common with conversation analysis and its focus on the coordinated actions of speakers and hearers in social interactions and relationships. Gittell asserts,

> Relational Coordination theory sheds light on the relational work process that underlies the technical work process, arguing that coordination is not just the management of interdependence between tasks – it's also the management of interdependence between the people who perform those tasks. RC theory reveals the inter-subjectivity of the coordination process, paying close attention to the quality of communication and relationships among participants, as well as to the technical requirements of the work.
>
> *(Gittell 2012)*

The problem of intersubjectivity is a primary focus of phenomenological philosophy (Husserl 2001) and its operationalization in sociology through the work of Harold Garfinkel (1967) and Harvey Sacks (1992).

We turn next to a description of three different, but related, language-based initiatives designed to change the conversations and the organizational culture of a large medical school.

Putting sociolinguistics to work: the Relationship-Centered Care Initiative at the Indiana University School of Medicine

In January 2003, armed with a theoretical background in language and social interaction, organizational tools that had their roots in attention to language and culture, and generous funding from the Fetzer Institute in Kalamazoo, MI, we set about to change the nature of the conversations that were occurring at the Indiana University School of Medicine, the largest in North America. The Relationship-Centered Care Initiative (RCCI) and its outcomes have been described elsewhere (Inui et al. 2006; Cottingham et al. 2008; Inui et al. 2008; Williamson et al. 2011). In this chapter, we focus on three specific areas in which we used Appreciative Inquiry and Relational Coordination to change the nature of the conversations in the day-to-day life of the organization: faculty development, admissions, and the generational differences in the use of social media. For each, we provide a case example that includes a brief background, the organizational challenge, intervention strategy, and outcomes achieved. Our goal is to be illustrative, not exhaustive, in our discussion and where possible to make the link between organizational behavior and sociolinguistic thinking.

Case 1: Faculty development, 'the physician as patient'

Much of the teaching that is done in medical school, especially in the first two pre-clinical years, takes place in the classroom and uses a standard lecture format. Although this model is based upon a time-honored tradition, there is evidence in medicine and other clinical disciplines that it is a poor way to communicate information and skills (Davis et al. 1995). Scholarship on what has been termed the informal, or 'hidden', curriculum of medical education (Hafferty and Franks 1994) suggests that students learn as much by what they see their instructors do on the wards and in the clinic as they do in the classroom. Recognition of the power of the hidden curriculum has led to calls for reform in the content and process of what is taught in the medical school curriculum (Hafferty et al. 2011). Unfortunately, faculty who were trained in the traditional lecture format do not necessarily have the skills of small group process and role modeling that medical education reform requires. Helping faculty develop the appropriate language and behaviors to teach in new ways is a challenge in most medical schools including Indiana University School of Medicine.

A particularly difficult concept for medical students to grasp, given their age and relatively good health, is what it means to suffer from illness, disease, and loss. Lectures about suffering, as an abstract concept, do not convey the experience of learning first hand from patients or, in this case, faculty role models who have been patients. We were interested in giving a diverse group of faculty with responsibilities for teaching first- and second-year medical students an opportunity to learn about experiential teaching using peer-to-peer storytelling and a technique known as teaching by parallel process (role modeling), based on the work of Marvel (1991) and others (Markakis et al. 2000). Our goal for the session was to change the conversations faculty would first have among themselves and then, by parallel process, with students about the nature and experience of suffering.

The idea for the faculty development session was simple. We started with the notion of inviting several high profile physician faculty members, including the dean, an executive associate dean, a department chair, and a division chief (all of whom had had life-threatening illnesses and had become patients) to tell their stories in a three-hour faculty development workshop. All agreed, and at the suggestion of the dean, the spouses of each were contacted and also agreed to participate. To illustrate differences in perspectives and language, each couple was asked to write, but not share, a one-page description of what it was like to be a patient or the spouse of a physician who had become a patient. The workshop opened with each couple reading their description, for the first time, in front of their spouse and an audience of 30 clinician educators. The workshop received Institutional Review Board (IRB) approval so that its content could be videotaped and used for education and research purposes. Below is a partial transcript of the opening descriptions from one of the couples, Bill and Mary Tierney (names used with permission).

> *Physician/patient's opening statement*
> About 25 days after I was hired as Division Chief [in General Internal Medicine], I was diagnosed with Stage 3, non-Hodgkins Lymphoma … Right around the end of my last treatment, my wife had an abnormal mammogram … and for reasons to this day I don't really understand, it bothered me more waiting to get her biopsy results than it did getting my own diagnosis. I realized that for the entire time I was being treated for Lymphoma that I had completely ignored the effect that my condition had on her. And she had completely not transmitted

> any of that [anxiety] other than just caring about how hard it had been on her. And I realized that waiting for the biopsy must have been a lot easier than being told that I had cancer and being treated for it. We never talked about prognosis; the prognosis wasn't terribly good at the time. It just opened my eyes to how insensitive I had been to the effect my condition had on her. I was just completely unprepared for how much different it was for a family member than it was for the person with the actual condition.

> *Spouse's opening statement*
> It is common knowledge that Pablo Picasso had his Blue Period. It is not common knowledge that I had what I label my 'guilt period'. The first instance of guilt occurred about 10 seconds after Bill revealed to me that he had been diagnosed with Stage 3 Lymphoma. What can possibly happen in a flash of 10 seconds that can set up a pattern of feelings of guilt? The answer in this case is just words. Those words were, 'Oh no. Please don't leave me now. We have too much time left. I will be alone.' Then the words were gone and my mind turned to Bill's awful illness and ordeal. I was left with the reality that my first thoughts were of myself and not of Bill's impending struggle. Other instances of guilt become my companion throughout the next 2 years. With the exception of one instance, none of them were uttered out loud. I remember accompanying Bill to his first chemo treatment and thinking, 'okay, I can do this.' But later for subsequent treatments, [I didn't go] and I felt glad and then guilty … I did not want to watch that bright red medicine go into him … Some months later I attended a high school reunion without Bill … I had so much fun talking with old friends and just being away. When I returned home Bill asked, 'How was the reunion?' and I said, 'It was so much fun. I haven't had so much fun in a long time.' As soon as I said that 'bang' guilt, big time. Guilt is not a good companion. It eats away at you and it's isolating but I lived with it and it was my truth. It's now 5 years later and I'm okay with how I felt at the time.

Many points could be made about these two opening statements. For our purposes, it is worth noting that both the physician/patient and his spouse made assumptions and were aware of things they didn't express to one another until the evening of the workshop. For Bill, it was the assumption that his spouse's silence was a measure of empathic witnessing and support, whereas for Mary the same silence, with the one exception of returning from a reunion with old friends, represented guilt for not doing enough or thinking too much about her own needs. Interestingly, both felt that they had neglected the suffering of the other which produced unstated feelings of guilt. In terms of teaching and learning using parallel process, this pair of narratives offered both Bill and Mary, *and* the audience, powerful insights into the role of language, tacit assumptions, and interpretation in shaping experience. Further, sharing their narratives transformed their understanding of an important life event and deepened their relationship.

As was true for Bill and Mary, each of the other three couples' descriptions held similar drama and strong emotions. After a brief opportunity for workshop participants to comment and ask clarifying questions of the couples, each of the presenters became a facilitator for a small group session in which workshop participants were invited to share their own experiences of suffering, either their own or witnessing the suffering of others. The idea was to use parallel process to 'immerse' participants in doing the same activity for themselves that they had just seen modeled. The small group discussions were quite poignant and experiences of tragedy, loss, and witnessing surfaced and were shared among small group members.

There were no trainees in the workshop but there was a professor from a nearby university who had had a very negative experience in communicating with a fourth-year medical student during a recent hospitalization. The professor was a cancer survivor and reported that after a cursory look at her medical record, the fourth-year student casually said, 'I see here you're a cancer survivor and you haven't had a recurrence yet?' So incensed was she at the language used by the student that she called the dean of the medical school and complained bitterly about the student's insensitivity. The dean's response was to first apologize and then invite her to join the workshop to see how faculty members were learning to teach humanistic skills. The professor agreed to do so.

Sitting among a group of four physicians and a behavioral scientist, the professor tearfully described the pain and suffering she had experienced as a result of the student's casual use of language and what she interpreted as his disregard for her lived experience. In response, group members provided comfort and shared their own stories of suffering, many of which came from their own training and described situations in which their emotional needs were disregarded by their clinical instructors. For example, one faculty member described how as a fourth-year medical student she was asked by an attending physician to conduct cardio pulmonary resuscitation (CPR) on a patient who several other residents had already tried unsuccessfully to resuscitate. As she began a clearly futile process the rest of the team left the room and moved on to see their next patient. She was overwhelmed by feelings of loss, doubt, shame, and abandonment, yet there was never any discussion of the death or any opportunity for team members to work through their feelings about what had happened. Hearing these stories in her small group, the professor was able to acknowledge the fact that what the trainee actually needed was better guidance and coaching in how to have a conversation with a cancer survivor and not a failing grade or punishment for failing to keep his patient's needs at the center. At the same time, creating the conditions for this conversation had made faculty members acutely aware of the need for better teaching in this domain.

There were three concrete outcomes from this particular conversation. First, the professor emailed the dean the day after the workshop and asserted that the humanities weren't being taught at her university; they were, instead, being taught and embodied at the Indiana University School of Medicine, a 180-degree turnaround from her initial experience as a patient. Second, on the basis of her experience in the workshop, and her deeper understanding of the intent and motivation to change the nature of the conversation in educating students about suffering, the professor volunteered to become adjunct medical school faculty and help teach the interviewing portion of the Introduction to Medicine course to first-year students. Third, while we do not have follow-up data on how, and to what extent, faculty changed their behavior on the basis of the workshop, we know from comments at the conclusion of the workshop and emails and anecdotes from participating faculty that many felt that they had gained skills and insight into teaching by example, not by edict.

Case 2: Changing conversation in admissions committee interviews

> I'll never forget my medical school interview even though it was 27 years ago. I was interviewed by two admissions committee members who interrogated me, machine gun style, about whether I thought I was 'tough enough' to become a doctor and whether women should even become doctors if they were going to have children and raise families.
>
> *(Reflection of a senior faculty member, 2010)*

> I just wanted to take this opportunity to thank you for taking time out from your busy schedule to interview me today for the incoming class at Indiana University School of Medicine. I also wanted to thank you for making the interview process so relaxed and conversational. Truthfully, I could not have asked for a better experience in beginning my pursuit of becoming a doctor.
>
> *(Letter from a medical school applicant, 2011)*

Admission to medical school begins the long process of professional socialization that culminates in becoming a physician. While the White Coat Ceremony or the Dean's convocation may mark the 'official' beginning of medical school, it is the admission interview that gives the successful applicant their first exposure to the core values and expectations of the institution where they will spend a minimum of their next four years. Researchers have investigated the criteria admission committees use to select candidates and how the interview is weighted, but little is known about the conversations that actually transpire between applicants and admissions committee officers and how they affect recommendations to accept or reject (Elam et al. 2002).

With permission of all 26 admissions committee members (ACMs), 13 teams each composed of two interviewers, and approval from the Indiana University (IU) IRB, we designed a novel experiment to address this question using a 'standardized student', in this case an actress who played the role of an aspiring medical student who was randomly placed into the sequence of genuine applicants scheduled for interviews. The unannounced standardized student was coached on the role she was to play, and was given fictitious credentials and a narrative describing her interest in medicine and the fact that she had had an institutional action which involved underage consumption of alcohol as a freshman in college. She also carried a concealed digital audio recorder with which to record her interviews for later transcription and analysis. None of her interviews was flagged as being 'fake' by admissions committee officers despite their being invited by the study investigators to identify the simulated interviewee. Within the limits of training, the standardized applicant's story was exactly the same from interview to interview. In this way we were able to hold the simulated student's performance relatively constant and look at variations in the questioning style of the interviewer(s). In other contexts, standardized patients, (SPs), have been used extensively in assessing clinical and communication competencies of physicians and the technique has proven to be a valid method of assessment (Beaulieu et al. 2003). Below, we present transcribed fragments from three Standardized Applicant (SA) interviews with admissions committee members (ADM) from different interviewing teams each inquiring about the administrative action. For ease of understanding, the admissions committee member is identified as INT and the standardized student as ST.

Interview Team # 1

INT: I noticed on your resume there was a little problem that you had at some time-back at USI (University of Southern Indiana) of with drinking in the dorm or something//what was that all about]
ST: Oh yeah Um,
→ INT: I mention that not because, I wanna bring it up
ST: (little laugh)
INT: but because the way the committee works (lengthy pause)
ST: (lengthy pause) Right
INT: they're going to ask me about this

Interview Team # 2

INT: The-one thing I have to clear up-(can I) get to it?
ST: Okay
INT: is your self-reported institutional action
ST: Oh um-hmm
→ INT: Is that like it was when you were, a young, naive student
ST: Oh definitely

Interview Team # 3

→ INT: Okay, um okay (whispered) Okay, in college you were cited for alcohol abuse in the dorm (2) (laughs) So tell us about it.

In analyzing these three interview fragments it is clear that there was wide variation in the interviewing styles used by the admissions committee members (ACMs). In the first example, the interviewer asks the standardized student about her institutional action but hedges his statement by saying that it is not necessarily his interest that is driving the question but the committee at large that will question him if he does not. This is a classic example of a question that 'passes the buck' in terms of the intent of the question, which is to learn if the applicant is at risk for problem drinking. Example 2 illustrates the use of a leading question, one that hints at the type of answer being searched for. In this instance, the interviewer hints at the preferred answer in characterizing the institutional action as having happened 'when you were, a young, naive student', an assertion with which the standardized student readily agrees. In example 3, the interviewer asks in a neutral way for the standardized student to explain the institutional action, neither hinting at a preferred answer nor turning the motivation for the question as having come from another source.

In addition to the interview itself, each interviewing team makes a recommendation to the committee at large about whether to accept or reject the applicant. Two of the teams had an interviewer who was aware of the identity of the simulated student, leaving 11 teams who voted. On the basis of their interview with the standardized student presented above, 7 of the 11 teams strongly recommended that the applicant be admitted to the medical school. However, 4 of the teams recommended equally strongly that she be denied admission. In reviewing the transcripts of the recorded interviews it became clear that the way in which the questions were being asked of the SA was associated with the recommendation to accept or reject. Teams that used leading questions that treated the institutional action as the minor indiscretion of 'a young, naive student' were much more likely to recommend admission than teams that used neutral questions and carefully assessed what the student had learned from her actions. These teams were more likely to recommend rejection.

The final step in changing conversations among admissions committee members was to feed back the information that had been gathered from their standard student interviews in the spirit of quality improvement. Committee members were quite shocked that there was only 64 percent agreement on recommendations to admit or reject the 'same' standardized student. As a result, a half-day workshop with skills practice was designed to help committee members standardize the format for asking questions. Results to date have been encouraging and preliminary data from subsequent standardized student interviews suggest rates of agreement that are in the 85–90 percent range.

Case 3: Changing conversations about the use of social media: the two cultures

In his 1959 essay, *The Two Cultures and the Scientific Revolution*, the noted scientist and novelist C.P. Snow argued that there was a gulf in language and understanding between science and art and that the two cultures were incommensurable with one another, despite the fact that there are common words and phrases used by scientists and artists to describe their work. A decade later, the literary critic George Steiner suggested a similar gap in describing the relationship between everyday speech and the language of mathematics (Steiner 1998). More recently, variations, if not divisions, in language use and understanding have been described by sociolinguists in terms of age (Eble 1996), gender (Tannen 1990), and race (Erickson and Schultz 1982). An interesting variation on this theme, with implications for medical education, is the distinctive use of social media by the so-called 'millennial' generation of children born at beginning of the 1980s.

It is widely known that the 'Millennials', who include medical students, residents, and to some degree fellows and junior faculty, are almost constantly engaged in using social media. In a two-part series entitled 'Digital Natives, Digital Immigrants', Marc Prensky (2001a, 2001b) makes the case that there is a digital divide that separates Millennials from Generation Xers or Baby Boomers. According to Prensky, Millennials are 'Digital Natives', surrounded by digital media to such an extent that their language and very brain structures may be different from those of previous generations. Digital natives are used to receiving and processing information from multiple sources instantaneously. They use skills like parallel processing and multitasking to analyze situations and data. Another major difference is that they prefer to view graphics *before* reading a text rather than after which is more characteristic of Baby Boomers and Gen Xers. They also prefer random access (like hypertext) rather than being bound by linear search strategies. Millennials function best when networked with others; they thrive on instant gratification and frequent rewards. And, they prefer games to 'serious' work (Prensky 2001a, 2001b).

In contrast, those born before the advent of the digital age reveal their non-native status through a 'Digital Immigrant Accent' that manifests itself in a number of ways. For example, digital immigrants would rather print out a digital document to edit it rather than editing it online. They prefer to communicate via phone rather than texting or other forms of communication such as instant messaging. Digital immigrants are often stymied by reading directions for how to use digital media step by step and finding themselves frustrated by their preferred approach. Digital natives, by contrast, are intuitive users of digital media and devices and use trial and error methods until they hit upon a workable solution. Digital immigrants fear that the 'costs' of using digital technology (e.g., learning to use software or digital devices and the tendency to play games when there is serious work to do) outweigh the benefits (Prensky 2001a, 2001b)

To better understand the divide between digital natives and digital immigrants in medical education we as co-authors (EC, a fourth-year medical student and RF a senior faculty member and administrator) designed a *Gedanken*, or thought, experiment, in which we independently responded to the following open-ended question about social media: 'What is your experience of how medical students use social media in the formal and informal curriculum of the medical school?' We report the results as a dialog below.

EC: Very little of our *formal* medical education utilizes social media. Rather, it is used widely in student run organizations. Many have their own social media pages where events, photos, comments, links, etc., are updated by student leaders periodically. Medical students in general are highly motivated to participate in and lead service-oriented events despite their heavy course loads and demanding clinical duties. Social media provides an efficient vehicle for keeping in touch with fellow students.

RF: Students' use of social media is something of a black box for me. I don't use it much myself and don't really have a clear idea of what others see in it. I do notice that in teaching sessions almost every student has a mobile device that they refer to from time to time during lectures. From what I can see they appear to be surfing or texting rather than taking notes. It sometimes feels disrespectful because their attention seems to be split between the lecture material and other unrelated activities and paying attention to the lecture material.

EC: In the past, a typical strategy for communicating among students was hallway bulletin boards, often overflowing with advertisements for social events, service projects, apartments for rent, furniture for sale, and myriad volunteer opportunities that might be available. A few years ago, the school implemented advanced lecture-recording technology that allows lectures to be streamed on line thus obviating the need to be physically present for classes. This makes flyers, bulletin boards and other analog methods of reaching out to students outdated and obsolete.

RF: Many of us were trained in an era in which class attendance was mandatory and we as faculty got to know our students, and the students got to know one another extremely well. With online streaming of lectures and the number of contact hours being reduced there is a sense of lost opportunity to create campus community, at least in a physical sense. I assume that if I don't see students physically present in classes that they are 'blowing off' the opportunity to learn in community and get to know one another as colleagues and friends, something that I found extremely useful in my own training and feel is important to professional growth and development.

EC: Another old-fashioned means of communication is telephone phone calls. With the advent of text messaging, one can skip the pleasantries and go straight to the point. No more, 'Hello, how are you? I'm fine, thanks for asking. Say, do you have a minute so I can tell you about volunteering at the student clinic?' A typical text message instead says, 'Volunteer at the clinic tomorrow. Be there at 9am.' To a busy person, this is an ideal way to communicate. Unfortunately, text messages are not very personal and consequently are not very powerful ways to persuade a friend to give up her Saturday to volunteer at the student clinic.

RF: I use the telephone a lot in my professional life and prefer it to text messaging and email. If I want to get something done quickly I almost always pick up the telephone and make a call. While the telephone doesn't provide as much paralinguistic information as being face-to-face I find that I am better able to judge the other person's willingness to help and negotiate with them if I can hear their voice rather than just read their words.

EC: E-mail is a wonderful tool to use when messages need to be disseminated to a large group of people in a very small amount of time, with near perfect reliability. The trouble is that every organization understands this principle and sends out e-mails on a regular basis. As a student, I get 20–30 messages a day from various student interest groups, volunteer opportunities, school announcements, class assignments, and personal messages. Many of those messages were completely irrelevant to me. After a while I started missing important messages because they were getting lost in the midst of all the unimportant ones. Since then, a negative attitude toward e-mail solicitation seems to have grown among the student body.

RF: I am responsible for the professionalism curriculum at the medical school and often need to contact students about professionalism issues. While most students are responsive to my emails I also find that some students don't respond which I interpret as a sign of unprofessional behavior. Like many faculty I assume that the average medical student is a lot more conversant with technology than I am and that a lack of email response somehow shows a lack of interest and/or motivation. The irony is that I get 80–100 emails a day and if I don't respond immediately (which is nearly impossible to do) I'm getting inquiries about whether I'm okay and if there is anything wrong!

EC: A website is another way to disseminate information to the public, and when the website traffic is high this strategy is quite effective. However, few students actually check the school's website with any frequency.

RF: We post information about school policies, a calendar of events, and dates to remember on our official website. In addition, there is a weekly electronic newsletter, SCOPE, which goes out to the entire student body with additional articles of interest and important information about the campus community. It is disappointing to learn that few students, when queried, report availing themselves of these resources.

EC: For medical students, social media is a great way to keep in touch with others because of our busy schedules. We seldom have enough time to devote to maintaining our many relationships the old-fashioned way, and have become very reliant on social media to keep us connected to friends and events. As long as we stay mindful about protecting patient privacy and guarding our behaviors in these very public forums, social media can be a very valuable tool for many different purposes.

RF: I worry that social media is creating a world of instant messaging that is diminishing students' ability to reflect on their education, learn in community, and deepen their appreciation of what it means to serve. It seems inconceivable to me that deep meaning can be conveyed in 160 characters or less.

As you will no doubt have observed, Dr. Chen's reflections on the use of social media in medical education were quite different from mine. Many of her observations focused on the positive potential for social media to enhance learning and make the process of education more effective. For example, as a Baby Boomer, where I might be put off by the directness of tweeting, Dr. Chen stresses its efficiency in an otherwise very crowded cognitive space. And, while I prefer the traditional classroom (with all eyes on me), Dr. Chen stresses the time saved in travel plus the ability to either slow down or rewind portions of a lecture that seem particularly salient and important as distinct advantages of social media. Finally, where I see the use of social media as a potential threat to professionalism, Dr. Chen sees it as a tool for expanding connections and communication. In essence, although we may be referring to the same words when we use the term social media, these terms have vastly different meanings for us. As sociolinguists who study language in context, it is precisely the sorts of differences in perspective and experience that characterize Millennials' and other's understanding of social media that create distinctive communities of use. Medical educators who are primarily digital immigrants populate one community; Millennials the other.

While we don't think that the digital revolution has created nearly as great a divide as Steiner or Snow argue, we do think that there are significant differences in experience and understanding that are well worth exploring in terms of their implications for medical education. And, as has been true for the study of language change, it is worthwhile considering where the edge of the water might be in terms of meaningful dialogue among Millennials, Gen Xers, and Baby Boomers all working toward a common goal of improving medical education.

In our small thought experiment we learned that as senior faculty, who are mostly Gen Xers or Baby Boomers, we don't really know or understand the full breadth of how social media are and will continue to be used by trainees. Efforts to set standards and policies for social media use are helpful, but may be so narrow as to exclude the positive potential social media have for those who use it most. We learned that our own values for what counts as professional behavior (such as having to be physically present for a class) may have to be modified in light of the evidence about educational effectiveness. We learned that it is important to continue to set high expectations for professional behavior and to give those who experience lapses the opportunity to grow and learn from their mistakes. Finally, and we believe most importantly, we learned that it is critical to look for opportunities to have generation-spanning dialogues that are respectful of Millennials' attitudes and values and at the same time allow for other generations to speak meaningfully about potential risks that may inhere in the moment or lie just over the digital horizon.

Summary and Conclusion

We began this chapter by considering different units of analysis that can be used to study language. Our point of departure was to ask whether it is possible, using principles of applied sociolinguistics, to change the nature of entire conversations in a large bureaucratic organization and in so doing change its culture.

We, like other theorists, recognize that organizations are more than bricks and mortar; they are also the embodiment of the moment-by-moment and day-to-day human activities that go into creating what they produce, be it widgets or wellness. We believe that by transforming the types of conversations that occur in an organization, ipso facto, one has changed the organization. Guided by the principles of Appreciative Inquiry, Relational Coordination, and the theories of linguists such as Sapir and Whorf, we set out to change the conversations about education, candidate selection, and generational differences in a large medical school. By most objective standards, we succeeded in transforming a number of crucial conversations and in essence the culture of our organization (Suchman et al. 2004; Litzelman and Cottingham 2007; Cottingham et al. 2008; Inui et al. 2008; Williamson et al. 2011).

As scientists, what we learned in the process is that Appreciative Inquiry holds great potential to bring about meaningful, long-lasting positive change in the conversations that take place in a complex organization such as an academic health science center. As educators, we learned that it is possible to create a safe space for conversations to occur between physician/patients and their spouses and, in turn, to use the cognitive and linguistic assumptions and presuppositions visible in those conversations to teach faculty about experiential learning as an educational tool. As admissions officers, who act on behalf of the public and are entrusted with selecting the next generation of physicians, we learned that variations in the ways applicants were questioned was a source of unwanted variation. Using detailed sociolinguistic transcriptions from taped interviews with a standardized applicant allowed us to change the awareness of admissions committee members of the impact of their own linguistic practices on the type and quality of data they gathered and the decisions made on that basis. Finally, as authors from different generations with a common interest in language, social media, and professionalism, we were able to conduct an experiment that led to a deeper and fuller understanding of the differences that exist between digital natives and digital immigrants. The surprising finding here was the trap of assuming that because one shares the same words and vocabulary that the meaning of events and behaviors is the same. Medical students may use social media a great deal more than their teachers and in ways far different than their teachers might have imagined. In a digital world, physical presence may play less of a role than it did in previous generations. It is important to remember that one's physical absence does not necessarily signal a lack of interest, motivation, or respect. It may just be the most efficient way students have to get what they perceive their task as medical students to be – to learn as much as possible in as short a time as possible. Technology, like language itself, is neither good nor bad; it is how and for what purposes it is used that determines its value.

Language, whether communicated face to face or digitally, will continue to be embedded within and, in many respects, define organizational culture. Close attention to language use in organizational contexts can produce surprisingly useful insights. Taking the next step of applying those insights in the service of change is both a challenge and an opportunity. As a basic social science, linguistics is a natural home for understanding the origins and development of language. As an applied science, sociolinguistics and conversation analysis are natural disciplines to transform the types of conversations and uses of language among speakers and hearers, to improve the quality of individual and organizational lives.

Related topics

Organizational culture change; social media; medical school admissions; Appreciative Inquiry; Relational Coordination.

Further reading

Cooperrider, D., Whitney, D. and Stavros, J. (2007) *Appreciative Inquiry Handbook* (2nd edn), San Francisco, CA: Berrett-Koehler.

Hafferty, F.W. and Casellani, B. (2011) 'The two cultures of professionalism: sociology and medicine', in J.M.B. Pescosolido, J. McLeod, and A. Rogers (eds) *The Handbook of Health, Illness & Healing: Blueprint for the 21st Century*. New York: Springer: 201–219.

Inui, T.S. (2003) *A Flag in the Wind: Educating for Professionalism in Medicine*, Washington, DC: Association of American Medical Colleges.

May, N.B., Becker, D., Frankel, R., Haizlip, J., Harmon, R., Plews-Ogan, M., Schorling, J., Williams, A. and Whitney, D. (2010) *Appreciative Inquiry in Health Care: Positive Questions to Bring Out the Best*. Brunswick, OH: Crown Custom Publishing.

References

Beaulieu, M.D., Rivard, M., Hudon, E., Saucier, D., Remondin, M. and Favreau, R. (2003) 'Using standardized patients to measure professional performance of physicians.' *International Journal for Quality in Health Care* 15(3): 251–259.

Bushe, G. R. and A. F. Kassam (2005) 'When is appreciative inquiry transformational: a meta-case analysis.' *Journal of Applied Behavioral Science* 41(2): 161–181.

Carter, C. A., Ruhe, M. C., Weger, S., Litaker, D., Fry, R. E. and Stange, K. C. (2007) 'An appreciative inquiry approach to practice improvement and transformative change in health care settings.' *Quality Management in Health Care* 16(3): 194–204.

Cooperrider, D., (ed.) (2001) *Appreciative Inquiry: An Emerging Direction of Organization Development.* Champaign, IL: Stipes Publishing.

Cooperrider, D. and D. D. Whitney (2005) *Appreciative Inquiry: A Positive Revolution in Change.* San Francisco, CA: Berrett-Koehler Publishers.

Cottingham, A. H., Suchman, A. L., Litzelman, D .K., Frankel, R. M., Mossbarger, D. L., Williamson, P. R., Baldwin, D. C., Jr. and Inui, T. S. (2008) 'Enhancing the informal curriculum of a medical school: a case study in organizational culture change.' *Journal of General Internal Medicine* 23(6): 715–722.

Davis, D. A., Thomson, M. A., Oxman, A. D. and Haynes, R. B. (1995) 'Changing physician performance. A systematic review of the effect of continuing medical education strategies.' *Journal of the American Medical Association* 274(9): 700–705.

Dyrbye, L. N., Massie, Jr., F. S., Eacker, A., Harper, W., Power, D., Durning, S. J., Thomas, M. R., Moutier, C., Steele, D., Sloan, J. and Shanafelt, T. D. (2010) 'Relationship between burnout and professional conduct and attitudes among US medical students.' *Journal of the American Medical Association* 304(11): 1173–1180.

Eble, C. (1996) *Slang and Sociability*. Chapel Hill, NC: Chapel Hill Press.

Elam, C. L., Stratton, T. D., Wilson, J. F. and Scott, K. L. (2002) 'How admission committees decide: influence of committee members' experience and applicants' academic characteristics.' *Academic Medicine* 77(10 Suppl): S26–28.

Erickson, F. and J. Schultz (1982) *The Counselor as Gatekeeper*. New York: Academic Press.

Garfinkel, H. (1967) *Studies in Ethnomethodology*. Englewood Cliffs, NJ: Prentice Hall.

Ginsburg, S., Regehr, G. and Lingard, L. (2003) 'The disavowed curriculum: understanding student's reasoning in professionally challenging situations.' *Journal of General Internal Medicine* 18(12): 1015–1022.

Gittell, J. H. (2002) 'Relationships between service providers and their impact on customers'. *Journal of Service Research* 4(4): 301.

——(2009) *High Performance Healthcare: Using the Power of Relationships to Achieve Quality, Efficiency and Resilience.* New York: McGraw-Hill.

——(2012) 'Relational Coordination theory.' Retrieved December 19, 2013, from: http://rcrc.brandeis.edu/about-rc/relational%20coordination.html

Hafferty, F. W. and R. Franks (1994) 'The hidden curriculum, ethics teaching, and the structure of medical education.' *Academic Medicine* 69: 861–871.

Hafferty, F. W., Brennan, M. and Pawlina, W. (2011) 'Professionalism, the invisible hand, and a necessary reconfiguration of medical education.' *Academic Medicine* 86(11): e5.

Helms, A. S., Perez, T. E., Baltz, J., Donowitz, G., Hoke, G., Bass, E. J. and Plews-Ogan, M. L. (2012) 'Use of an Appreciative Inquiry approach to improve resident sign-out in an era of multiple shift changes.' *Journal of General Internal Medicine* 27(3): 287–291.

Hojat, M., Vergare, M. J., Maxwell, K., Brainard, G., Herrine, S. K., Isenberg, G. A., Veloski, J. and Gonnella, J. S. (2009) 'The devil is in the third year: a longitudinal study of erosion of empathy in medical school.' *Academic Medicine* 84(9): 1182–1191.

Husserl, E. (2001) *The Shorter Logical Investigations*. New York: Routledge.

Inui, T. S., Cottingham, A. H., Frankel, R. M., Litzelman, D. K., Mossbarger, D., Suchman, A., Vu, T. R. and Williamson, P. R. (2006) 'Educating for professionalism at Indiana University School of Medicine: feet on the ground and fresh eyes.' In D. Wear and J. Aultman (eds) *Professionalism in Medicine: Critical Perspectives.* New York: Springer Publishers.

Inui, T. S., Cottingham, A. H., Frankel, R. M., Litzelman, D. K., Suchman, A. L., and Williamson, P. R. (2008) 'Supporting teaching and learning of professionalism – changing the educational environment and students' "navigational skills".'In R. L. Cruess, S. R. Cruess and Y. Steinert (eds) *Teaching Medical Professionalism.* New York: Cambridge University Press.

Karnieli-Miller, O., Taylor, A. C., Cottingham, A. H., Inui, T. S., Vu, T. R. and Frankel, R. M. (2010) 'Exploring the meaning of respect in medical student education: an analysis of student narratives.' *Journal of General Internal Medicine* 25(12): 1309–1314.

Karnieli-Miller, O., Vu, T. R., Holtman, M. C., Clyman, S. G. and Inui, T. S. (2010) 'Medical students' professionalism narratives: a window on the informal and hidden curriculum.' *Academic Medicine* 85(1): 124–133.

Karnieli-Miller, O., Vu, T. R., Frankel, R. M., Holtman, M. C., Clyman, S. G., Hui, S. L. and Inui, T. S. (2011) 'Which experiences in the hidden curriculum teach students about professionalism?' *Academic Medicine* 86(3): 369–377.

Litzelman, D. K. and A. H. Cottingham (2007) 'The new formal competency-based curriculum and informal curriculum at Indiana University School of Medicine: overview and five-year analysis.' *Academic Medicine* 82(4): 410–421.

Markakis, K. M., Beckman, H. B., Frankel, R. M., Holtman, M. C., Clyman, S. G., Hui, S. L. and Inui, T. S. (2000) 'The path to professionalism: cultivating humanistic values and attitudes in residency training.' *Academic Medicine* 75(2): 141–150.

Marvel, M. K. (1991) 'Improving clinical teaching skills using the parallel process model.' *Family Medicine* 23(4): 279–284.

Prensky, M. (2001a) 'Digital natives, digital immigrants, part I.' *On the Horizon* 9(5): 1–6.

——(2001b) 'Digital natives, digital immigrants, part II: Do they really think differently?' *On the Horizon* 9(6): 1–6.

Rossi-Landi, F. (1983) *Language as A Work and Trade*. South Hadley, MA: Bergin & Garvey.

Sacks, H. (1992) *Lectures on Conversation*, edited by G. Jefferson. Cambridge: Blackwell.

Santen, S. A., Holt, D. B., Kemp, J. D. and Hemphill, R. R. (2010) 'Burnout in medical students: examining the prevalence and associated factors.' *Southern Medical Journal* 103(8): 758–763.

Shendell-Falik, N., Feinson, M. and Mohr, B. J. (2007) 'Enhancing patient safety: improving the patient handoff process through appreciative inquiry.' *Journal of Nursing Administration* 37(2): 95–104.

Snow, C. P. (1959) *The Two Cultures*. Cambridge: Cambridge University Press.

Steiner, G. (1998) *Language and Silence: Essays on Language, Literature and the Inhuman*. New Haven, CT: Yale University Press.

Suchman, A., Williamson, P., Litzelman, D. K., Frankel, R. M., Mossbarger, D.L. and Inui, T.S. (2004) 'Towards an informal curriculum that teaches professionalism: transforming the social environment of a medical school.' *Journal of General Internal Medicine* 19(5 Pt 2): 501–504.

Tannen, D. (1990) *You Just Don't Understand: Women and Men in Conversation*. New York: William Morrow.

Wear, D., Aultman, J. M., Varley, J. D. and Zarconi, J. (2006) 'Making fun of patients: medical students' perceptions and use of derogatory and cynical humor in clinical settings.' *Academic Medicine* 81(5): 454–462.

Whorf, B. (1940) 'Science and linguistics.' *Technology Review* 42(6): 229–231.

Williamson, P. R., Baldwin, D.C. Jr., Cottingham, A. H., Frankel, R., Inui, T. S., Litzelman, D. K., Mossbarger, D. L. and Suchman, A. L. (2011) 'Transforming the professional culture of a medical school from the inside out.' In A. L. Suchman, D. Sluyter, and P.R. Williamson (eds) *Leading Change in Healthcare: Transforming Organizations Using Complexity, Positive Psychology and Relationship-Centered Care*. Oxford: Radcliffe Publishers.

19

Communication skills training for resident physicians

A physician-educator perspective

Benjamin Blatt, Noemi Alice Spinazzi, and Larrie Greenberg

Introduction

Communication between physicians, patients, and families represents a significant challenge in a busy clinical environment. Over the past 50 years, a discipline devoted to communication has evolved within medicine and medical education, resulting in a large body of research and commentary. This work is reflected in international consensus statements (Simpson et al. 1991; Makoul and Schofield 1999) and has influenced accreditation bodies for undergraduate (medical school) and graduate (residency) medical education, leading to communication education as an expectation for doctors-in-training (Association of American Medical Colleges 1999; General Medical Council 1993; Workshop Planning Committee 1992). The Liaison Committee on Medical Education (LCME), made up of representatives from the Association of American Medical Colleges and the American Medical Association, is responsible for medical school accreditation, and oversees all medical schools in their development, implementation, and evaluation of the undergraduate curriculum. At the graduate level a similar role is played by the Accreditation Council for Graduate Medical Education (ACGME). A review of the literature suggests that the major focus of communication skills teaching has been at the undergraduate (medical student) education level (Aspegren 1999). Though the ACGME has also put forward an expectation for communication skills education for residents, residency programs have been slow to develop programs in this area. Graduate and undergraduate medical education are administered separately, and thus there are gaps in the continuity of curricula at these two levels. Our goal in this chapter is to review the state of the art of communication education in graduate medical education. Residency programs in all specialties throughout the US are grappling with how to best ensure that doctors are competent and empathic communicators.

The specific purposes of this chapter are (1) to provide an overview of the evolution of thinking about doctor–patient communication in the medical world and how this has translated into resident education, (2) to review current research and practice (including our own at Children's National Medical Center (CNMC) and George Washington University (GWU)), and (3) to provide a vision for the future of communication skills in the education of physicians.

Medical communication skills training in the US: a brief history

Communication has not always been a central focus of clinical care. In the 1960s and 1970s physician–patient communication began to gain more attention from patients, doctors, and medical educators. Patients, empowered by consumerism and Internet access, voiced their need to understand and be understood. The medical community responded to this need and to the growing body of research that underscores the importance of communication to patient outcomes (Kaplan et al. 1989; Stewart 1995). To review just a few of the research milestones, in the 1970s Barbara Korsch showed a positive relationship between pediatricians' communications skills and parents' satisfaction (Korsch et al. 1968). In the 1980s, Kaplan and Greenfield demonstrated that effective patient–physician communication influences medical outcomes such as blood pressure and diabetes control (Kaplan et al. 1989). Also in the 1980s, Howard Beckman recorded doctor–patient interactions and reported that, on average, doctors interrupted patients after 18 seconds of the interview, inhibiting patients from conveying important problems which then never got addressed (Beckman and Frankel 1984). From the 1970s until today, Debra Roter (Roter and Larson 2002) explored doctor–patient interactions using the Roter Interaction Analysis System (RIAS) to classify and quantify the characteristics, emotional and linguistic, of medical communication. The research of these and many other pioneers energized a communication movement within medicine. Some educators founded organizations like the American Academy on Physician and Patient and the Bayer Institute for Health Care Communication to teach and promote communications education. Others like Stephen Cole, Mack Lipkin, and Suzanne Kurtz authored textbooks on the subject (Cohen-Cole 1991; Lipkin et al. 1995; Kurtz et al. 1998). Cole's and Kurtz's texts were designed for teaching basic medical communication skills to novice trainees. Lipkin's text is an extensive review of the medical interview for a more expert audience, and covers faculty development and research as well as a general interviewing framework.

The work of these and many others has shaped current thinking about clinician–patient communication. The evidence that evolved from their work supports two core precepts of the field. The first is that communication matters to patient care. As noted above, effective interpersonal and communication skills correlate with improved patient outcomes; ineffective skills correlate with medication errors and malpractice suits (Levinson et al. 1997). The second is that communication skills can be taught and learned. Prior to the medical communication movement, how a physician communicated was frequently termed 'bedside manner'. It was sometimes conceptualized as an innate personality trait – some had it, some didn't. If it was susceptible to any development and nurturing, this happened through the apprenticeship of the physician-in-training with an experienced physician. Current evidence, however, indicates that trainees can learn to improve their communication proficiency through specialized communication skills training (Aspegren 1999; Kaplan et al. 1997). Communication skills are as teachable and improvable through deliberate practice as traditional medical skills such as lumbar puncture, paracentesis, or ultrasound examination (Lipkin 1996). Some trainees will become more proficient than others, but almost all can achieve an acceptable level of competence. The importance of ensuring that all trainees reach this level of competence is underscored by how often they will have to implement these skills during their lifetime of practice. The medical interview, the vehicle for clinician–patient communication, is the most common procedure that a clinician performs (Lipkin 1996). During their careers, doctors complete 160,000 to 300,000 interviews.

Given the importance of effective communication to the practice of medicine, it is understandable that every American medical education, licensing, and accreditation organization considers it to be essential (Rider and Keefer 2006). On the undergraduate level, medical students must demonstrate communications competence with standardized patients on the National Board of Medical Examiners Clinical Skills Examination in order to receive licensure. On the graduate level, the Accreditation Council for Graduate Medical Education has included communication as one of their six core competencies. Every US resident is expected to learn and to be able to demonstrate effective communication skills.

To fully understand the expectations of the ACGME in educational terms, it is necessary to digress and review the paradigm shift that has occurred in graduate medical education – the competency movement. Until a few decades ago, graduate medical education resembled an apprenticeship. Residents watched faculty and more advanced peers model skills, and then, under supervision, performed the skills themselves. If in the eyes of their supervisors, the residents performed adequately, they advanced. This system was haphazard. In assessing residents supervisors failed to use common standards and objectives. The competency movement made standards and objectives more explicit (Rider et al. 2007). It broke clinical practice down into content domains called competencies. Communication, patient care, and professionalism, for example, are three of the six ACGME competencies. Under each domain the ACGME required measurable behaviors (behavioral objectives) and a clear definition of the methods to be used to measure each behavior. For example, under the communications competency, effectively communicating with patients from different cultures might be such a behavioral objective and the method chosen to assess it might be an interaction with a standardized patient (an actor carefully trained to simulate a patient role). The close linkage of performance assessment to measurable behaviors that must be systematically evaluated in a standardized way is at the heart of the paradigm shift.

Under each domain the ACGME listed a few subdomains, but left it to individual residency programs to define specific measurable behaviors and choose methods of evaluation. The ACGME wanted a collaborative process in which they would provide the overarching framework, leaving individual programs to decide upon the details which fit best within their local context. Communications experts across the US also banded together to fill in the details. For example, in 2003 a group of 16 physicians in the Harvard Macy Program for Physician Educators came together in the Kalamazoo consensus conference (Makoul 2001) to advance the process and defined 20 specific, measurable communications behavior objectives (Rider and Keefer 2006).

The competency movement clarified residency education by providing a content framework and mandating measureable behaviors within each competency. It did not, however, address developmental sequence – which behaviors should be taught when during the years of a residency program. Ideally, programs should be vertically integrated – learners should be taught skills that build upon each other in increasingly sophisticated levels. Milestones and entrustable professional activities are the terms educators are currently using to address vertical integration. Applied to the communications competency, a beginning level milestone might be: residents when taking a history should be able to effectively respond to a patient's fears as well as medical concerns. A more advanced level milestone: residents should be able to effectively address physical, psychosocial, and spiritual distress in an end-of-life conversation. Linked to each milestone is an evaluation method that defines competence (e.g., the resident must demonstrate the ability to address 10 predefined critical items in an end-of-life discussion with a standardized patient). Milestones are competence dependent, not time dependent. It may take one resident longer to achieve a milestone than another. Ultimately, milestone competence in communications and other patient care tasks must come together so that residents can integrate them, in order to perform the aforementioned entrustable professional activity (EPA). For example, to perform a procedure on a patient (like inserting a central line), a resident must be able to competently get informed consent, communicate with a nervous patient and family, and insert the central line, performing all the critical steps on the procedure checklist. An EPA is a terminal outcome of the education process – a skill complex that a doctor is mentor-certified to be able to perform without supervision (ten Cate and Scheele 2007).

Establishing milestones and entrustable professional activities is the latest mandate on the ACGME agenda and is in an early pilot phase in a few residency programs. Establishing behavioral objectives for the communication competency is further along (the ACGME competencies initiative began in 2002). Despite these mandates from external accrediting bodies, it is our impression that many residency programs, which far outnumber medical schools, still do not have a formal communications curriculum and do not comprehensively evaluate resident skills in this area. Of those residencies that do have communications curricula, some have published descriptions of their efforts, but few have attempted to study the effect of these teaching efforts on residents' skills. A major purpose of this chapter is to present the work of those who have performed such studies in order to summarize the current state of knowledge about the kinds and the effectiveness of communications education at the graduate medical education level. We will first review our personal experience with interventions to improve residents' communications competency, which we started in the 1970s and 1980s and continues until now. We will then review the experience of others as published in the recent literature.

The George Washington University (GWU) experience

One of us (LG) began work in teaching communication skills to residents in 1980. In this summary of our experience, we will review the programs we developed and our teaching and evaluation methods in three areas: crisis communication, telephone communication, and communication around difficult experiences.

Crisis communication

The purpose of our first program (Jewett et al. 1982) was to increase the competence of residents in crisis counseling skills with parents whose child faced a potentially fatal illness. The participants in this program were 24 second- and third-year residents during their oncology rotation. Instead of practicing their skills on a real family, which would have been unethical, they counseled 'simulated parents' (SPs) – in this case, professional counselors trained to portray the parent role authentically. The counselors were also trained to evaluate the residents using a checklist and to give residents feedback on their communication skills.

During week one of the program, residents informed the 'parents' that their child had leukemia. After this videotaped baseline encounter, the 'parents' broke role and gave the residents feedback on their communication skills. This feedback constituted the intervention to improve residents' counseling skills. During week four, the residents repeated the same encounter with a different simulated family.

The effectiveness of the intervention was determined by comparing the residents' baseline performance with their post-intervention week four performance. Residents also rated the effectiveness of the program by completing a questionnaire. Results were as follows: (1) residents improved in providing critical information; (2) residents improved in the clarity of information they provided to the SPs; (3) residents' interpersonal skills on average improved.

The program was assessed as being effective to extremely effective by all of the residents. This study only looked at short-term outcomes – no attempts were made to reassess the residents' skills later.

In reality, residents would not counsel parents with a child with leukemia as this is done by experienced oncology attending physicians or fellows. They could apply the principles they learned about communicating a difficult diagnosis, however, to less demanding bad news scenarios in which they often would play a part, such as informing parents and children of a diagnosis of diabetes or other chronic illness.

The purpose of a second program (Greenberg et al. 1995) was to teach residents crisis counseling skills for a different, but equally challenging, scenario: informing standardized parents that their child had come to the emergency department (ED) dead on arrival. To establish a baseline 27 residents were videotaped informing standardized parents that their child had died suddenly. They then received the intervention: feedback from the SPs instructing them on (1) what content to convey based on a consensus checklist derived from a survey of pediatric ED physicians, and (2) how they communicated the information. Four to ten weeks later the residents again encountered standardized parents in a second case scenario. Residents' pre- and post-intervention communication skills performance were compared using the Gibb Trust Scale and National Board of Medical Examiners Patient Perception Questionnaire (PPQ).

Residents showed improvement in two categories of the Gibbs instrument: Distrust/Trust, Dependent/Independent but no differences on the PPQ. As in the previous study, there were no attempts to assess residents' skills long term. We were impressed by the effectiveness that utilizing SPs represents as a method to teach residents crisis counseling skills.

A third program focused on pediatric intensive care unit fellows (post-residency trainees) (Vaidya et al. 1999). Because the children they care for are seriously ill, intensive care fellows give bad news every day despite never having received formal instruction in this type of communication. The purpose of this program was to train intensive care fellows to communicate to family about a seriously ill child admitted to a pediatric intensive care unit (PICU). All seven pediatric fellows assigned to the PICU at Children's National Medical Center participated. The 'giving bad news' curriculum was conducted over the course of a day. In the morning each fellow interacted with an SP (pre-test) followed by feedback (the intervention); in the afternoon, each interacted with a second SP (post-test). The SP cases evolved, with each child becoming more gravely ill during the course of the day. The intervention, feedback from the SP after the first case, focused on residents' verbal and non-verbal performance.

We evaluated the fellows' performance in five categories: communication skills, content issues, support systems, interventions, and patient perceptions. Fellows demonstrated improvement in mean scores of these five categories and the overall combined scores of all categories.

We were impressed with how realistically SPs can simulate real-life experiences in different contexts and improvement in fellow performance supports their effectiveness as teachers. In retrospect, because of the small number of fellows in this program, qualitative analysis might have offered additional insights and ideas for program improvement.

Telephone communication

Counseling patients by telephone is an integral part of practice, but educators have described few curricula to teach residents telephone communication. One of the authors (LG) and a colleague developed a self-directed learning curriculum in the form of an interactive CD-ROM to teach pediatric residents telephone management skills (Ottolini and Greenberg 1998). The CD-ROM was designed to respond to residents' typed-in questions, activating the voice of a simulated parent. The scripts used represented the 10 most common reasons parents call pediatricians. To study the effectiveness of the CD-ROM program, 24 residents were randomized either to use the computer-based program (experimental group) or to read information about the 10 scenarios (control group). The telephone skills of residents in both groups were tested both prior to and after their instructional interventions. The testing occurred in two half-day sessions during which residents answered calls with an advice nurse. Unbeknownst to the residents, standardized parents called them twice during the pre-intervention and post-intervention sessions. The standardized parents were actors specially trained to simulate real parents and to present the same case in the same way each time. These 'stealth' parents allowed us to present residents with identical challenges, thus constituting a test that was not confounded by patient differences. We recorded the phone conversations and assessed the residents in nine communications categories: identifying information, clarifying the chief complaint, determining the severity and duration of the chief complaint, ascertaining the child's appearance (how sick), home therapy, associated symptoms, illness exposure, pertinent medical history, and the emotional tone of the caller.

In comparing intervention and control residents, we found that post-test scores were higher in the computer group than the reading group. Interpersonal skills improved modestly in both groups on the PPQ. All of the residents rated the experience positively in almost all aspects.

The results of this study supported the effectiveness of the CD-ROM as an effective means to teach residents telephone communications skills. It also provided an efficient means to teach a complicated subject, since it did not require faculty time. Though there is considerable initial expense in its creation, once developed, the CD-ROM can be used repeatedly without additional cost. This study also highlights the effectiveness of stealth standardized parents as a means of evaluation. Since residents don't know they are not real patients, they are a more authentic means of assessment than traditional standardized parents. Of all simulation methods, we believe that assessing health outcomes with stealth standardized patients comes nearest to the 'holy grail' of measuring real patients' health outcomes.

Communication around difficult experiences

Violence is a major public health issue among American youth, leading to a high homicide rate in adolescents aged 15–19 years. Counseling adolescents and young adults about violence prevention is one way to address this problem, and educators at the Children's National Medical Center (CNMC) have developed a violence counseling training program for physician trainees (Abraham et al. 2001). The purpose of this study was to evaluate the effectiveness of the CNMC training program in teaching trainees to detect and counsel potentially violent teens. At the beginning of a 1-month adolescent medicine rotation, the program was presented in the form of a 3-hour workshop to half the trainees (intervention group); the other half (control group) were asked to read a standard manual on violence prevention.

During the last week of the rotation all trainees were assessed in encounters with a 'stealth' standardized patient who presented to the clinic with a complaint of a persistent headache. Participants did not know that they were not seeing a real patient. The SPs were blinded to whether trainees were in the control or experimental group. If during the interview the trainee probed about the headache to determine if there was a psychosocial problem underlying the chief complaint, the SP revealed that she had been threatened by a group of peers at her school and fearing for her safety, carried a knife in her purse.

To assess the intervention and control groups, the adolescent standardized patients completed the PPQ questionnaire for evaluating trainee communication skills. The intervention group demonstrated higher scores for interpersonal skills and showing interest than controls. They also outperformed controls in seeking to uncover other violence in the SPs' lives as well as identifying and managing the violence-related scenario.

This study demonstrated that a relatively brief intervention may have a positive impact on trainees' skills in violence identification and management. As in the previously described work in telephone communication, this study also demonstrated the value of stealth standardized patients in assessing communication skills.

Recent residency training programs

Over the past seven years one of us (BB) developed and implemented two specialized communications training programs for residents: CREATE and Relationship Express. In 2006 we developed the Cross Residency Experience for ACGME Training and Education (CREATE) program to train residents to communicate effectively in six challenging situations: Bad News, End of Life, Angry Patient, Informed Consent, Bad Result, and Cultural Difference. CREATE sessions are structured as 2-hour workshops, each following the same pattern: a DVD-guided section followed by skills practice with standardized patients. The DVD first shows a patient presenting a complaint, then summarizes principles of communication relevant to the patient's complaint, and finally shows an experienced clinician using these principles to communicate with the patient. In the second part of the workshop residents apply the communications skills they have just seen modeled to encounters with standardized patients. They receive detailed feedback from faculty, fellow residents, and SPs.

Relationship Express is a basic communications program designed for residents in specialties that are particularly time-pressured. We have used it most extensively with the residency program in anesthesia. The workshops train residents in six basic communication objectives that can be accomplished within a 10-minute interview.

The experience of others: review of the current literature

We initiated a search of the medical literature from 1995 to the present to assess what articles from the United States or Canada had been published on teaching and evaluating resident communication skills. In consultation with an information specialist we used three search engines: Medline, PubMed, and Google Scholar. On Medline, a search with keywords '*residents AND communication AND skills*' yielded 518 results; '*communication AND teaching AND residents AND outcomes*' yielded 23 results; '*counseling and teaching and residents*' yielded 98 results; '*medical error AND communication skills*' yielded 8 results; and '*medical error AND communication skills AND residents*' yielded 2 results. On PubMed, a search with the keywords '*communication skills training residents*' yielded 616 results. On Google Scholar, a search of the literature since 1995 using the keywords '*residents communication skills training*' was performed to identify any articles that may have been missed by the previous searches on the aforementioned scientific databases. This search yielded over 14,000 results. Using Google filters to sort the search results, we then narrowed the search results to around 500 articles. The vast majority of search results consisted of baseline assessments of residents' communication skills or attitudes toward communication skill training without an intervention or follow-up. Since these studies did not describe any educational intervention, they were not selected for further review. In contrast, 39 studies described educational interventions aimed at improving residents' communication skills and met our inclusion criteria. We summarized these studies in Table 19.1; please see Appendix 19.1 at the end of this chapter for full reference information for the studies in the order in which they appear in the table. For each study, the following were recorded: the title of the article; the goals and objectives of the study (if stated); the teaching methods used in the educational intervention; the evaluation methods used; the number of hours included in the educational intervention; how many participants were involved in each study; the study's results (the effect on residents' communication skills); and our comments. Data were recorded in the table either as direct quotations from the studies themselves, as paraphrasing of the authors' comments, or as summaries of the study findings.

The 39 studies included in Table 19.1 focused on a diversity of communications skills as indicated in the following list, in order of frequency:

Bad news, end of life, palliative care	14
General communication skills/mixed skills	9
Behavioral change (tobacco, alcohol, obesity)	7
Bad result/medical error	3
Empathy	2
Communication about sexual matters	2
Other (interaction of communication with procedural skills; understanding the Kalmazoo communication model through film and video)	2
Total	39

Programs also used a great variety of teaching methods, including lecture, role play, standardized patient practice, video clips from TV shows and movies, trigger tapes, online interactive teaching programs, and feedback from patients and nurses. Diversity also characterized study length, ranging from 30-minute feedback sessions to all-day retreats to 4-week electives.

Some researchers studied residents from multiple specialties; most, however, studied residents from single specialties. Pediatrics was far and away the most represented specialty (11/39 studies); others represented in much smaller numbers were ob-gyn, psychiatry, internal medicine, surgery, emergency medicine, otolaryngology. Specialties from which we did not find papers included anesthesia, neurology, neurosurgery, dermatology, and urology.

Most studies fit the following design: (1) baseline evaluation of the participants' communication skills or of the participants' confidence in their own skills; (2) an intervention; (3) a post-intervention evaluation. The majority of studies (18) evaluated the outcome of their intervention right after the completion of the curriculum; 3 studies administered the evaluation within a week; 5 within one month of completion of the educational intervention. The majority of studies that met the inclusion criterion (26) measured their outcomes within just one month after completion of the communication skills training program. Ten studies collected outcome data more than one month after completion of the educational intervention (6 weeks–1 year later); of those ten, 3 compared short term (within one month) and long term

Table 19.1 Summary of studies on communication skills training programs

	Type of program	*Stated goals*	*Evaluation methods*	*Length/ # of residents*	*Evidence of improvement in residents' communication skills?*	*Additional notes*	*Kirkpatrick Classification*
1	Video feedback technique to enhance communication skills training	To evaluate a brief teaching intervention comprising the video feedback linked to a one-hour didactic and role-play teaching session on pediatric residents' communication with a simulated patient (SP)	Simulated interviews evaluated through RIAS and compared to the initial interviews. Dimensions of successful communication (N=38 mutually exclusive categories) were identified. Three adherence-related problem-solving skills were coded, including use of problem-solving probes, problem-solving assistance, and partnership and support. A self-assessment questionnaire is also included.	4 hours/ 28	Simulated encounters increased in length of time ($p<0.001$) in post-training sessions. This increase is accounted for almost entirely by an increase in patient talk ($p<0.05$). The number of open-ended questions increased ($p< 0.001$), as well as areas of active partnership building and problem solving.	Intervention is innovative and intuitive. Majority of residents found the feedback session helpful in improving clinical skills. Improvement in use of open ended questions and empathy is greater for females.	1 & 2
2	Teaching communication skills using the integrated procedural performance instrument (IPPI): A randomized controlled trial	To determine whether immediate feedback on communication and interpersonal skills in videotaped IPPI scenarios would lead to improvements of these skills in further IPPI scenarios. To assess whether any improvements in communication skills occurred at the expense of the participants' technical skills	Participants' technical skills were assessed through validated assessment scales—a 26-item checklist and a 5-item lobal rating scale. Communication and interpersonal skills were assessed through a validated scale including overall communication ability, empathy, coherence, verbal, and nonverbal expression.	30 min/ 16 residents 16 med students	Participants in the feedback group outperformed control group on every item of the communication scale—overall score, empathy, coherence, verbal, and nonverbal expression—in the 2 IPPI scenarios following intervention ($P< 0.05$). No difference in scores for technical skills post-intervention were demonstrated (checklist: experimental mean: 64% vs control: 59%, $P = 0.40$).	Small sample size. No significant difference in technical skills in the IG vs. the CG, both scored lower on the second IPPI (possibly due to a harder scenario). From personal experience with sim center models, it is easier to perform procedures on a model than on a real person, and one wonders if the same improvement in communication skills could happen without worsening technical skills in real life scenarios (i.e., external validity of the findings).	1 & 2
3	A Controlled Trial of a Short Course to Improve Residents' Communication With Patients at the End of Life	To evaluate a short course to improve residents' communication skills delivering bad news and eliciting patients' preferences for end-of-life care	Communication skills were evaluated using audio-recorded encounters with standardized patients before and after intervention. Physicians delivered bad news and discussed patients' treament preferences.	16 hours/ 56	Residents attending the course demonstrated significant increase in overall skill ratings in the delivery of bad news, with specific improvement in information giving and responding to emotional cues. Although cumulative scores for discussions about patient treatment preferences did not increase, residents demonstrated enhanced skills including discussing probability, presenting clinical scenarios, and asking about prior experience with end-of-life decision making. It is a relatively short, intensive course that is shown to improve the end-of-life communication skills of U.S. medical residents.		2

	Type of program	*Stated goals*	*Evaluation methods*	*Length/ # of residents*	*Evidence of improvement in residents' communication skills?*	*Additional notes*	*Kirkpatrick Classification*
4	Using television shows to teach communication skills in internal medicine residency	To assess the efficacy of cinemeducation (television shows) for teaching communication skills using the Kalamazoo model. Primary endpoint was self-rated understanding of the Kalamazoo model on communication. Secondary endpoint was the self-rated comfort levels of residents in three challenging clinical scenarios	Baseline self-reported assessment (on level of confidence with various communication skills based on Kalamazoo consensus statement) was completed by the residents. A similar post intervention assessment was administered. Residents filled out a satisfaction survey at the end of intervention.	1 hour (part of the weekly teaching sessions)/ 64 (43 responded)	Not tested	Residents indicated improved understanding of an evidence-based model and increased comfort levels in applying such a model in clinical practice. Furthermore, residents' understanding of the seven essential competencies in the Kalamazoo model also improved and they reported improved comfort levels in three challenging clinical scenarios (all p< 0.005 to p< 0.001).	1
5	Improving Residents' End-of-Life Communication Skills with a Short Retreat: A Randomized Controlled Trial	To study the effect of a day-long communication skills training retreat on enhanced performance, confidence with end-of-life conversations, and residents' ability to respond to patient emotions	All participants were evaluated pre- and post-intervention with two 10-minute conversations with SPs. A trained faculty member observed conversation and provided feedback. Communication competence was evaluated through recorded conversations using validated rating tools and palliative care expert judgement. Participants completed questionnaires before and after skills evaluation. The surveys included personal experiences with EOL care, formal teaching and/or rotation in palliative care, and self-reported confidence to perform communication tasks.	5 hours retreat (plus SP interviews and post-interview feedback time)/ 49 Baseline data includes responses from all residents randomized to one of the groups (control n = 28, retreat n = 21)	Retreat group improved total score with marginal significance (p= 0.07) for "breaking bad news". Adjusting for gender (male versus female) and residency track (primary care versus other), the retreat group had significantly higher post-intervention scores than control (p = 0.046). For discussing direction of care, neither group improved total score but the retreat group's post-intervention total score was significantly higher than control. Neither group improved significantly over time with respect to general interviewing or task-related skills. The retreat group improved significantly (32.4% improvement) in responding to emotion; adjusting for gender and residency track, there was a significant group-by-time interaction (p<0.05).	Retreat group showed significantly higher self-assessed preparation to tell about new, life threatening diagnoses compared to its preretreat assessment and to control. No other significant between-group differences were found.The results are less impressive due to limited size/power. The differences between IG and CG are marginal, and many categories lacked pre and post difference in IG scores.	1 & 2
6	Randomized Trial of Teaching Brief Motivational Interviewing to Pediatric Trainees to Promote Healthy Behaviors in Families	To determine the effect of training on MI skills of pediatric trainees, as measured using a standardized coding system applied to videotaped visits with SPs. Using an RCT design, the study hypothesizes that training and subsequent tailored, written feedback would improve skills.	A set of OSCEs developed to assess trainee skill, consisting of 3 clinical scenarios (stations) in which SPs portrayed parents of children with asthma in a 12-minute segment of a visit. MITI 2.0 was used to score the OSCEs plus 2 global ratings of residents' styles regarding empathy/ understanding and MI spirit. The % MICO, defined as the proportion of all resident communication behaviors coded as open questions, reflections, or MI-adherent behaviors, was used to quantify change. A convenience sub sample (N=8) from both arms provided 10 audiotapes of patient visits after training to assess the ecological validity of OSCE-derived skill assessments.	2 4.5-hour workshops. Evaluation by OSCE clinical scenarios 3 times, adding ~ 2 hours/ Sample (n=16) predominantly female (75%), representative of residency program	Trained residents demonstrated increased skill (%MICO score) at 3 months compared with control. At 7 months, %MICO scores increased 16% to 20% (P<.02) across all OSCE stations. Study findings showed good ecological validity.	Solid study. The question is, does evidence support the assumption that good MI skills translate into better patient skills and better outcomes? Rubak S., Sandbaek A., Lauritzen T., Christensen B. "Motivational interviewing: a systematic review and meta-analysis". Br J Gen Pract. 2005;55(513):305-312.	2

	Type of program	Stated goals	Evaluation methods	Length/ # of residents	Evidence of improvement in residents' communication skills?	Additional notes	Kirkpatrick Classification
7	Human Emotion and Response in Surgery (HEARS): A Simulation-Based Curriculum for Communication Skills, Systems-Based Practice, and Professionalism in Surgical Residency Training	To examine a pilot human factors curriculum during a 2-year period, one component of a comprehensive 5-year curriculum spanning core competencies of interpersonal and communication skills, systems-based practice, and professionalism and using low- and high-fidelity simulation techniques	Empathy and caring skills evaluated using 8 brief video vignettes to prompt resident responses to common communication challenges. Each video vignette consisted of a narrated case introduction and a video clip of patient speaking. Surgery residents were given 90 seconds to respond in writing to each vignette. Each resident observed and responded to two vignettes before and two after the training sessions. Pre- and post-vignettes were alternated by cohort. Vignette responses were coded using a 5-point scale.	6 hrs for empathy and communication skills/ 27 PGY1s and 15 PGY2s	Analyses of video vignette tests indicated significant improvement in empathic communication for PGY1 ($p=0.001$) and PGY2 ($p=0.004$).	Analysis focused narrowly on doctor-patient communication skills. It tested whether the residents improved in the targeted areas, though the way such improvement was assessed was indirect (in writing, as opposed to via observation of actual interpersonal interactions).	2
8	eLearning to enhance physician patient communication: A pilot test of "doc.com" and "WebEncounter" in teaching bad news delivery	To test the effectiveness of eLearning tool "doc.com" in facilitating essential communication competency learning for giving bad news. Hypothesis: adding a web-based practice and feedback session with a SP (WebEncounter) would further enhance knowledge, skills, and self efficacy	Before the first WebOSCE exercise, interns completed a brief questionnaire about the quality of their medical school training in breaking bad news. Each WebOSCE was scored by research coordinator present. A post intervention questionnaire assessed participants' confidence in delivering bad news.	10-minute OSCEs followed by feedback, plus the time for completing doc.com module/ 55 (18 responded to self efficacy pre and post surveys)	Borderline significant: mean scores on the checklists were similar between 3 randomized groups at baseline. The doc.com + WebOSCE group gained the most from the intervention, and a simple ANOVA comparing the mean changes almost significant ($p=0.053$). A linear trend across the three groups, assuming that adding components should increase the effect, was significant for mean change, $p=0.018$.	Significant positive trend, showing that adding the online practice component WebEncounter enhanced our residents' abilities to employ effective communication skills in giving bad news.	2
9	Effect of Multisource Feedback on Resident Communication Skills and Professionalism: A Randomized Controlled Trial	To test the effect of multi-source feedback, including self-assessment and tailored coaching on resident communication skills and professionalism	Patients rate MD performance in 10 areas of communication and professionalism (5 ordinal response options). Parents asked to provide qualitative feedback about what they liked most and what they would change about the care they received from resident during hospital stay. For the nurse evaluation, items related to effective communication, timeliness of completing tasks, responsibility and accountability, effective care planning, being sensitive and empathetic, establishing rapport, respecting confidentiality, demonstrating honesty and integrity, communicating effectively with staff, treating staff with respect, completing tasks reliably, accepting suggestions graciously, anticipating postdischarge needs, and being a team member. Qualitative comments were also collected from nurses. Residents were contacted to complete Web-based self-assessment survey.	Coaching session ~30 minutes/ 36 (18 & 18)	Parent ratings increased for both groups. While parent ratings increased more for the multi-source feedback group, differences between groups were not significant. Nurse ratings increased for the multisource feedback group and decreased for control. Between-group difference in change was significant for effective communication, timeliness of completing tasks, and demonstrating responsibility and accountability.		3

	Type of program	Stated goals	Evaluation methods	Length/ # of residents	Evidence of improvement in residents' communication skills?	Additional notes	Kirkpatrick Classification
10	Structured Teaching versus Experimental Learning of Palliative Care for Surgical Residents	To test a structured curriculum in palliative care for surgical residents	Outcomes measured in 3 domains: 1) core knowledge, 2) palliative care communication skills, 3) resident perceptions of palliative care, including self-confidence. Palliative care communication skills were assessed through validated OSCEs with 2 standardized family members of a patient in surgical ICU experiencing a protracted postop course with several complications. Residents were instructed to address end-of-life needs and potential withdrawal of life-sustaining interventions, and code status. 2 trained clinical raters (1 physician and 1 surgical ICU nurse) evaluated residents' OSCE interactions on a 10-point Likert scale. Standardized family members and residents themselves provided ratings on the same scales. Intervention and comparison groups underwent a survey on residents' perceptions of palliative care (BEFORE OSCE in the comparison group and after for the intervention group, as OSCE itself may have been an intervention).	Structured curriculum=6 hour dedicated palliative care teaching over 2.5 days/ 6 postgraduate yr-2 residents (intervention) and 6 postgraduate yr-5 residents (comparison)	The study finds the opposite: NO improvement in residents' communication skills. Note that communication skills were only a small part of the whole curriculum.	The fact that 2 groups (novice vs. veteran residents) BEGAN with similar scores before intervention makes results questionable: if comparison in the study is the effect of the curriculum as compared to effect of clinical experience, then one would expect that BEFORE the educational intervention the inexperienced group should have lower scores than experienced group. The lack of difference between curriculum and experience is surprising, and could have been faults with curriculum itself (extra readings in the busy lives of residents without ensuring homework was completed).	1 & 2
11	End-of-Life Care: A Retreat Format for Residents	To develop a curriculum teaching internal medicine resident end-of-life communication: 1) elicit patient's values and preferences, 2) communicate bad news, 3) discuss preferences for nutrition and hydration, ventilator withdrawal, and resuscitation, 4) prescribe opioids using different routes of administration, 5) recommend appropriate symptom management treatment	Quantitative and qualitative measures to evaluate the retreat. EPEC pre/post questions and faculty-generated questions, including both multiple-choice format and problem-solving short answers.	1- day retreat/ All year-2 internal medicine and family medicine residents and geriatric fellows from a community hospital. Number NOT provided	Residents' attitude and knowledge assessed on multiple choice only. The results show NO IMPROVEMENT in the multiple choice questions on communication skills (p:0.092, see notes section).	A"LISTEN" acronym that may be put forth a helpful teaching aid to palliative care communication skill teaching. While there was no significant change in communication skills, the measurement (8-item multiple choice questions) may be inappropriate and cannot be meaningfully compared to OSCE or real interaction. Overall not a well-done study with unclear writing.	1

	Type of program	*Stated goals*	*Evaluation methods*	*Length/ # of residents*	*Evidence of improvement in residents' communication skills?*	*Additional notes*	*Kirkpatrick Classification*
12	The Palliative Care Clinical Evaluation Exercise (CEX): An Experience-Based Intervention for Teaching End-of-Life Communication Skills	Initial phase of a larger project to teach/reinforce palliative care communication skills among internal medicine residents. Palliative Care CEX piloted among year-1 residents to assess feasibility and perceived educational value	The perceived educational value of the CEX was measured along several dimensions: overall educational value, quality of preceptor teaching, educational impact of the exercise, and obstacles to learning. As a secondary outcome, limited measurements of residents communication skills as perceived by the residents themselves and by the faculty observers were also obtained. Immediately before the discussion, the Palliative Care Clinician (PCC) administered a brief six-item scale in which residents rated their competence in conducting bad news and code status discussions, and the adequacy of their prior training in end-of-life communication skills. During the intervention, the PCC recorded the type of discussion: bad news, code status, or both along with the amount of time taken for each aspect of the intervention. Various characteristics of the patients were also documented. PCCs also measured the degree to which discussions met explicit quality criteria derived from existing instruments and a review of literature on end-of-life communication skills. PCCs documented sitting down, making eye contact, avoiding medical jargon, as well as subjective evaluation of criteria such as appearing empathetic. A research assistant contacted the residents after they completed the Palliative Care CEX to administer a structured telephone survey of 33 items designed to assess residents perceptions of the ease of completing the Palliative care CEX and the educational value of the exercise. At the end of their first year, we administered a 20-item questionnaire that assessed their attitudes about the educational value of the exercise. Residents who did not complete the Palliative Care CEX received a separate seven-item, open-ended questionnaire that assessed perceived barriers to completing the CEX, and their perceptions of end-of-life communication training. Copies of the questionnaires are available from the authors on request.	Discussions averaged 49.5 min, divided among prediscussion counseling, resident– patient discussion, and post discussion feedback/ 44	NO: This study limited itself to testing the residents' perception of the program. A majority of residents perceived training in end-of-life communication skills to be an unmet educational need and rated the educational value of the Palliative Care CEX highly. The intervention improved residents' self-rated competence in conducting discussions with seriously ill patients, consistent with the outcomes of other experience-based training programs in end-of-life communication skills.	This study was a Kirkpatrick level 1 only study. Hence, there is no evidence that the intervention makes any difference in the residents' skills.	1

	Type of program	*Stated goals*	*Evaluation methods*	*Length/ # of residents*	*Evidence of improvement in residents' communication skills?*	*Additional notes*	*Kirkpatrick Classification*
13	Breaking bad news in obstetrics and gynecology: educational conference for resident physicians	To educate OB/GYN residents about communicating poor prognoses through a panel discussion and patient educators teaching	Two-phase evaluation including resident feedback about the format, content transferability across clinical situations, and an open-ended question, "what feedback do you have about this conference?" invited general critiques. 3 panelists' feedback obtained via a telephone call.	Not specified: time for the panel discussion and for questionnaire completion/ 12	No: Study did not test changes in the residents' communication skills. The study listed residents' feedback, which was unanimously positive. They indicated willingness to pay more attention to the partners and family members while delivering bad news and learning the value of staying in touch after giving bad news. They appreciated the opportunity to "practice giving bad news" with the panelists and indicated the information transferable to other situations. Panelists expressed appreciation for being able to tell their stories and be of benefit to residents. While they acknowledged discomfort with revisiting their painful experiences, this was balanced by the sense of being helpful. All of the panelists indicated that they would do it again.	Not a trial. This method has potential to be tested in a formal trial exploring Kirkpatrick 2 and above.	1
14	Teaching Sexual History-Taking Skills Using the Sexual Events Classification System	To test whether combining Sexual Events Classification System interview with other validated educational methods (e.g., SP interviews and competency-based scoring assessments) would improve residents' abilities to sexual history taking skills	Residents completed anonymous survey to assess the usefulness of the experience after the course.	Not specified: most likely a few hours/ 7	N/A	This article describes a teaching method that has been used for years and assessed residents' changes in attitudes and self confidence in performing sexual history interview. Residents reported perceived improvement in skills, and responded positively to the intervention.	1
15	Assessing Residents' Communication Skills: Disclosure of an Adverse Event to a Standardized Patient	To assess communication skills in disclosure of poor outcome to SPs and compare performance before and after teaching. Hypothesis: formal training on disclosure of adverse outcomes would improve resident performance	14 OB/GYN residents (PGY-2 to PGY-5) evaluated in a 2-station OSCE (goals: obtaining patient history/counseling and discussing an adverse outcome). In each history/counseling station, an evaluation grid was developed. For the disclosure meeting, residents were evaluated using a checklist extracted from adverse event disclosure guidelines developed by Canadian Patient Safety Institute. The assessment measured whether residents were able to follow suggested guidelines. The residents then participated in a workshop on disclosure and were retested.	2-hour workshop/ 14	YES: Mean score improved after the workshop. Analysis using Student t test showed significant differences in mean scores.	This study demonstrates that OSCE is an effective way to evaluate residents' communication skills and identify deficits. Residents exhibited significant improvement on a disclosure OSCE after formal teaching in disclosure interview.	2

	Type of program	*Stated goals*	*Evaluation methods*	*Length/ # of residents*	*Evidence of improvement in residents' communication skills?*	*Additional notes*	*Kirkpatrick Classification*
16	Linking a Motivational Interviewing Curriculum to the Chronic Care Model	To pilot-test a curriculum for a Primary Care Internal Medicine residency program that links motivational interviewing (MI) training to the self-management support (SMS) component of the chronic care model. The aim is to address residency training deficits in health behavior counseling	Preliminary qualitative assessments of curriculum with the goal of continuously improving the curriculum. Learners completed anonymous evaluations after didactics, practicum, and at the completion of residency. Residents discuss this curriculum during group feedback sessions with faculty.	Modules ranged from 3-8 hours each per week. 155 hours total including clinical time for practicing these skills/ 30	Only subjective reports: "Faculty directly observed residents during clinical encounters using MI and SMS skills to work more collaboratively with patients and to improve patient readiness for self-management goal setting."	A complex intervention curriculum. Residents report improved understanding of the CCM, increased confidence with assisting patients in health behavior change, and more awareness of socioeconomic obstacles, increased SMS engagement when working with health coaches, and improved patient–physician collaboration. Faculty directly observed residents during clinical encounters.	1 (no hard data shown)
17	Three Scenarios to Teach Difficult Discussions in Pediatric Emergency Medicine: Sudden Infant Death, Child Abuse With Domestic Violence, and Medication Error	To educate EM residents and fellows on the communication skills to engage in difficult discussions when caring for children in an emergency department setting	Feedback of the 96 residents who participated in simulations. Included with each of the three scenarios are three assessment tools combining a scenario specific critical action checklist and a global competency scale. Assessment tools not validated, but are used to assist in providing feedback to learners.	Not specified; three scenarios took place at different times during the year/ 96	n/a	Description of a teaching method and learner's feedback, but do not assess curriculum efficacy. There are 14 pages of appendices alongside the article with evaluation scales and scenario outlines for others to replicate/ incorporate the program at their own institutions.	1

	Type of program	Stated goals	Evaluation methods	Length/ # of residents	Evidence of improvement in residents' communication skills?	Additional notes	Kirkpatrick Classification
18	Evaluation of an Evidence-Based Tobacco Treatment Curriculum for Psychiatry Residency Training Programs	To evaluate the Rx for Change in Psychiatry curriculum, developed for psychiatry residency programs and focused on identifying and treating tobacco dependence among individuals with mental illness	Attendees completed a voluntary pre- and post- survey and a 3-month follow-up survey. Attitudes regarding barriers to addressing tobacco use were assessed. In the first year, a systematic chart review (N 1,204 medical charts) covering 3-month timeframe 3- months prior to and following the training. Behaviors including tobacco use assessmented.	4 hours/ 55	The percent of patients that residents reported asking about smoking remained unchanged from pretraining to 3-month follow-up: 39% and 41% respectively, p 0.967. However, significant increases were found in residents' reports of advising their patients who smoke to quit (28% to 55%, p 0.002), assessing their patients' readiness to quit (19% to 48%, p 0.001), providing assistance with quitting (26% to 50%, p 0.004), arranging follow up (8% to 28%, p 0.010), and providing cessation referrals (3% to 19%, p 0.003). No significant changes were found over time among the untrained residents. Among the residents who were trained, consistent with their self reports, significant improvements were found in their advising smokers to quit, assessing readiness to quit, assisting with quitting, and arranging follow up (p 0.05 in all cases).	Note that level 3 outcomes (application of the skills learned in the program into everyday practice) were self-reported, as opposed to measured by independent reviewers. Training effect can be conceptualized by increase in number of patients seen by residents who received attention to their tobacco use. Curriculum resulted in significant changes in residents' knowledge, attitudes, confidence, and behaviors for treating tobacco dependence among patients with mental illness. Changes pre- to posttraining were sustained at 3-month follow-up. Very positive perception of the training program and its utility.	1 & 3
19	Obesity Prevention in Pediatrics: A Pilot Pediatric Resident Curriculum Intervention on Nutrition and Obesity Education and Counseling	To implement and evaluate an "Obesity Prevention in Pediatrics" curriculum incorporated into an existing pediatric residency program's year-2 community rotation	Attitudinal questionnaires, multiple-choice knowledge examinations and a pre-established checklist of desired skills and behaviors were used to assess the curriculum's effect on participants' ability and willingness to manage obese or at-risk pediatrc patients and their families.	not specified/ 6	Residents' level of knowledge (measured by scores on the multiple-choice examinations) tended to improve significantly following participation in the curriculum. Residents' subjective responses to the attitudinal surveys, both individually and as a group, also tended to describe a significantly higher level of comfort and perceived competency ($p=0.016$) in the nutrition counseling and weight management of obese and at-risk children and adolescents and their parents at the conclusion of the curriculum.	The use of direct observation of the residents is described here. However, the results of the checklists are not discussed anywhere else. Unfortunately, they did not comment on the checklist results and did not design a pre and post intervention observed doctor-patient encounter coded with the checklist.	1

	Type of program	Stated goals	Evaluation methods	Length/ # of residents	Evidence of improvement in residents' communication skills?	Additional notes	Kirkpatrick Classification
20	Resident Physicians' Competencies and Attitudes in Delivering a Postnatal Diagnosis of Down Syndrome	To assess obstetrics/ gynecology and pediatric residents' knowledge about Down syndrome and comfort in counseling parents with a newborn child with Down syndrome. And to evaluate similarities and differences between the two specialties.	The intervention was evaluated with 1) a situational inventory administered before and after the intervention that assessed physicians' perceived confidence and competence in assisting and supporting families and their discomfort in potentially interacting with parents of children with Down syndrome; 2) a cognitive inventory to assess physicians' knowledge of the most important aspects of Down syndrome; and 3) a module satisfaction scale that asked viewers to assess the CD-ROM format and the accuracy and comprehensiveness of the information presented.	not specified/ 30 first- and second-year residents specializing in either obstetrics/gynecology (10) or pediatrics (20).	N/A (communications skills were not actually tested before or after).	Overall, first and second year residents improved significantly on both content and comfort level measures and recommended the use of this module for all levels of medical education. 28 of the 29 participants became more comfortable with these situations, and 26 residents improved on the knowledge tests. (P< .001). No significant differences in knowledge improvement were found between the 15 second-year residents and the 14 first-year residents. Pediatrics residents voiced a significantly greater need for this information and training than did obstetrics–gynecology residents. Residents in pediatrics showed greater improvement in comfort level than did residents in obstetrics– gynecology.	1
21	Preparing Residents to Counsel About Smoking	To evaluate the effects of an innovative, multicomponent, theory-based educational intervention for pediatric residents on prevention of tobacco use and counseling for cessation.	A pre-post test design was used to evaluate the effects of an educational program on residents' attitudes and their self-reported tobacco use prevention and cessation counseling practices. Baseline data were collected at the beginning of the training session using a 39 item questionnaire. Follow-up data were collected with a similar questionnaire 3 mo after intervention. Using a 5-point Likert scale, residents reported how often they asked about smoking status, provided counseling, handed out written materials, referred patients to a specialist or program, and made a follow-up plan for (1) children and adolescents who do not smoke, (2) adolescents who smoke, and (3) parents who smoke. Residents also reported how frequently they applied Motivational Interviewing principles by assessing the patient's or parent's perception of how important it is to quit smoking and their ability to quit.	3 hour symposium and 1-hour "booster session" held 6 weeks after initial symposium/ 46 residents in the Pediatrics and combined Medicine/Pediatrics training program [however, only 32 (69.6%) completed both baseline and the 3-month follow-up surveys].	Frequency of counseling increased significantly after the educational intervention (but it should be noted that the application of skills learned in the program in everyday practice was self-reported, not measured by independent reviewers). Use of the MI principles (assessment of importance of quitting, and assessment of confidence to quit smoking) also increased significantly: the standardized effect size was 0.57 for change in overall frequency, 0.66 for assessing importance, and 0.78 for assessing confidence, representing a medium-sized effect on these measures.	Among potential mediators of improved counseling, confidence in one's own ability to counsel increased significantly, while perceived importance of counseling and perceived effectiveness of counseling showed no significant change. Feeling inadequately trained decreased substantially: 66.7% of residents agreed that this was a barrier for them at baseline and 28.1% claimed it as a barrier at follow-up. ($p = 0.07$)	1 & 3

	Type of program	Stated goals	Evaluation methods	Length/ # of residents	Evidence of improvement in residents' communication skills?	Additional notes	Kirkpatrick Classification
22	Improving the Patient, Family, and Clinician Experience After Harmful Events: The 'When Things Go Wrong' curriculum	To develop, implement and assess an educational progam that addresses the human dimensions of error using separate tracks for faculty physicians and trainees to improve communication skills for disclosure and apology	The evaluation method used was a comparison of a baseline anonymous assessment of learner experiences, attitudes, and perceptions about medical error, and a post-intervention survey focusing on the same aspects.	not specified/ 154 trainees (108 third-year medical students; 46 medical and surgical residents)	No (communications skills were not actually tested before or after). Study's results focused on the learners' perception of the program. After participating in the curriculum, surveyed participants indicated that the session would affect their own practice as clinicians, independent of their level of training (79% of trainees).	NOTE: this is a very thought provoking, well written and stimulating article, even though the study itself lacks statistical analyses and rigorous research methodology. It is worth reading because of the questions it raises.	1
23	Communicating Bad News – A Pediatric Department's Evaluation of a Simulated Intervention	To determine if pediatric residents and ED fellows could improve their ability to counsel and inform SPs about bad news	Each participating trainee was videotaped and observed twice while communicating bad news to the SPs. In the first interview, SPs assessed the trainee's baseline skills. The second interview, which occurred 4-10 weeks following intervention, was evaluated in the same manner, and results were compared to baseline. Outcome measures included a 30-point content checklist of information that should be provided to parents of a child who was DOA; and two scales to assess interpersonal skills: the Gibb trust scale and the NBME Patient Perception questionnaire (PPQ). At the beginning of each session, trainees completed a self-assessment questionnaire to determine previous experience in giving bad news.	not specified/ 28	There was statistically significant improvement in 2 general content categories: communication and follow up. There was a significant difference in total content score but not in essential issues. Trainees demonstrated an improvement in counseling skills from the first to the second interview in 2 categories of the Gibb's checklist (trust/distrust: $p = 0.0113$; and dependent/independent: $p = 0.0411$). No significant differences were found in the PPQ.	Trainees' comfort level before the intervention was less than midrange but increased significantly after the interactions, suggesting that actual role playing with and feedback from the SPs contributed to increased comfort level. Unexpected finding: statistically positive correlation among content scores and counseling skills: a higher score on PPQ and/or Gibb was correlated with higher total content score (authors hypothesized that as confidence with content increased, the trainee could redirect more attention to interpersonal skills).	2
24	Educating New Resident Physicians in Death Notification (research brief, not a true article)	Not stated, but the objective seems to be to determine if a one hour lecture on death notification improves residents' performance in death notification	On the afternoon of the same day as the lecture, both the intervention and control groups participated in a 12 minute simulated death notification. Each resident was given a death scenario and asked to inform the survivors. The evaluators scored each performance as excellent, satisfactory, or unsatisfactory.	1 hour/ 36	The 2 groups had similar death notification experience (apart from the intervention) and had enrolled in similar residency programs. The death notification lecture group performed significantly better in the scenario than did the non-lecture group ($p = 0.023$).	This was a prospective randomized trial. The authors suggest that an ACLS course is an ideal setting for teaching new physicians death notification skills. This was not a full article; rather, it was a research brief in Academic Medicine from 1999.	2

	Type of program	*Stated goals*	*Evaluation methods*	*Length/ # of residents*	*Evidence of improvement in residents' communication skills?*	*Additional notes*	*Kirkpatrick Classification*
25	A Communication Assessment and Skill-building Exercise (CASE) for First-year Residents (a brief under the Residency Programs Curriculum heading in Academic Medicine, 2002- not a full article)	To create opportunities for (1) teaching essential interviewing and communication skills to trainees at the beginning of residency, (2) assessing resident skills and confidence with specific types of interview situations, (3) developing faculty teaching and assessment skills, (4) encouraging collegial interaction between faculty and new trainees, and (5) guiding residency curricular development	Residents' performances at each station were analyzed, and individual profiles were created for each resident. All residents and faculty completed evaluations of the exercise.	50 minutes - 1 hour/ 26	N/a: there was no pre-post intervention comparison.	This was not a study, just a report. Residents reported learning important skills, receiving valuable feedback, and increasing their confidence in dealing with certain types of stressful communication situations in residency. The residency program director found individual resident performance profiles valuable for identifying learning issues and for guiding curricular development. Time constraints were the most frequently cited area for improvement.	1
26	Teaching Physicians How to Break Bad News – a one day workshop to teach pediatric residents	To increase the competency of pediatric residents in crisis counseling skills with parents whose child has a potentially fatal illness. The objective of the project were: 1) to provide instruction to the residents in critical information to discuss with parents during the first interview; 2) to provide instruction and give feedback on interpersonal and communication skills; and 3) to evaluate the program's effectiveness in improving information giving and interpersonal skills.	One 1.5 hour session occurred during the first week of the rotation and the second occured in the last week. Immediately following the interview portion of the session, the residents filled out and scored a checklist that gave them immediate feedback on the proportion of critical information he/she imparted to the parents. SPs also completed checklists: one concerning their feelings during the session and one rating the clarity of the information that the resident imparted. At the end of each session the SPs and the residents completed an evaluation form about the session. The resident's performance on the "critical" information checklist, the clarity of critical information checklist, and the SPs' trust and feelings checklists were used as evaluation metrics.	4 hours/ 24 second and third year pediatric residents	Critical Information Giving: There was a significant imporvement after the intervention in the proportion of critical information discussed with SPs: 65% post vs. 55% pre, $p<0.05$. Clarity of Information Giving: 68% of residents improved, the other 32% worsened, no p value provided. Interpersonal Skills: 68% of the residents were rated as having an overall acceptable positive level of interpesonal skills (15/22) in the first interview. In the second interview this number increased to 86% of residents (19/22); no p-value provided. Instruction appeared to have the most impact on the residents' listening skills.	1) The responses of parents and physicians on the checklist were significantly related (r: .83, $p< 0.001$). 2) Residents rated the program between effective and extremely effective, and deemed it highly applicable or applicable to their present work and future careers. 3) The authors suggest that the decline in performance observed in a number of residents could be attributed to fatigue, interference with other responsibilities, and personality differences with the SPs, all of which could be encountered in real life practice and must be accounted for by the resident in order to have an effective crisis counseling session with any family.	1&2

	Type of program	*Stated goals*	*Evaluation methods*	*Length/ # of residents*	*Evidence of improvement in residents' communication skills?*	*Additional notes*	*Kirkpatrick Classification*
27	Improving Emergency Medicine Residents' Approach to Patients With Alcohol Problems: A Controlled Educational Trial	To improve emergency medicine residents' knowledge and practice in screening and intervening with patients presenting to the ED with alcohol problems, and to assess whether emergency medicine residents' attitudes and beliefs, perceptions of role responsibility, and self-efficacy influence their knowledge and performance.	Residents completed anonymous surveys at baseline and 1 year after intervention, testing current practice, perceptions of self-efficacy, role responsibility, current attitudes and beliefs, and provider readiness to change approach to patients with alcohol problems (all responses were in the form of Likert scales). Residents also completed the Brief Substance Abuse Attitude Scale (SAAS) testing their attitudes toward substance-abusing patients. The primary outcome variable was change in practice, as measured by a review of medical records: for each resident, 20 ED records with preselected targeted diagnoses were reviewed for evidence of screening, intervention, and referral before and after the intervention. Improvements in practice were measured by the increase in proportion of patients screened and counseled over time and compared between the intervention and control groups.	4 hours: 90-minute didactic program, 30-minute video, and a 2-hour skills-based workshop 36 (17 in the intervention group and 19 in the control group)	The intervention group had a significant increase in the practice of screening and brief intervention as measured by ED record review. Although the intervention group started with a lower baseline value, their improvement was significant both within their group and between groups. (P<.001 for both comparisons). No improvement was noted in the control group over time.	This intervention teaches counseling and screening communication skills. However, the study tested not improved counseling skills but how frequently residents apply them to their practice. Results: Significant differences between the intervention and control group were only found for 2 items: the intervention group showed greater improvement in their ability to assess patients' readiness to change and a decrease in their perceived lack of (1) resources available to refer patients and (2) available role models. The intervention group also had a significant increase in overall knowledge scores (p<0.001).	1 & 3

	Type of program	Stated goals	Evaluation methods	Length/ # of residents	Evidence of improvement in residents' communication skills?	Additional notes	Kirkpatrick Classification
28	Development of a Communication Curriculum for Emergency Medicine Residents	To teach and assess communication and interpersonal skills (CIPS) for emergency medicine (EM) residents and to report strengths and weaknesses in residents' performance and their reactions to the curriculum.	A CIPS checklist consisting of 22 skill items in five categories (basic interpersonal skills, efficient information gathering, healthcare team communication, ongoing patient/family communication, and empathy) filled out by the 2 faculty observers, the SP, and the residents was the primary evaluation tool. Residents also provided feedback on the curriculum through voluntary and anonymous surveys.	About 1 hour: introductory session, 10-15 minute SP encounter, 10–15 min videotape review, and 10-15 minute feedback session/ 26 (10 PGY-I residents, 8 PGY-2s, and 8 PGY-3s)	The pilot examined strengths and weaknesses in residents' CIPS as a group. It did not compare the residents' performance before and after the intervention.	This study is observational and retrospective of EM residents' CIPS performance during a single SP encounter assessed by a CIPS checklist. Resident performance gaps were identified as skills performed less than 85% of the time. Residents demonstrated the highest performance in Basic Interpersonal Skills 98.4% (CI 96.5–100.2%) followed by Efficient Information Gathering 94.9% (CI 89.9–99.8%), Healthcare Team Communication 71.2% (CI 61.8–80.5%), and On-going Patient/Family Communication 70.2% (CI 61.6–78.8%). They demonstrated the lowest performance in Empathy 33.9% (CI 27.1–40.6%). Residents rated their overall experience favorably. NOTE: the SP was a fellow resident and faculty was present in the room during the SP encounter, which likely affected how realistic the encounter was to the residents.	1

	Type of program	*Stated goals*	*Evaluation methods*	*Length/ # of residents*	*Evidence of improvement in residents' communication skills?*	*Additional notes*	*Kirkpatrick Classification*
29	Pretraining and Posttraining Assessment of Residents' Performance in the Fourth Accreditation Council for Graduate Medical Education Competency: Patient Communication Skills (RCT)	To teach surgical residents to incorporate patient centered communication skills into their practice, including providing information and education, emotional support, transition, and continuity of care; involving family and friends; and respecting patient values and preferences.	Before the intervention, residents completed an anonymous survey on their awareness of communication skills and participated in a simulated encounter in which they had to inform a patient about either a breast cancer or rectal cancer diagnosis. The SP graded the resident on 2 scales: a case-specific content checklist (a 13-item yes/no checklist of communication content specific to that cancer) and the Master Interview Rating Scale (MIRS). Following the educational program, residents completed a second SP encounter that was graded according to the content checklist and the MIRS.	About 3 hours: Two 10-15 minute resident/ SP encounters, a 90 minute workshop, and a 30 minute role-playing session/ 30	The posttest median score of 11.0 (84%) was significantly higher than the pretest score of 8.5 (65%) (P=.005). No signfiicant differences were found between scores in the rectal cancer and breast cancer scenarios. There was no significant difference in the total MIRS score pre- and post-test; however, there was significant improvement in the "support systems" sub-category (P=.03).	The study's design is standard, with pre and post intervention SP encounters scored with checklists. There was significant improvement in the content checklist (however, it is not clear whether this checklist was previously validated or was one made up by the authors). Residents showed no significant improvement in total MIRS score, and significant improvement only in one subset. These results are therefore not compelling. Possible explanations for this discrepency proposed by the authors: 1) case-specific skills may be easier to learn through checklists, while other communication skills (e.g., demonstrating empathy) are more complex; 2) the MIRS may be more subjective and scores may be biased because non-orthogonal categories are evaluated separately; 3) some variables tested by the MIRS are dependent on confidence with clinical knowledge rather than communication skills; and 4) Inter-rater variability, while non-significant, may have nonetheless affected the results.	2

	Type of program	Stated goals	Evaluation methods	Length/ # of residents	Evidence of improvement in residents' communication skills?	Additional notes	Kirkpatrick Classification
30	Improving empathy and relational skills in otolaryngology residents – a pilot study	To develop an empathy training protocol to improve interpersonal skills and to evaluate interpersonal skills of residents.	At baseline and at study completion, residents completed 5 self-report measures: (1) the Balanced Emotional Empathy Scale (BEES); (2) the Jefferson Scale of Physician Empathy; (3) the Neurobiology of Emotions Assessment (developed by the authors) assessing knowledge of the neurobiology and physiology of emotions; (4) the Ekman Facial Decoding Test, assessing accuracy in identifying emotions revealed by subtle facial cues; and (5) the Consultation and Relational Empathy (CARE) measure. Patients also rated the physicians on the CARE measure at baseline and upon training completion.	4.5 hours: Three 90-minute empathy and relational skills training modules/ 11	There were statistically significant improvements in residents' knowledge of the neurobiology and physiology of empathy ($P = .008$, large effect size) and in self-reported empathy with patients ($P = .01$, small to medium effect size). Although not significant, patient ratings of residents' empathy also increased.	The residents' performance was evaluated by real patients. This is a research brief more than a true article; the authors provide limited data and do not back up all statements with data (e.g., the authors state that patients' ratings of the residents improved, but do not provide data or p values). Residents' ability to decode subtle facial expressions of emotion (Ekman Test), their self-reported ability to empathize with their patients (Jefferson Scale) and with other people (BEES), and patients' ratings of physician empathy (CARE) all increased in the predicted direction, but none of these effects achieved statistical significance.	1 & 3
31	Evidence of improved knowledge and skills after an elective rotation in a hospice and palliative care program for internal medicine residents	To test whether a clinical elective improves measures of knowledge and skill in palliative care issues.	The outcomes measured were: knowledge and skill in managing pain and common symptoms of advanced disease, communication skills with patients about goals of care and death, knowledge of palliative care, and appropriate use of hospice programs. Knowledge in these target areas was assessed with a questionnaire administered at the beginning and end of the rotation. Communication skills were assessed using a videotaped interview with an SP, which was evaluated using the SEGUE criteria developed and validated by Makoul. Residents also completed a written assessment of the rotation.	4 weeks/ 25 (but only 17 filled out the post-test assessment)	All residents were able to accomplish the specific tasks of the SEGUE instrument (Set the Stage, Elicit Information, Give Information, Understand the Patient's Perspective, and End This Visit). However, variability among residents was detected in the debriefing of the videotape where approaches, choices of words, and effects could be evaluated. According to qualitative reports, residents demonstrated improved communication and interviewing skills across the course of the rotation in response to repetitive exposure to similar communication challenges (but this was not captured with any objective instrument).	This article focuses more on describing the rotation's curriculum than it does outlining the objective evaluation of its effectiveness. There was a 10 percent improvement in knowledge ($p < 0.05$), but the study lacked a control group. Qualitative review suggested the residents found the rotation valuable, but because it was an elective, this rotation was prone to selection bias towards residents who already display appropriate attitudes. The instrument used to assess changes in knowledge was not previously validated.	1 & 2

	Type of program	Stated goals	Evaluation methods	Length/ # of residents	Evidence of improvement in residents' communication skills?	Additional notes	Kirkpatrick Classification
32	Teaching Error Disclosure to Residents: A Curricular Innovation and Pilot Study	To assess change in perceived preparedness to disclose medical errors. The goal was to compare change in obstetrics/ gynecology residents' self-efficacy in disclosing medical errors after a formal educational session.	Residents completed an anonymous postintervention survey that assessed change in perceived preparedness to disclose medical errors. The curriculum was assessed based on self-efficacy regarding the skills used in disclosure, self-efficacy regarding response to emotion, and the perceived usefulness of the curriculum.	4 hours/ 15 fourth year OB GYN residents	After the session, residents considered themselves more prepared for the following: knowing what to include in and how to introduce error discussions, dealing with a patient's emotional reaction, responding to a patient's questions regarding how an error occurred, and recognizing one's own emotions when discussing medical errors ($P < .05$ for all). Residents believed that they would be likely to use the skills learned in the remainder of residency and in their future career.	The study only looked at residents' perception of the intervention and changes in their confidence.	1
33	Breaking bad news education for emergency medicine residents: A novel training module using simulation with the SPIKES protocol	To educate and improve physician's confidence and competence in delivering bad news and notification of death by teaching and practicing a six-step process that focuses on gathering information, transmitting the medical information, providing support, and summarizing the information.	All participants were asked to fill out the evaluation sheets after the workshop. A course survey evaluated the activity as a whole and the quality and usefulness of each session on a 5-point Likert Scale. There was also a self-efficacy form that included items similar to the SPIKES forms.	5 hours/ 14	N/a	The study only looked at residents' attitudes, not their actual skills. The participants thought that patient care would improve after this educational experience with a mean Likert score of 4.79 (out of 5). The overall usefulness of the course was scored 4.73. Among the participants, 43% thought that the session with simulation scenarios was the most useful, as compared to role play (14%) and lectures (7%), and 36% found all the sessions equally useful. All the participants agreed that the course should be continued as part of their annual regular academic activity.	1
34	Improving Pediatric Residents' Alcohol and Other Drug Use Clinical Skills: the Use of and Experiential Curriculum	To assesss whether pediatric residens' knowledge and attitudes about AOD (alcohol and other drugs) issues would change significantly after participating in an experiential-based AOD curriculum; and whether their clinical skills in AOD issues would improve after completing such curriculum.	An OSCE was developed to measure clinical behavior skills: residents conducted 3 interviews with SPs in various AOD scenarios, performing all 3 interviews before and after the completion of the curriculum. Residents also took a written test on their knowledge in various AOD-related issues before and after completion of the curriculum. Residents also rated their interest, competence, satisfaction and knowledge in AOD- related clinical issues on a 5 point Likert scale.	4 or 5 half days/ 44 first and second year pediatric residents (15 of these were in the control group)	After adjusting for pretest scores and race, the intervention group showed a significant increase in written test scores as compared to the control group ($p=0.0001$). There were also significant differences between intervention and control groups in all three scenarios. Residents' self-ratings did not differ between groups.	This study is a little old. The authors looked at pre- and post- test scores as well as between group scores, thus having 2 types of control for their intervention. More information about the curriculum itself would have been useful.	1 & 2

	Type of program	Stated goals	Evaluation methods	Length/ # of residents	Evidence of improvement in residents' communication skills?	Additional notes	Kirkpatrick Classification
35	Sexual Communication Skills in Residency Training: The Robert Wood Johnson Model	To assess the feasibility and impact of implementing an educational model of human sexuality training with medical residents from different specialty and subspecialty backgrounds.	The workshop used an audience-response feedback system for evaluating responses and providing feedback to the participants on key questions. At the conclusion of the workshop, a brief posttest evaluation was provided where participants were asked to rate their overall level of satisfaction with the material provided as well as changes in their perceived comfort and ability in sexual interviewing. A 6-month follow-up of a very limited sample of participants was also performed: residents were contacted by email approximately 6 months after the workshop and asked questions concerning changes in their practice.	5.5 hours (one half-day workshop)/ 46 residents belonging to a variety of specialties (however data is available only on 34)	N/a	Before the workshop, 46% of respondents stated that they rarely or never discussed sexual issues with their patients, though more than 90% agreed that sexual problems can have a major impact on quality of life and 74.5% stated that it was moderately to very important to know about a patient's sexual health. 92.8% of the participants rated the workshop presentations as moderately or highly informative and very interactive; 67.4% stated that they attained greater awareness of sexual problems. 52% reported that the workshop helped them develop comfort and skill in sexual history taking, and 41% rated themselves as moderately improved in this area.	1
36	Evaluation of an Educational Intervention To Encourage Advance Directive Discussions between Medicine Residents and Patients	To evaluate an educational intervention focused on teaching internal medicine and medicine-pediatric residents and interns skills to discuss advance directives.	The intervention was evaluated by auditing the charts of admitted inpatients 10 days prior to and 5 days subsequent to the intervention to determine if there was a documented DNR discussion between the patient and the resident or intern.	1-1.5 hours (standard morning rounds)/ 8 internal medicine and medicine– pediatric residents and interns	No: Seventy-nine records of patients assigned to the eight physicians who attended the intervention were reviewed before and after the intervention. Before the intervention, 32% of the patients had a documented advance directive discussion while 34% of the patients had a discussion after the intervention. This 2% increase in frequency of discussion was not statistically significant. There was no significant correlation between attending the intervention and having the discussion with the patient.	This study is not of very high quality (having a very small sample size and assessing change in a very short period of time). Additionally, only minimal details about the educational intervention are provided.	2

	Type of program	Stated goals	Evaluation methods	Length/ # of residents	Evidence of improvement in residents' communication skills?	Additional notes	Kirkpatrick Classification
37	Teaching Pediatric Residents to Provide Emotion-Laden Information	To determine whether simulation with immediate videotape feedback is an effective teaching technique to improve pediatric residents' skills in communicating emotion-laden information to parents.	The participants' performances on the first and fourth sessions were rated and compared to determine improvement. Additionally, 10 private pediatric practitioners who participated in one of the two rated simulated sessions without receiving the training acted as a control group. Videotapes were independently reviewed by 2 blinded raters using 3 scales: the interview attributes questionnaire [IAQ]; the communication behavior coding scale [CBCS]; and the specific parameter coding scale [SPCS].	not specified/ 22 PGY-2 pediatric residents	A t test analysis of individual items on the 3 scales revealed no significant dfferences in the IAQ scale, significant and near significant differences in the CBCS scale (specifically in the use of reinforcement, use of reassurance, and number of questions asked about the parents' understanding of the child condition). On the SPCS, the only significant or near significant difference was on how frequently and accurately the etiology was discussed and how frequently and accurately ambulation and intelligence were discussed.	No P values were provided.	2
38	Enhancing parent–provider communication in ambulatory pediatric practice	To evaluate the effectiveness of a brief intervention to enhance interpersonal communication skills by pediatric and internal medicine/pediatric residents with parents of children seen in ambulatory practice. The objectives were to increase residents' use of empathy, positive affect, support, and collaboration with parents.	Medical visits with residents were audio-taped and parents were asked to complete questionnaires regarding their perception of the visit immediately after. The target outcomes in this investigation were represented by utterances concerning positive affect, empathy/reassurance, and partnership. Data from the audio-tapes was coded and analysed, and the communication subscale of the Parents' Perceptions of Primary Care measure (P3C) was used to assess parents' perceptions of the visit. Parents also completed the Parent Medical Interview Satisfaction Scale (PMISS).	1–1.5 hours/ 28 residents	Most of the interpersonal utterances were stable or increased over time, with the use of reassurance/optimism increasing significantly ($p < .01$). The total amount of interpersonal communication utterances increased over time ($p = .03$) Results of the P3C showed that both pre-and post-intervention, parents perceived residents as communicating well, with no change over time ($T = .42$, NS). Parents were significantly more satisfied with the care their children received following the intervention ($p < .01$).	This intervention was evaluated with real patient opinions and probably has the greatest external validity.	3
39	Teaching Interviewing Skills to Pediatric House Officers	To assess the interviewing skills of pediatric interns compared with those of PL2s, PL3s and clinical faculty, and to evaluate the effect of a short course in interviewing on the interns' communication styles.	Interviews were videotaped to evaluate physician-patient interaction, data gathering, hypothesis formation and provision of therapy education, reassurance, support, and anticipatory guidance. Participants interviewed SPs at the beginning of their rotation and again at the end of the rotation, videotapes of their interviews were used to evaluate their performance. The interns' performances were also compared with those of five practicing members of the clinical faculty.	1.5 hr + 30 minute feedback session/ 13 pediatric interns (8 in the study group, 5 in the control group)	Data-gathering ability increased significantly; the focus of attention shifted from a more disease-oriented to a more patient-oriented interview; less direct, less leading questions were used to obtain data; and more support and reassurance were provided post-intervention. Members of both the intervention group and the control group improved significantly and approached the proficiency level of practicing pediatrician after completeing the rotation (p values between 0.06 and 0.5).	This article is from 1978.	2

(> 1 month) outcomes. Seven studies did not specify how soon after the completion of the curriculum they tested their outcomes.

Of the 39 studies, 36 reported successful outcomes; 3 reported that their educational intervention had no effect on residents' attitudes, knowledge, or communication skills. One study, which we did not include in our survey, described their educational intervention in depth, reported measuring outcomes, but did not actually publish their outcomes.

In analyzing the study outcomes, we classified them using Donald Kirkpatrick's four levels evaluation model (Kirkpatrick 1975): level 1: the learners' reaction to the training program; level 2: the degree to which participants acquired the intended communication skills; level 3: the degree to which participants applied what they learned during the educational intervention in their everyday practice; and level 4: changes in patient outcomes as a result of the patients' physician undergoing communication skill training.

Twenty-five studies measured level 1 outcomes. Level 1 studies can be divided into two outcome categories: those studies that evaluated the learner's perception of the curriculum and its effectiveness, and those that compared the participants' confidence in their own skills and self-assessments before and after the educational intervention. Nineteen studies measured level 2 outcomes (evaluating the degree to which participants acquired the intended communication skills), most using Objective Structured Clinical Exams (OSCEs) with standardized patients and a few using written exams. OSCEs were scored using a disparate array of checklists and scales, some created by others (and psychometrically validated previously) and some created by the authors themselves. No two studies used the same scale, thus making comparisons across studies impossible. Six studies measured level 3 outcomes (evaluating to what degree participants applied what they learned during the educational intervention in their everyday practice). Typically these used retrospective chart reviews to determine whether the residents applied the target communication skills (e.g., discussing advanced directives, smoking cessation counseling). Two studies obtained feedback from the patients themselves regarding the study participants' performance. No study measured level 4 outcomes (i.e., changes in patient outcomes as a result of the patients' physician undergoing communication skill training).

Summary and Future Directions

Though educators have documented extensive efforts to teach residents communication skills (since 1995 over 500 articles have been published), relatively little has been done to assess the effectiveness of these efforts. In addition to our own published work, we found 39 articles on teaching residents communication skills which contained an intervention and an evaluation of that intervention. In only 21 of the 39 did researchers use objective measures (Kirkpatrick levels 2, 3); in the rest they relied exclusively on resident perception to assess the effectiveness of their programs. Researchers also used very different methods to teach their residents and evaluate their programs. Because of the paucity of high level evaluations and the diversity in methods, it is difficult to use this research to draw conclusions about how best to achieve resident competency in communication skills.

Program diversity, however, has a positive side. Efforts of individual educators resulted in a rich creativity in addressing a difficult educational challenge. Within the 39 papers are some particularly exciting and innovative approaches. In the otolaryngology paper, for example, the authors built a program based on mirror neuron research (Riess et al. 2011). In it they trained residents in relational skills using exemplar videos of difficult interactions which displayed real-time physiologic responses, allowing residents to see the degree to which doctor and patient were discordant or concordant. In addition they assessed at a high level, using real patients to rate their residents pre- and post-intervention. In another example, Daetwyler et al. trained residents using an interactive online program called Doc. Com and assessed the program using live resident interactions with web-based standardized patients (Daetwyler et al. 2010). In a third example the authors used the sophisticated verbal interaction analysis method we cited in the Background section, the Roter Interaction Analysis System (RIAS), to code their residents' performance in a pre-test and post-test (Roter et al. 2004).

Innovations of the sort we just summarized and the need for program integration suggest important directions for the future of communications skills teaching and evaluation in graduate medical education. To advance the field we believe that five areas deserve special attention: (1) application of new evidence-based knowledge about how we learn and communicate; (2) application of new technologies; (3) integration and coordination within and across programs; (4) faculty modeling and reinforcement, and (5) implementation of better ways to study our efforts.

Using neurophysiology research in communications teaching, as exemplified in the ENT study, is a good example of the application of new knowledge. It is our belief that we will incorporate neurophysiology more and more as the field advances, providing a hard science base for our education efforts. In addition, new knowledge is steadily becoming available based on studies that provide supporting evidence for theories of how we learn. Deliberate practice theory (Ericsson et al. 1993), for example, which charts the path to expertise, is supported by a growing body of research, as is Self-Determination theory (Kusurkar et al. 2011), which explains learner motivation. These and other evidence-based constructs need to be applied to our programs.

New technologies also need to be considered for application to our programs. The ENT experience reported above would have not been possible without methods that allow us to measure relationship physiology in real time and use it to create better communicators. Other researchers are also developing means to dynamically measure non-verbal factors (e.g., changes in body position, facial expressions, and mirroring behavior) as well as verbal factors in doctor–patient communication and use them to improve performance (Pentland 2010). New technology, we believe, will also help us better implement verbal interaction analysis which requires labor-intensive work from trained coders. Also, we believe we will develop even more sophisticated online teaching programs and increase the capacity through the Web to interact with standardized patients asynchronously and on demand.

Integration and coordination within and across the continuum of medical education is another important step in advancing communication education. Diversity is a necessary first phase in the development of a new field. The next necessary phase is integration – how to bring together what we have learned to best teach residents to be communications competent. Integration across programs – using similar teaching and evaluation methods – provides a common language for researchers and allows them to perform more statistically powerful evaluations. Equally important, however, is vertical integration within programs and, ultimately, across the medical student–resident–practicing physician continuum. Currently, we believe there is very little integration of communications skills teaching between medical school and residency. Reasons include different administrative systems for medical schools and residency programs and the multiplicity of different approaches offered in the literature. In addition, we believe there is little vertical progression in such teaching within the years of residency. Vertical integration is a current major focus for graduate medical educators. As noted previously, it is framed in terms of the question, 'What developmental sequence of milestones and entrustable professional activities should be set for residents to define their pathway from novice to physician capable of independent practice?'

Faculty modeling is still another essential to furthering the communication competence of residents. If faculty do not reinforce communications concepts between formal educational interventions and, even more importantly, model exemplary communication skills, it is unlikely that residents will implement their communications training. Absence of faculty modeling may stem from the failure of the promotions and tenure system to reward such behavior. It also may stem from lack of faculty skills, which underscores the need for concerted efforts toward faculty development.

In addition to advancing teaching methodology, another goal for the future is to raise the level of evaluation of our teaching efforts. A number of obstacles exist, including small numbers in residency programs limiting statistical power, limited resident availability because of duty hour restrictions, and the difficulties of measuring long-term outcomes.

With small numbers of residents in any one program, it is difficult to conduct randomized control trials with enough statistical power to detect differences between intervention and control groups. This leaves training programs with limited options. Banding together to increase the number of residents in the study pool is one approach. Another is to use qualitative analysis, which does not depend on large numbers of study participants. Qualitative analysis, for example, could explore narratives from residents and their patients about their communication encounters, looking for themes to help explain successes and failures.

Resident duty hour restrictions are another barrier to quality evaluation and also to teaching communication skills. The ACGME, to preserve patient safety and resident health, limits the time (total and consecutive hours) residents are available for patient care and education activities. Duty hour restrictions make adding special time slots for communication teaching unworkable. A related challenge is the difficulty of using the same resident cohort over time because of interruption due to vacation, dispersion to different hospitals, and maternity leave. Though it entails compromises, the most viable approach to time limitations is creatively to find ways to incorporate communication skills teaching into the existing schedule. This might require distilling a 2–3-hour workshop into a one-hour session so it will fit into the one-hour noon conference that is a standard part of the regular schedule.

Still another barrier to better evaluation is the difficulty of conducting high Kirkpatrick level studies – studies that measure ultimate patient outcomes. Long-term effect and patient care impact are two of the ultimate outcomes for medical education. We want residents to communicate well not just at the end of a workshop, but throughout their careers. Also, we want our residents to communicate well enough to make a difference in the health and well-being of their patients. Measuring long-term outcomes is difficult, especially when there is so little funding available in this area. Such measurement requires more researcher time and effort and is therefore expensive. It also requires multiple participations from highly stressed populations – residents caring for large numbers of sick patients and sick patients worried about their illnesses and their lives. Adding to the challenge are inadequate resources to assist with data collection and entry, and no protected time for faculty.

Ways around some of the obstacles to measuring patient impact do exist. As we saw before, a number of studies used simulation methodology to approximate it. They were able to assess resident communication skills with standardized patients. SPs can offer residents a broad spectrum of communication challenges: e.g., interacting with a patient from another culture, giving bad news, talking about a medical error. Simulations, however, though very realistic, may not be identical with what happens in real life. Using 'stealth' SPs comes closer to reality, but observing residents' interactions with real patients is critical.

As is evident from our review, graduate medical education has been turning increasing attention to communication teaching and has developed many creative approaches. The challenge for the future is to increasingly apply neurophysiologic advances and new technology, to develop our faculty into better role models, to perform higher level evaluation of our programs, using the results to better our efforts, and to move from a phase of diversity into a phase of integration. Integration, when done well, will provide future doctors with a progressive curriculum of communication education that ensures their ability to talk with patients in a manner that addresses both their human and their medical needs.

Related topics

Resident; communication; evaluation; research methodology; doctor–patient relationship.

Further reading

Lipkin, M., Putnam, S.M., and Lazare, A. (eds) (1995) *The Medical Interview: Clinical Care, Education and Research,* New York: Springer Verlag.

Makoul, G. (2001) 'Essential elements of communication in medical encounters: the Kalamazoo consensus statement', *Academic Medicine*, 76: 390–393.

References

Abraham, A., Cheng, T.L., Wright, J.L., Addlestone, I., Huang, Z., and Greenberg, L. (2001) 'Assessing an educational intervention to improve physician violence screening', *Pediatrics,* 107: e68.

Aspegren, K. (1999) 'Teaching and learning communication skills in medicine: a review with quality grading of articles Best Evidence Medical Education (BEME) Guide 2', *Medical Teacher,* 21: 563–570.

Association of American Medical Colleges. (1999) *Contemporary Issues in Medicine: Communication in Medicine*, Washington, DC: Association of American Medical Colleges.

Beckman, H.B. and Frankel, R.M. (1984) 'The effect of physician behavior on the collection of data', *Annals of Internal Medicine*, 101(5): 692–696.

Cohen-Cole, S.A. (1991) *The Medical Interview: The Three-Function Approach*, St. Louis, MO: Mosby Year Book.

Daetwyler, C.J., Cohen, D.G., Gracely, E., and Novack, D.H. (2010) 'eLearning to enhance physician patient communication: a pilot test of 'doc.com' and 'WebEncounter' in teaching bad news delivery', *Medical Teacher*, 32(9): e381–e390.

Ericsson, K.A., Krame, R.T., and Tesch-Römer, C. (1993) 'The role of deliberate practice in the acquisition of expert performance', *Psychological Review*, 100(3): 363–406.

General Medical Council. (1993) *Tomorrow's Doctors: Recommendations on Undergraduate Medical Education*, London: General Medical Council.

Greenberg, L.W., Ochsenschalger, D., O'Donnell, R., Mastruserio, J., and Cohen, G. (1995) 'Communicating bad news: a pediatric department's evaluation of a simulated intervention', *Pediatrics,* 103: 1210–1217.

Jewett, L.S., Greenberg, L.W., Champion, L.A.A., Gluck, R.S., Leikin, S.L., Altieri, M.F., and Lipnick, R.N. (1982) 'The teaching of crisis counseling skills to pediatric residents: a one-year study', *Pediatrics,* 70: 907–911.

Kaplan, C.B., Siegel, B., Modill, J.M., and Epstein, R.M., (1997) 'Communication and the medical interview', *Journal of General Internal Medicine*, 12: S49–S55.

Kaplan, S.H., Greenfield, S., and Ware, J.E. Jr. (1989) 'Assessing the effects of physician–patient interactions on the outcomes of chronic disease', *Medical Care*, 27(3): S110–S127.

Kirkpatrick, D.L. (1975) 'Techniques for evaluating training programs', in D.L. Kirkpatrick (ed.) *Evaluating Training Programs*, Alexandria, VA: ASTD.

Korsch, B.M., Gozzi, E.K., and Francis, V. (1968) 'Gaps in doctor–patient communication', *Pediatrics*, 42: 855–871.

Kurtz, S., Silverman, J., and Draper, J. (1998) *Teaching and Learning Communication Skills in Medicine*, Abingdon: Radcliffe Medical Press.
Kusurkar, R.A., ten Cate, T.J., Van Asperen, M., and Croiset, G. (2011) 'Motivation as an independent and dependent variable in medical education: a review of the literature', *Medical Teacher*, 33: e242–e262.
Levinson, W., Roter, D.L., Mulloly, J.P., Dull, V.T., and Frankel R.M. (1997) 'Physician–patient communication: the relationship with malpractice claims among primary care physicians and surgeons', *Journal of the American Medical Association*, 277: 553–559.
Lipkin, M. (1996) 'Sisyphus or Pegasus? The physician interview in the era of corporatization of care', *Annals of Internal Medicine*, 124: 511–513.
Lipkin, M., Putnam, S.M., and Lazare A. (eds) (1995) *The Medical Interview: Clinical Care, Education and Research*, New York: Springer Verlag.
Makoul, G. (2001) 'Essential elements of communication in medical encounters: the Kalamazoo consensus statement', *Academic Medicine*, 76: 390–393.
Makoul, G. and Schofield, T. (1999) 'Communication teaching and assessment in medical education: an international consensus statement', *Patient Education and Counseling*, 37(3):191–195.
Ottolini, M.C. and Greenberg, L. (1998) 'Development and evaluation of a CD-ROM program to teach residents telephone management', *Pediatrics*, 101: e2.
Pentland, Alex. (2010) *Honest Signals*, Cambridge: Massachusetts Institute of Technology.
Rider, E.A. and Keefer, C.H. (2006) 'Communications skills competencies: definitions and a teaching toolbox', *Medical Education*, 40: 624–629.
Rider, E.A., Nawtoniak, R.H., and Smith, G.D. (2007) *A Practical Guide to Teaching and Assessing the ACGME Core Competencies*, Marblehead, MA: HCPro.
Riess, H., Kelley, J.M., Bailey, R., Konowitz, P.M., and Gray, S.T. (2011) 'Improving empathy and relational skills in otolaryngology residents – a pilot study', *Otolaryngology – Head & Neck Surgery*, 144 (1): 120–122.
Roter, D. and Larson, S. (2002) 'The Roter Interaction Analysis System (RIAS): utility and flexibility for analysis of medical interactions', *Patient Education and Counseling*, 46: 243–251.
Roter, D.L., Larson, S., Shinitzky, H., Chernoff, R., Serwint, J.R., Adamo, G., and Wissow, L. (2004) 'Use of an innovative video feedback technique to enhance communication skills training', *Medical Education*, 38: 145–157.
Simpson, M., Buckman, R., and Stewart, M., (1991) 'Doctor–patient communication: the Toronto consensus statement', *BMJ*, 303: 1385–1387.
Stewart, M.A. (1995) 'Effective physician–patient communication and health outcomes: a review', *Canadian Medical Association Journal*, 152: 480–492.
ten Cate, O. and Scheele, F. (2007) 'Competency-based postgraduate training: can we bridge the gap between theory and clinical practice', *Academic Medicine*, 82: 542–547.
Vaidya, V.U., Greenberg, L.W., Patel, K.M., Strauss, L.H., and Pollack, M.M. (1999) 'Teaching physicians how to break bad news: a one day workshop using standardized parents', *Archives Pediatrics & Adolescent Medicine*, 153: 419–422.
Workshop Planning Committee. (1992) 'Consensus statement from the workshop on the teaching and assessment of communication skills in Canadian medical schools', *Canadian Medical Association Journal*, 147(8): 1149–1152.

Appendix 19.1: Literature review references (in order in which they appear in Table 19.1)

1 Roter, D.L., Larson, S., Shinitzky, H., et al. Use of an innovative video feedback technique to enhance communication skills training. *Med Educ*. 2004; 38: 145–157.
2 Moulton, C.A., Tabak, D., Kneebone, R., Nestel, D., MacRae, H., LeBlanc, V.R. Teaching communication skills using the integrated procedural performance instrument (IPPI): a randomized controlled trial. *Am J Surg* 2009; 197(1): 113–118.
3 Alexander, S.C., Keitz, S.A., Sloane, R., Tulsky, J.A. A controlled trial of a short course to improve residents' communication with patients at the end of life. *Acad Med.* 2006; 81: 1008–1012.
4 Wong, R.Y., Saber, S.S., Ma, I., Roberts, J.M. Using television shows to teach communication skills in internal medicine residency. *Med Educ.* 2009; 9: 9.

5 Szmuilowicz, E., el-Jawahri, A., Chiappetta, L., Kamdar, M., Block, S. Improving residents' end-of-life communication skills with a short retreat: a randomized controlled trial. *J Palliat Med.* 2010; 13: 439–452.
6 Lozano, P., McPhillips, H.A., Hartzler, B., Robertson, A.S., Runkle, C., Scholz, K.A., et al. Randomized trial of teaching brief motivational interviewing to pediatric trainees to promote healthy behaviors in families. *Arch Pediatr Adolesc Med.* 2010; 164(6): 561–566.
7 Larkin, A.C., Cahan, M.A., Whalen, G., Hatem, D., et al. Human emotion response in surgery (HEARS): a simulation-based curriculum for communication skills, system-based practice, and professionalism in surgical residency training. *J Am Coll Surg.* 2010; 211: 285–292.
8 Daetwyler, C.J., Cohen, D.G., Gracely, E., Novack, D.H. eLearning to enhance physician–patient communication: a pilot test of 'doc.com' and 'WebEncounter' in teaching bad news delivery. *Medical Teacher.* 2010; 32(9): e381–e390.
9 Brinkman, W.B., Geraghty, S.R., Lanphear, B.P., et al. Effect of multisource feedback on resident communication skills and professionalism: a randomized controlled trial. *Arch Pediatr Adolesc Med.* 2007; 161(1): 44–49.
10 Bradley, C., Webb, T., Schmitz, C., Chipman, J., Brasel, K. Structured teaching versus experiential learning of palliative care for surgical residents. *Am J Surg.* 2010; 200: 542–547.
11 McFarland, K.F., Rhoades, D.R. End-of-life care: a retreat format for residents. *J Palliat Med.* 2006; 9: 82–89.
12 Han, P.K., Keranen, L.B., Lescisin, D.A., Arnold, R.M. The palliative care clinical evaluation exercise (CEX): an experience-based intervention for teaching end-of-life communication skills. *Acad Med.* 2005 Jul; 80(7): 669–676.
13 Romm, J. Breaking bad news in obstetrics and gynecology: educational conference for resident physicians. *Arch Women Ment Health.* 2002; 5: 177–179.
14 Donald, C., Fidler, D.C., Petri, J.D., Chapman, M. Teaching sexual history-taking skills using the sexual events classification system. *Academic Psychiatry.* 2010; 34: 353–356.
15 Posner, G., Nakajima, A. Assessing residents' communication skills: disclosure of an adverse event to a standardized patient. *J Obstet Gynaecol Can.* 2011; 33: 262–268.
16 Abramowitz, S.A., Flattery, D., Franses, K., Berry, L. Linking a motivational interviewing curriculum to the chronic care model. *J Gen Intern Med.* 2010; 25(Suppl 4): 620–626.
17 Overly, F.L., Sudikoff, S.N., Duffy, S., Anderson, A., Kobayashi, L. Three scenarios to teach difficult discussions in pediatric emergency medicine: sudden infant death, child abuse with domestic violence, and medication error. *Simul Healthc.* 2009; 4: 114–130.
18 Prochaska, J.J., Fromont, S.C., Leek, D., Hudmon, K., Louie, A.K. Evaluation of an evidence-based tobacco treatment curriculum for psychiatry residency training programs. *Acad. Psychiatry.* 2008; 32(6): 484–492.
19 Gonzalez, J.L., Gilmer, L. Obesity prevention in pediatrics: a pilot pediatric resident curriculum intervention on nutrition and obesity education and counseling. *J Natl Med Assoc.* 2006; 98: 1483–1488.
20 Ferguson, J.E., Kleinert, H.L., Lunney, C.A., Campbell, L.R. Resident physicians' competencies and attitudes in delivering a postnatal diagnosis of Down syndrome. *Obstet Gynecol.* 2006; 108(4): 898–905.
21 Scal, P., Hennrikus, D., Ehrlich, L., Ireland, M., Borowsky, I. Preparing residents to counsel about smoking. *Clin Pediatr.* 2004; 43: 703–708.
22 Bell, S.K., Moorman, D.W., Delbanco, T. Improving the patient, family, and clinician experience after harmful events: the 'when things go wrong' curriculum. *Acad Med.* 2010; 85(6): 1010–1017.
23 Greenberg, L.W., Ochsenschlager, D., O'Donnell, R., Mastruserio, J., Cohen, G.J. Communicating bad news: a pediatric department's evaluation of a simulated intervention. *Pediatrics.* 1999; 103: 1210–1217.
24 Pollack, M. Educating new resident physicians in death notification. *Acad Med.* 1999; 74: 721.
25 Roth, C.S., Watson, K.V., Harris, I.B. A Communication Assessment and Skill-building Exercise (CASE) for first-year residents. *Acad Med.* 2002; 77: 746–747.
26 Vaidya, V.U., Greenberg, L.W., Patel, K.M., Strauss, L.H., Pollack, M.M. Teaching physicians how to break bad news: a 1-day workshop using standardized parents. *Arch Pediatr Adolesc Med.* 1999; 153: 419–422.

27 D'Onofrio, G., Nadel, E.R., Degutis, L.C., et al. Improving emergency medicine residents' approach to patients with alcohol problems: a controlled educational trial. *Ann Emerg Med.* 2002; 40: 50–62.
28 Sullivan, C., Ellison, S.R., Quaintance, J., Arnold, L., Godrey, P. Development of a communication curriculum for emergency medicine residents. *Teaching and Learning in Medicine: An International Journal.* 2009; 21(4): 327–333.
29 Chandawarkar, R.Y., Ruscher, K.A., Krajewski, A., Garg, M., Pfeiffer, C., Singh, R., et al. Pretraining and posttraining assessment of residents' performance in the Fourth Accreditation Council for Graduate Medical Education Competency. *Arch Surg.* 2011; 146(8): 916–921.
30 Riess, H., Kelley, J.M., Bailey, R., Konowitz, P.M., Gray, S.T. Improving empathy and relational skills in otolaryngology residents – a pilot study. *Otolaryngol Head Neck Surg.* 2011; 144(1): 120–122.
31 Von Gunten, C.F., Twaddle, M., Preodor, M., et al. Evidence of improved knowledge and skills after an elective rotation in a hospice and palliative care program for internal medicine residents. *Am J Hosp Palliat Care.* 2005; 22: 195–203.
32 Bonnema, R.A., Gosman, G.G., Arnold, R.M. Teaching error disclosure to residents: a curricular innovation and pilot study. *Journal of Graduate Medical Education.* 2009; 1(1): 114–118.
33 Park, I., Gupta, A., Mandani, K., Haubner, L., Peckler, B. Breaking bad news education for emergency medicine residents: a novel training module using simulation with the SPIKES protocol. *J Emerg Trauma Shock.* 2010; 3: 385–388.
34 Kokotailo, P.K., Langhough, R., Neary, E.J., Matson, S.C., Fleming, M.F. Improving pediatric residents' alcohol and other drug use clinical skills: use of an experiential curriculum. *Pediatrics.* 1995; 96: 99–104.
35 Rosen, R. et al. Sexual communication skills in residency training: the Robert Wood Johnson model. *Journal of Sexual Medicine.* 2006; 3(1): 37–46.
36 Furman, C.D., Head, B., Lazor, B., Casper, B., Ritchie, C.S. Evaluation of an educational intervention to encourage advance directive discussions between medicine residents and patients. *J Palliat Med.* 2006 Aug; 9(4): 964–967.
37 Wolraich, M., Albanese, M., Reiter-Thayer, S., Barratt, W. Teaching pediatric residents to provide emotion-laden information. *J Med Educ.* 1981; 56: 438–440.
38 Hart, C.N., Drotar, D., Gori, A., Lewin, L. Enhancing parent–provider communication in ambulatory pediatric practice. *Patient Educ Couns.* 2006; 63: 38–46.
39 Farsad, P., Galliguez, P., Chamberlin, R., Roghmann, K.J. Teaching interviewing skills to pediatric house officers. *Pediatrics.* 1978; 61(3): 384–388.

20

Teaching medical students to become discourse analysts

From conversational transcripts to clinical applications

Mei-hui Tsai, Feng-hwa Lu, and Richard M. Frankel

Introduction

In patient-centered communication (McWhinney 1989; Roter 2002), one of the main goals in outpatient interviews is for doctors to gather a full perspective of patient problems, which leads doctors to propose diagnoses and treatment plans. This process is often hindered by two common communication problems: 'patients with hidden agendas' and 'doctor–patient non-concordance'. The former refers to situations where patients consciously or subconsciously avoid stating the reason for their visit at the beginning of their interaction with the doctor (Barsky 1981; Beckman and Frankel 1984: 692). It has been hypothesized that some patients prefer to postpone voicing their concerns until the end of the encounter. As well, patients may keep their concerns unstated as a 'test' of the clinician's care for them, and look for other help, that is, doctor-shopping (Barsky 1981: 495) if they do not find the current visit helpful. The second case, 'doctor–patient non-concordance', describes a situation where doctors do not always share the same perspective as their patients regarding their principal problem(s) (Freidin et al. 1980; Burack and Carpenter 1983), especially when the problems are psychosocial in nature. This situation also suggests that doctors tend to take the problems initially presented by patients as the principal ones.

To avoid these communication problems, medical educators (Levinson 1987; Billings and Stoeckle 1999) recommend the use of 'open questions', i.e., questions which encourage patients to reveal all the problems they have which include symptoms, pressures, concerns, or expectations. With a full spectrum of concerns, the doctor can identify patients' underlying principal problems and thus make diagnoses and a treatment plan that are more accurate (i.e., evidence-based) and appropriate (i.e., responding to the patients' concern and expectations), both of which contribute to achieving 'patient-centered' outcomes. Unfortunately, this interview skill does not seem to be well practiced, according to two well-cited reports. In their study of 74 doctor–patient interviews, Beckman and Frankel (1984) found that 69 percent of the time (51 out of the 74 encounters), doctors interrupted a patient's problem presentation by directing the interview to a specific topic. In only one of these 51 cases was the patient offered the chance to complete his/her problem presentation. On average, this interruption took place 18 seconds after patients began their problem presentations. The above results are somewhat surprising as patient-centeredness has been urgently called for since the 1950s (Wooden 1958), followed by the biopsychosocial model proposed by Engel (1977) and most recently by the Institute of Medicine report (2001) which identified patient-centered care as one of six dimensions of quality in medical care. The '18th second' interruption point has been so widely cited by academic and popular writers[1] that we would expect this to have led to a change in behavior. Frustratingly, in a larger-scale follow-up study by Marvel et al. (1999), the period before doctors interrupted patients increased only minimally fifteen years later. Among the 264 medical interviews they analyzed, only 28 percent of the patients completed their initial problem presentation. For the other cases, 24.6 percent of the primary problems were unsolicited and 45.5 percent were redirected to other topics. This redirection took place at a mean of 23.1 seconds after patients began problem presentation. The researchers also found that doctors who had fellowship training in communication skills were more likely to allow patients to complete their initial problem presentation (44 percent vs. 22 percent).

Two conclusions can be drawn from the above discussion. First, although health professionals are aware that it is rare for patients to completely present their problems at the beginning of the interview, little improvement in this situation has been achieved. Second, evidence suggests that education can make a difference in doctor communication behavior. Among the items that appear on most checklists for evaluating medical communication and interpersonal skills (Iramaneerat 2007), open questions have been emphasized by many medical educators as an important means of encouraging patients' problem presentation (Levinson 1987; Billings and Stoeckle 1999). An immediate issue to be addressed here is how open questions can be taught to avoid the prevalent phenomena of doctors' early interruption and redirection in order to achieve the goal of patient-centeredness.

In 2006, two researchers based at National Cheng Kung University ('NCKU' hereafter), Taiwan, started a new communication course for fourth-year medical students, 'Outpatient Communication and Interview Skills'. This course was 'new' in two senses. As biomedical science is the primary focus of course work in most medical schools in Taiwan, there is only one 36-hour required communication course offered at NCKU. While this current course offers an additional elective option, it also features the integration of specialties from two fields, an MD in Family Medicine and a PhD in linguistics, and utilizes research-informed content from discourse analysis (e.g., Tsai 2006) and its community-based conversation data as teaching material.

In this 36-hour course of 18 weeks, a three-hour training session is devoted to improve students' use of open questions. The significant effects of this approach, as evident from students' contrastive performance in their two videotaped interviews with a standardized patient before and after the training session, are documented elsewhere (Tsai et al. 2013). Here, we introduce this innovative pedagogy by demonstrating: (1) how community-based research findings from discourse analysis can be integrated in teaching communication skills of medical students in Taiwan; (2) how conversational transcripts facilitate a bottom-up teaching approach; and (3) how this bottom-up approach transforms students from discourse analysts to professional medical communicators.

The need for a community-based clinical communication course

The term 'community-based' communication course refers to the design of teaching materials that closely reflect the authentic professional workplace settings where learners will practice in the future. For decades, Western medicine has been the mainstream practice in Taiwan. As is true in most Western societies, training and practice start with a focus on the scientific and biomedical aspect of disease and the training of doctors' communication skills is generally neglected in the formal curriculum. The adoption of Western medicine in Taiwan is 'alien' for most elderly people, the biggest patient population, in two senses. A majority of the textbooks used in medical schools are from English-based publishers (e.g., Wiener et al. 2001; Bickley and Szilagyi 2003; Billings and Stoeckle 1999). Practically, every Taiwanese medical resident or intern carries the portable *Pocket Medicine* (Sabatine 2007) with them on their hospital rounds. The classroom language is mainly Mandarin, the official language of Taiwan. These two foci pose a language barrier, as most of the elderly population – especially those aged 70 or older – are monolingual and speak the local dialect Southern Min, which is seldom used by the younger generation.

The lack of formal curriculum and community-based Chinese textbooks in clinical communication hinders cross-generation interaction between young doctors and elderly patients. To start a history-taking with the literal Taiwanese translation *'Guo kin-a-jit e-tang wi-li tso siann-mi?'* or *'Li hi-bang gun kin-a-tsit an-tsuann ka li pang-bang?'* for the English expressions 'What can I do for you today?' and 'How do you hope I might help you today?' may sound awkward for some elderly patients who are not used to the mindset of seeing healthcare interaction as a customer service encounter. To encourage patients' reflective thinking with *'Li kam-kak tsia-e bun-te si siann-mi guan-in tso-sing-e'* ('What do you think is the cause of your problems?') may not be effective for elderly patients who tend to see doctors as all-knowing and able to identify causes of health problems. The use of teaching material based on first-hand practical experience (e.g., from senior doctors) or studies that integrate social, cultural, and professional aspects of interactional norms (e.g., ethnography of communication, Hymes 1964) can better facilitate students' learning of communicative competence for healthcare purposes.

The study of medical discourse and transcripts

In teaching communication skills to medical students, the use of integrated approaches with scholars from fields such as discourse analysis is becoming popular (Frankel and Beckman 1993; Hodges et al. 2008; Roberts and Sarangi 2005). The study of medical discourse uses detailed transcripts of audio or videotaped medical conversations. Such transcripts, either in a script style (e.g., Excerpt 1) or column style (Excerpt 2), represent written versions of the doctor–patient conversation, displaying conversational features such as silences, repetitions, word searches, interruptions, and the prior or post-context of a current utterance. The transcript is thus a technical representation of the spoken data. Based on linguistic evidence, medical discourse analysts examine how healthcare providers achieve their daily professional tasks by talking to patients, and how the nature of such an institutionalized conversation is different from everyday talk (ten Have 1989).

The findings from these studies offer insights into potential sources of or solutions to irregular or difficult communication (Mishler 1984: 64–65). For example, Maynard (1993) studied pediatricians' conversational strategies in delivering the diagnosis of developmental disabilities to a child's parents. The author found that the use of a circuitous conversational strategy, the 'perspective-display series', helped establish a doctor–parent agreement in their perception regarding the child's abnormal status and made the physician's subsequent diagnosis and treatment plan relevant and legitimate.

In summary, one of the ultimate goals of discourse analysis of professional communication lies in applying its findings, grounded in meticulous linguistic analysis of data collected from the workplace, to improve the professional's communicative competence in managing daily routine and difficult communication.

A bottom-up teaching approach

Among the various teaching approaches, social constructivism stands out for its philosophy of student-centered and collaborative learning situated in social contexts (Vygotsky and Cole 1978; Davis et al. 1974). In this research, we use the term 'bottom-up approach', in contrast to a top-down or teacher-centered one, to encapsulate the philosophy of social constructivism wherein knowledge is dynamically and interactively constructed by students themselves, that is, students as the knowledge 'constructors' and teachers the 'facilitators' of this construction process. The teachers' tasks include designing materials and activities, engaging students, and confirming or modifying the knowledge constructed by students during the activities. In contrast to teachers' monologues in traditional lectures, class activities include teacher–student dialogues, group discussions, observations and analysis, role plays, and so on. The material includes any observable forms such as video clips, conversation transcripts, and written descriptions of communicative events.

The process of knowledge construction in a bottom-up approach starts with students' analytical, reflective, and critical thinking in response to the material presented to them. In this process, students reflect on their personal background and previous knowledge, organize their thoughts, and formulate their point of view on the current topic at hand. This process relies on what the students find to be meaningful – the essential ingredient in successful learning (Yelon 1996).

Open questions in the medical interview

This section describes how community-based data collection and research findings from discourse analysis can be used in teaching Taiwanese medical students' use of open questions. To gain a better understanding of what counts as open questions in the medical interview context, Tsai (2006) conducted a linguistic analysis of open questions, including defining 'open', and identifying three categories and six sentential forms of open questions. This analysis was based on two sources: a literature review (Tsai 2006: 37–62) of existing frameworks describing open questions, including the widely cited coding categories by RIAS,[2] and 30 first encounters between elderly patients (average age of 75) and nine family medicine physicians. The data were collected in a teaching hospital in southern Taiwan and the main language used in the interaction was the local dialect Southern Min (Tsai 2006: 7–10; cf. Table 20.1 and Excerpt 2). The main findings of Tsai (2006) include the following:

1 Two core senses of open questions 'non-directive/indefinite' and 'revealing/ventilating' (2006: 38).
2 Three categories of open questions: general, biomedical, and psychosocial (2006: 39–41; see Table 20.1).

3 Six sentential forms of general and biomedical open questions (2006: 99–116; see Table 20.2). One important note from Tsai (2006: 115–132) is that the form of open questions is not confined to 'Wh-questions'. Some yes–no questions (e.g., 'do you have any other problems'), statements (e.g., 'tell me' or 'let me hear'), and short phrases ('any other' and 'and') also achieve the speech act of open question in appropriate contexts.

The above principles are based on frameworks by international scholars and are also enriched by attention to local context. The data serve as authentic teaching materials in three ways. First, the interaction is situated in the local workplace and conducted in the community language that students will practice in the future. The written transcripts or audio dialogues serve as additional language learning material for most students whose command of the local language is generally limited. Third, the word-by-word representation of spontaneous verbal interaction, in contrast to planned dialogues, and the research-informed typical conversational patterns give students a sense of the reality of what they will encounter in future professional practice (e.g., monolingual and illiterate elderly patients). Teaching materials that include these features are community-based and thus more salient compared to interview textbooks based on a foreign language and culture.

Table 20.1 Three categories of open question*

General open questions: range covers all possible patient problems	1-1 What problems bring you here today? *Kin-a lai si siann-mih mun-te?* 1-2 Why are you here today? *Kin-a lai si an-tsuann?* 1-3 Do you have any other problems? *Kam ko-u ki-tha-e mun-te?*
Biomedical open questions: range covers all possible biological or physical states	2-1 What symptoms do you have? *Li u siann-mih tsing-thau?* 2-2 What is your discomfort? *Li u siann-mih bo-song-khuai?* 2-3 What physical problems do you have? *Li u sann-mih moo-penn?*
Psychosocial open questions: range covers the patient's psychological or social problems, e.g., lifestyle, significant social events, concerns, expectations and desire	3-1 How do you hope I might help you today? *Li hi-bang gun kin-a-tsit an-tsuann ka li pang-bang?* 3-2 What changes have there been in your life recently? *Tsue-kin sing-ua kam u sann-mih pen-hua?* 3-3 Is there anything bothering you recently? *Tsue-kin kam-u te huan-lo sann-mih tai-tsi?* 3-4 This sleeping problem is quite annoying, right? *Tse bo-ho-khun e bun-te hoo li tsiok huan-lo honn?* 3-5 Is there any reason that you live by yourself? *Kam-u sann-mih guan-in. kak-ki tsit-le tua?*

Source: Revised from Tsai (2006: 40–2).

Note

* Most of the examples cited here are translations of Southern Min data in which the distinction between 'general' vs. 'biomedical' is clear in Chinese, but may not have an appropriate English equivalent. To maintain the distinction, some of the English translations may sound inauthentic for native speakers.

Table 20.2 Six forms of open questions

Forms	*Examples*
1.Wh-Q	1-1 What brings you here today? [general] 1-2 How are you suffering from pains/discomfort? [biomedical] 1-3 What pains/discomfort do you have? [biomedical]
2.Yes–no Q	2-1 Is there anything I can do for you today? [general] 2-2 Do you have any other problem? [general] 2-3 You have some problems? [general]
3.Indefinite enumeration	3-1 Do you have anything like hypertension, diabetes? [biomedical] 3-2 Do you have hypertension, diabetes, or anything like that? [biomedical]
4.Sentential fragment ('any other')	4-1 Any other problems? [general] 4-2 Anything else? [general] 4-3 What else? [general]
5.Statement ('tell me')	5-1 Tell me all the problems you have. [general] 5-2 Let me hear all the symptoms you have. [biomedical]
6.Continuer marker ('and')	6-1 And? [general] 6-2 Then? [general]

Source: Revised from Tsai (2006: 99–100).

Course design: teaching goals and plan

Following Miller's (1990) framework for assessing health professional's clinical skills/competence/performance (cf. Table 20.3), we set up four goals for an 18-week elective course. The second column in Table 20.3 displays the four levels of students' learning 'open questions': knowledge, competence, performance, and action.

The three-hour session on open questions is scheduled during weeks 9 and 10. The evaluation of this session is based on students' use of open questions in weeks 4 and 14, that is, before and after the teaching (cf. Tsai et al. 2013 for the teaching effects of this session). Table 20.4 provides details of the three-hour teaching plan for the unit 'open questions', including class activities, teaching material, the specific goals of each activity, and the corresponding general goals stated in Table 20.3.

Table 20.3 Learning goals

KNOW (Knowledge)	Students KNOW WHY open questions are important at the beginning of the information gathering stage and KNOW WHAT open questions are.
KNOW HOW (Competence)	Students KNOW HOW to use open questions.
SHOW HOW (Performance)	Students SHOW HOW open questions are used by themselves, fellow students, and visiting staff.
DOES (Action)	Students USE open questions in their interview with standardized patients.

Source: Based on Miller (1990: S63).

Table 20.4 Teaching plan – open questions

Time	*Activities*	*Goals*
35:00	1. STs* watch a clip from the film *Erin Brockovich** and respond to the following questions: 1a. What were the five pieces of information presented by the Robinson couple and in what sequence? 1b. Among the five pieces, which is the most important but difficult to bring up? 2. STs analyze the dialogue transcript (Excerpt 1) and respond to the following questions: 2a. What are the conversational clues to signal people's hesitation in bringing up their main concerns? 2b. How does this interaction resemble similar problems in doctor–patient communication?	STs KNOW WHAT the importance of open questions is at the beginning of the information-gathering stage. 1. People tend to delay their most important concern until the end of an interaction. The first presented problem may thus not always be the primary one. 2a. Speakers' hesitation in bringing up their primary concerns is evidenced by the fact that such information tends to be introduced later by others and preceded by pauses or hedges (lines 15–18 in Excerpt 1). 2b. Patients with hidden agendas, i.e., stating their main concern later (lines 22–24 in Excerpt 1)
25:00	3. TR* shows Figure 20.1 and explains the macro versus micro patterns of gathering information and asks: 3a. Which way do they consider better to get a full range of patient problems at the beginning of the interaction? 3b. What kind of questions can they try? What are some examples?	STs KNOW WHAT the functions of open questions are. 3a. A macro pattern helps doctors to get an overall picture of all problems the patient has at the beginning of the interview and helps doctors decide what the principle problems are. 3b. Open questions, such as 'What can I do for you today?'
20:00	4. TR gives three groups of open questions from Table 20.1 and asks: 4a. How are the three categories of questions different from each other? 4b. How can they be used for different purposes?	STs KNOWS HOW: 4a. Open questions have different scopes and functions and some are more open than others. 4b. General open questions are more useful than biomedical and psychosocial questions in gathering a full range of patient problems.
20:00	5. TR provides transcripts of medical interviews by senior doctors (Excerpt 2) and asks: 5a. Which utterances work as open questions? 5b. How are they used in different contexts? 5c. How many pieces of patient problems (in Excerpt 2) are solicited by the doctor's use of open questions?	5. STs SHOW HOW to make and use open questions, and HOW they help solicit all possible patient problems. 5a. Open questions can come in different sentential forms (cf. Table 20.2). 5b. Open questions in a full form tend to occur earlier in an interview (e.g., 'What brings you here today?') and those in shorter form later (e.g., 'Anything else?' 'And?'). 5c. The more open questions doctors used, the more likely they will get a full picture of patient problems.
20:00	6. TR gives more examples of open questions (Table 20.2) and asks STs to analyze how they work differently.	6. Reinforce STs' KNOWledge of open questions.
30:00	7. TR provides transcripts of students' interviews with standardized patients videotaped in week 4 and asks: 7a. How many open questions are used and what are they? 7b. How much information is collected when open questions are used versus not used?	7. Students KNOW HOW and SHOW HOW they are aware of the following common problem that most beginners have experienced – starting the information-seeking stage with a micro pattern (cf. Figure 20.1).

Time	*Activities*	*Goals*
30:00	8. Two STs play the roles of the doctor and patient and start the information-seeking stage. One student observes the interview and takes note of instances of open questions used by the doctor.	8. STs SHOW how open questions are used by others and then they USE open questions in their own interviews.

Notes

***ST = Student; *TR = Teacher**

**Erin Brockovich* (2000; dir. Steven Soderbergh) depicts how an untrained legal assistant (Erin Brockovich) single-handedly helped residents of a California community in suing a power company that was responsible for water pollution that caused illness among the residents. In this clip (00:53:40–00:55:26), the Robinson couple visit Erin and talk about the unusual things they have experienced and their concerns.

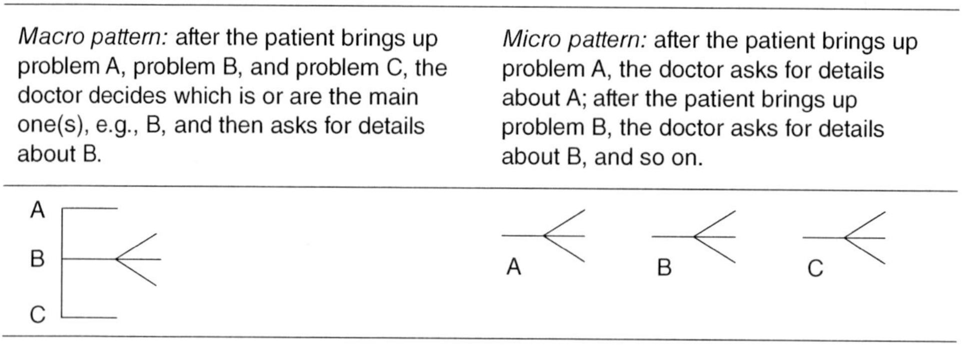

Figure 20.1 Macro vs. micro patterns in soliciting patient problems

Teaching materials and approach

In this section, we discuss how conversational transcripts from authentic doctor–patient interviews and movie dialogues are used as the main teaching material to cultivate learners' sensitivity to language use, and how the bottom-up teaching approach transforms students from discourse analysts to professional medical interviewers.

Excerpt 1: Erin Brockovich (00:53:40–00:55:26)[3]

1	Wife:	Excuse me. Are you Erin Brockovich?
2	Erin:	Yeah.
3	Husband:	I'm Tom Robinson. This is my wife Mandy.
4	Erin:	Hi.
5	Husband:	We used to live across the street from the Jensens. I think you know Donna.
6	Erin:	Yeah.
7	Husband:	Um … PG&E bought our house last year. (Showing pictures of chickens) The vets said they had a bunch of tumors and stuff. You can see they couldn't really walk.
8	Erin:	How many were born like this?
9	Husband:	Uhh … twelve or thirteen or so.

	10	Wife:	Yeah. When Donna told us about you and what you told her about the chromium. We figured that might have something to do with this too.
	11	Erin:	Yeah. It might … I'm really … may I keep this?
	12	Husband:	Yeah.
	13	Erin:	Okay, great. Thank you so much. I really appreciate it.
	14	Wife:	Umm … uh, there's something else too.
	15		(pauses for 2 seconds)
	16	Erin:	What?
→	17	Husband:	Um.. t's:::um … um..well..um..Mandy here has had five miscarriages…
→	18		(pauses for 3 seconds)
	19	Erin:	I'm so sorry.
	20	Wife:	I figured it was something I did … uh … like when I smoked marijuana, maybe …
	21	Husband:	(The wife turns to the husband) hh::
→	22	Wife:	or took birth control pills. But umm then Donna said that you thought that this chromium might be to blame for her problems. So I figured …
→	23		(pauses for 4 seconds)
→	24	Wife:	Maybe it wasn't just me.

Excerpt 2: G174B3J1G100000049
Mr. Ko (74M, accompanied by his son); Dr. Ong (31M, third-year resident)

Line	*Time*	*Doctor (31-year-old, male, third-year resident)*	*Patient (74-year-old, male)*
1.	00:00		(the patient was seated, the son just entered the room)
2.	00:03	is he your son? *I si lin hau-senn o?*	
3.	00:04		right, *tioh,*
4.	00:05	ok:, …umm::, wish you good, I'm Dr. Ong. *honn:, ...enn::,li-ho, gua si W i-su,*	
→5.	00:08	what problems bring you here today::? *kin-a-jit lai, u siann-mih bun-te leh?*	

Line	*Time*	*Doctor (31-year-old, male, third-year resident)*	*Patient (74-year-old, male)*
6.	00:11		/? .. ? / main problem is the…the hand trembles, it feels weak, /? .. ?/ */?..?/tsu-iau si khuann tsit-e..tshiu e-tshuah, bo-lat, /? .. ?/*
7.	00:15	.. your hand trembles?= *.. tshiu e-tshuah hio?=*	
8.	00:16		=yeah yeah,= *=tioh tioh,=*
9.	00:17	=is it one hand or both hands which are trembling? *=kan-tann tsit-ki tshiu nia iah-si nng-ki tshiu?*	
10.	00:18		=both hands, both hands, /this hand/.. is /better/, *=nng-ki tshiu, nng-ki tshiu,/tsit-tshiu/.u khah./ho tsit-kua/,*
11.	00:21	I see:: = *honn::*	
12.	00:22		=umm, this joint yeah, … this joint.. does not bend, *=enn, tsit-e kuan-tsat honn, ... tse kuan-tsat ..uan be loh-khi,*
13.	00:27	.. what? .. your finger joints do not bend, *.. hann? ..uan be loh-khi,*	
14.	00:28		they don't bend, *uan be loh-khi,*
→15.	00:30	= if you have any other problems, tell me all about them *=a na u ki-tha-e bun-te tso li kong*	
16.	00:31		.. as for other problems, I don't have any, *.. ki-tha-e long bo siann-mih bun-te,*
17.	00:32	. .I see:, about your trembling hands, did you .. = *.. hoonn:, tshiu e tshuah u .. =*	

Line	*Time*	*Doctor (31-year-old, male, third-year resident)*	*Patient (74-year-old, male)*
18.	00:35		= if I were to mention anything else, that would be .. when I urinate, it does not function normally, /??/, *=tioh-si .. sio-pian bo tsing-siong, /??/,*
19.	00:37	how did it function abnormally? *sio-pian an-tsuann bo tsing-siong hann?*	
20.	00:39		sometimes .. /? . ?/ / (I) feel like peeing/, but sometimes (I) don't, *u-si-a../?.?/ /tsit-tiam-a siunn-beh pang-jio/,u-si-a iu-koh bo,*
21.	00:43	I see:,= *honn;,=*	
22.	00:43		=(I) can't hold my pee, *=jio long kim-be-tiau,*
→23.	00:45	=I see, and? *=an-ne honn, koh-lai leh?*	
24.	00:47		well .. nothing else, *tioh .. ki-tha long-bo siann-mih,*
25.	00:49	have you ever been treated anywhere? *ah li u ti to-ui khuann-kue hann?*	

Transcripts as teaching materials

The transcripts used in this course come from three sources. One-third are from interviews between students and a standardized patient, conducted before and after the training, and the interviews are partially transcribed by the students themselves. Two-thirds represent interactions between visiting staff or residents of family medicine with their first-visit elderly patients collected in Tsai's study (e.g., 2006). Occasionally, scripted dialogues from feature films or videos for teaching communication skills are used when appropriate materials are unavailable from our collection.

The use of transcripts facilitates the bottom-up teaching of interview skills in the following way: compared to video viewing, the use of transcripts is easy to operate and provides an easy-to-access context of verbal interaction. In column style, transcripts present a holistic picture of individual speakers' verbal participation. Line numbers help in locating targeted utterances. A transcript hardcopy in hand provides the pre- and post-contexts of the targeted utterances under analysis, such as the patient's next-turn response to the doctor's use of a specific open versus closed-ended question. In contrast, the use of video material is more cognitively demanding on both students and teachers, because it operates linearly and requires extra time for repeated back and forth replay. Furthermore, students may concentrate better on the single signal, that is, the written words on the transcripts, in contrast to the audio and video signals from video clips.

Second, word-by-word details, such as hesitations, word searches, and overlapping, facilitate micro observations and cultivating students' sensibility with regard to fine and delicate language use. In our teaching of the prevalent pattern of patients with hidden agendas and conversational signs of this pattern (activities 1 and 2 in Table 20.4), we asked students to identify: (1a) the five pieces of information presented by the Robinson couple and the sequence of their occurrence; and (1b) the piece of information that was the most important but difficult to bring up. With a quick look at the transcript, most students identified the information sequence: chickens with tumors that were unable to walk (line 7), the relationship between the tumor and the toxicant chromium (line 10), the wife's five miscarriages (line 17), the wife's smoking marijuana and taking birth control pills (lines 20–22), and the relationship between the miscarriage and chromium (lines 22). Consensus was high (80 percent) regarding the information in either lines 20 or 22 as the most important but difficult to bring up.

We then asked students: (2a) to identify the conversational clues to signal hesitation in bringing up main concerns, and (2b) to identify how the sequence from the film resembles similar problems in doctor–patient communication. This activity was designed to guide students to be sensitive to: (A) discursive signs of raising difficult topics, e.g., the husband speaking on his wife's behalf (line 17) and the couple's silences and hesitations (lines 15, 17, and 18); and (B) the fact that people often delay their important concerns until the end of an interaction, that is, patients with hidden agendas.

Third, transcripts also helped sharpen medical students' analytical thinking in exploring the 'semantic', 'syntactic', and 'pragmatic' aspects of language use. For example, in activities 4 and 5, students discuss how three groups of questions randomly selected from Table 20.1 are different from each other (4a), which utterances from Excerpt 2 work as open questions (5a), how they are used in different contexts (5b), and how many patient problems are solicited by each (5c). When students see the differences among general, biomedical, and psychosocial open questions, they become aware of the concept of 'semantic scope'. Their awareness of 'syntactic form' is also heightened when students identify that a yes–no question (e.g., 'do you have any other problems?'), a statement (e.g., 'if you have any other problems, tell me all about them' in line 15), or a short phrase (e.g., 'and?' in line 23), all achieve the same function as the most typical 'wh-interrogative' (e.g., 'what problems bring you here today?' in line 5). Students learn to appreciate the pragmatic aspect of language choice when they are shown that doctors' increased use of open questions improves the likelihood that they will get a full picture of the patient's problems, as patients are not always aware of or may neglect other health issues unless explicitly encouraged. Mr. Ko, for example, did not think of any other problem ('as for other problems, I don't have any' line 16) when Dr. Ong said, 'if you have any other problems, tell me all about them' (line 15). This probe did prompt him to mention his urine problem later in line 18 ('if I were to mention anything else, that would be ... when I urinate, it does not function normally'). With the use of three open questions (lines 5, 15, 23) and one open response ('I see' in line 11, cf. Beckman and Frankel 1984: 694), Dr. Ong collected three patient problems by the 47th second of the interview (i.e., hand trembling, joints that fail to bend, urine problem) and was assured that the patient did not have any other issues beyond these (line 24).

A fourth function of using transcripts is that they facilitate students' reflective assessment of their interview skills. The process of students' transcribing and analyzing their interview with patients (i.e., activity 7), provides an opportunity to reflect on verbal behavior. For example, some students commented on their rude interruption of the patient's problem presentation by changing the topic they wished to explore and their overuse of discourse markers such as *henn* or *hio* 'well, umm', which they saw as signs of nervousness or lack of confidence.

An alternative source of transcripts for teaching communication skills is feature films or videos. Movie clips are widely used in teaching the bio-psycho-social-spiritual aspects of health care (Alexander et al. 2007). Although many micro features of spontaneous conversations, such as word search and repetitions, may not be present in such planned forms, discursive mechanisms such as word choices, silences, and relevant contexts are nevertheless efficiently preserved. Such transcripts are especially useful for teaching difficult communication, for example, a bad news delivery or end-of-life communication (DiBartolo and Seldomridge 2009), since collecting spontaneous examples of such events might be difficult and pose ethical dilemmas (Tsai forthcoming). The powerful emotional stress and dramatic tension depicted in movies also serve as efficient teaching material to engage students in discussing the communication issues that are involved.

Transformation from discourse analysts to professional medical interviewers

Our use of conversational transcripts to implement a bottom-up approach is described in the following sequence with the four learning goals stated in Table 20.3. The process starts with students reviewing the transcripts, formulating communication principles or strategies that will then be confirmed or modified by the teacher, and practicing these skills. Our ultimate goal is to transform students from 'discourse analysts' to 'professional medical interviewers'.

1 KNOW WHY: Students observe transcripts to experience and locate existing communication difficulties, and thus appreciate the importance of using open questions (e.g., activities 1–3, Table 20.4).
2 KNOW HOW: Students analyze transcripts of medical interviews of visiting staff or residents, identify scopes and forms of open questions, and formulate patterns in using open questions; thus, students connect the forms of open questions with the functions that they achieve (e.g., activities 4, 5, 6).
3 KNOW HOW and SHOW HOW: Students examine transcripts of their interviews with a standardized patient conducted in Week 4, reflect on and evaluate their use of open questions (e.g., activity 7).
4 DOES: Students practice the use of open questions (e.g., activity 8).

Given the student-centeredness of a bottom-up approach, knowledge of open questions is constructed via students' analytical, reflective, and critical thinking in response to the material presented to them, which includes transcripts of medical interviews conducted by students or senior doctors. The process is *analytical* in the sense that it requires students to organize their thoughts on the conversational data, *reflective* in that it relies on students' personal background and previous knowledge about communication, and *critical* in that it encourages students to come up with a meaningful point of view on or a manageable solution to the communication issues at hand, for example, how to avoid doctor–patient non-concordance. The knowledge of the three semantic categories, six sentence forms, and pragmatic functions of open questions constructed in this way is thus personalized, practical, substantive, and durable.

In this knowledge construction process, students are trained to be discourse analysts. During each activity, the teacher facilitates this process, and confirms or modifies the knowledge constructed by the students. The above process in teaching open questions is therefore bottom-up – from students to teachers.

As with most student-centered approaches, the primary drawback of the bottom-up approach is that it is time-consuming and thus less applicable to content-based courses. This problem is balanced by the following higher principles and goals of this current course. Cultivation of communication skills relies more on practice than knowledge and students' sense of achievement in constructing knowledge on their own overrides the amount of knowledge that they generate. The process of how to independently generate knowledge benefits learners more than the actual amount of knowledge does, since learning is a lifelong endeavor and knowledge is constantly changing.

While the unique feature of word-by-word details makes discourse transcripts a valuable pedagogical tool, it may also make it less practical in two ways. First, the transcribing process is cumbersome and time-consuming and the exhaustive details may seem extravagant for some, especially for medical students. With some editing, details irrelevant to the teaching goals can be eliminated. The time-consuming nature of transcribing spoken conversation can be reduced by advanced sound-recognition technology. The current report, however, is meant to demonstrate how discourse researchers can turn the transcripts they have at their disposal into valuable pedagogical materials for teaching professional communication.

Does this teaching approach and content help to make students professional communicators in terms of their use of open questions? The following gives a simplified account of the impact of this training (cf. Tsai et al. 2013).

Our evaluation is based on the 27 students' performances in their two videotaped interviews with a standardized patient before and after this three-hour training session. We identified all instances of the three open question types used during each interview before and after the teaching, coded the question types (open questions versus elaborating questions) used by the doctor as the first, second, and third questions in the information-seeking sequence, and tested their occurrence statistically. The results show significant changes in the students' performance in the following ways:

1 The contrast between a total of 94 occurrences of open question before the training and 197 after suggests that after the training students are more aware of the use of open questions and more willing to use them (i.e., the 'action' part, Table 20.3).
2 The use of general and psychosocial open questions (e.g., 'Do you have any other problems?' and 'Is there anything bothering you recently?') significantly increased after the training ($p < 0.05$).
3 The biased interview pattern of the micro approach (cf. Figure 20.1) observed before the training, which assumed that patients came for biomedical problems and that they mentioned their primary concern first – was replaced after the training by a macro approach that invited patients to bring up all possible problems. Evidence for this change includes the following two patterns:

   a There was a significant preference ($p < 0.05$) for using a general open question to a biomedical open question to start the information-seeking stage after the training (e.g., 'What problems bring you here today?' versus 'What symptoms do you have today?')

b After the training, there is a significant decrease ($p < 0.05$) in the use of elaborating questions in the second and third question positions (e.g., 'How long did this headache last?') that targeted details of an already mentioned problem. Such usage discourages patients from bringing up all possible problems early in the interaction.

Conclusion

To improve medical students' communication skills, an innovative pedagogical design combining expertise from medical education and discourse analysis was developed. Among the communication skills used in outpatient interviews, the use of open questions is recommended to solicit a full spectrum of a patient's problems and address two prevalent communication issues: patients with hidden agendas and doctor–patient non-concordance. The teaching approach and content of this innovation feature a bottom-up approach that engages students as the knowledge constructors of open questions and integrates community-based conversational transcripts and research-informed discourse findings as the primary teaching modalities. The teaching content is research-informed by discourse studies that combine both international and local professionals' communicative norms about the use of open questions. The use of authentic data of doctor–patient interviews, collected in the local workplace and conducted in the local dialect, gives students a sense of the reality of their future professional practice. Such teaching content draws a contrast to those adopted by most communication courses at medical schools in Taiwan, which rely on textbooks tailored to Western society and culture.

The classroom activities consisting of analyzing conversational transcripts lead to the four teaching goals for students: *knowing what* the importance of open questions is, *showing what* open questions are, *showing how* to use them, and *practicing* their use. The use of word-by-word transcripts also helped facilitate the bottom-up teaching process by providing easy-to-access contexts of verbal interaction, facilitating micro analytical observations of conversational features, cultivating students' sensitivity to language use, and encouraging students' reflective assessment of their interview skills through the analysis of transcripts from their own encounters. This three-hour training session heightened students' awareness and sensitivity to the use of open questions and also helped change their behavior, that is, transforming them from discourse analysts to professional medical communicators.

This report demonstrates how training in discourse analysis, data collection, and evidence from discourse research can be applied to the teaching of medical students' interview skills. This approach adds to the important trend in medical education of integrating academic work with professional communication practice, that is, language for a specific purpose (Bhatia 2012). Although the use of transcripts is beneficial in many ways, the task of transcribing itself and the time needed to appreciate the fine points of language use in medical encounters by 'listening to one's self perform' remains a challenge for future studies.

Acknowledgments

The researchers are indebted to the support provided by the National Science Council and the Ministry of Education in Taiwan. They are also grateful for the help given by Andy Noonan, an English Language Fellow at National Cheng Kung University, for his expertise in teaching.

Related topics

Open questions; doctor–patient communication; medical education; bottom-up teaching approach; discourse transcripts.

Notes

1 By December 2011, the '18th second' interruption point had at least 374 citations (cf. the ISI Web of Knowledge) and by popular writers such as Pink (2005: 110).
2 RIAS: Roter Interaction Analysis System. http://www.riasworks.com
3 The dialogue in Excerpt 1 is extracted from the website http://www.imsdb.com/scripts/Erin-Brockovich.html and modified by the details of the dialogue from the DVD section 00:53:40 to 00:55:26 of *Erin Brockovich*, published by the Universal Studios, Universal City, California, and distributed by the agent Deltamac (Taiwan) Co., Ltd. in 2000.

Further reading

Maynard, D.W. (1993) 'The perspective-display series and the delivery and receipt of diagnostic news', in D. Boden and D. Zimmerman (eds) *Talk and Social Structure*, Berkeley, CA: University of California Press. (Maynard demonstrated how pediatricians' use of the circuitous conversational strategy 'the 'perspective-display series' helped establish a doctor–parent agreement in their perception regarding the child's abnormal status and made the physician's subsequent diagnosis and treatment plan relevant and legitimate.)

Roberts, C. and Sarangi, S. (2005) 'Theme-oriented discourse analysis of medical encounters', *Medical Education,* 39: 632–640. (Via the approach of theme-oriented discourse analysis, this paper demonstrated how language constructs medical professionals' daily practice.)

Tsai, M.H. (2006) *Opening Hearts and Minds: A Linguistic Framework for Analyzing Open Questions in Doctor–patient Communication,* Taipei, Taiwan: The Crane Publishing Company. (This book described what 'open questions' are in the context of medical interviews, including their sentential forms and pragmatic functions.)

References

Alexander, M., Pavlov, A., and Lenahan, P. (2007) 'Lights, camera, action: using film to teach the ACGME competencies', *Family Medicine,* 39: 20–23.

Barsky, A.J. (1981) 'Hidden reasons some patients visit doctors', *Annals of Internal Medicine*, 94: 492–498.

Beckman, H.B. and Frankel, R.M. (1984) 'The effect of physician behavior on the collection of data', *Annals of Internal Medicine*, 101: 692–696.

Bhatia, V. (2012) 'Disciplinary and professional boundaries in LSP: issues, challenges and insights', paper presented at the Third Conference of the Asia-Pacific LSP and Professional Communication Association: Crossing Boundaries: Working and Communicating in the Asia Pacific Region, the Marshall School of Business at USC, March.

Bickley, L.S. and Szilagyi, P.G. (2003) *Bates' Guide to Physical Examination and History Taking,* Philadelphia, PA: Lippincott Williams & Wilkins.

Billings, J.A. and Stoeckle, J.D. (1999) *The Clinical Encounter: A Guide to the Medical Interview and Case Presentation,* St. Louis, MO: Mosby.

Burack, R.C. and Carpenter, R.R. (1983) 'The predictive value of the presenting complaint', *Journal of Family Practice,* 16: 749–754.

Davis, R.H., Alexander, L.T., and Yelon, S.L. (1974) *Learning System Design: An Approach to the Improvement of Instruction,* New York: McGraw-Hill.

DiBartolo, M.C. and Seldomridge, L.A. (2009) 'Cinemeducation: teaching end-of-life issues using feature films', *Journal of Gerontological Nursing,* 35: 30–36.

Engel, G. L. (1977) 'The need for a new medical model: a challenge for biomedicine', *Science,* 196: 129–136.

Frankel, R.M. and Beckman, H.B. (1993) 'Teaching communication skills to medical students and house officers: an integrated approach', in J.M. Clair and R.M. Allman (eds) *Sociomedical Perspectives on Patient Care*, 211–222, Lexington: University Press of Kentucky.

Freidin, R.B., Goldman, L., and Cecil, R.R. (1980) 'Patient–physician concordance in problem identification in the primary care setting', *Annals of Internal Medicine*, 93: 490–495.

Hodges, B.D., Kuper, A., and Reeves, S. (2008) 'Discourse analysis', *British Medical Journal*, 337: 570–572.

Hymes, D, (1964) 'Introduction: toward ethnographies of communication', *American Anthropologist*, 66: 1–34.

Institute of Medicine (2001) 'Crossing the quality chasm: a new health system for the 21st century', Washington, DC: National Academies Press.

Iramaneerat, C. (2007) 'A validity study of a communication skills assessment of medical residents', unpublished thesis, University of Illinois at Chicago.

Levinson, D. (ed.) (1987) *A Guide to the Clinical Interview*, London: W. B. Saunders.

McWhinney, I. (1989) 'The need for a transformed clinical method', in M. Stewart and D. Roter (eds) *Communicating with Medical Patients*, Newbury Park, CA: Sage Publications.

Marvel, M.K., Epstein, R.M., Flowers, K., and Beckman, H.B. (1999) 'Soliciting the patient's agenda: have we improved?' *Journal of the American Medical Association*, 281: 283–287.

Maynard, D.W. (1993) 'The perspective-display series and the delivery and receipt of diagnostic news', in D. Boden and D. Zimmerman (eds) *Talk and Social Structure*, Berkeley, CA: University of California Press.

Miller, G.E. (1990) 'The assessment of clinical skills/competence/performance', *Academic Medicine: Journal of the Association of American Medical Colleges*, 65: S63–67.

Mishler, E.G. (1984) *The Discourse of Medicine: Dialectics of Medical Interviews*, Norwood, NJ: Ablex Publishing.

Pink, D.H. (2005) *A Whole New Mind: Moving from the Information Age to the Conceptual Age*, New York: Riverhead Books.

Roberts, C. and Sarangi, S. (2005) 'Theme-oriented discourse analysis of medical encounters', *Medical Education*, 39: 632–640.

Roter, D. (2002) 'Three blind men and an elephant: reflections on meeting the challenges of patient diversity in primary care practice', *Family Medicine*, 34: 390–393.

Sabatine, M.S. (2007) *Pocket Medicine: The Massachusetts General Hospital Handbook of Internal Medicine*, Philadelphia, PA: Lippincott Williams & Wilkins.

ten Have, P. (1989) 'The consultation as a genre', in B. Torode (ed.) *Text and Talk as Social Practice*, Dordrecht: Foris Publications.

Tsai, M.H. (forthcoming) 'Movie dialogues as discourse data in the study of forecasting mechanism in medical bad news delivery', *Communication & Medicine*.

Tsai, M.H. (2006) *Opening Hearts and Minds: A Linguistic Framework for Analyzing Open Questions in Doctor–patient Communication*, Taipei, Taiwan: The Crane Publishing Company.

Tsai, M.H., Lu, F.-H., and Frankel, R.M. (2013) 'Learning to listen: effects of using conversational transcripts to help medical students improve their use of open questions in soliciting patient problems', *Patient Education and Counseling*, 93(1): 48–55.

Vygotsky, L.S. and Cole. M. (1978) *Mind in Society: The Development of Higher Psychological Processes*, Cambridge, MA: Harvard University Press.

Wiener, C.M., Kasper, D.L., Braunwald, E., Hauser, S., Longo, D., Jameson, J.L., and Fauci, A.S. (2001) *Harrison's Principles of Internal Medicine*, New York: McGraw-Hill.

Wooden, H.E. (1958) 'Patient-centered cardiac care', *Hospital Progress*, 39: 80–82.

Yelon, S.L. (1996) *Powerful Principles of Instruction*, White Plains, NY: Longman.

21

Exploring communicative interactions between visitors and assisted-living residents with dementia

Boyd Davis, Margaret Maclagan, and Dena Shenk

Introduction

Although deaths from Alzheimer's disease between 2000 and 2008 rose by 66 percent, according to the Alzheimer's Association (2011), the 5.4 million Americans who have this condition live from four to eight and some as long as 20 years after their diagnosis, with near-astronomical projections for costs of care (Alzheimer's Association 2011). Indeed, Tschanz et al. (2011) project that the current world estimate of 26.6 million cases will grow to 106.2 million by 2050, and caution researchers that a 'significant proportion' will progress slowly through the disease. Care-giving techniques take on new weight given this information: in addition to safety and cleanliness, social interaction and communication play crucial roles in how the person with dementia is positioned (Sabat 2008) and their identity maintained or reframed (Beard et al. 2009). Formal caregivers for persons with dementia in residential settings, the focus of this discussion, are minimally trained at best, particularly in the needs the residents have for social engagement, and, by typically talking over or across their patients or restricting interaction to task instructions, provide instrumental care to the disease, rather than to the person (Davis and Pope 2010). The development of site-evaluated materials and training in dementia-sensitive communication techniques which can be used by family members, volunteer visitors, and formal caregivers is badly needed; to date, it has not been possible to obtain a formal and sustained on-site evaluation of the impact of training materials on staff–resident interaction other than by informal observation and student/trainee anecdotes.

Staff conversation with assisted-living residents is often the primary means residents have for social engagement and social interaction. However, direct observation in nursing homes by a number of researchers, including Allen-Burge et al. (2001: 215), find that 'the major portion of interactions consisted of ineffective communication, facts/opinions, *and questions*' (emphasis ours). Sustaining and managing conversations with persons who have dementia often requires training, which ideally will include staff-level reinforcement and periodic brush-up sessions (Davis and Smith 2011), about language and dementia. Learning to provide sensitive and effective communication has the potential to decrease dementia-related challenging behaviors (Smith and Buckwalter 2005), including agitation (Chenoweth et al. 2009), and to promote lucidity (Normann et al. 2002). Although the extent to which psychosocial interventions such as communications training or cognitive reframing can affect dementia-compromised behaviors is debated, their trend is positive (Vasse et al. 2010; Vernooij-Dassen and Downs 2005; Vernooij-Dassen et al. 2011).

Not all communication, however, is helpful. Questions are particularly chancy, because of their multiple roles in conversation, as noted over 30 years ago by Esther Goody (1978). Steensig and Drew (2008) outline five research traditions for questioning: the grammatical and syntactic perspective; the perspective from interaction, including indirectness and directness and their implication for politeness theory; the perspective on what questions do or perform; the developmental perspective from the standpoint of language acquisition; and an emphasis or theme on the 'constraining' force of questions. All these perspectives are potentially helpful in considering discourse with people with dementia. In this chapter, we focus mainly on an interactional perspective. James (2008: 6) has commented, 'Questions are as poisonous to the well-being of people with dementia as radiation is to the health of newborn babies.' While that may be a bit overstated, no question is entirely innocent. Yet much of the conversation directed toward persons with dementia (PWD) consists of questions, usually in an effort by the unimpaired conversation partner to find a topic which can be sustained for several turns.

This discussion reports on our finding that in the absence of a specific training sequence, both volunteer visitors and nurse aides, the unlicensed support staff who provide roughly 80 percent of the hands-on care, tend to pepper communication with one question after another. Indeed, they often inadvertently choose question types that close down conversations rather than open them up. Unfortunately, we have seldom been legally permitted to record conversations between formal caregivers and residents in assisted living communities in North Carolina: administrators of secure-care and assisted living residences have been strongly concerned about potential ramifications for resident and staff retention. Although we both suggest and offer training programs and materials, we are usually not able to evaluate their ultimate effectiveness by recording interactions between PWD and staff or volunteers subsequent to such training. Instead, we must depend on personal observation without recordings, data gathered by students, or informal reports from staff administrators. In this chapter we therefore focus on studies we have carried out with nurse aide trainees at a local community college who use our materials for training prior to their clinical experience with patient care, and with university students who interact with PWD as part of their courses in gerontology. Insights from the questions asked by students/trainees and the responses these questions receive from PWD can provide guidance for developing and expanding training programs that enhance caregivers' interactions with those they care for. Data collected from student interactions with PWD over the last decade have made us aware of both the prevalence and the problems inherent in question–answer routines, particularly with certain question types.

We will begin by providing general background into conversation with people with dementia and move to a more specific focus on questions and answers. We follow this with a review of three dementia-care conversation techniques which were developed for training materials used with both university students and nurse aide trainees. We then offer highlights of what we have learned so far about question types and the responses they elicit, from two pilot studies on questions. We next look at questions and responses in an ongoing study of conversations with PWD, focusing particularly on 'Maureen Littlejohn', which includes data involving pre-professional graduate students in conversations with her. Finally, we will identify several implications for training and education in dementia care conversation.

Background

Conversing with people with dementia

As Alzheimer's disease progresses, language problems increase. Semantic content diminishes, although pragmatics and syntax are less affected (Ripich and Terrell 1998; Dijkstra et al. 2002). But the 'self' persists. In their discussion of how language is tied into presentation and maintenance of self, Fazio and Mitchell (2009: 40) cite nearly two decades of work by Sabat and by Harré, singly, together, and with other colleagues, to show that 'losses in aspects of selfhood might be traced to dysfunctional social interaction rather than solely the neuropathology of the disease'. Awareness of self and place can be identified in conversations with persons in early-stage dementia and also with persons in later stages who can still communicate orally (Clare 2010). Even as the disease continues, storytelling, poetry, and life writing can be used: these techniques, all of which involve conversational interaction, show 'ongoing and creative efforts to cope with dementia as a manageable disability' (Ryan and Schindel-Martin 2011: 212).

Conversation entails interaction: Smith and Buckwalter (2005) underscore the importance for people with dementia of social interaction which decreases their sensory deprivation and social isolation. They recommend reminiscence keyed to sensory cues such as memory books, or personalized videotapes of family pictures. Bourgeois et al. (2010: 8) identify augmentative and alternative communication tools that are being adapted and used to support 'language expression and comprehension/memory support for persons in middle-stage dementia'. These include memory wallets and memory books. Maclagan and Grant (2011) illustrate how persons who have been trained in strategies for conversational maintenance are able to use such tools to elicit interaction and co-construct personal stories even when the person with dementia can no longer offer new information.

Multiple reviews of research on implementing communication techniques are available. Vasse et al. (2010) conducted a systematic review of 721 studies to identify 19 interventions; McGilton et al. (2009), reviewed 598 manuscripts to find a set of six studies focused on improving outcomes through training healthcare staff, particularly paraprofessionals. Both reviews include studies by Tappen, Burgio, and Dijkstra and their colleagues. Tappen et al. (2001) compared the impact of conversation alone, exercise alone, and conversation with exercise on resident communication performance. They found conversation alone to have the most beneficial effect for the PWD, not just on social interaction but also on the coherence and informativeness of the conversation offered by the impaired partner. Burgio et al. (2002) list repetitive demands and verbal outbursts as parts of the challenging behaviors that staff must deal with in working with persons with dementia. His team taught aides to use both behavior management and communication skills, including both verbal and non-verbal skills, such as eye contact, or announcing single activities. This study illustrates how agitation and some challenging behaviors can be diminished through psychosocial techniques that include conversational interaction. Dijkstra et al. (2002:70) included a review of nurse aide discourse with persons in different stages of dementia. They found that nurse aides used more facilitative techniques, including fewer questions, with people in early-stage dementia and suggest that perhaps they considered 'question asking to be a facilitative strategy for late-stage dementia residents who appear to be less talkative'. However, our pilot studies of the use of questions in moderate and late moderate dementia suggest that is not the case.

Questions

When an untrained person is not sure what to do in a conversation with a person who has dementia, they typically ask a question, because that is what they would do to start a conversation with somebody who has no cognitive impairment. However, such a person who is unused to talking with persons with cognitive impairment often neglects to wait a little bit longer for the answer, and will start asking question after question. Occasionally an unimpaired person will neglect to present any kind of backchannel feedback, and will depend almost totally on a question–answer exchange. Questions are an essential component of ordinary conversation, but not all question types are equal. Some take longer than others to answer. People with dementia take longer than controls to answer questions, and they take longer to answer some questions than others, indicating that some questions are more difficult for them to respond to than others. Tag questions are easiest to respond to, followed by *yes/no* questions, and so-prefaced questions; wh-questions (questions beginning with *who what where when why how)* are hardest (Davis et al. 2011).

A constant barrage of direct questions to PWD, whether intended or not, becomes a power play that baffles, confuses, and embarrasses recipients who may no longer have the ability to present what the questioner may consider to be an appropriately speedy and informative response. The question-asker has the power to sanction or ratify the answer, and to reposition the recipient, which can result in malignant social positioning (Sabat et al. 2004). Such negativity impedes the efforts of PWD to maintain self-esteem and facets of identity.

Identifying the impact of questions: nurse aide trainees and university students

In 1998, Davis began collecting conversational interviews with PWD and worked over the next three years to study the ongoing transcriptions to develop interventions that could help PWD sustain conversational interaction. As the transcripts multiplied, other researchers joined in the task of analyzing them for what PWD retained that could be used and expanded, as opposed to what PWD had lost (Davis 2005a). Three preliminary interventions were demonstrated and evaluated in staff training, conference workshops, and longitudinal projects with gerontology and nursing professionals. From 2005 to 2009, supported by funding from the National Alzheimer's Association, Davis, Smith, Shenk, and other researchers developed, implemented, and evaluated materials for training in dementia care communication targeting second-language and low-literacy nurse aides. This allowed us to refine the conversational interventions, particularly regarding question–answer routines, and in 2006, to start using the same materials with university students.

The three conversational intervention techniques are *go-aheads*, *quilting* (Moore and Davis 2002), and *indirect questions* (Davis 2005b, 2011). All three interventions involve releasing power to the cognitively impaired person, which is different from most doctor–patient discourse (Ainsworth-Vaughn 1997), therapeutic discourse (Ferrara 1994), or the pragmatics of interpersonal discourse in health care (Davis 2011). Our training materials, used for both nurse aide trainees and gerontology students, emphasize the importance of using facilitative and supportive techniques to support as natural a conversation as possible.

- A *go-ahead* is a two-syllable backchannel or continuer, such as *Uh-huh, Mmm-hmm*, or *Oh really*! Go-aheads encourage conversation partners to continue what they were saying and are used naturally by most speakers in any conversation. We encourage the use of two syllables because many PWD have attentional issues as well as hearing impairments, and there is a better chance of being heard if the unimpaired speaker says *mmm-hmmm* instead of just *mmm*. We use an intonation contour chart to model four ways to say *mmm-hmmm*.

- *Quilting* co-constructs a small narrative: an unimpaired partner repeats or paraphrases information back to the impaired speaker, as a way of eliciting additional details which can then be woven into a short story concerning the impaired speaker. Paraphrase or repetition by the unimpaired partner, which we depend on for quilting, is called diaphonic repetition by Perrin et al. (2003), who consider that it can have four functions: (a) the immediately prior talk of the interlocutor has been correctly heard and interpreted, (b) a confirmation request function, (c) a positive reply function, signaling agreement, (d) a negative reply function, signaling disagreement, based on exchange structure and prosody (intonation, speech rate, register, key). We typically model the technique and ask the students to practice it in pairs, with these instructions:

> Listen to the conversation for a phrase that sounds like it could be part of a larger story. Often that phrase will be formulaic, used to evaluate an event, or to give an especially memorable detail.
>
> Repeat the speaker's full phrase or sentence slowly, as if it were important, and then pause.
>
> Record the detail as a reminder for future conversation.
>
> Return to that detail in the next conversation you have, and phrase it as a statement.

- *'Indirect' questions* are presented as statements with a question-contour: *you like that shirt?;* as tag-questions: *you like that shirt, don't you?;* or as so-prefaced *yes/no* questions: *So, you have two sisters* (Davis 2005b). They may be closed or open-ended, and we recommend also trying some open-ended comments such as *Tell me about your favorite breakfast*. Students are encouraged to avoid direct (wh-) questions such as *What do you ...?* Calling these recommended question types 'indirect' allows persons with little knowledge of grammatical terminology a way to distinguish them from 'direct', which they understand from elementary school as *who–what–where–when* questions. After modeling the technique, we ask students to create dialogues in pairs without using 'direct' questions, with one acting as a visitor and the other as a resident, with the following instructions:

> Find out something about the resident's childhood.
> Learn something about the resident's family, probably in childhood.
> Discover something about the resident's hobbies/favorite holiday/vacation spot.

We have some indication of the impact of the minimal training curriculum in dementia care communication that we offer university students. Beginning in 2006, the Interdisciplinary Gerontology Program at the University of North Carolina-Charlotte has required a communication-based service-learning component in its undergraduate introductory gerontology course, offered each semester (Hancock et al. 2008). Before beginning their visits to assisted living and dementia-care communities, students are given an hour's training in conversing with older people, emphasizing the three basic conversational techniques mentioned above. Working singly or in pairs, students hold and record conversations with persons with dementia, which are then transcribed and deposited in the *Carolinas Conversations Collection*, a password-protected web portal supported for delivery at the

Medical University of North Carolina by the National Libraries of Medicine (http://carolinaconversations.musc.edu/about/).

At the end of the course, students assess each other's reports on their use of the three interventions. Table 21.1 represents student assessments of interactions between roughly 200 students and 76 assisted living residents during spring 2006 to fall 2010 (many residents were recorded several times, often by pairs of students). *Go-aheads*, for instance, were tried by multiple students with every resident, with improved interaction; fewer students tried quilting and indirect questions, but found slightly more 'greatly improved' interactions.

Student evaluations suggested that even one hour of training improved their conversations with residents with dementia. Comments such as the following, from a student in 2008 who tried all three techniques, were typical:

> Go-aheads were most often used, which tied the circumstances [together]. Indirect questions were used, because *direct questions puzzled our conversation partner*. Quilting was used several times to stimulate conversation. Both student partners were mindful of the training conducted in class. *With direct questions, our conversation partner was so nervous/worried that he could not properly express his ideas*. [Italics ours]

Responses from the nurse aide trainees are similar to those from the university students. The nurse aide trainees use the same materials as the university students for communication training, but have been asked to respond to the communication materials as a whole rather than to the specific interventions. Interestingly, roughly a fourth of their responses concern the quilting intervention, with comments such as the following from this 2009 trainee:

> Having personal experience with a parent who had Alzheimer's disease it was probably hardest on me to see the memory decline. Not realizing it at the time during the onset of her memory loss I used the quilting technique. I can attest that it does work, and it definitely eased some of her frustrations to communicate effectively. It also required incredible patience to cope with the memory decline. The quilting technique will definitely help us all give good care to the memory impaired.

Only a few nurse aide trainees report using any of the variations for 'indirect questions', for reasons such as the one offered below by a 2009 trainee:

> I found the communication module on Moodle to be helpful, especially the section on how to better communicate with patients with Alzheimer's or Dementia. For example, it was mentioned that it's best to use open-ended or indirect questions versus direct questions. For some people, this would obviously be a better way to start a conversation. However, for me, this is a bit counterintuitive. Prior to nursing school, I was in the business world for nearly two decades, and over the years I have become somewhat programmed to be more direct and straight to the point. So, I will need to remember this as I continue to work with patients who have cognitive issues.

Comments such as this last one suggest that a more intensive training about question types and the responses they elicit is needed, and it will have to focus directly on what apparently does seem counter-intuitive for both university students and health services trainees. This can perhaps best be achieved by demonstrating the delay in reply to different question types, which we analyze below in the two pilot studies, and by demonstrating the amount of

Table 21.1 Undergraduate students' evaluations of three communication techniques

Intervention	*#Interactions*	*#Residents*	*Worsened interaction*	*Helped interaction*	*Improved interaction*	*Greatly improved interaction*
Go-ahead	168	76	5	23	134	6
Quilting	120	52	4	23	81	11
'Indirect' questions	104	56	5	29	57	13

information (lexical and idea density) produced in responses to different question types, even by highly fluent PWD.

Pilot studies on questions: more formal investigations of question types

We soon recognized from the transcripts of interactions with PWD that question–answer routines were more important in dementia-care communication than either we had realized or that the literature had emphasized. Accordingly, we developed two pilot studies to explore responses to three different closed questions plus an open question and to an unexpected wh-question.

Pilot study 1

In study 1, Talking while Sitting, the researcher asked four scripted questions during facilitative natural conversations with 14 persons who were sitting comfortably in their own residence. One of the questions was an unexpected wh-question, *What did you have for breakfast?*; the others were *Do you like roses? You like that shirt, don't you?* and *So, you had two sisters*? The participants comprised 7 with high probability of dementia and 7 with low probability. Figure 21.1 shows question types and pauses by those with high and low probability of dementia:

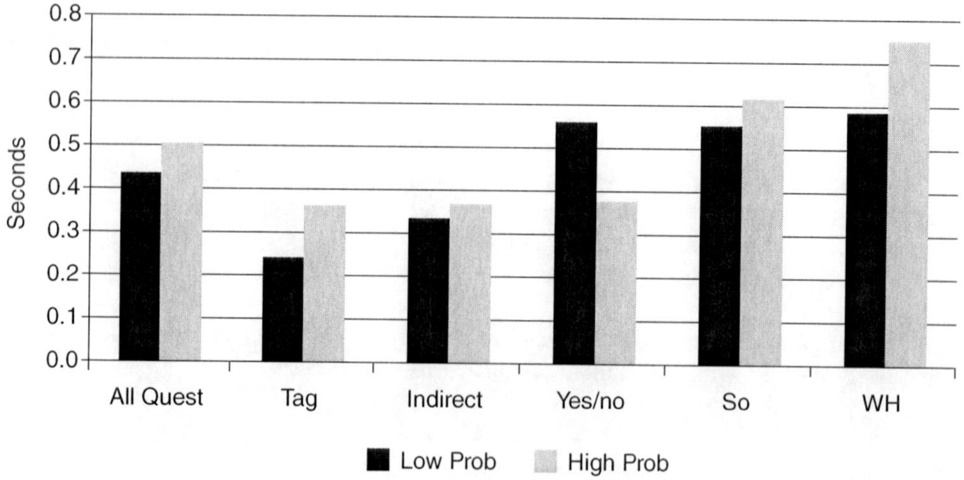

Figure 21.1 Average pause times before responding to questions. (Participants were responding to questions while seated in their own residence.)

Pauses were greater in responses by participants with high probability of dementia, particularly before responding to the wh-question. Those with low probability of dementia paused longer before *yes/no* questions because they provided more information, rather than just giving a simple 'yes' or 'no'.

Pilot study 2

In study 2, we examined the impact of the sudden unexpected question on persons engaged in facilitative natural conversation with the researcher while walking on a GAITRite® carpet (Davis et al. 2011). Again, persons were divided into those with and without early moderate or moderate dementia. In earlier research, Davis and Maclagan (2009) discussed research that finds pauses often signal time for planning and processing. Using Praat phonetics software (Boersma and Weenink 2011), we analyzed pause length between question and answer (compared to other turn-related pausing) to discriminate among question types. Not surprisingly, while walking and talking, the unexpected wh-question caused a slow-down for all participants, but especially so for those with dementia or with high risk of dementia, as seen in the length of pause in seconds before the response and/or the presence of 'stalls': hesitations, *oh, ah,* optional phrases, reformulations, pauses (indicated by time in seconds and –), and then an answer:

What did you have for breakfast? – –
.536 I had – –
.611 some – – –
1.103 a banana, with milk.

Figure 21.2 displays the pauses for turns and for wh-questions by cognitive impairment.

Pilot studies 1 and 2 are described in more detail in Davis et al. (2011). They showed that whether walking or sitting while conversing, persons with cognitive impairment took longer to answer wh-questions, and had longer 'stalls'.

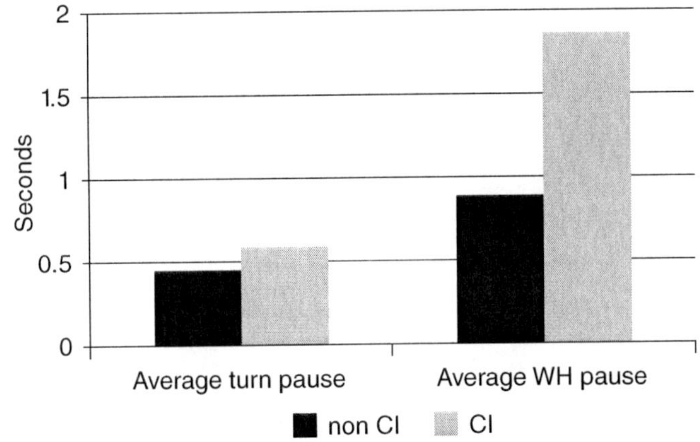

Figure 21.2 Average overall pause times between turns and before responses to wh-questions according to cognitive status. (Participants answered questions while walking.)

Case study: conversations with assisted living residents

The findings we report here are part of a larger and ongoing study where we investigate how paraprofessionals, volunteers, and novice caregivers initiate conversation-based relationships with persons with dementia, and the extent to which they do or do not depend on questions to drive their conversations. To do this, we recruited eight graduate students enrolled in either a Master's degree or a graduate certificate program in gerontology, to visit and record interactions with four residents in a special care assisted living community for people with dementia. Two students individually visited each resident five times, so that each resident received a total of 10 visits. Seven of the students were women; one was a man. Their ages ranged from 24–35. Three of the students, Lorene, Susie, and Ella, had received the minimal communication training in one of their previous courses; the rest had received no training (see Table 21.2).

The four residents visited by the students were all women in their eighties with a diagnosis of probable dementia of the Alzheimer's type. None had been formally screened for dementia, because this is not a requirement for people in assisted living. They were informally staged and assigned to units in the assisted living community according to their functional abilities and the degree of care they required. Two of the women, Littlejohn and Grande, were in the least care unit and were able to participate in conversation, with Littlejohn being less impaired than Grande. Hall was in the intermediate care unit and was less able to initiate conversational turns. The fourth resident was in the greater care unit, and barely spoke, though she appeared to participate in conversations non-verbally. Because of the non-verbal nature of her interactions, we do not report on interactions with her in the following analysis.

The conversations all took place in the residents' own rooms. They were recorded on digital recorders (Olympus DS 5000 or similar) and transcribed using Transcriber (available as free software under GNU General Public License, http://trans.sourceforge.net/en/presentation.php), which allowed the transcript and the sound files to be time aligned. Pauses were automatically calculated by LaBB-CAT corpus analysis software (Fromont and Hay 2008).

Results

Overview of the conversations

Our analysis of the results from conversations between the six student volunteers and the three verbal residents moves from the general to the more detailed. We start with an overview of the conversations between the six students and their partners, the three verbal residents.

Table 21.2 Amount of training for graduate student conversation partners

Resident	*Unit*	*Student*	*Prior student training*
Maureen Littlejohn	1	Lorene	Minimal overview in graduate summer course on dementia
		Mina	None, but has carework experience
Anna Grande	1	Susie	Minimal training in undergraduate gerontology course
		Aidan	None, but has carework experience
Barbara Hall	2	Ella	Minimal training in undergraduate gerontology course
		Jacie	None, but has read some training materials

We look first at the amount of language produced, then at the students' use of different question types and, finally, at the idea density in the responses by the two most verbal residents. Table 21.3 shows the total length of the six conversations and the total number of words spoken by the resident in each conversation. We also give the time and number of words spoken by the resident in the first conversation in the series.

From Table 21.3 it is clear that the residents produced different amounts of language overall and that they responded differently with the different students. As might be expected, Ms Littlejohn, who was the least impaired, sustained the interaction for the greatest time – but only with one of the students, Lorene. She also produced the greatest overall number of words in interactions with Lorene. It is a mistake to assume that persons with dementia are equally happy to talk with any visitor or staff member, or that any visitor is equally happy to talk with any person with dementia. Immediately, it is clear that the way the students conducted their conversations mattered greatly, and their success was keyed to their skills with handling questions and sustaining the resident's topic as well as to their listening skills, usually identified by go-aheads and overlaps. Students who asked too many of the wrong question type found their conversations grinding to a halt.

Overall, the six students asked 747 questions in their 30 conversations with the three residents, out of a total of 3,440 student conversational turns. Students differed widely in their percentage of turns containing a question: 39 percent of Aidan's turns were questions; 22 percent of Jacie's; 21 percent of Susie's; 19 percent of Ella's; 17 percent of both Lorene's and Mina's (see Table 21.4).

Table 21.3 Length of conversations (minutes:seconds) and number of words spoken by the residents in all conversations and also in the first conversation

		Overall		*Conversation 1*	
Resident	*Student*	*Duration (min:sec)*	*# Resident words*	*Duration*	*# Resident words*
Ms Littlejohn	Lorene	123:52	13,403	35:56	4,573
	Mina	49:31	6,280	13:47	1,724
Ms Grande	Susie	95:46	3,745	34:28	1,397
	Aidan	75:11	3,813	12:57	1,026
Ms Hall	Jacie	107:03	4,450	12:40	623
	Ella	62:52	2,574	10:36	454

Table 21.4 Number of student and resident turns and number and percentage of student turns that were questions

		# turns			
Resident	*Student*	*Resident*	*Student*	*# Questions*	*% Questions*
Ms Littlejohn	Lorene	1,174	1,126	187	17%
	Mina	241	233	39	17%
Ms Grande	Susie	647	650	136	21%
	Aidan	505	520	202	39%
Ms Hall	Jacie	435	444	96	22%
	Ella	424	467	87	19%
Total		3,426	3,440	747	

Just as important as the number of questions is the number of different types of questions the students asked the residents over all the conversations, shown in Table 21.5. Our pilot studies had helped us identify the question types that caused the greatest delay in preparing an answer. The easiest, or quickest to answer, is the tag question but it was actually the least used. The next easiest type of question for the residents to respond to is the *yes/no*, which made up 57 percent of all questions asked by the students. The hardest question type to answer is the wh-question, and that, unfortunately, was the second most common type of question asked by all of the students. Mina, the student who elicited the fewest conversational turns from her impaired partner, had received no training about communication or the interventions, including the focus on questions. She asked the smallest percentage of the relatively easy *yes/no* questions and more than half of her questions, 54 percent, were the difficult wh-questions. In effect, all those wh-questions shut down her impaired conversation partner, who ended their last interaction by suggesting that Mina find someone else with whom to talk.

Questions in this dataset: their impact on responses

Our next goal was to investigate whether specific question types elicited responses with particular characteristics that would enable us to recommend using one type over another. The question types recommended in the materials for trainees and university students, the so-prefaced, *yes/no*, and indirect questions elicited more responses, but although they took longer to answer, wh-questions usually received more detailed answers than other question types, particularly if they were in any sense open-ended or did not require specific recall of events or persons.

In order to examine responses to questions in more detail, we looked at idea density in the responses by Ms Littlejohn and Ms Grande to the four students who interacted with them. Idea density (ID), the number of propositions or ideas per sentence-like utterance (Kintsch 1974) was found to be a highly important predictor in the Nun Study (Snowdon et al. 1996).

Table 21.5 Different types of questions asked in the conversations. Percentages are given for the most common question types

		Tag	*Yes/no*	*So*	*Wh-*	*Other*	*Total*
Ms Littlejohn	Lorene	0	95 48%	40 24%	42 21%	10	187
	Mina	0	14 36%	3 8%	21 54%	1	39
Ms Grande	Susie	4	96 71%	2 1%	32 24%	2	136
	Aidan	0	114 56%	17 8%	59 29%	12	202
Ms Hall	Jacie	1	61 64%	10 10%	22 23%	2	96
	Ella	0	50 57%	17 20%	20 23%	0	87
Total		5	430 57%	89 12%	196 26%	27	747

Diaries written by members of a community of nuns when they were in their twenties, which were high in idea density predicted greater cognitive or brain reserve; those with low density were associated with poorer cognition in later life and greater chance of AD pathology identified after death (Snowdon et al. 1996; Riley et al. 2005). Reed et al. (2010: 1) found that ID in language samples taken later in life can also be used as a 'predictor of future cognitive decline'.

CPIDR (Computerized Propositional Idea Density Rater) was used to assess the propositional or idea density of responses to questions. CPIDR, a software program (Brown et al. 2007) was originally developed to analyze schizophrenic/schizaphasic language production. Its output is based on part-of-speech tagging, dividing the number of verbs, adverbs, adjectives, prepositions, and conjunctions by the total number of words. When tested against human raters, 'it agrees with them better than they agree with each other' (Brown et al. 2008: 540). For this analysis we used CPIDR to calculate idea density scores on whole turns rather than on arbitrary ten word sequences used in many studies, including Brown et al. (2007).

Idea density varies from 0 to 1, with scores closer to 1 showing responses that were phrased more succinctly. Ms Littlejohn's idea density was highest with Lorene at 0.524. It was slightly lower with Mina, at 0.465. Ms Grande's idea density was slightly higher with Susie (0.396) than with Aidan (0.353). Figure 21.3 separates the idea density according to question type and shows that, as expected, Ms Littlejohn's responses had a higher idea density and were thus more succinct than Ms Grande's for most question types and her responses were more succinct to Lorene than to Mina.

The highest idea density is from Ms Grande's responses to *so* questions, a question type recommended in training. However, where Lorene asked Ms Littlejohn 40 *so* questions, Susie only asked Ms Grande two, so Ms Grande's high score is not very reliable. Overall, Ms Littlejohn responded more efficiently than Ms Grande. Part of this is due to Ms Littlejohn's greater fluency (sustained by her use of formulaic phrases and colloquial expressions) and part of this is because she received a full range of question types and apparently liked many

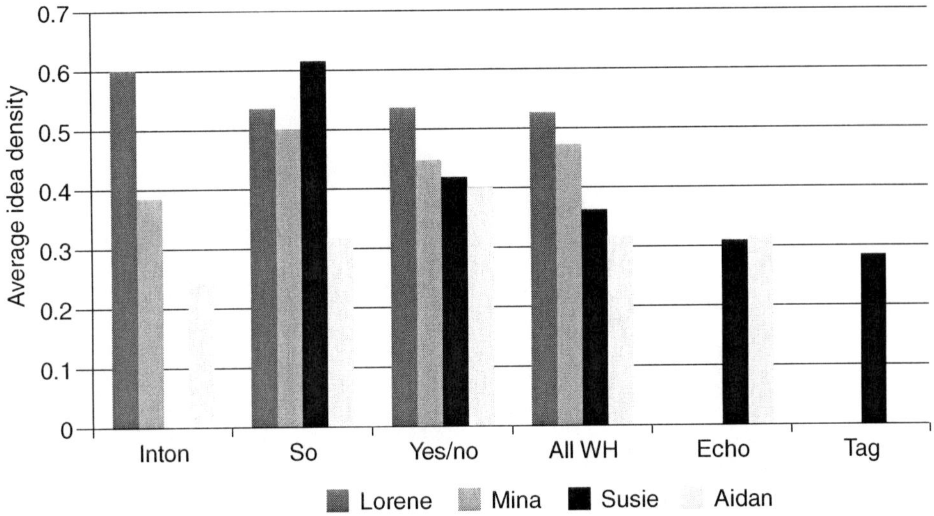

Figure 21.3 Idea density according to question type. Lorene and Mina were interacting with Ms Littlejohn and Susie and Aidan with Ms Grande

of the topics, particularly in engagement with Lorene. Figure 21.3 clearly shows that, although some questions elicited responses with higher ID, one student in each pair consistently elicited higher quality language from both Ms Littlejohn and Ms Grande, across all question types, and in each case, that student had received some minimal training in dementia care communication, including the go-ahead, quilting, and 'indirect' question interventions.

Maureen Littlejohn's language production was the highest of the group; indeed, her fluency was the highest of anyone living in her unit and her production speed and retained pragmatic skills in conversation gave the initial impression that she had little if any cognitive impairment. She has been able to function well as a person with mild or early moderate dementia as long as she does not have to work with finances or find her way around outside the secure unit where she lives. In a separate study, Davis and Maclagan (2011b) have begun to identify the high number of multi-word expressions, formulaic phrases, and repeated stories/story fragments that account for a considerable amount of her fluency. Table 21.6 displays her average idea density together with the average number of ideas and words per utterance.

Table 21.6 shows that responses with the greatest number of ideas do not always have the highest idea density. *Where* questions had the second highest number of ideas per response at 17.2, but the lowest idea density (0.366). This shows that they often included extra or irrelevant material. Table 21.6 also shows the wide range of standard deviations in Ms Littlejohn's responses. This reflects the variation in the length of her utterances as well as the variation in their content. Responses to *so* questions, for example, varied from a simple *yes* or *no* with an idea density score of 0 to a response with an idea density score of 0.447 that referred to her bird feeder: *Well uh they won't hang around if there is not any feed so I see a little ol' bird out there now but uh we'll we'll take care of that at some point in time*. Similarly, in response to *So you grew up on a farm*, Ms Littlejohn responded *Yeah we uh we had a farm uh that land had been in the family for years* which had an idea density of 0.235 even though it was relatively succinct. As Chand et al. (2010: 6) note, low scores for idea density often 'reflect vague and repetitious expression' as shown in Ms Grande's response *that's the trouble* with an idea density score of 0.25 to Aidan's question *Well do you have anything else you have to do today?*

Table 21.6 Maureen Littlejohn's responses to both Lorene and Mina analyzed by CPIDR, sorted by average idea density

Question type	*Total*	*Average idea density*		*Average number of ideas*		*Average number of words*	
		Mean	*sd*	*Mean*	*sd*	*Mean*	*sd*
Which	2	0.61	0.008	20	2.8	33	4.3
How	21	0.587	0.165	9.1	10.2	18	22.6
Indirect	11	0.565	0.287	4.7	4.1	8.75	8.2
So	27	0.538	0.29	10.0	31.2	19.4	25.5
Yes/no	101	0.522	0.2	8.8	7.7	16.2	14.5
Wh-What	27	0.485	0.169	8.1	8.3	15.4	15
Who	6	0.46	0.29	9.4	13.2	17.8	25.3
When	1	0.367	–	11	–	30	–
Where	5	0.366	0.24	17.2	29.1	30	43.7

Idea density analysis shows clearly that Ms Littlejohn's responses are more succinct than those of Ms Grande. It also shows how different types of question are responded to. Because it can be calculated automatically by CPIDR, idea density is a relatively quick method of identifying the extent to which someone with dementia is still able to provide clear and succinct responses to questions.

Implications

Asking questions about questions raises even more. Future research needs to focus on episodic questions that ask for detailed memories (*What did you have for dinner last night?*) as opposed to semantic questions that ask for more general information (*What do you like to eat?*), since many of the student questions combine the two types. It could be useful to look more closely at idea density in topics the impaired person introduces, as opposed to those introduced by the student volunteers, usually by means of a question. The interactional aspects of these conversations are crucial, particularly as they show the retention of pragmatics and politeness (Temple et al. 1999; Davis 2005b; Hamilton 2008). We have found some instances of the impaired person's seeming to take the perspective of the other, and additional instances of the use of extenders (Maclagan et al. 2008) by persons with impairments to collaborate with unimpaired conversation partners by getting them to finish the utterance.

When Heritage (2002: 314) examined how nurses designed questions in an open context, he found that 'regardless of the specific aims of questioning, the ways in which questions are designed unavoidably serve to index particular relationships between questioner and respondent'. That is, of course, what we have been quietly identifying throughout this discussion, and it is clearly what we need to re-emphasize and expand in the training we have been offering to our trainees and our university students. Communications training can also impact staff attitudes toward dementia and impact on direct care services for persons with dementia (Kristiansen et al. 2006). Such training will become even more necessary with the increasing number of direct care workers such as nurse aides (Arkin 2011). We see clear implications for developing materials for family, volunteers, and staff training about when to ask questions and what types to avoid, under which conditions (Davis and Smith 2011). We are currently evaluating materials and training that include our findings from the pilot studies, such as the dialogues or role plays in Table 21.7 which model facilitative conversation – and the avoidance of wh-questions – while walking.

Table 21.7 Sample talking–walking dialogues illustrating facilitative conversation

Do this!	*Not this!*
You are walking down the hall with Ms Green. You say: 'I'm glad we're walking to breakfast. I like scrambled eggs, don't you?'	You are walking down the hall with Ms Green. You say: 'I'm glad we're walking to breakfast. What did you eat yesterday?'
'It's nice to see everybody up and about. Having a shower will feel good, and we'll find a towel.'	'It's nice to see everybody up and about. Where's your bath towel? What did you do with it?'
'Everybody seems to like playing games. My favorite game is ____. Maybe you like that also?'	'Everybody seems to like playing games. What game did you play last night?'

Summary

In this chapter we have highlighted the growing importance of care giving for people with Alzheimer's disease and the increased need for developing greater understanding of conversational techniques and components, particularly question-asking. It is in conversation that much social interaction and social engagement takes place for persons with dementia, which can help reduce agitation or some problem behaviors, and it is also a primary means of maintaining social identities. However, the constraining impact of question-asking is poorly understood.

We note in passing several ways that researchers categorize questions, such as open vs. closed, and focus on 'indirect' vis-à-vis direct wh-questions, interrogatives beginning with *who, what, where, when, why,* and *how.* We explain the importance of using pauses before the response to identify question difficulty (Davis and Maclagan 2011a), and summarize two pilot studies with talking while sitting and talking while walking, each of which used facilitative natural conversation with four scripted questions, one of which was an unexpected wh-question. Not surprisingly, persons either diagnosed with dementia or screened as having a high probability of dementia paused longer before answering any question and especially so before answering any wh-question.

Our analysis examined the impact of questions on interactions between residents with dementia and conversation partners with minimal or no training in conversational techniques for dementia care communication. The detailed analyses were carried out on conversations by undergraduate student volunteers who were asked to use three specific conversational techniques in conversations with people with dementia. One of the techniques was the replacement of direct questions by indirect and *so,* questions. Conversational interactions were first analyzed in terms of the number of words and turns and whether a student volunteer used go-ahead signals (backchannel feedback) instead of peppering the resident with questions, the typical act of a person who has not been trained in conversing with older persons, particularly those with dementia. We tabulated the frequency of question types in this dataset. The computerized program, CPIDR, analyzed each response to each question type for number of words and idea density. These were tabulated according to question type and compared for the two most fluent residents. We see a number of future directions including the expanded investigation of resident responses to semantic as opposed to episodic questions, and how the interactional aspects of the conversations allow a focus on pragmatics and politeness, the importance of phatic commentary and the manipulation of fillers and extenders. Finally, we end where we began, with a call for the development and testing of materials and training for volunteers, staff, and family members on dementia care communication.

Related topics

Alzheimer's disease; care giving; questions; communication skills training.

Further reading

Blatt, Benjamin and Greenberg, Larrie. 'Communication skills training for resident physicians: a physician-educator perspective'. (Chapter 19 in this volume.)

Dijkstra, K., Bourgeois, M., Petrie, G., Burgio, L., and Allen-Burge, R. (2002) 'My recaller is on vacation: discourse analysis of nursing-home residents with dementia'. *Discourse Processes*, 33, 53–76.

Sabat, S., Johnson, A., Swarbrick, C., and Keady, J. (2011) 'The "demented other" or simply "a person"? Extending the philosophical discourse of Naue and Kroll through the situated self'. *Nursing Philosophy*, 12, 282–292.

Small, J. and Perry, J. (2005) 'Do you remember? How caregivers question their spouses who have Alzheimer's disease and the impact on communication'. *Journal of Speech, Language, and Hearing Research*, 48, 125–136.

References

Ainsworth-Vaughn, N. (1997) *Claiming Power in Doctor–Patient Talk*. Oxford: Oxford University Press.

Allen-Burge, R., Burgio, L., Bourgeois, M., Sims, R., and Nunnikhoven, J. (2001) 'Increasing communication among nursing home residents'. *Journal of Clinical Geropsychology*, 7, 213–230.

Alzheimer's Association. (2011) *Facts and Figures 2011*. http://www.alz.org (accessed 19 November, 2011).

Arkin, S. (2011) 'Service learning students as Alzheimer treatment providers'. *Topics in Geriatric Rehabilitation*, 24, 1–22.

Beard, R., Knauss, J., and Moyer, D. (2009) 'Managing disability and enjoying life: how we reframe dementia in personal narratives'. *Journal of Aging Studies*, 23, 227–235.

Boersma, P. and Weenink, D. (2011) Praat: doing phonetics by computer [Computer program]. Version 5.3.03. Accessed 21 November 2011 at: http://www.praat.org/

Bourgeois, M., Fried-Olsen, M., and Rowland, C. (2010) 'AAC strategies and tools for persons with dementia'. *The ASHA Leader*, 16 March, 8–11.

Brown, C., Snodgrass, T., Covington, M., Herman, R., and Kemper, S. (2007) 'Measuring propositional idea density through part-of-speech tagging'. Poster presented at Linguistic Society of America, January, Anaheim, CA. Accessed 21 November 2011 at: http://www.ai.uga.edu/caspr/

Brown, C., Snodgrass, T., Kemper, S., Herman, R., and Covington, M. (2008) 'Automatic measurement of propositional idea density from part-of-speech tagging'. *Behavior Research Methods*, 40, 540–545.

Burgio, L., Stevens, A., Burgio, K., Roth, D., Paul, P., and Gerstle, J. (2002) 'Teaching and maintaining behavior management skills in the nursing home'. *The Gerontologist*, 42, 487–496.

Chand, V., Baynes, K., Bonnici, L., and Farias, S. (2010) *Analysis of Idea Density (AID): A Manual*. UC-Davis Center for Mind and Brain. Accessed 1 December 2011 at: http://mindbrain.ucdavis.edu/labs/Baynes/idea-density-alzheimers-disease

Chenoweth, L., King, M., Jeon, Y., Brodaty, H., Stein-Parbury, J., Norman, R., et al. (2009) 'Caring for aged dementia care resident study (CADRES) of person-centred care, dementia-care mapping, and usual care in dementia: a cluster-randomized trial'. *The Lancet Neurology*, 8, 317–325.

Clare, L. (2010) 'Awareness in people with severe dementia: review and integration'. *Aging and Mental Health*, 14, 20–32.

Davis, B. (ed.) (2005a) *Alzheimer Talk, Text and Context: Enhancing Communication*. New York: Palgrave.

——(2005b) 'So, you had two sisters, right? Questions and discourse markers in Alzheimer's discourse'. In B. Davis (ed.) *Alzheimer Talk, Text and Context: Enhancing Communication*. New York: Palgrave, 128–145.

——(2011) 'Interpersonal issues in health discourse'. In M. Locher and S. Graham (eds) *Interpersonal Pragmatics*. Berlin: deGruyter Mouton.

Davis, B. and Maclagan, M. (2009) 'Examining pauses in Alzheimer's discourse'. *American Journal of Alzheimer's Disease and Other Dementias*, 24, 141–154.

——(2011a) 'Pauses, placeholders and fillers in Alzheimer's discourse: glueing relationships as impairment increases'. In N. Amiridze, B. Davis, and M. Maclagan (eds) *Fillers and Placeholders in Discourse and Grammar*. Amsterdam: John Benjamins.

——(2011b) 'Exploring characteristics and functions of retained story fragments in talk by persons with probable MCI/early, moderate and later dementia: a corpus-based investigation'. Dementia and Dialogue Conference Presentation, Pennsylvania State University, April.

Davis, B. and Pope, C. (2010) 'Institutionalized ghosting: language use in the process of erasing the body with Alzheimer's'. *Language Policy*, 9, 29–44.

Davis, B. and Smith, M. (2011) 'Dementia care communication in residential facilities: intersections of training and research'. In P. Backhaus (ed.) *Communication in Elderly Care*. New York: Continuum, 20–39.
Davis, B., Maclagan, M., Karakostas, T., Liang, S., and Shenk, D. (2011) 'Watching what you say: walking and talking in dementia'. *Topics in Geriatric Rehabilitation*, 27(4), 268–277.
Dijkstra, K., Bourgeois, M., Petrie, G., Burgio, L., and Allen-Burge, R. (2002) 'My recaller is on vacation: discourse analysis of nursing home residents with dementia'. *Discourse Processes*, 33, 53–76.
Fazio, S. and Mitchell, D. (2009) 'Persistence of self in individuals with Alzheimer's disease'. *Dementia*, 8, 39–59.
Ferrara, K. (1994) *Therapeutic Ways with Words*. Oxford: Oxford University Press.
Fromont, R. and Hay, J. (2008) 'ONZE Miner:Development of a browser-based research Tool'. *Corpora* 3(2), 173–193. See also http://onzeminer.sourceforge.net/
Goody, E. (1978) *Questions and Politeness: Strategies in Social Interaction*. New York: Cambridge University Press.
Hamilton, H. (2008) 'Language and dementia: sociolinguistic aspects'. *Annual Review of Applied Linguistics*, 28, 91–110.
Hancock, C., Shenk, D., and Davis, B. (2008) 'Integrating gerontology service-learning students as members of a research team'. In P. Lan Lim (ed.) *Service Learning and Gerontology Education*. New York: Hampton Press.
Heritage, J. (2002) 'Ad hoc inquiries: two preferences in the design of "routine" questions in an open context'. In D. Maynard, H. Steenstra and H. van der Zouwen (eds) *Standardization and Tacit Knowledge: Interaction and Practice in the Survey Interview*. New York: Wiley Interscience, 313–333.
James, O. (2008) *Contented Dementia: 24-Hour Wraparound Care for Lifelong Well-being*. London: Vermillion.
Kintsch, W. (1974) *The Representation of Meaning in Memory*. Hillsdale, NJ: Lawrence Erlbaum.
Kristiansen, L., Hellzen, O., and Asplund, K. (2006) 'Swedish assistant nurses' experiences of job satisfaction when caring for persons suffering from dementia and behavioral disturbances: an interview study'. *International Journal of Qualitative Studies on Health and Well-Being*, 1, 245–256.
McGilton, K., Boscart, V., Fox, M., Sidani, S., Rochon, E., and Sorin-Peters, R. (2009) 'A systematic review of the effectiveness of communication interventions for health care providers caring for patients in residential care settings'. *Worldviews on Evidence-Based Nursing*, 6, 149–159.
Maclagan, M. and Grant, A. (2011) 'Care of people with Alzheimer's disease in New Zealand: supporting the telling of life stories'. In P. Backhaus (ed.) *Communication in Elderly Care*. New York: Continuum, 62–89.
Maclagan, M., Davis, B., and Lunsford, R. (2008) 'Fixed expressions, extenders and metonymy in the speech of people with Alzheimer's disease'. In S. Granger and F. Meunier (eds) *Phraseology: An Interdisciplinary Perspective*. Amsterdam: John Benjamins, 175–186.
Moore, L. and Davis, B. (2002) 'Using repetition techniques to help elderly communicators'. *Geriatric Nursing*, 23, 262–266.
Normann, H., Norberg, A., and Asplund, K. (2002) 'Confirmation and lucidity during conversations with a woman with severe dementia'. *Journal of Advanced Nursing*, 39, 370–376.
Perrin, L., Deshaies, D., and Paradis, C. (2003) 'Pragmatic functions of local diaphonic repetitions in conversation'. *Journal of Pragmatics*, 35, 1843–1860.
Reed, B., Chand, V., Baynes, K., Bonnici, L., and Farias, S. (2010) 'Is idea density in late life a marker of cognitive reserve? Effects on cognitive decline'. Poster presented at the Alzheimer's Research Symposium, UC Berkeley, CA. June 28.
Riley, K., Snowdon, D., Desrosiers, M., and Markesbery, W. (2005) 'Early life linguistic ability, late life cognitive function, and neuropathology: findings from the Nun Study'. *Neurobiology of Aging*, 26, 341–347.
Ripich, D. and Terrell, B. (1998) 'Patterns of discourse cohesion and coherence in Alzheimer's disease'. *Journal of Speech and Hearing Disorders*, 53, 696–735.
Ryan, E. and Schindel-Martin, L. (2011) 'Using narrative arts to foster personhood in dementia'. In P. Backhaus (ed.) *Communication in Elderly Care*. New York: Continuum, 193–217.

Sabat, S. (2008) 'Positioning and conflict involving a person with dementia: a case study'. In F.M. Moghaddam, R. Harré, and N. Lee (eds) *Global Conflict Resolution through Positioning Theory*. Springer: New York, 81–93.

Sabat, S., Napolitano, L., and Fath, H. (2004) 'Barriers to the construction of a valued social identity: a case study of Alzheimer's disease'. *American Journal of Alzheimer's Disease and Other Dementias*, 19, 177–185.

Smith, M. and Buckwalter, K. (2005) 'Behaviors associated with dementia'. *American Journal of Nursing*, 105, 40–52.

Snowdon, D., Kemper, S., Mortimer, J., Greiner, L., Wekstein, D., and Markesbery, W. (1996) 'Linguistic ability in early life and cognitive function and Alzheimer's disease in late life. Findings from the Nun Study'. *Journal of the American Medical Association*, 275, 528–532.

Steensig, J. and Drew, P. (2008) 'Introduction: questioning and affiliation/disaffiliation in interaction'. *Discourse Studies*, 10, 5–15.

Tappen, R., Williams, C., Barry, C., and DiSesa, D. (2001) 'Conversation intervention with Alzheimer's patients: increasing the relevance of communication'. *Clinical Gerontologist,* 24, 63–75.

Temple, V., Sabat, S. and Kroger, R. (1999) 'Intact use of politeness in the discourse of Alzheimer's sufferers'. *Language and Communication*, 19, 163–180.

Tschanz, J., Corcoran, C., Schwartz, S., Treiber, K., Treen, R., Norton, M., et al. (2011) 'Progression of cognitive, functional, and neuropsychiatric symptom domains in a population cohort with Alzheimer dementia: the Cache County dementia progression study'. *American Journal of Geriatric Psychiatry*, 19, 532–542.

Vasse, E., Vernooij-Dassen, M., Sijker, A., Rikkert, M., and Koopmans, R. (2010) 'A systematic review of communication strategies for persons with dementia in residential and nursing homes'. *International Psychogeriatrics*, 22, 189–200.

Vernooij-Dassen, M. and Downs, M. (2005) 'Cognitive and behavioural interventions for carers of people with dementia' (Protocol). *Cochrane Database of Systematic Reviews 2005,* Issue 2, Art. No. CD005318.

Vernooij-Dassen, M., Draskovic, I., McCleery, J., and Downs, M. (2011) 'Cognitive reframing for carers of people with dementia'. *Cochrane Database of Systematic Reviews 2011,* Nov. 9, Art. No. CD005318.

22 Healthcare team communication

Melinda M. Villagran and Paula K. Baldwin

Introduction

Communication is central to the study of healthcare teams because social interaction creates and sustains team structures and processes. Ideally, members of effective healthcare teams engage in communication to share timely, culturally, and linguistically appropriate health information to achieve team goals. The structure of the healthcare team is typically physician-directed and hierarchical, but optimal patient care requires dynamic and deliberative dialogue among a wide variety of healthcare professionals, patients, and caregivers, using appropriate sociolinguistic practices (Jones and Stubbe 2004). Information dissemination, problem solving, coordination, and affiliation among members of high performing teams are achieved through reflexive, ongoing interaction and shared decision-making (Jones and Stubbe 2004).

Communication also has direct links with patient health outcomes resulting from team-based patient care (Kuziemensky et al. 2009). Interdisciplinary healthcare teams seek to deliver coordinated care through a complex maze of roles, structures, regulations, and contexts with the goal of achieving optimal health outcomes for patients. Recent healthcare reforms place a strong emphasis on use of inter-professional collaboration to achieve cost-effective health outcomes for patients, but all too often health organizations manifest fragmentation and turbulence that limit the capacity for optimal team functioning. Moreover, the complex nature and high demands of health environments require coordination among team members trained in differing aspects of patient care (Kuziemsky et al. 2009), but clinicians do not typically receive formal team communication skills training as part of their medical education.

Contemporary research related to healthcare team communication focuses on two main areas: individual communication skills training for clinicians, and clinician cultural competency. Unfortunately, much of this work fails to tie individual communication skills to the co-creation of team communication, and fails to fully explicate the links between team-based structural and procedural communication processes that improve patients' health outcomes (Epstein and Street 2007). Research does suggest that ineffective communication among healthcare professionals can result in medical errors, uninformed patients, and missed opportunities to maximize treatment options and health outcomes (Epstein and Street 2007), but specific strategies for effective communication are not particularly generalizable because they rely on contextual issues of each interaction (LWP 2009).

Recent increases in the prevalence of healthcare teams may be related to more and better communication technologies used by health professionals. Face-to-face interpersonal interactions are now coupled with tools such as electronic medical records, cell phones, and web portals to share information and deliver care. These issues highlight the need to better understand how team communication processes among healthcare providers impact successful healthcare delivery.

This chapter explores historical and current conceptions of healthcare team communication as supported by the sociolinguistic and organizational communication perspectives from the Language in the Workplace Project (LWP 2009). Several critical team communication issues, current contributions and research regarding healthcare teams, applicable research methods for healthcare teams, and recommendations for practice and future directions are discussed. Although the structure and functions of healthcare teams varies greatly, most healthcare teams share the ultimate goals of delivering high quality care to improve health outcomes for patients.

Defining teams

Organizational scholars have long suggested the future of the global workplace will be comprised of interconnected teams (Dodd 2008). Unlike groups that may be comprised of autonomous individuals working concurrently on some task or goal, teams represent a system of interconnected individuals with unique roles, working collaboratively to attain a common goal (Ilgen 1999). Healthcare teams work interdependently to accomplish positive outcomes that are attributed to the team effort, as opposed to any one member's contribution.

Healthcare teams are distinct from the more general concept of teamwork, which can be used in a broader sense to discuss care provided by more than one member of an organization. Teamwork implies the existence of a functional team, but many studies on teamwork have found remarkably little structure, coordination, or integration among professionals involved in patient care (O'Leary et al. 2010). Specifically, research on the potential for team communication in operating rooms, intensive care units, and general medical units found although physicians were generally positive in their teamwork assessments, nurses felt communication and true collaboration with physicians was suboptimal or nonexistent (Joint Commission 2007; Nicotera and Clinkscales 2010; O'Leary et al. 2010). Some healthcare professionals reported a lack of shared decision-making about team processes among members. Specifically, nurses often served as a liaison between physicians and patients, but generally did not feel empowered to define or perform this role. Since a lack of teamwork among healthcare professionals is associated with more medical errors, and less favorable patient outcomes, a greater emphasis on team training, and the integration of teamwork into more structured healthcare teams could be beneficial (Joint Commission 2007; O'Leary et al. 2010).

Current conceptualization of team communication

Much of the literature on organizational communication struggles to acknowledge differences between *organization*-as-noun, which conceptualizes the structure of organization as a being or entity in-and-of-itself, and *organization*-as-verb, which focuses on relevant processes and activities that constitute a team (Putnam and Nicotera 2010). Similarly, despite a growing body of research on teams in the healthcare context much of this research overlooks differences among *team*-as-noun (an entity or being in which members work together to achieve a shared goal), *team*-as-adjective (a special type of cognition, attitude, or behavior among persons on a team), and *team*-as-verb (discursive and regulatory actions performed to achieve a shared goal).

Team-as-noun research generally focuses on outcomes achieved through the efforts of a seemingly monolithic team, and tends to minimize the importance of discursive practices within the team. *Team*-as-noun research may also examine the juxtaposition of the healthcare team versus an individual healthcare worker, to determine whether teams are more effective than individuals seeking to achieve the same goal. Comparative research on the effectiveness of teams versus individual healthcare professionals is performed with the assumption that team coordination is achieved through interaction, but team interactions may be difficult for healthcare providers who are used to working more independently.

Team-as-adjective research examines components, characteristics, and classifications of teams. This type of study explores the extent to which team characteristics such as team efficacy or team composition affect team interactions and goal achievement. By considering the personal and professional backgrounds of members, health organizations can seek the best configurations to maximize effective communication (Kozlowski and Bell 2003).

Team-as-verb research recognizes the dynamic processes of communication within a team, and seeks to reveal how team processes are enacted in support of collective goals. This type of research places the greatest emphasis on the communicative constructions of roles, relationships, and behaviors among members.

Historical perspectives

In the past, physicians, nurses, technicians, and administrators have often functioned autonomously in healthcare settings, based on the rules of varying hierarchical structures, professional identities, and personal discursive practices (Ledema 2007). In the last decade however, some health delivery systems such as the US Military Health Service and the Veteran's Healthcare Administration, have shifted away from an individual healthcare provider model toward team-based systems of coordinated care. Not surprisingly, increases in the implementation of team-based approaches to health care have brought about more research conducted to explore issues related to team processes and outcomes (Crabtree et al. 2010). Team researchers have produced volumes of work on various aspects of teams, including team structures, contexts, and overall team functioning (Mathieu et al. 2008).

Some research demonstrates how team-based health care can have significant implications for the type of care provided to patients, as well as the practice infrastructure that supports patients and providers across the continuum of care (Fields et al. 2010). In the healthcare context, team-based approaches to patient-centered care can produce improved health outcomes for patients, and reduced costs for health organizations, but the body of evidence regarding specific team outcomes is still limited (Fields et al. 2010). Newer team models may draw from the research on communication among interdisciplinary healthcare teams (IDT) in palliative care settings, which have proven to improve patient safety, satisfaction, and health outcomes during the last two decades (Hearn and Higginson 1998). The IDT model of care has been successful in health care because it increases the potential for coordinating patient care across medical subspecialties and professional roles. When teams are adopted as part of efforts to improve patient safety however, the focus on communication among team members is often minimized in favor of assessments of issues such as commitment to safety, attitudes toward stress, and knowledge of how to report adverse events (Sexton et al. 2006).

Critical issues and topics

Healthcare team communication often seeks to leverage information and resources for patient care across a variety of subspecialties. From a systems perspective, each team operates as a set of interrelated or interacting components, with 'formal and informal connections and relationships among its components' (Cushman and Craig 1976: 41), and shaped by necessity from the particularly specialized discourse of the healthcare profession itself (Candlin and Gotti 2004). Across time, team structures are constituted by regularities, patterns, traits, and values enacted through discourse among the members (Katz and Kahn 1978). Each specialized aspect of team functioning is a necessary element in the delivery of comprehensive patient health care, so team members' training and professional expertise, medical subspecialties, academic backgrounds, and professional affiliations shape the nature and goals of interactions.

Specialization and classification

A recent comprehensive analysis of team classification research found three underlying constructs impacting healthcare team communication across a myriad of team taxonomies and types: skill differentiation, authority differentiation, and temporal stability (Hollenback et al. 2012). Each team construct offers the opportunity for successful team communication, but also may contribute to miscommunication or conflict among members. Team skill differentiation is 'the degree to which members have specialized knowledge or functional capacities that make it more or less difficult to substitute members' (Hollenback et al. 2012: 94). The interdisciplinary composition of healthcare teams creates differentiation among members based on professional and personal training and experiences. Divergent language seeking to stress power based on skill differentiation was evident in data from Nicotera and Clinkscale's (2010) study of nurses at the nexus of healthcare teams:

> The comment is made, 'I am an RN. Get a tech to do certain things.' [it] used to be RNs working side-by-side with the techs. They should be helping each other … They do not work as a team. They need to understand that this is not 'my patient' or 'your patient,' it is 'our patient.'

Authority differentiation in teams refers to 'the degree to which decision-making responsibility is vested in individual members, subgroups of the team, or the collective as a whole' (Hollenback et al. 2012: 94). Authority differentiation is a major factor in healthcare teams because of laws and professional conventions, which mandate physicians' decision-making authority as leaders in the healthcare process. Like skill differentiation, authority differentiation may be stressed in team discourse aiming to reinforce power structures among team members (Nicotera and Clinkscale 2010). Marin et al.'s (1994) study of conflict among healthcare teams provided illustrations of conflict arising from boundaries for patient interaction based on authority differentiation. Among nurses in this study, patient advocacy communication was:

> 'a no win situation because someone would end up a victim, the doctor or the patient'
> 'you're damned if you do, damned if you don't'
> 'you want to make sure the patient knows what is going on, but you're not the doctor. It'd probably be a real sticky situation'
> 'As a patient advocate ... it's important to tell them [patients] what their rights are'... but 'it would get me into trouble with the surgeons.'

The temporal stability of a team is defined as, 'the degree to which team members have a history of working together in the past and an expectation of working together in the future' (Hollenbeck et al. 2012: 94). Temporal stability is a significant threat to communication effectiveness among healthcare team members because of the multi-organizational, multi-disciplinary, and multi-functional nature of health care. For example, physicians may routinely work with a healthcare team in a hospital for a period of time, but may not be present in the hospital when the physician does not have patients at the facility. Moreover, hospital staff members who work in shifts around the clock may be members of different teams based on their work schedule. Specialists who are members of a team delivering care for a specific disease, or to a specific patient population, would not be included if the same team cares for a variety of patients with a variety of diseases.

Synergy development

Researchers have identified five stages of development of a team, each of which impacts the quantity and type of communication among the members (Dodd 2008). In the first phase individuals come together to form a structural group, but members may lack information or confidence in a shared vision for the group's long-term goals. Team members begin seeking information from other members regarding the roles, expectations, and intended outcomes of their efforts. In the second phase, team members become more familiar with each other, and communicate about past conflicts or concerns that might inhibit the team's effectiveness. The third phase occurs when team members gain experience working together as a team. In this phase, team members begin to develop their own normative process for healthcare delivery as a team, and also begin to form expectations about individuals' personal and professional strengths and weaknesses as a team member. Peak performance of the healthcare team occurs in the fourth phase of team development, when an increase in trust among members fosters shared decision-making and open communication to achieve team goals. The final phase of development is characterized by highly productive and innovative team functioning where members with specialized responsibilities work together at peak efficiency. Teams operating at this level have relational and professional knowledge of each member, drawn from experience working as a team. Ad hoc teams working together for short periods may find it difficult to attain peak efficiency because of undefined roles and a lack of trust in the skills of individual members (Dodd 2008).

Benefits from team-based care may come from the synergistic nature of systems. All systems have synergy, which means the components interact in such a way that team interactions produce care that could not be produced by any one component of the system. Thus far, healthcare team researchers have not definitively identified the best way to maximize synergy through a particular team structure. Instead, the structure and management of individual teams seem to be contingent on the nature of the organizational and regulatory environment, and the specific goals of the team for patient care.

Interconnected interpersonal interactions

Interconnected interpersonal interactions are the central mechanism through which teams are constituted, but few interventions directly evaluate interactions among team members (Epstein and Street 2007; Jones and Stubbe 2004). Despite a 2008 call from the Institute of Medicine to, 'train residents in how to hand over their patients using effective communications,' few medical education programs place a strong emphasis on team communication skills as part of resident education (Institute of Medicine 2008). Despite the lack of team communication training, Kuziemsky et al. (2009) found healthcare team structures are constituted through interactions among members who work together to achieve two core communication goals: internal interactions among team members and external interactions on behalf of the team. Internal communication shaped and reinforced the team's identity, climate, and cultural norms regarding practices for implementation of policies and procedures. The extent to which individual team members felt empowered in their team roles was contingent upon internal interactions that bolstered mutual respect and shared decision-making among members. External interactions were more likely to focus on issues of workflow and interagency agreement regarding team decisions. Team climate was created by task and relational communication among internal and external parties, and climate was positively associated with team members' perceptions of their teams' quality, and patients' perceptions of the quality of care provided by the team (Mohr et al 2011). Although task climate may be relevant in considering the quality of team functioning, patients' perceptions of the team's relational climate may have a greater impact on quality of care measures (Mohr et al. 2011).

Boundaries

Teams coexist to achieve shared goals for their patients and membership is informally shaped by boundaries between internal and external forces. There are four general types of team boundaries, each of which has implications for communication between and among members. *Physical team boundaries* include the physical location of teams, the physical technology or equipment used to support team interaction, and any other physical tool or structure used to create secure team interactions. Teams may be co-located in a hallway or wing of a building, or they may use specific software to gain access to team-related tasks and discussions. Some technological channels of communication create impenetrable boundaries that connect team members, and separate the team from the external environment. Computer programs with password protection, for example, are useful only to the extent that all team members have access and knowledge of the program. Members may use face-to-face communication more often for interactions, or may coordinate care using an electronic medical record system. Virtual teams are not bound by any formal or geographical boundaries, but rather work together using technology such as videoconferencing systems or Internet-based communication portals.

Problematic physical boundaries for interdisciplinary healthcare teams may include a lack of access to the same paging system or records system to share information and coordinate care (O'Leary et al. 2010). *Linguistic team barriers* refer to specialized language used among members of the team in interactions with each other. *Systemic boundaries* dictate the rules that regulate interaction among members. Systems are often tied to the professional titles and levels of experience of each team member. The system of medical education, for example, dictates the nature of communication among medical residents, attending physicians, and other hospital staff. Ineffective team system boundaries are a source of consistent miscommunication. Examples of ineffective systems boundaries are teams with unclear role specialization, overlap of responsibilities among members who do not communicate, and a lack of a common communication channel to share information. *Psychological boundaries* restrict communication among team members due to stereotypes or prejudices held by individual members (Ledema 2007). For in-patient teams, research suggests regularly scheduled interdisciplinary rounds can be an effective way to overcome communication barriers that lead to miscommunication among teams (O'Mahony et al. 2007). Increased collegiality and information sharing during interdisciplinary rounds also contributed to reduced lengths of stay for patients.

Current contributions and research

Member communication creates healthcare team structures that vary based on the team's goal and the resources available to contribute to the formation and maintenance of the team. For example, many teams draw on individual expertise of members and extend across formal medical professional roles, medical specialties, and types of care. Diverse roles and dispersed boundaries among members increase the importance of streamlined and timely communication among all members.

Implementation of interdisciplinary teams

Some teams function as a unit within a larger organization, such as a hospital or clinic. This type of team may be comprised of individuals who work for the same organization, but whose functional role in the organization is shared among team members. An example of this is the approach of the patient-centered medical home (PCMH) or patient-aligned care team, which has recently been implemented by the US Military Health Service and Veteran's Administration. The PCMH has been implemented to care for diverse patient populations including those in primary care, mental health clinics, and among the homeless veteran population. The PCMH moves from a model of one physician caring for one ill patient, to a team-based model where a consistent group of providers care for patients by providing healthcare information, promoting prevention, and treating patients. Similar to the nursing model utilized for decades in the US, a PCMH is built by combining aspects of teamwork and patient-centered communication, and includes patients and family members as co-equal partners in their healthcare team and care. The team-based infrastructure of the PCMH means practice patterns across patients can be assessed because the same team serves a whole practice. A key aspect of the PCMH team is that each member plays a specialized role in the total care infrastructure. By shifting responsibility for certain tasks away from the physician to other team members, patients receive more care from more team members, but this shift requires coordinated and regular communication among team members.

Kuziemsky et al.'s (2009) study on interdisciplinary team communication found six core team processes: care planning, information exchange, teaching, decision-making, negotiation, and leadership. Of primary concern was the extent to which external information was shared among team members, and whether members felt empowered to negotiate and advocate for a particular decision or care plan. When teams engaged in shared decision-making and negotiation based on equal access to information, leaders were more likely to emerge in particular instances based on expertise and formal role expectations. Some evidence suggests the synergistic nature of teamwork can help healthcare professionals to make better decisions and reach more accurate conclusions than would be made by any one team member (Hearn and Higginson 1998). External communication processes are highly important to gain information and services from care partners including nursing homes, home health agencies, and medical specialists.

Multi-team systems

Successful healthcare delivery often requires multi-team systems where individuals communicate with members of their own team, and collectively communicate with members of other teams to achieve a collective goal (Zaccaro et al. 2011). A hospital multi-team system might be comprised of teams of nurses, physicians, technicians, and hospital administrators that are both independent from other teams, and interdependent upon other teams within the larger healthcare structure. Gray defines inter-organizational collaboration such as that required by multi-team systems as 'the process through which parties who see different aspects of a problem can constructively explore their differences and search for solutions that go beyond their own limited vision of what is possible' (1989: 5). Teams who work together typically require some level of deliberate negotiation and adjustment among members to create mutual goals, make decisions, and gain consensus on the teams' goals and plan of action. All team members must develop shared meanings by using a common language that reflects the diversity of contributing disciplines and organizational types to achieve a common goal of patient well-being.

Team research trends

Research examining all types of healthcare processes often takes place in the academic medicine context. Traditionally, the culture of health care places a greater value on technical proficiency among individuals over interpersonal skills competence. Medical education systems in the US teach and reward individual excellence and individual mastery of medical knowledge and skills, whereas group skills are rarely rewarded. Students receive grades, choose medical specialties, and ascend through their medical education based on individual achievement, and receive little or no training on team-based approaches to health care. Recently, however, renewed interest in practice-based research has spurred an increase in team-building activities during medical residency. Training and education meant to support the conduct of practice-based research may also provide new opportunities to conduct research on aspects of team communication and team functioning in the healthcare context.

Programs with successful research cultures among medical residents report a few common elements that mirror essential components of healthcare teams. First, scholarly activity must be viewed as valuable based on mentoring and modeling from other residents and program leaders. Like healthcare delivery teams, resident scholarship teams must be empowered to define team roles, and to engage in shared decision-making. Formal curricular activities also must include training and experience in the conduct of research, and there must be a team-like support system in place to mentor and assist residents in the research process (Seehusen and Weaver 2009).

Recent research examines the relationship between knowledge and skills gained from practice-based research teams during the medical residency, and attitudes toward participation in healthcare teams for patient care. These findings reveal similarities between the uncertainty experienced among residents regarding practice-based scholarship, and uncertainty among residents regarding shared patient care in healthcare teams. In the context of medical education, both types of teams provide opportunities for research on team-based care planning, information exchange, teaching, decision-making, negotiation, and leadership. In addition, research that assesses team processes and outcomes resulting from team training could provide valuable clues about attitudes and skills among clinicians who participate in team education programs. For example, a recent study examined the extent to which medical students trained in shared decision-making among teams successfully integrated their own communication of medical information and data with the preferences and values of patients and other clinicians on the healthcare team.

Many US health delivery organizations, such as the Joint Commission, the Institute for Healthcare Improvement, the National Quality Forum, and the Accreditation Council for Graduate Medical Education, have cited the importance of teamwork in health care (Baker et al. 2008). The National Defense Authorization Act of 2001 requires the Department of Defense to deliver team training through the Health Care Team Coordination Program, and the Joint Commission recommends all hospitals establish team training programs. These programs offer several new opportunities for research on team processes. For example, the US Department of Defense (DoD), in conjunction with the Agency for Healthcare Research and Quality (AHRQ), developed a comprehensive research protocol to assess healthcare team processes among DoD medical professionals. TeamSTEPPS, which stands for Team Strategies and Tools to Enhance Performance and Patient Safety, is the result of a multi-year research and development project by DoD and the AHRQ. The TeamSTEPPS curriculum is accompanied by a set of measures that tap into team members' attitudes toward team structure, leadership, mutual support, situation monitoring, and communication (Baker et al. 2008).

A recent analysis of team processes after TeamSTEPPS training examined communication in three high stress labor and delivery units. A combination of didactic training and simulated team activities were used to help participants learn, practice, improve, discuss, and receive feedback on necessary communication skills among team members. In labor and delivery teams, the combination of didactic training with in-situ communication-based simulation exercises led to a 37 percent improvement in perinatal morbidity (Riley et al. 2011). Studies involving didactic and simulation activities could provide formative research for expanded studies of teams engaged in other areas of patient care.

Recommendations for practice

Communication processes among team members serve different functions with a variety of impacts. For instance, research has demonstrated that well-organized patient-centered medical teams had a positive impact on racial and ethnic health disparities through enhanced access to the range of health providers (Beal et al. 2007). Research suggests in some instances minority patients are just as likely as Caucasians to have care when needed, receive preventive screening, and have chronic conditions managed appropriately when they receive care through a patient-centered team model.

Contexts

Communication is contextually bound, so the context of healthcare team communication often dictates the nature of team discourse in a given setting. Recent research examined multiple types of information sharing among team members within the context of an Emergency Room (Thomas et al. 2010). An example of this may be observed in the communication processes that occur with an Emergency Room team in the instance of an infant emergency resuscitation. Information about the event is shared as well as current status of the infant. The communication interaction as to the most likely cause of the distress and probable best course of action is manifested through observations, impressions, opinions, and questions. The team process work using verbal and nonverbal cues and these communication channels result in a team-coordinated intervention for the infant. However, differentiation of communication process is distinguished by the quality of the communication interactions of the team and the eventual outcomes of these processes in the context within which it occurs.

Processes

Team processes are rooted in collaboration among members (LaFasto and Larson 2001), so healthcare teams must be mindful of the process of their interactions. Communication in collaborative teams involves team building, respectful negotiation, conflict management, containment of negative behaviors, and workplace design to facilitate collaboration (Larson and LaFasto 1989). Additional attributes associated with successful team collaboration include willing participation of members, shared planning and decision-making, shared responsibilities and shared power based on knowledge or expertise (Henneman et al. 1995). For healthcare team collaboration to be effective, members must feel safe to communicate with team members to manage conflict and solve problems (LaFasto and Larson 2001).

Outcomes

Kuziemsky et al. (2009) outlined several patient outcomes resulting from team communication processes including reintegration to the family and home environment, adherence to treatment recommendations, communication satisfaction, and achievement of optimal health goals. Team communication processes were also linked to family caregivers' satisfaction with patient care, and caregivers' facilitation of discharge planning.

Future directions

Several innovations for improved team communication in healthcare settings are currently changing the nature of how healthcare teams organize, and interact on behalf of patients. Current trends include increased use of interdisciplinary teams (IDT) ; reflexive practice; situation, background, assessment, recommendation (SBAR); and e-health communication technology to facilitate team interactions. First, use of an interdisciplinary team in hospice end-of-life care is mandated by Federal law (Health Care Financing Administration 1983), and the utility of IDT is increasingly apparent. Medicare requirements dictate regular IDT meetings in order to develop holistic plans of care (Baldwin et al. 2011). In this setting, scholars have applied another model for interdisciplinary collaboration (Bronstein 2003) which demonstrates five main components similar to Dodd's (2008) model: interdependence between the team members, professional activities created by the team inception, flexibility, collective goal ownership, and reflection on the team processes to address patient and family care.

Second, use of 'reflective practice,' where discourse is contextualized (Schon 1983), can create an environment where the experiences and knowledge of the healthcare team members dictate the analysis, problem-solving, and therefore, solutions for the interdisciplinary communication strategies. Reflective practice provides the opportunity for internal and external feedback (Jones and Stubbe 2004), giving scholars a window into the contextual factors of the dynamic team interactions. The use of reflective practices can also serve to overcome the limitations of the communication audit process of diagnosis and prescription (Downs 1988) by allowing input by the practitioners themselves, in this case, healthcare team members. Implementing reflective practices to improve healthcare team communication strategies can serve to reduce the distance between theory and application (Jones and Stubbe 2004).

Third, the SBAR mental model framework is an increasingly popular communication tool in the US and Great Britain to improve patient safety and healthcare team communication

(Haig et al. 2006). SBAR – situation, background, assessment, and recommendation – was originally developed for use by flight crews in the US Navy. It was later imported into the healthcare field by employees of Kaiser Permanente to provide a routine structure for patient handoffs between shifts at hospitals (Haig et al. 2006). The goal is to limit extraneous and repetitive information during team interactions, and focus on four key issues that highlight necessary actions by team members. The following example comes from the Institute for Healthcare Improvement, and emphasizes the basic content and structure of SBAR:

- *Situation*: 'Dr. Jones, I have a 55 Y/O Man who looks pale, sweaty and is complaining of chest pressure'
- *Background*: 'He has a history of HTN, admitted for GI Bleed received 2 units, last crit two hours ago was 31 his vital signs are: BP 90/50, Pulse 120'
- *Assessment*: 'I think he's got an active bleed and we can't rule out an MI but we don't have a troponin or a recent H&H'
- *Recommendation*: 'I'd like to get an EKG and labs and I need for you to evaluate him in right away.'

SBAR offers several potential benefits to improve team communication. First, SBAR may help reduce medical errors caused by ineffective team communication by providing a routine and expected structure for team interactions. Second, the cognitive load of team members delivering information in a patient handoff or meeting may be reduced as use of SBAR becomes a routine practice over time. Routinization means using the framework diminishes uncertainty regarding which information needs to be conveyed to a team member caring for the same patient.

Fourth, and finally, team members are increasingly connected through virtual channels intended to improve interaction among team members, but certain mediated communication channels may actually serve to limit the need for interpersonal contact to achieve group goals. For example, providers now share information about patients using asynchronous communication such as electronic medical records (EMR) to coordinate care and medical decision-making. The proliferation of EMR facilitates virtual teamwork by allowing each team member to contribute to the record based on their individual task roles, and their individual experience with the patient. The running record can then be shared virtually among team members as a way to update each team member on the patient's progress and current health status. Research suggests virtual teams may experience less conflict and a higher level of performance than teams who communicate via face-to-face communication.

Related topics

Healthcare teams; organizational culture; interdisciplinary health care.

Further reading

A Healthcare-Delivery System for the Next Generation (2006) RCHE Publications. Paper 49. http://docs.lib.purdue.edu/rche_rp/49 (White paper based on summit covering important trends in health care such as clinical and business intelligence, efficiency and effectiveness of care, and personalized healthcare delivery.)

Ellingson, L.L. (2002) 'Communication, collaboration, and teamwork among health care professionals'. *Communication Research Trends*, 21(3): 1–44. (A thorough review of the emergent field of health communication regarding dyadic collaborations and teamwork trends.)

Nembhard, I.M. and Edmonson, A.C. (2006) 'Making it safe: the effects of leader inclusiveness and professional status on psychological safety and improvement efforts in health care teams'. *Journal of Organizational Behavior*, 27: 941–966. (The importance of leader inclusiveness within cross-disciplinary teams helps in overcoming existing power differentials allowing better collaboration.)

Office of Rural Health and Primary Care. Rural Health Advisory Committee Work Group (2009) *Rural Health Care: New Delivery Model Recommendations*. St. Paul, MN: ORHPC. (The challenge of healthcare delivery in rural resource-challenged areas offers unique opportunities for interdisciplinary teams to provide quality health care to rural patients.)

World Health Organization (2008) *Primary Health Care: Now More Than Ever*. The World Health Report. Geneva: WHO. (Responding to globalization of healthcare needs, teams are a critical part of providing primary health care.)

References

Baker, D., Krokos, K., and Amodeo, A. (2008) 'TeamSTEPPS teamwork attitude questionnaire manual. Agency for Healthcare Research and Quality. Online. Available http://teamstepps.ahrq.gov/abouttoolsmaterials.htm (accessed 11 September, 2011).

Baldwin, P., Wittenberg-Lyles, E., Oliver, D.P., and Demiris, G. (2011) 'An evaluation of interdisciplinary team training in hospice care'. *Journal of Hospice and Palliative Nursing*, 13(3): 172–182.

Beal, A.C., Doty, M.M., Hernandez, S.E., Shea, K.K., and Davis, K. (2007) *Closing the Divide: How Medical Homes Promote Equity in Health Care.* New York: The Commonwealth Fund.

Bronstein, L.R. (2003) 'A model for interdisciplinary collaboration'. *Social Work*, 48: 297–306.

Candlin, C.N. and Gotti, M. (2004) Special Issue: Intercultural discourse in domain-specific English. *Textus: English Studies in Italy*, 17(1): 5–16.

Crabtree, B., Nutting, P.A., Miller, W.A., Stange, K., Stewart, E., and Jaén, C.R. (2010) 'Summary of the National Demonstration Project and recommendations for the patient-centered medical home'. *Annals of Family Medicine,* 8: s80–90.

Cushman, D.P. and Craig, R.T. (1976) Communication systems: interpersonal implications. In G.R. Miller (ed.) *Explorations in Interpersonal Communication*. Beverly Hills, CA: Sage.

Dodd, C. (2008) *Managing Business and Professional Communication*. Boston, MA: Pearson.

Downs, C.W. (1988) *Communication Audits* (3rd edn). Glenview, IL: Scott Foresman.

Epstein, R.M. and Street, R.L., Jr. (2007) *Patient-Centered Communication in Cancer Care: Promoting Healing and Reducing Suffering*. NIH Publication No. 07-6225. Bethesda, MD: National Cancer Institute.

Fields, D., Leshen, E., and Patel, K. (2010) 'Driving quality gains and cost savings through adoption of medical homes'. *Health Affairs,* 29(5): 819–826.

Gray, B. (1989) *Collaborating: Finding Common Groups for Multiparty Problems*. San Francisco, CA: Jossey-Bass.

Haig, K., Sutton, S., and Whittington, J. (2006) 'SBAR: Shared mental models for improving communication among clinicians'. *Joint Commission Journal on Quality and Patient Safety,* 23: 167–175.

Health Care Financing Administration: Medicare Program Hospice Care: Final Rule (AMPHCFR): Health Care Financing Administration, Agency for Health Policy Research. Federal Register December 16, 1983.

Hearn, J. and Higginson, I.J. (1998) 'Do specialist palliative care teams improve outcomes for cancer patients? A systematic literature review'. *Palliative Medicine*, 12: 317–332.

Henneman, E., Lee, J., and Cohen, J. (1995) 'Collaboration: a concept analysis'. *Journal of Advanced Nursing*, 21: 103–109.

Hollenbeck, J.R., Beersma, B., and Schouten, M.E. (2012) 'Beyond team types and taxonomies: a dimensional scaling conceptualization for team description'. *Academy of Management Review*, 37(1): 82–106.

Ilgen, D.R. (1999) 'Teams embedded in organizations: some implications'. *American Psychologist*, 54: 129–139.

Institute of Medicine. (2008) *Resident Duty Hours: Enhancing Sleep, Supervision, and Safety.* Washington, DC: Institute of Medicine Press.

Joint Commission (2007) Sentinel event statistics. Online at: http://www.jointcommission.org/SentinelEvents/Statistics/ (accessed January 31, 2012).

Jones, D. and Stubbe, M. (2004) 'Communication and the reflective practitioner: a shared perspective from sociolinguistics and organizational communication'. *International Journal of Applied Linguistics,* 14(2): 185–211.

Katz, D. and Kahn, R.L. (1978) *The Social Psychology of Organizations*. New York: Wiley.

Kozlowski, S.W.J. and Bell, B.S. (2003) Work groups and teams in organizations. In W.C. Borman, D.R. Ilgen, and R.J. Klimoski (eds) *Handbook of Psychology: Industrial and Organizational Psychology* (Vol. 12: 333–375). Hoboken, NJ: Wiley.

Kuziemsky, C.E., Borycki, E.M., Purkis, M.E., Black, F., Boyle, M., Cloutier-Fisher, D., et al. (2009) 'An interdisciplinary team communication framework and its application to healthcare "e-teams" systems design'. *BMC Medical Informatics and Decision Making*, 9: 43.

LaFasto, F. and Larson, C. (2001) *When Teams Work Best: 6000 Team Members and Leaders Tell What It Takes to Succeed.* Thousand Oaks, CA: Sage.

Larson, C. and LaFasto, F. (1989) *Teamwork: What Must Go Right/What Can Go Wrong*. Newbury Park, CA: Sage.

Ledema, R. (ed.) (2007) *The Discourse of Hospital Communication: Tracing Complexities of Contemporary Health Organizations*. Basingstoke: Palgrave Macmillan.

LWP. (2009) *Language in the Workplace Project: Research*. Wellington: School of Linguistics and Applied Language Studies, Victoria University of Wellington. http://www.victoria.ac.nz/lals/lwp/research.aspx

Marin, M.J., Sherblom, J.C., and Shipps, T.B. (1994) 'Contextual influences on nurses' conflict management strategies'. *Western Journal of Communication*, 58: 201–228.

Mathieu, J.E., Maynard, M., Rapp, T., and Gilson, L.L. (2008) 'Team effectiveness 1997–2007: a review of recent advancements and a glimpse into the future'. *Journal of Management*, 34: 410–476.

Mohr, D.C., Young, G.J., Meterko, M., Stolzmann, K.L., and White, B. (2011) 'Job satisfaction of primary care team members and quality of care'. *Official Journal of the American College of Medical Quality*, 26: 18–25.

National Quality Forum. (2006) A national framework and preferred practices for palliative and hospice care quality: a consensus report. December. http://www.qualityforum.org/Publications/2006/12/A_National_Framework_and_Preferred_Practices_for_Palliative_and_Hospice_Care_Quality.aspx (accessed February 19, 2011).

Nicotera, A.M. and Clinkscales, M.C. (2010) 'Nurses at the nexus: a case study in structurational divergence'. *Health Communication,* 25: 32–49.

O'Leary, K.J., Ritter, C.D., Wheeler, H., Szekendi, M.K., Brinton, T.S., and Williams, M.V. (2010) 'Teamwork on inpatient medicine units: assessing attitudes and barriers'. *Quality and Safety in Health Care*, 19: 117–121.

O'Mahony, S., Mazur, E., Charney P., Wang, Y., and Fine, J. (2007) 'Use of multidisciplinary rounds to simultaneously improve quality outcomes, enhance resident education, and shorten length of stay'. *Journal of General Internal Medicine*, 22: 1073e9.

Putnam, L.L. and Nicotera, A.M. (2010) 'Communicative constitution of organization is a question: critical issues for addressing it'. *Management Communication Quarterly,* 24: 158–165.

Riley, W., Davis, S., and Miller, K. (2011) 'Didactic and simulation nontechnical skills team training to improve perinatal patient outcomes in a community hospital'. *Joint Commission Journal on Quality and Patient Safety,* 37(8): 357–364.

Schon, D. (1983) *The Reflective Practitioner: How Professionals Think in Action*. New York: Basic Books.

Seehusen, D.A. and Weaver, S.P. (2009) 'Resident research in family medicine: where are we now?' *Family Medicine,* 41(9): 663–668.

Sexton, J.B., Helmreich, R.L., Neilands, T.B., Rowan, K., Vella, K., and Boyden, J. (2006) 'The safety attitudes questionnaire: psychometric properties, benchmarking data, and emerging research'. *BMC Health Services Research*, 6: 44.

Thomas, E., Williams, A., Reichtman, E., Lasky, R., Crandall, S., and Taggert, W. (2010) 'Team training in the neonatal resuscitation program for interns: teamwork and quality of resuscitations'. *Pediatrics,* 125: 539–546.

Zaccaro, M., Marks, M., and DeChurch, L. (2011) *Multiteam Systems: An Organization Form for Dynamic and Complex Environments.* London: Routledge.

23

The interpenetration of communicative contexts

Examples from medical encounters

Aaron V. Cicourel

Introduction

A researcher's decision to tape-record conversation or discourse creates a contextual frame that limits what is to be identified as relevant data, their organization, and the kinds of analysis and inferences to which these data will be subjected. Research on conversation and discourse varies considerably in the extent to which an investigator will describe the circumstances of taping a conversation and her or his involvement with those taped. Similar conditions exist in other types of research on social interaction. For example, in field research, a participant observer must be sensitive to the fact that elicitation procedures can force informants to become aware of issues or conditions about which they normally are not aware or may be aware of only in the local context of everyday settings. Silverstein (1981) notes that much if not most of what is of interest to researchers is beyond the informant's ability to articulate meanings, in ways we would like or expect. The researcher's questions can create contextual frames that may not be consistent with informants' everyday practices. A similar problem exists in laboratory experiments of social interaction where status and role relations are foci of attention. The investigator's and subjects' conceptions of status and role relations are contingent on implicit and formally defined notions of 'context' created for the experimental occasion. We seldom know the extent to which simulated social relations reflect or are contrary to the kinds of experiences subjects have in their everyday encounters.

While many researchers will agree that talk and some notion of 'context' shape each other as part of an emergent process that changes through time and space, not all students of language use will concede that ethnographic material, participant attributes, and patterns of social organization that are constitutive of talk need to be included in studies of the structure of conversation or discourse. For example, conversation analysts (Sacks et al. 1974; Schegloff 1987) prefer to focus on such things as sequential organization, and how that organization creates local contextual elements in conversation. The researcher's use of social categories in any analysis must be linked to participants' recognition of the categories as integral to the events being studied. This research attitude can result in a very formal type of analysis. Linguistic approaches to discourse analysis (Brown and Yule 1983) also minimize the role of ethnographic and organizational conditions that can also result in a formal analysis of utterance sequences. What remains unclear is the extent to which the decision to tape or use particular materials includes or excludes explicit and tacit knowledge about reported and unreported ethnographic conditions, participant attributes, and patterns of social organization that can selectively shape subsequent analysis. The researcher can exercise considerable discretion in what the reader will be shown or told about 'context'.

The content of conversation or discourse material can be made to appear rather transparent when we use brief, formal or informal exchanges among people we do not know, who interact in settings described in a limited way, or when we use casual, mundane everyday conversations among friends during informal exchanges. When the research analyst is working in her or his own society, and the reader is expected to be from the same society, it is especially convenient to use brief, formal or informal mundane conversations. The investigator's ability to comprehend these exchanges is assumed to be self-evident and is seldom if ever an aspect of the analysis. But if a fuller analysis of participants' conversation and ethnographic understandings about activities, objects, and ideas is desired, and that understanding presupposes prior social experience, and/or technical, scientific, or professional training, then other strategies besides a completely local analysis must be employed.

Verbal interaction is related to the task at hand. Language and other social practices are interdependent. Knowing something about the ethnographic setting, the perception of and characteristics attributed to others, and broader and local social organizational conditions becomes imperative for an understanding of linguistic and non-linguistic aspects of communicative events.

In the present chapter, I discuss several settings within a larger organizational bureaucracy that contribute to two senses of 'context' that are routine aspects of conversational interaction in all everyday environments. One use of the term 'context' includes an institutionalized framing of activities. In traditional social science theorizing, it is customary to speak of group-derived prescriptive norms that pressure and/or channel people with designated titles, presumed competencies, duties or responsibilities into certain physical spaces at certain times in order to engage in a finite number of specifiable activities. Within this institutionalized context or framing of activities, emergent processes of talk appear that create a more narrow view of 'context' in the sense of locally organized and negotiated interaction.

The extent to which the investigator knows about the institutionalized and everyday events that participants and analysts categorize by the use of specific terms varies. For example, the analyst of particular settings may or may not be present when speech events are recorded. Within this more narrow sense of 'context', therefore, the analysis of a tape and transcript may or may not begin with the investigator's direct experience with the ethnographic setting in which the speech events were recorded.

When the investigator knows little or nothing about the speech event and the event is rather short-lived and apparently not viewed as part of or influenced by existing institutionalized or bureaucratic activities, what gets identified as context can be more easily located in the talk said to be attended by the participants. The investigator can begin her or his analysis by examining the way the conversation is initiated, the way intonation and stress are used, the content of lexical items and phrases, the occurrence of pauses or hesitations, turn-taking moves, and the way topics are introduced, sustained, and altered or changed. The focus of attention can become the sequential organization of conversation material that presupposes that participants, investigator, and reader all share a common knowledge base that is largely tacit or unstated but which becomes partially articulated by the way the investigator begins to make claims about the categories to which the participants are said to be attending. The investigator and reader presumably can each examine the same data and make claims and counter-claims about the clarity and substance of the analysis.

The methodological strategy of using local talk as the source of information in the narrow sense of context can be self-serving by the way the researcher not only ignores prior and current organizational or institutional experiences of participants, but by the kinds of data that are presented for analysis. For many students of language and social interaction, therefore, the notion of context need not include references to the participants' and researcher's personal, kin, and organizational relationships and other aspects of complex or institutionalized settings. Casual, fleeting speech events, however, are often constrained and guided by normative institutionalized features that we associate with encounters in public places described in general but vivid terms by Goffman (1959, 1963, 1971) among others. These brief exchanges can also carry considerable cultural and interpersonal 'baggage' for participants because of long-term social relationships unknown to or unattended by the investigator. The investigator who examines a speech event can therefore be forced to attend to its several senses of context narrowly or broadly because of the kinds of data presented to the reader.

The present chapter is identified explicitly with the view that both a broad and local sense of context are needed for the study of language use. The focus on discourse in the pages that follow should not be construed as being relevant only to conversational material, but also applies to the study of single utterances. I examine a complex environmental setting in order to underscore the importance of context at different levels of analysis. The following pages begin with a conversation in which three people emerge as speakers. Subsequent sections provide the reader with a brief overview of the organizational settings and the ethnographic circumstances in which the data were obtained. After investigating additional speech events, I close the chapter by illustrating how both immediate and other aspects of context must be taken into account if we are to understand language and social interaction in everyday life. The focus of this chapter, therefore, differs from but also builds on conversation and discourse theorists concerned primarily with the structural features of conversation such as turn-taking, side sequences, topicalization, coherence, and related notions. It is important to locate the analysis of language and social interaction in a wide variety of social activities that are implicitly and explicitly known to the participants and investigator.

A routine conversation

The speech event presented in Example 1 can be viewed as a routine conversation between three unidentified people who will be identified below.

Example 1: A conversation between three physicians

1 PA: (?) (low voice level) Is this the same one (we?)
2 (ya?) did yesterday?
3 IDA: No. This is the eye lady.
4 PA: (?)
5 IDA: Cellulitis
6 PA: Oh.
7 IDA: With group A strep..in shock
8 PA: In shock. (Slight rise in voice level) How about that.
9 IDA: I[t?] was gonna be more interesting [if she didn't
10 MR: [I'm(?)

IDA: have bacteremia but (laughing and voice level
increasing) now she's had [bacteremia so
MR: [There's a little, there's
little (voice level increases) problem with that
that I'll, will go into more as far
IDA: Yeah.
MR: how much shock she really [was in,
IDA: [was in, right
MR: compared to what [abrupt shift] she's a liver lady.
you know, an' I don't know what her blood pressure sits
at. [It may not be real high to [start with.
IDA: [Right. [Right.
PA: So she didn't have peripheral, evidence of shock
really? [Just a low blood pressure.
MR: [No, she wasn't, she wasn't ever clamp, you
know
PA: Uh huh
MR: clamped down *or* flushed or anything
PA: OK
MR: I can .. and, and she doesn't
[abrupt shift] one thing that argues
against a lot of neuropathy, you know, from diabetes, for
one, she's only had it for three years, but two, you know,
her neuro exam an' her an' her peripheral vascular exams,
is really normal, is normal sensory, good pulses distally,
and stuff, and I just have a hard time,
PA: Yeah
MR: there'd be a lot of sy-sympathetic, you know
PA: Right
MR: phone calls.
IDA: Have they got sinus films on yer yet?

Notes: Each dot between words = one second. The brackets indicate points of overlap in the exchange.

Telling the reader that three physicians are involved is an initial attempt at penetrating what is occurring in this encounter. Lines 1–12 strongly suggest that the participants are engaged in a discussion regarding the medical condition of some other party. The investigator's control over when and what material will be shown to the reader can, therefore, vary considerably and can create different interpretive frames. Saying that three physicians (they also could be other healthcare providers) are talking implies that they are probably in a medical facility of some kind, but there is no indication of precisely what kind or part of a healthcare facility they are in. Nor can we be sure if the patient is nearby, is an inpatient or an outpatient. We know nothing about the physicians' gender or personal characteristics nor their specialties. Nor do we know if this information is relevant to the analysis.

The opening lines (1–8) of Example 1 do not mention the term 'physicians' nor is there any indication in lines 1–3 that a 'patient' is involved. Having identified the three participants as 'physicians', we can also say that they are talking about a 'patient' who has been dubbed the 'eye lady', for some unstated reason, or a patient who is experiencing difficulty with her eye.

Although the content of lines 1–3 of Example 1 ('Is this the same one [we?] [ya?] did yesterday? No. This is the eye lady.') does not suggest a healthcare facility, physicians, a patient with eye problems, and the term 'cellulitis' in line 5 might be recognizable enough to send us to a medical dictionary as we begin our analysis. Alternatively, we might seek help from informants or examine further sequences of conversation in the hope that other lexical items, phrases, prosodic features of the talk, or thus far unstated non-verbal perceptions might increase our understanding of this encounter. For example, notice the remark by IDA in line 7 ('group A strep .. in shock'), which could refer to an infection. The comment or observation by PA in line 8 ('In shock. How about that.') could be interpreted as expressing interest in the categories supplied by IDA and perhaps mild surprise. The subsequent remarks by IDA in lines 9, 11, and 12 of Example 1 ('I[t?] was gonna be more interesting if she didn't have bacteremia but now she's had bacteremia so') suggest that PA and IDA are both familiar with the terms 'cellulitis', 'group A strep', 'in shock', and 'bacteremia'.

The significance the analyst attributes to particular utterances or to their sequential order, and claims about the participants' perception and understanding of a speech event, are often the result of examining subsequent utterances (Sacks et al. 1974). If we do not invoke institutional and local socio-cultural details with which to identify the participants of conversation, the analysis of meaning is nearly impossible.

I will now abruptly shift my mode of analysis by telling the reader something about the participants in Example 1 and about how the data were obtained. The setting is generally known to the reader and investigator alike because of a commonsense understanding of categories such as 'patient', 'healthcare facility', 'medical center', 'hospital', and 'medical school'. Stating that the talk is in a medical setting does not tell the reader that there is medical talk taking place nor who is doing the talking and with what credentials. But claiming the participants in a given speech event are physicians talking about a particular (technical sense of) 'patient' orients us to categories we associate with particular members of a medical setting and a basis for making claims about the use of these categories in their talk. The term 'patient', for example, is used in at least two ways in this chapter.

For the reader of this chapter, the term 'patient' probably implies a commonsense notion of someone who is not feeling well or is 'sick'. For the healthcare expert, however, the term 'patient' can activate thoughts about someone with neurophysiological, biochemical, and psychopathological symptoms and conditions that are part of an extensive technical compositional semantics and clinical as well as mundane experiences. For the most part, the term 'patient' will be used in the second sense just noted. Thus, even mundane terms such as 'eye lady' (line 3, Example 1) and 'she's a liver lady' (line 19, Example 1) imply an activation of technical knowledge and experiences that are part of complex socially organized activities.

The research setting and types of participants

The case material I present in this chapter represents a small portion of data from field research in two teaching hospitals. The material is part of routine institutionalized bureaucratic activities that are typically associated with healthcare delivery in Western countries. My observations and tape-recording of activities mostly involved physician–patient, physician–physician, or physician–technician interaction, and also include extensive field notes about the settings and the participants.

The medical settings observed are typical of teaching hospitals but are not necessarily representative of other clinic or hospital settings in which there is an absence of House Staff (interns, residents, and training fellows). The inclusion of House Staff adds hierarchical relationships and hence additional bureaucratic conditions that differentiate teaching from non-teaching hospitals. Additional details about organizational conditions, the influence of status and role relationships, and the expertise or background knowledge associated with such designations will be provided as the chapter unfolds.

The range of speech events in these settings can be diverse and can include a quick exchange of greetings, brief exchanges of gossip or rumors about patients, or staff, and discussion about the local baseball or football team's fortunes. There also can be brief and lengthy exchanges between physician and patient, technical discussions among physicians and between physicians and nurses or technicians, and somber or emotionally charged exchanges between family members and healthcare personnel. The exchanges can occur in a variety of settings such as the patient's room, in a clinic examining room, a hall or corridor, an empty elevator, the cafeteria, at the X-ray facility, the nurses' station, or a laboratory.

Over a period of months, I observed and then began to tape-record various clinical exchanges. These exchanges included outpatient clinics where patients may be seen initially or as a follow-up from prior visits or inpatient service. I also accompanied the resident or attending physician on ward rounds, or visits to the X-ray facility, to daily laboratory rounds, and to weekly grand or teaching rounds where cases of unusual interest are presented before attendings (one or more physicians qualified to supervise residents) from the county and residents from several hospitals.

The ethnographic activities alluded to above obviously provided many opportunities to express my ignorance about medicine and to ask questions of different experts. The field research was facilitated by my official connection with a school of medicine. Knowing some of my informants independently of the research setting because of committee activities in the School of Medicine made participation in the research setting easier and enabled me to ask many 'dumb' questions as a non-medical specialist. But familiarity with the settings can also create problems. For example, my colleagues sometimes forgot that I am not a physician and spoke to me as if I were fully capable of understanding technical matters that were discussed. I often pretended to seem informed in order to not disturb the speech event, but later would have to ask for help.

My ethnographic experiences, consultations with people called 'physicians', and occasional uses of a medical dictionary enabled me to take a number of liberties in describing the material in Example 1. I can tell the reader that there is a female inpatient located in a medical teaching hospital with an eye problem as well as additional difficulties associated with the technical terms 'group A strep' (line 7), 'shock' (line 7), and 'bacteremia' (line 11). I rely on the reader's commonsense understanding and my use of expert informants to claim that the physicians are talking about someone with an infection and perhaps something more serious (as may be evident by the references to 'shock' and 'bacteremia'). Less transparent here is the remark by IDA (lines 9–12) that the case would have been more interesting if the patient did not have bacteremia.

Re-examining the conversation in Example 1

The exchange in Example 1 does not state that the three participants are attached to a healthcare facility of some kind nor is there any mention of a patient. The conversation begins in line 1 with the introduction of a topic ('Is this the same one ... ') and a reference to some object or someone that had something done to it the day before.

In the second section above, I alluded to the possible content of lines 1–7 of Example 1. An analyst might choose to ignore further discussion of content at this point and instead could focus on who speaks first and how someone responds, identifying turns, the selection of next speaker, topicalization, side sequences, adjacency pairs, registers used, topic and comment, deictic, anaphoric, metaphoric, and metanymic expressions, to mention some familiar aspects of the study of language in social interaction.

The opening question by PA ('Is this the same one [we?] [ya?] did yesterday?') in line 1, Example 1, can be seen as topicalizing an unidentified but particular type of object that other participants presumably recognize as fitting into a specific subset of a general category. We can subsequently categorize this object as a 'patient' in the technical sense by assuming the participants are healthcare providers of some kind. The response by IDA in line 3, Example 1, rejects a particular subset of the unidentified hypothesized category but does allude to another subset by stating 'This is the eye lady.' In lines 5, 7, and 12 of Example 1, IDA seems to clarify the hypothesis about the category 'patient' by describing particulars such as 'cellulitis', 'group A strep', 'in shock', and 'bacteremia'.

The opening question by PA in line 1, Example 1, might also be loosely interpreted as one part of an adjacency pair (e.g., question–answer sequence) in which the second part consists of the 'No' of line 3 by IDA. Perhaps this type of analysis might be stretched even more if we ignore the 'No' of line 3 and the 'Oh' of line 6 and say that the second part of the adjacency pair consists of fragments from lines 3, 5, 7, and possibly 12 of Example 1. To paraphrase the exchange, PA's question in line 1, 'Is this the same one (we?) (ya?) did yesterday?' is answered by IDA in lines 3, 5, 7, and possibly 12 ('No. This is the eye lady', 'Cellulitis', 'With group A strep ... in shock', and 'now she's had bacteremia'). If we go beyond this loose illustration of sequential analysis, we can ask how much local context is the analyst required to construct in order to convince herself or himself and the reader that the interpretations being claimed are adequate for some sequence of text?

What counts as 'relevant ethnographic details'?

I observed the exchange in Example 1 as well as other exchanges involving this patient. Consequently, I can assert from my notes that PA turned directly to IDA when posing the question about the 'same one' in line 1. The speech event can be further clarified by noting that PA refers to a Pathology Attendant who is the Chief of the Microbiology Laboratory, and IDA is the Infectious Disease Attending. MR is the infectious disease Medical Resident for the rotation period during which the event occurred.

The exchange reported in Example 1 occurred after MR and IDA had both interviewed the patient and had discussed the case. Their participation in the encounter reported in Example 1 had already been anticipated because of the expected earlier exchange. PA is the expert here and methodically examines a series of small slips of paper each morning at 11:00 a.m. in which new or additional information about a patient's cultures is noted. IDA is also an expert about microbiological aspects of each patient, particularly the clinical ramifications of the case. By addressing IDA, PA asks the responsible clinical expert about the case in order to contextualize the laboratory findings. There are other people in the corner of a large room (which is actually one part of the suite in which the microbiology labs are located). There often is a fourth-year medical student doing a month's rotation in infectious disease cases, a pathology resident who assists PA with laboratory details including the cultures for each patient, slides, and petrie dishes to be examined that morning, an infectious disease resident from pediatrics, and one or two teaching fellows.

In a teaching hospital, IDA may begin with a few comments on the case but normally turns it over to MR for the details. After this, PA first examines the slide or cultures and either directly describes the morphology of the organism(s) or invites the medical student or fellow or a resident to tell the group what organism(s) is/are involved. PA then invariably gives the group additional information about the nature of the organism, the kinds of disease and/or symptoms associated with the laboratory findings, and the patient's likely prognosis with different types of treatment.

The opening line of Example 1, therefore, assumes coherence by reference to a presumed activity done with thus far unidentified others the day before. As noted above, the unidentified others in the present case are the MR and IDA. The response by IDA in line 3 shifts the topic to someone called 'the eye lady'. The inaudible comment by PA in line 4 of Example 1 could have been a request for details about the case. IDA provides one detail ('cellulitis'). From my watching his facial expression and hearing the intonation of his voice ('Oh' in line 6), I infer that the term is of interest to PA. When IDA provides additional information about the patient, PA repeats the last phrase ('in shock') and with a slightly rising voice level seems to be expressing mild surprise ('How about that'). Then IDA, in lines 9, 11, and 12, refers to how much more interesting the case would have been if the patient had not had 'bacteremia' ('I[t?] was gonna be more interesting if she didn't have bacteremia but now she's had bacteremia so'). MR, however, in lines 10 and 13–17 ('There's a little, there's little problem with that that I'll, will go into more as far how much shock she really was in') seems to be questioning the patient's 'shock' and these doubts are related to the issue of bacteremia with or without shock.

The remark by IDA in line 18 of Example 1 repeats the last two terms used by MR and adds 'right' as if to support MR's observation. Earlier, I was with IDA and MR when the two discussed the case and knew that there were doubts expressed (in two separate medical histories) by other physicians about the patient's 'shock'. MR's completion of his remark from line 17 (stated as 'compared to what' in line 19) was followed by an abrupt shift in the topic. Presumably the patient's 'shock' was to be contrasted with an unstated something else ('compared to what') when MR decided to abruptly shift the topic to the patient's liver ('she's a liver lady, you know'). So in addition to being 'the eye lady' of line 3, the metaphor shifts to that of 'liver lady'. The reader's technical knowledge may be strained by the phrase 'a liver lady'. My participation in the setting tells me we have a patient with a current eye problem and a prior liver problem attributed to a history of alcohol abuse.

On the basis of previous conversations with informants, I can report that one clinical sign of shock is very low blood pressure. MR's remark in line 21 ('It may not be real high to start with') refers to the time of admission for the patient when her blood pressure was observed to be low but where no one (including the patient) was aware of her normal blood pressure. The inference of possible shock, therefore, can be problematic depending on the patient's normal blood pressure. IDA had contributed to MR's remarks through their previous conversations the day before, and the 'Right' uttered twice by IDA in line 22 could signal agreement with the present observation by MR and/or IDA's prior contribution. After reading the transcript, however, IDA reported that the intent of saying 'Right' twice was to hurry MR into expediting his delivery and remarks.

In lines 23–24, PA provides some clarification of the patient's alleged shock by his 'declarative–interrogative' that the patient apparently 'didn't have peripheral, evidence of shock really? Just a low blood pressure'. Although appearing to be a question, PA's remarks are spoken authoritatively through the use of a somewhat 'matter of fact' or 'self-confident' intonation and the mildly assertive nature of the content. There is also the ethnographic element that he is the primary expert here and can be indirectly asserting this expertise by his remarks in lines 23–24.

MR's rambling remarks in lines 25–36 of Example 1 address several possible topics that presuppose background in clinical medicine. For an attending, MR's remarks can become the basis for an organizational assessment of the resident or novice in infectious diseases. As non-medical specialists, students of language use in social interaction, we can only superficially assess the import of the material in Example 1 unless we seek the help of informants and have access to the kind of ethnographic information provided thus far.

Expanding the ethnographic context

I have presented a partial description of the way the selection of different ethnographic or organizational settings and types of speech events or social interaction can affect the analyst's interpretation of the research materials presented to a reader. In this chapter, I have ignored several administrative, professional, and technical matters that affect how patients are admitted into a medical setting, are diagnosed, and treated by different healthcare delivery personnel.

The present case involves a 48-year-old white female whose chief complaint was recorded in her admission history and physical examination as 'swelling of the left eye'. Additional details can be found in Cicourel (1987). Of interest here is her primary diagnosis of 'periorbital cellulitis' or what was described as a 'right-upper-lid abscess with periorbital cellulitis'. My informants helped me translate this last phrase into an infected, swollen-shut left eye, that seemed highly inflamed to me, with purplish coloring of the skin around the eye that was apparently caused by blood seeping into the skin. The patient's left side of her face was swollen as well as her eye and ear. There was pus oozing out of the area of the eyelids.

I accompanied MR when he first went to the medical ward to see the patient. Before interviewing the patient, MR went to the nurses' station to review the patient's chart. As is often the case with infectious disease patients, an attending physician other than IDA usually will see a patient admitted to the medical service. In the present case, two attendings had interviewed the patient and had ordered laboratory tests before asking for an infectious disease consultation. The results of these tests were reported in the chart. MR's infectious-disease-oriented interview of the patient, therefore, was in part influenced by his having had access to the patient's medical chart. MR's questions, therefore, reflect aspects of these prior experiences.

In addition, this interview is influenced by his prior medical school training. The medical student's knowledge of infectious diseases can be traced to one or two courses (depending on the quarter of semester basis of the medical school) in microbiology. I attended some of the lectures in microbiology and also interviewed the director of the course, who is also PA in the conversation of Example 1. With the help of informants, it is possible to trace aspects of the basic science concepts and clinical medicine experience medical students are exposed to before they enter an intern or residency program. Knowing something about the physician's prior experiences in medical school and as a House Officer can provide the analyst and reader with possible aspects of the background knowledge tacitly or explicitly assumed or employed during a speech event. I do not have time to present all of the content of my interview with PA in his role as the microbiology course director, but instead will provide the reader with a few highlights that can be linked to the conversation in Example 1.

Trying to trace the kinds of basic and clinical science concepts that medical students and House Staff are exposed to before they attain the status of 'attendings' is not meant to imply that such codifiable knowledge is the primary source of background necessary for the diagnostic reasoning and treatment directed at patients. In my work on medical communication and diagnostic reasoning, I have stressed the importance of tacit clinical experience and the everyday understanding of mundane social interaction as aspects of a world presumed to be known in common but not necessarily examined reflexively by participants in the medical or any other area of life (Cicourel 1982, 1986, 1987). I call the reader's attention, however, to the necessity of incorporating systematically codified knowledge (textbooks, detailed lectures, laboratory practices, apprentice-like experiences) into our understanding of bureaucratic and non-bureaucratic language use and social interaction. Inasmuch as sociolinguistics tends to address various kinds of everyday events in which the analyst can 'pass' as an expert because of her or his background in language use and social interaction, the analysis of content is often viewed as fairly straightforward. By calling the reader's attention to the role of multiple ethnographic and/or organizational settings and informants, I underscore the complexity of the term 'context' or 'local' and more abstract senses of culture or social organization for understanding language use and social interaction.

According to the microbiology course director during an interview obtained early in my research and noted above, students should remember the following:

Example 2

'... what are the important bacteria, and, in terms of human
disease, and what are their unique microbiologic
characteristics ... The streptococci can be differentiated
into the hemolytic ones and the non-hemolytic ones and
green ones. Those that are alpha-hemolytic make green
colonies. And among the beta-hemolytic ones we have the
group A strep, which is really the only accepted cause of
bacterial pharyngitis ... The streptococci are in chains,
the pseudomonas and the enterobacteriaceae are gram negative
rods, and they look a lot alike on the gram stain ...
And if you look at the streptococci for a minute, the group
A strep, is able to cause sore throats primarily because of
the M protein ...
... what are the unique microbiologic characteristics that
permit me to recognize this organism, let's say right out
of the blood culture bottle like you've seen us do up
there? ... Did this patient have cellulitis, or lymphangitis?
Yes. Well, then it's probably a group A strep ...

The technical remarks by the pathologist made during the interview conducted before the completely independent laboratory conversation of Example 1 refer to the clinical consequences medical students are expected to remember from courses in microbiology. The references to 'streptococci' (line 3), 'beta-hemolytic ones' (line 6), and 'group A strep' (line 7) in Example 2 are directly related to the 'sore throats' of line 12 and are a significant aspect of the diagnostic reasoning employed in the present case. Notice the reference to 'cellulitis' and its association with 'group A strep' in lines 17–18. The pathologist's remarks provide clear evidence of prior training on the part of physicians that plays a role in job-related speech events. Such training may be important not only to participants, but also to the analyst's understanding of medical communication and semantic aspects of diagnostic reasoning in the case under review and in medical settings generally.

The concepts mentioned by the pathologist in Example 2 are not merely aspects of textbook knowledge associated with prior training, but are also part of a medical student's laboratory experiences with the microorganisms noted in Example 2. Without this background knowledge based on studying textbooks, listening to lectures, and working in a laboratory setting, it would be rather difficult for a participant to display her or his group membership in the conversation of Example 1. In the case of a medical resident, there will have been prior experiences as an intern in which aspects of the material in Example 1 will have been discussed.

Another source of background knowledge that can influence speech events in medical settings is the way that novice physicians are exposed to an initial lecture (also given to them as a written handout) when they begin their training. The following lines are from lecture notes developed by an infectious disease attending physician. I quote selectively from the written handout given to the House Staff.

Example 3

'I. Septicemia – microbial agents in the bloodstream ...

B. One is led to the diagnosis of bloodstream infection by a **sudden change** in clinical state ...

All sorts of organisms can cause hypotension, but, **in the absence of hypoxia (pneumonia) or heart failure,** gram-negative bacteremia with endotoxemia is by far the most common cause of sustained hypotension ...

D. Other causes of infectious shock

3. Streptococcal shock (group A strep), often in the absence of bacteremia, associated with soft tissue infections (usually severe) ... '

Of interest are references to 'microbial agents in the bloodstream' (line 1), 'the diagnosis of bloodstream infection by a **sudden change** in clinical state' (lines 2–4), and 'organisms [that] can cause hypotension' such as 'gram-negative bacteremia with endotoxemia' (lines 5–7). A sudden change in clinical state can be a drop in blood pressure (hypotension), which in turn can be linked to the release of bacteria or endotoxins in the bloodstream that can lead to shock. The most succinct remark can be found in lines 10–13 of Example 3 because it comes fairly close to the case described in Example 1. The patient was found to have group A strep and bacteremia as noted by IDA in Example 1. The case revealed bacteremia but MR claimed the patient may not have been in shock. The presence of shock was never confirmed. The remarks contained in Example 3 and given to House Staff at the two hospitals in which I conducted my research directly associate this background material to specific aspects of the exchange in Example 1.

I will close this section by quoting a brief excerpt from MR's original interview with the patient. The interview occurred prior to the speech event reported in Example 1.

Example 4

I wanna take (?) your blood. (?) blood pressure (?)
(.....) (mumbling) A lot of people get, bacteria
in their blood, and ya get uh shock. [Low monotone
intonation] When your blood pressure goes down
because it means (?) the bacteria releases certain
toxins, depending on (?) area (?) [raised intonation]
Has your, blood pressure always run kind of on the low
side, ma'am?

Before MR and I entered the ward to see the patient, MR had reviewed the patient's chart and was aware of the two prior medical histories therein and hence was also aware of the suspected diagnosis of bacteremic shock. MR was also aware of many other medical facts and hypotheses about the patient's condition. MR's explanation (only partly shown here) to the patient about her medical problems (linking a drop in blood pressure to a prior release of 'certain toxins') can be linked directly to the prior medical histories that existed in the patient's chart, the infectious disease attending's written handout, and the pathologist's description of what medical students should remember of their coursework in microbiology. In turn, all of these matters, plus MR's interview with the patient, had an effect on the remarks by PA, IDA, and MR in Example 1.

Concluding remarks

The chapter has presented a few of the large number of interpenetrating medical events that form the local context for language use and social interaction in any given encounter. I have sought to discuss the topic of local context in terms of those cultural and organizational constraints, normative expectations, and immediate conditions that surround local speech events as they unfold.

The notion of interpenetrating medical communicative contexts seeks to place the local mutual shaping of talk and context into a framework that incorporates structural and processual aspects of social organization and reasoning during social interaction. The medical setting I chose as the point of departure for the present chapter was the source of a conversation between three physicians. The material presented in Example 1 can be subjected to different types of interpretation, contingent on the analyst's orientation to language use and social interaction and the extent to which the notions of background and context are employed.

The local interaction in Example 1 is intended to call the reader's attention to outside organizational experiences or institutionally guided and constrained social interaction and/or speech events that are directly relevant to the way local exchanges are likely to occur. For example, the interaction described in Example 1 can be linked to the microbiological aspects of medical education (Example 2) and the lecture on Septicemia (Example 3) given to the House Staff at the beginning of the medical academic year. All social interaction and/or speech events presuppose and are informed by analogous prior forms of socially organized experiences.

The analyst's decision to describe the materials in Example 1 as an exchange between three healthcare delivery workers or professionals creates a cultural context for the analyst and reader and simultaneously calls attention to the use of social categories that hopefully can be attributed to participants' recognition of their relevance for the speech event being examined. The analyst's decision to focus on particular sociolinguistic notions (topicalization, turn-taking, speech act categories, coherence, types of deixis, frozen expressions, preferred sequences, etc.) rather than the interrelationship between discourse and culture or the interrelationship between discourse and linguistic theory, can trigger different expectations on the part of the reader.

Telling the reader that the three participants in Example 1 are physicians, that the exchange took place in a hospital microbiology laboratory while they were discussing a patient with suspected bacteremic shock, and preparatory to examining the patient's blood cultures, creates a cultural context within which the analyst and reader can understand what transpires. Our understanding deepens when the physicians are identified as a pathology attending, an infectious disease attending, and an infectious disease medical resident. Not only are the expressive style and the content observed contingent on organizationally constrained status and role relationships that can influence who speaks first, whose views will be influential or will prevail vis-à-vis action to be taken, but the analyst's and reader's ability to comprehend the significance of broader and local socio-cultural issues may require extensive consultation with medical experts.

The present case actually began with MR and the researcher going to the nurses' station of a university medical center medicine ward to examine the medical chart of a patient suspected of having bacteremic shock. MR was performing an organizational obligation of initiating a consultation requested of the Division of Infectious Diseases.

The material from the microbiology course presented above reflects information medical students are expected to know, and the excerpts from the lecture given to new House Staff reflect the kinds of training experiences a novice like an intern or resident physician is likely to possess when reading a patient's chart and then interviewing the patient.

By the time the case reached the microbiology laboratory rounds depicted in Example 1, the patient had also been interviewed by IDA; MR and IDA had discussed the case in some detail; IDA had interviewed the patient; and IDA had consulted the patient's chart, added to it, and had consulted two standard textbooks on microbiology.

The analysis of material in Example 1, the excerpts on the microbiology course (Example 2), the infectious disease attending's lecture notes for new House Staff (Example 3), and the fragment from MR's interview with the patient (Example 4) represent a small part of a complex set of interpenetrating contexts. In the present chapter, I have documented only minimally the way informants helped me understand organizational conditions, local speech events and social interaction, the meaning of complex concepts, and procedures from basic and clinical medical science and practical experiences. I have, however, employed several types of ethnographic and textual materials in order to underscore what I have characterized as unavoidable aspects of organizational and local constraints and processes that are integral to rethinking 'context'.

A nagging issue that undoubtedly remains for many readers is the familiar one that an infinite regress can occur whereby the observer presumably must describe 'everything' about a context. Such a demand is of course impossible to satisfy because no one could claim to have specified all of the local and larger socio-cultural aspects of a context. Observers or analysts, like participants of speech events, must continually face practical circumstances that are an integral part of all research or everyday living. As researchers, we obviously privilege some aspects of a context while minimizing or ignoring other conditions. The observer is obligated to justify what has been included and what has been excluded according to stated theoretical goals, methodological strategies employed, and the consistency and convincingness of an argument or analysis. Meaning and understanding in everyday life are contingent on cognitive and linguistic activities, that is a knowledge of how to use language structures that we call metonyms, metaphors, and other imaginative constructions associated with particular lexical items, phrases or utterances, and personal experiences. Therefore, some specification of the environmental conditions in which these language practices emerge, are embedded, and evolve should guide the researcher's depiction of context. I have tried to indicate some of the conditions that can be identified in a medical setting to illustrate the way different senses of the term 'context' can be pursued conceptually and empirically.

Acknowledgments

Parts of this chapter were initially presented at the Invited Session 'Rethinking "Context": Language as an Interactive Phenomenon, Part I' (Society for Linguistic Anthropology and General Anthropology Division), American Anthropological Association annual meeting, Philadelphia, PA, December 1986. A version of the paper appeared in the *Social Psychology Quarterly.* The present version has been expanded slightly and further revised. I am grateful to Charles Davis and Elizabeth Ziegler for their invaluable support and advice, and to Sandro Duranti, Charles Goodwin, Douglas Maynard, Hugh Mehan, James Wertsch, and two anonymous referees for their helpful substantive suggestions on earlier drafts. Douglas Maynard also provided very useful editorial suggestions.

Related topics

Diagnostic reasoning; medical education; cognitive sociology; situated interpretation; context.

Further reading

Cicourel, A.V. (1973) *Cognitive Sociology,* Harmondsworth: Penguin.

——(1980) 'Three models of discourse analysis: the role of social structure', *Discourse Processes* 3: 101–132.

Duranti, A. and Goodwin, C. (1992) *Rethinking Context: Language as an Interactive Phenomenon,* Cambridge: Cambridge University Press.

References

Brown, G. and Yule, G. (1983) *Discourse Analysis,* Cambridge: Cambridge University Press.

Cicourel, A. (1982) 'Language and belief in a medical setting', in H. Byrnes (ed.) *Contemporary Perceptions of Language: Interdisciplinary Dimensions,* Washington, DC: Georgetown University Press.

——(1986) 'The reproduction of objective knowledge: common sense reasoning in medical decision making', in G. Bohme and N. Stehr (eds) *The Knowledge Society,* Dordrecht: Reidel Publishing.

——(1987) 'Cognitive and organizational aspects of medical diagnostic reasoning', *Discourse Processes* 10: 346–367.

Goffman, E. (1959) *The Presentation of Self in Everyday Life,* Garden City, NY: Doubleday Anchor Books.

——(1963) *Behavior in Public Places,* New York: Free Press.

——(1971) *Relations in Public,* New York: Basic Books.

Sacks, H., Schegloff, E.A., and Jefferson, G. (1974) 'A simplest systematics for the organization of turn-taking for conversation', *Language* 50: 696–735.

Schegloff, E.A. (1987) 'Between macro and micro: contexts and other connections', in J. Alexander, B. Giesen, R. Munch, and N. Smelser (eds) *The Micro-Macro Link,* Berkeley, CA: University of California Press.

Silverstein, M. (1981) *The Limits of Awareness* (Sociolinguistic Working Paper 84), Austin, TX: Southwest Educational Development Laboratory.

24

Mental healthcare professionals' role performance

Challenges in the institutional order of a psychiatric hospital

Branca Telles Ribeiro, Diana de Souza Pinto, and Claudio Gruber Mann[1]

> *Nilma*: I got in the ward, not thinking much, two patients were having sex. I admit that, I've been here for a while. ..... then I put my hands up and said 'what's happening here?' (laughter) (...) but that was the only reaction I had. Then they left and I didn't know what to say, either 'you can't do this' or 'can do this but not (here).' You're not ready when it happens, you know it happens, yet you don't expect to see it .....

Introduction

This chapter discusses how a group of psychiatric professionals perceive and respond to patients' sexual activities when they are confined to a psychiatric institution. In this study, Mental Health Care Professionals (MHCP) from the Institute of Psychiatry of the Federal University of Rio de Janeiro (Brazil) express their perceptions and positions regarding the sexuality of psychiatric patients. The study lies at the intersection of the fields of mental health and applied linguistics (Ribeiro 1994; Pinto et al. 2005; Ribeiro and Bastos 2005). It assumes that professional discursive practices are constructed by an institutional order as described by Sarangi and Roberts (1999). The data derive from a multidisciplinary focus group discussion of mental health professionals (doctors, psychologists, nurse technicians, among others) which examined various views as to sexuality, mental health, and HIV/AIDS. This focus group was part of an umbrella research project, the Interdisciplinary Project in Sexuality, Mental Health and AIDS (PRISSMA – *Projeto Interdisciplinar em Sexualidade, Saúde Mental e AIDS*) that designed the Brazilian intervention program for the prevention of HIV infection for psychiatric patients with acute mental problems, held at the Institute of Psychiatry at the Federal University of Rio de Janeiro.

The following questions emerge when analyzing the interaction from a discourse perspective: What interactional challenges do mental health professionals face when they encounter sexual practices in a psychiatric clinic? How do they perform their professional roles discursively in light of the institutional order? How do they balance personal reasoning and judgment in the absence of relevant guidelines regarding sexual conduct? Three institutional roles emerge in this focus group discussion: the manager and protector, the official enforcer and guard, and the counselor. These professionals also display ambiguity and tension in performing such roles. These are the issues we will examine in this chapter.

Our data analysis is based on the interactional perspective of role performance (Sarangi 2010) and situated identities. It addresses Goffman's (1974) classic question 'what's going on here and now?' when sexual practices are perceived by professionals as being inappropriately performed in a clinical setting. The concepts of schema and frame (Tannen and Wallat 1993), footing (Goffman 1981), and positioning (Harré and van Langenhove 1991) will be used to discuss how professionals configure their roles to relate to personal and institutional expectations regarding their expertise.

HIV/AIDS in mental health: clients' sexuality and vulnerability

Studies have shown that the HIV/AIDS epidemic has affected the most vulnerable members of society (Bastos and Szwarcwald 2007; Sánchez and Bertolozzi 2007). Individuals with Severe Mental Illness (SMI, i.e., schizophrenia, schizoaffective disorder, bipolar disorder, and major depression with psychotic features) are no exception, presenting high HIV infection rates in urban communities around the world. In the United States, the prevalence of AIDS infected patients is in the range of 3.1 percent to 22.9 percent; in Europe, it is 6.5 percent; 1.9 percent in Asia; and 23.8 percent in Africa (Rosenberg et al. 2001; McKinnon et al. 2005). In the US, findings across samples suggest that seroprevalence varies with geographic concentration of HIV, presence of comorbid psychoactive substance use disorders, age and ethnicity; but rates are consistently high (Cournos 1996). According to Guimarães et al. (2007), the Brazilian psychiatric population rates are known to be 0.8 percent for HIV seroprevalence; 14.7 percent for Hepatitis B; 2.6 percent for Hepatitis C; and 1.1 percent for Syphilis. All these were higher when compared to the general population in the country (Ministry of Health of Brazil 2012).

Some specific factors seem to contribute to a greater vulnerability of the psychiatric population to HIV infection, such as difficulty in establishing stable relationships; social and economic disadvantages; frequent reports of sexual abuse; impaired critical assessment, especially in psychiatric events; hypersexuality; impulsivity; and low self-esteem; all of which can lead this population to fail to take precautions during sexual relationships (Cournos et al. 1991; Menon 1994).

Mental health care professional role performance at the Institute of Psychiatry

Our discussion will point to tension, ambivalence, and conflict in performing a given professional role; however, much of the difficulty may be due to the lack of institutional guidelines and/or protocols for dealing with sexual practices. These mental health care professionals often configure their roles following personal reasoning and judgments rather than institutional policies. The conflicted aspects of such role performances contribute to 'general instability and uncertainty, partly manifested at the interactional level' (Sarangi and Roberts 1999: 10). The analysis will illuminate how participants indicate local co-membership construction and highlight a common lack of interactional expertise: 'They show co-membership with each other saying in effect that (they) are all in this boat of uncertainty together' (Erickson 1999: 121). We will see that certain professionals take on certain specific footings (Goffman 1981) and positionings (Harré and van Langenhove 1991) which allow us to examine the ongoing process of role performance construction of this focus group.

The institutional order

Psychiatry is a nineteenth-century discipline. The asylum, a confinement institution where custody for 'the sick, the criminal and the vagrant' (Shorter 1997: 4) was provided, was a part of many villages in Europe in the nineteenth and early twentieth centuries. The notion that the institution by itself could cure patients, inspired by the Enlightenment philosophy, was revolutionary and helped established the psychiatric hospital as a curative center for psychological therapy. According to Goffman (1961), the traditional psychiatric hospital is an example of a *total institution*: an isolated enclosed social system whose primary aim is to control all aspects of inmates' lives, such as sleeping, eating and, for the purposes of our discussion, their sexual activities. The psychiatric hospital is 'a place established to care for persons thought to be at once incapable of looking after themselves and a threat to the community, albeit an unintended one' (1961: 15).

The Brazilian Psychiatric Reform (Hirdes 2009) is an anti-asylum movement founded on the belief that mentally ill individuals should have their human and citizens' rights respected.[2] However, institutionalization of the mentally ill is still common in Brazil although many question the efficacy and even safety of institutionalized treatment. As a result relevant questions surface in everyday psychiatric institutional practices: Is the hospital a place for the patient to be treated? How is this treatment conceived? Is it also a place where she or he should be protected? These questions have implications for how the institution positions patients. Are they perceived as temporarily deprived of their capacity to make their own choices or are they viewed as a citizen who needs to have their rights respected? If so, how to balance the need for treatment and the patient's right to have a healthy life, which should include, according to the World Health Organization (WHO),[3] the practice of their sexuality? To what extent might both treatment and protection coexist with sexual practices?

Defining the role of the institution has implications for how one deals with sex: if the institution is conceived as a place to keep patients away from society, and it is legally responsible for them, then sexual practices with others should not be allowed ('it's a problem,' says Denis, a medical intern) and zero tolerance should be the guideline. Control and repression would be key words here. On the other hand, if the institution is taken as a place where the 'mental health clients/citizens' will be treated and guided so as to make their own decisions responsibly, then prevention and counseling of HIV/STD (sexually transmitted disease) should be part of the institutional routine. In our analysis, we will see that professionals perform different institutional roles so as to assume different functions as they relate to patients' care: they may voice their firm concern in terms of their position regarding the role of the institution having to provide legal protection, or having to control, or provide treatment and care. Different footings emerge related to these roles.

The interactional order

As discussed by Sarangi and Roberts, 'Professional and institutional discourses share ways of constructing "truth" out of rhetoric and of developing rituals which both create and legitimate the practices of the profession and the institution. They also share conventions for the social distribution of knowledge and interests which account for the decision-making process' (1999: 16). During the focus group discussion, participants brought up professional concerns about the function of the institution. What happens when such rituals and discourse practices are not in sync? Often tension and ambivalence among professionals 'may work in a top-down way to transform the institutional order. It would lead to the realignments of professionals – repositionings – which would ultimately have implications for the institutional ethos' (1999: 18). Similar points were also noted in Candlin and Sarangi that emphasize the nature of hybrid roles proper of healthcare settings (2011: 17) with overlapping and confusing boundaries.

In the data analysis, we focus on professional concerns: what is expressed and contested in the discourse of this interdisciplinary team of mental healthcare professionals. We will examine transcribed segments from the audio-recorded focus group meeting where professionals discuss their clinical practice on an individual and institutional level, and how such practices are related to issues of sexuality in mental health clients. Our data analysis derives from interactional sociolinguistics (Erickson and Shultz 1982; Gumperz 1982, 1992). Particularly relevant are the concepts of *schema* and *frame* (Tannen and Wallat 1993) that have been used to refer to the organization of experience (Goffman 1974). As structures of expectation, schema and frame affect not only the way in which we interpret, remember, categorize, and revise what we know, but also what we say, how we mean it, how others hear it, and how we do things together linguistically and otherwise (Hoyle and Ribeiro 2002). Focusing specifically on talk and interaction, the notion of *footing* (Goffman 1981) highlights the alignment (position or stance) that mental healthcare professionals take toward one another and toward the content of their talk; alignments that can change from moment to moment and can be embedded at multiple levels. A shift in footing may signal a shift in social identity (e.g., the way professionals may position themselves vis-à-vis what they are saying) being made relevant through talk. In several cases, we will relate the notion of the speaker's footing (and alignment to self) to a moral and personal positioning (Harré and van Langenhove 1991) so as to capture personal attributes and reasonings and their potential effect on the group.

Frames and footings (Goffman 1974, 1981) capture shifts of context and participants' often conflicting and ambivalent alignments to what they are saying. Data analysis points to the tensions between professional and personal reasoning that suggest contradictions voiced throughout the focus group session. Prevention of HIV/AIDS and institutional policies regarding rights for clients/patients are some of the recurrent topics that emerge from talk and interaction.

Contextual information: the institute and the focus groups

The Institute of Psychiatry is located in a historical site with gardens that are often tended by the patients themselves. Since its foundation in 1938, the institute has been a teaching and research hospital that provides professional training and mental health policy at the national level. Since the 1990s, the institute has been a center for multidisciplinary studies in mental health and psychiatry. National research programs have been developed with major academic centers in Brazil.

In the PRISSMA Project (2002–2006), nine focus groups were conducted with professionals and patients in two adjacent psychiatric inpatient/outpatient institutions (the Institute of Psychiatry and Philippe Pinel). Focus groups were used to elicit key topics on content, format, delivery, and implementation of the intervention. The guiding topics/questions dealt with the sexuality of people with mental illnesses (experiences, representations, stigma, linguistic labels, actions, and norms related to risk behavior and prevention), the practice of sexuality inside and outside the institution, and the relationship between HIV/STD and mental illness (Pinto et al. 2007).

The focus group analyzed in this chapter lasted approximately 75 minutes. There were nine professionals (six females; three males) with different educational backgrounds who work in clinical assistance at the institute: two resident doctors, a psychologist, a social worker, two nurse technicians, a music therapist, a lab technician, and an occupational therapist (see Appendix 24.1 at the end of the chapter).[4] At the institute, these mental health care professionals participated regularly in multidisciplinary clinical teams at the time the data were collected. Senior psychiatrists led these clinical teams for a 90-minute meeting on a weekly basis. Most of these professionals have other part-time jobs. For this focus group analyzed in this chapter, the selection was based on those professionals whose functions were considered crucial to the management of the institutional routines of the institute. It is worth remembering that this focus group was formed for the purpose of the formative phase of the PRISSMA research which aimed to inform the creation/adaptation of a Brazilian intervention for the prevention of HIV infection in male and female clients of mental health services (day hospital and outpatient clinic), based on interventions already tested in other countries. Each group discussion was conducted by two researchers, here represented by a psychologist (Pedro) and a sociolinguist (Diana),[5] with prior experience mediating similar groups. Each group had an observer for non-verbal communication.

Tension and ambivalence in enacting professional roles

Two findings result from the analysis of this focus group discussion. First, participants recognize that sexual activities occur regularly. Second, there are no institutional guidelines to cope with many of the 'problematic' and 'complicated' situations. In the following sections, we indicate how mental health care professionals relate to these issues, which constitute an integral part of their professional lives.

Our initial research questions – what interactional challenges do mental health professionals face when they encounter sexual practices in a psychiatric clinic? How do they perform their professional roles discursively in light of the institutional order? – can now be more specific: Why do we have professional ambivalent and conflicting role performances? How do ambivalence and tension in role performance relate to the multiple and inherent purposes of such an institution (that is, to treat, care, and control)? How does the institutional order affect the interactional order?

Mental health care professionals acknowledge that there are sexual practices among patients at the institute, whether the wards are separated by gender (women's ward and men's ward) as most of the psychiatric institutions are, or mixed, which was the institutional routine from December 1997 until January 2003.[6] This finding is consistent with other studies (Pinto et al. 2007; Wainberg et al. 2007; McCann 2010); also, they stress that 'there used to be many problems' in the mixed gender wards.

In the following segment,[7] Wilma, a nurse technician, who had been working at the institute for 10 years at the time these data were collected, emphasizes that inpatient and outpatient sexual practices have always been part of the institutional routine.

Segment 1

Wilma: Not now, 'cause the wards are separated, male and female, but they've been mixed before, ok? And there were, ah ... many people that had sexual intercourse

> and this caused much trouble. (...) lots of sex. This has always happened here (... had sex in the) patio ..... (in the bushes), the tree, behind the bed, under it, they've always done it. The only thing is, when it changed to (the new) ward (...) They were separated, but it's still happening. Because there, in the male ward, men keep on having sex among themselves, the women there too, and when they get out of the ward, there are men and women together. So one has to (... be alert) all the time. [8]

In the next sections, we will see that despite the high frequency of sexual practices in the psychiatric hospital, institutional guidelines for coping with such situations are not provided. Consequently, the ways professionals approach patients in sexual encounters vary greatly.

The lack of institutional guidance, often criticized by focus group participants, leads each professional to the difficult decision of 'how to cope with sexuality among inmates'. Thus, these professionals have to turn to idiosyncratic and inconsistent solutions, grounded in their own schemas (Tannen and Wallat 1993). The data indicate that these 'moment-to-moment' (or ad hoc) responses range from prohibitions to leniency. Others denied or ignored sexual activities by inmates. Some claimed that no sexual activities occurred at the institute. In other words, mental health care professionals assume various footings, from repressing patients to counseling them. Although these professionals possess sound knowledge in their area of expertise (i.e., psychiatric care, mental health nursing, psychoanalytic psychology, etc.), they lack interactional knowledge (Sarangi 2005) to communicate what they know about sexual care to their patients and even to each other. In the words of a social worker,

Segment 2

Nilma: ..... and sometimes we don't really know how to deal with it [sex in the institution], what one is saying, the guy [the patient] is asking you one thing, what one is seeing there .....

The inclusive pronoun 'we' signals the group of professionals that, according to Nilma, is incapable (or at least reluctant) to approach such topics with patients. Before telling a story about her embarrassment when she discovered two patients having sex in the ward, Nilma admits that this group of professionals (herself included) is not prepared to face such situations. She further states her mixed feelings by adding that many demands come up: patients' questions to which she does not have an answer and scenes that she has to witness despite her inability to handle them. In the following sections, we will discuss data excerpts where these professionals explicitly admit their inability to approach the topic of sexuality with patients. When professionals have to cope with patients' sexual practices, they assume different footings and positionings, often related to specific functions of a psychiatric institution.

The perplexed professional. 'We don't know how to talk to the patient'

When mental health care professionals admit their lack of interactional knowledge in responding to sexual practices, an often performed footing is that of the 'perplexed professional'. Given the lack of guidance for dealing with patients' sexual activities, these professionals find themselves not knowing how to respond or address what they face. Without institutional guidelines or any type of protocol, professionals move back and forth between positions ('can't do this' or 'can do this but not (here)') as they talk to patients. They voice that they are not ready ('I didn't know if I would get out or if I would stay'). They also alternate between asking for immediate help from a nurse, an emotional response, and/or voicing the need to discuss such issues with peers, a more rational response.

In the following segments, the social worker Nilma and two nurse technicians, Wilma and Silvana, relate two (of the many) stories in which professionals are unwittingly positioned witnesses of a supposedly private scene. Again, we are reminded that the psychiatric hospital, as a total institution in Goffman's terms, is a social system where privacy is not maintained; rather, daily activities are carried out in the immediate presence of others.

Segment 3

Nilma: I got to the ward, not thinking much, two patients were having sex. I admit that, I've been here for a while. ..... then I put my hands up and said 'what's happening here?' (laughter) (...) but that was the only reaction I had. Then they left and I didn't know what to say, either 'you can't do this' or 'can do this but not (here).' You're not ready when it happens, you know it happens, yet you don't expect to see it ..... Then I called the nurse, I called the patients, and all.

Wilma: (that's right.) Call the nurse.
(laughter) [many participants]

Segment 4

Silvana: ..... We don't know how to talk to the patient. Once in the women's ward- men's ward, right? It used to be Ward 1, right? I was new to psychiatry. I open the door, and I didn't understand what was happening on the floor. (They'd pushed the beds aside), and I, yeah ... there was foot and head, hands ... it was all entangled, all entangled, and I stayed there, see, y'know? My colleague came to help me, screamed, right? and ... (big show) ... right? I stayed like that ... I I didn't know what to say. Sincerely- ... I was petrified. I didn't know if I would get out or if I would stay, right? My colleague came to help me. And after this, until today ... one of the patients who was in that nest, gave me a nickname, and whenever he sees me, he calls me by this nickname right next to my ear.

Nilma: Could you tell us?

Silvana: Yes. He calls me party pooper[9] (...)
(laughters) [many participants]

Lack of interactional knowledge is reiterated throughout this last segment directly positioning the group as well as the speaker ('We don't know how to talk to the patient', 'I didn't understand', 'I didn't know what to say'). This scene literally immobilizes the nurse technician 'I was petrified.' There is the use of negatives ('you're not ready', 'you don't expect to see it') contradicting prior expectations (Tannen and Wallat 1993) related to one's professional role. In Segment 3 Nilma provides an orientation to the patient grounded in ambiguity by stating alternative possibilities ('you can't do this' or 'can do this but not (here)'). While the professional seems to be paralyzed and responds emotionally, the patient seemed to know quite well what was going on. As the nurse technician states, the patient remembers this incident until today. In naming her a 'party pooper', he makes her revisit this complex event and her own lack of communicative competence in handling such an event. In both segments laughter occurs as a contextualization cue (Gumperz 1982) that often relieves tension in the group. It also works to create involvement among these professionals.

What is this institution for?

During the focus group discussion, different professionals brought up tensions regarding the function of the institution. Such tensions are clearly voiced by a second-year medical intern:

> *Segment 5*
>
> *Denis*: what are we thinking, is this [sex at the institute] a problem? If it is a problem, then are we thinking of zero tolerance in relation to sex, or if not, then we have to think, uhm ... of the best way (that intervention) can be done, uhm, in a preventive way ... right? Because, uhm ... (these are) almost opposite (positions) .... I would like to know how we will discuss this.

Some professionals present such issues as opposites. Two positions (enforcement of a 'no-tolerance' policy vs. prevention) are frequently voiced. It will be present in the different footings these professionals take as the discussion unfolds. Each footing relates to how they perceive the role of the institution. Personal reasoning and professional orientations will provide them some ad hoc guidelines as the data indicate.

As we see in Table 24.1, for some participants, the main institutional role is to protect. In this perspective, the institution functions as a place where the patient has to subscribe to a set of rules established by the professionals, being then closer to Goffman's characterization of a total institution, as previously discussed. As a consequence, patients are not positioned as responsible citizens, who can be accountable for their actions; rather, they are temporarily deprived of their civil rights.[10] Legal issues are raised as one of the main arguments for sustaining the institutional responsibility over the patient. The footing of the institutional manager and protector captures how some of these professionals may take this stance.

The institutional manager and protector

This footing reflects the role of the institution and its policies. When mental health care professionals speak from the protector footing, they refer to the hospital responsibility, accountability, and protection, particularly 'legal protection', as in the following two segments:

> *Segment 6*
>
> *Gustavo*: ..... there is a strong push for this thing of eroticism, of sexuality, but there isn't a push for being responsible towards sexuality. (...) and I think that here at the hospital, I think that it is, it is a bit difficult, because there is a- a legal question, because later the family, it ... (makes the hospital accountable) regarding this issue, regarding someone who gets an illness here, or else gets pregnant here, certainly it is- ... it falls truly on the hospital. At the hospital we have this role of ... we must protect those who come here for treatment, right? They must have some protection from the hospital regarding this issue, a legal protection.

Table 24.1 Relating professionals' perceptions of the institution to professional footings

Role of the institution	*Footing*
Legal protection	Institutional manager and protector
Protection/control	Guard and enforcer
Treatment and care	Counselor

Gustavo, a music therapist, starts by opposing locations in shared prior cultural knowledge, 'there' (the world outside the institution) with its 'strong push for this thing of eroticism' (depictured in the Brazilian culture) and its implicit lack of sexual responsibility, to 'here at the hospital' and its explicit legal obligations. Such contrastive deictic markers (there/here) establish a territorial difference. After delimiting the boundary of the institute, Gustavo refers to the point of view of the family if a sexual act (or at least one with consequences) occurs 'here'. In such circumstances, 'the family, makes the hospital accountable'.

Gustavo then takes a professional position: 'we have this role', 'we must protect'. He speaks from having a clear understanding regarding the performance of the protector's role. There is no ambiguity in his talk. It is direct and uses repetition for emphasis (Tannen 1989).

Gustavo: At the hospital we have this role of ... we must protect those who come here for treatment, right? They must have some protection from the hospital regarding this issue, a legal protection.

For this professional the notion of care, protection, and legal responsibility is clear. He speaks as an agent for others 'we have this role, we must protect … .' Here the notion of agency extends beyond the group to the institution: 'At the hospital we have this role of … .' If not, the consequences may be dire as indicated below:

Segment 7

Bruno: The hospital has a- some responsibility for this, right? Once the patient is admitted to the hospital, the hospital is responsible for him. If there is a pregnancy, then (...) if there is a pregnancy here inside the hospital ... oh, see ...

Silvana: There is a lawsuit.

(Several) lawsuits. [several voices at once]

The footing of the institutional manager often emerges in the group discussion, and frequently asserts the positions described above. We see the co-construction of situated professional identities being ratified and negotiated in talk and interaction. A related but somewhat different footing is introduced when professionals voice a very traditional stance, the authoritative footing of the guard and enforcer.

The guard and enforcer

As noted earlier, a key assumption in traditional psychiatry relates a cure to obedience and discipline. We will observe that professionals, despite their distinct competencies, refer to the inherent tension embedded in the assistance of mentally ill patients.

In each of the following segments, a related aspect to this footing emerges. For example, the nurse on duty must often assume the footing of guard/enforcer. Perhaps unsurprisingly, Bruno, a prior nurse technician, and today a lab technician, reports his rounds at night:

Segment 8

Bruno: Things got to a point that, when I had the night shift, things got to a point that I (...) at night, several (times) at night, I had to go there (...) to really get the patient out 'hey guy, come on, get up' ... (laughter).

'Things got to a point' refers to the sexual activity in the wards. It is up to Bruno to intervene by a direct command: 'hey guy, come on, get up' and separate the couples. However, we see internal tension when Bruno reflects on his actions: 'My God. So am I here to be a nurse or am I supposed to be a guard to prevent the patient ... from screwing? So I would stay ... I believed that I ... that wasn't it, I did not agree with that.' Conflicted embedded schemas are voiced by these professionals (to be a guard or a nurse?). The mediator, who is also a psychologist, voiced tension in taking a similar footing:

Segment 9
Pedro: you also had to scream, right? you also (...) right? You felt as if you were a traffic cop.

These excerpts capture how mental health care professionals view themselves and others when they are required to control sexual activities. They report on certain emotions (screams), and they perceive their performed role as repressive ('traffic cop', 'guard').

Sometimes we see professionals assuming an enforcer footing, then shifting to indicate their confusion as a perplexed professional, a frame lamination (Goffman 1974) in the segment below:

Segment 10 (full Segment 3)
Nilma: I got in the ward, not thinking much, two patients were having sex. ..... then I put my hands up and said 'what's happening here?' (laughter) (...) but that was the only reaction I had.

The social worker Nilma's first reaction is to gesture ('put my hands up') and then shout 'what's happening here?' After interrupting (and therefore intervening), she shifts to express her state of confusion 'that was the only reaction I had'. Sharing her conflicting expectations (Tannen and Wallat 1993) by providing contrasting information ('but that was the only reaction I had'), Nilma displays her internal tension at this encounter. Laughter provides a way to mitigate such conflict.

Mental health care professionals also position themselves as counselors. This footing signals their understanding of the institution: it is a place for treatment and care.

The counselor

Some professionals view education and prevention as strategies to counterbalance the unexpected encounters of sexual activity in the institution. Here again we can establish a relationship between the way professionals understand the function of the institution and their alignments towards this topic. Several times in this group discussion, mental health care professionals speak of a level of 'awareness' on the patient's part and the need to talk to the patient, rather than ignore that the patient has sex.

Segment 11
Gustavo: I think this issue of awareness, even for that patient who is not, is not able to control himself, I think that (...) there is something one could try to talk about, dialogue, show the ... (the points themselves), right? (...) even for those who can't quite uhm ... control (their instincts). I think that talk, in a way, it's

important (... y' know?) If one does not talk, of- ... closes one's eyes, that's a bit complicated. I think talk is always the best solution.

Pedro: So you say ... closing one's eyes ...

Gustavo: Yes, pretend that it's not happening, so, I think it needs to be discussed.

Talk often indicates social engagement. It is often the position of the mental health counselor. Talk implies a dialogue about certain 'points' (or topics). This kind of talk takes place within a relationship (a professional engagement with the patient) and as a discussion about the patient. Ignoring the needs of the patient 'can be problematic', according to Gustavo, a music therapist.

By providing guidance to younger peers, some professionals establish a footing of preceptor (Erickson 1999). They position themselves as clinically more experienced and interactionally competent in handling complex institutional situations. In the following segment, a senior psychologist suggests how to address couples who have sex at the institute.

Segment 12

Nadia: I'm thinking of a story here, of a trainee I had, who once cared for (some patients) ..... Just because he's [the patient is] crazy, does he have the right to do it [sex] at any time, because of his craziness? And do we keep reinforcing this, including this issue of craziness? I think not. At most, I think this discussion needs to take into account this issue, how does one live, that is, one understands one's sexual behavior, lives one's sexuality, how do we feel, in a way, as a woman and a member of society, one controls (one's own behavior), or not, right? ..... I said 'look, how do I ... I behave myself, how do I behave myself in life. ..... in a normal life, how do I behave, right?' (This) helps me create a more reasonable profile, see what I mean?

This professional advocates straight talk. Rather than validating 'craziness' (and therefore sex out of place), this psychologist advocates talking to the patient and pointing to proper behavior 'in a normal life'. Another footing seems to be embedded within the counselor stance: Nadia, the psychologist, frequently takes a mentoring footing as she questions the group 'do we keep reinforcing this, including this issue of craziness?' She assumes an unambiguous position 'I think not.' She advocates establishing standards that are common to all (mental patients and nonpatients alike) and raises rhetorical questions 'how does one live', 'how do we feel ... as a woman and a member of society'. In taking a clear stand, she declares 'look, how I behave myself in life ..... in a normal life.....?' In assuming a moral positioning (Harré and van Langenhove 1991) to model herself following 'reasonable criteria', i.e., 'a normal life', she demonstrates to others how to talk to patients: trying not to establish a difference between inside/outside the institution as a way to avoid discrimination.[11]

In this last segment, we see a nurse technician asserting to her peers a strong stance regarding how she addresses the patient:

Segment 13

Wilma: Yes, I will speak for myself, I don't know how it is, uhm, for other professionals. I talk straight with the patient. I say 'hey, you're gonna have

sex without condom, you can get AIDS.' I don't deceive them. Right now, I walked … passed by the room (where there is) someone who is HIV positive, I say, 'hey, watch out, ('cause there's) an HIV positive patient there,' I tell him even who the patient is, 'cause ah … to preserve that person. But I tell, I tell … (...) Because often the patient who is uhm hypersexualized, he is quite conscious, he is hypersexualized, but he is, most often, conscious, quite conscious, he knows quite well what he is doing.
{turning to the group and referring to Wilma}

Nadia: But this is the way she is.
Wilma: Yes. (...)
Guida: There are those who can't quite cope with this, right?
Wilma: Yes. But this is what I said, I'm speaking for myself.
Manuela: Yes ... no. That's right, it would be the ideal (response).

In the segment above, Wilma states clearly her own position towards sexual practices that might involve risk to the patient: she 'talks straight to the patient'. She embeds her warning bold on record (I say 'hey, you're gonna have sex without condom, you can get AIDS'). To stress her commitment as advisor/counselor, Wilma narrates a story that had just happened ('right now'). Though the patient may be hypersexualized, she repeats three times that the patient is 'conscious' and 'knows quite well what he is doing'. In asserting a way of handling such sexual behavior, she presents her own solution 'I will speak for myself.' Wilma's footing towards self relates to Harré and van Langenhove's (1991) distinction between personal and moral positioning. It is an intentional and explicit positioning, which has implications for others in the group. It is also a complex position as Wilma has embedded a prior conversation with a patient about a reference to a positive HIV patient, a potential ethical issue at the institute.[12] Two members of the group display their discomfort with such positioning; as indicated by Wilma: not everyone can 'quite cope with this' and this 'would be the ideal' (but implicitly stating that it would not be feasible).

Wilma asserts her footing as counselor regarding sexual practices in the institution. From the very beginning of the focus group session, she states: 'the patients talk about sexuality, they tell us very clearly what they like and what they don't like doing (regarding sex) (…) I think that only through education, can we do something.' She positions herself as a privileged listener, to whom patients talk frankly about sexual topics and behavior.

The institutional space to talk about sex: the workshop on sexuality

The institute hosts educational activities, including a Workshop on Health and Sexuality. In the focus group, various mental health care professionals refer to this workshop as the 'workshop on sexuality'. At the time data were collected, this 60-minute optional workshop was held every other week by two MHCP and was known as 'Claudio and Suely's workshop'. The male psychiatric nurse Claudio and the female social assistant Suely, who ran the workshop, were consultants for the Brazilian National Program on STD/AIDS between 2001 and 2007, conducting training for professionals countrywide. The workshop presented discussions on general health, and highlighted the importance of HIV/STD prevention. Patients often expressed their sexual feelings and concerns at the workshop.

In the following segment, the music therapist states clearly how mental health care providers perceive this space:

Segment 14

Gustavo: We always, whenever it's necessary, we always guide them, to basic care, whenever it's necessary, even because, with this activity headed by Claudio and Suely, somehow, it already solves many issues they bring up, that they could bring up, it already provides them with solutions. Get it?

Despite the mental health care professionals' varied footings, there is a common objective that they all share: to guide patients to the workshop 'whenever it's necessary'. When concerns about sexual activity arise (which happens frequently), professionals encourage patients to discuss them in this institutional space. This is seen as the privileged context where solutions will be provided since Claudio and Suely (who have worked at the institute for 20 years) are the experts on such matters.

According to Gustavo, the workshop can also anticipate solutions for future problems ('it already solves many issues they bring up, that they could bring up'). In some ways the workshop has had an unanticipated effect: it was created to educate patients and professionals to cope with complex situations regarding sex; yet it was soon transformed into the single institutional space where professionals and patients would bring up such complex topics to discuss, excluding such discussions from other team meetings and/or clinical encounters. Thus professionals in this institution would avoid engaging in patients' assistance and care for such matters and assign such responsibility to Claudio and Suely.

Segment 15

Guida: Because we come (to the patient), 'look, you've got a specific context to discuss the issue of sexuality, you go to the workshop, right?' There there's, there are some people who can't discuss uhm sexual issues with the patient. (voices). (... they say) 'you go to the workshop 'cause you discuss it there,' (''cause there are people there who will give you answers').

When professionals refer patients to the workshop ('you've got a specific context'), they often assume a counselor-related footing. The occupational therapist (Guida) acknowledges the patients' rights on expressing their sexuality, her own institutional responsibility in approaching the patient to discuss problems related to their illness ('Because we come to the patient and he expresses his difficulty in handling such issues. There there's, there are some people who can't discuss uhm sexual issues with the patient'). Rather than assuming the role of the counselors themselves, professionals refer patients to be assisted by two colleagues who are more knowledgeable and more interactionally competent to discuss sexual activities at the institute.

Summary: 'being in this boat of uncertainty together'

The analysis presented here discusses two dissonant points raised during the focus group discussion. First, mental health care professionals acknowledge the existence of sexual activities among patients/clients at the Institute of Psychiatry, which attest to what previous studies have already shown (Krumm et al. 2004; McKinnon et al. 2005). Second, professionals lack official guidelines for dealing with such activities. As a result, these professionals have developed their own set of responses that range from ignoring the activity to talking straight to the patient, assuming various alignments regarding patients' expression of their sexuality. One of the most prevalent footings, the perplexed professional, is caused by the lack of specific guidelines from the institution. Often these professionals feel confused and respond in a variety of ways to what is clearly perceived as unscripted behavior (screaming to the patients, calling the nurse, making intervening gestures, etc.). There is also tension regarding the role of the institution, which has implications on how sex is handled and on the various footings assumed by these professionals. The footing of institutional manager and protector relates to the institution as a place for legal protection. Hospital responsibility and legal protection particularly seem to guide professionals who assume this alignment. The guard and enforcer footings relate to the institution's protection and control function, according to which discipline and obedience are at stake. Finally, the counselor's footing captures key institutional functions related to treatment and care. When some mental health care professionals adopt this footing, they may talk straight to the patients about their sexual activities at the institute. The analysis has also indicated that the Workshop on Health and Sexuality conducted by two professionals is perceived as the official space where patients are usually referred to when they bring up sexual-related topics. When referring patients to this institutional activity, mental health care professionals also assume a counselor-related footing, since they ascribe part of their institutional task to other professionals, acknowledging herewith their lack of interactional knowledge to deal with sex-related topics and activities. What is particularly interesting in these data is that tension and ambivalence may work in a bottom-up way to transform the institutional order. It presents possible footings and repositionings that 'ultimately have implications for the institutional ethos' (Sarangi and Roberts 1999: 18). At this point in time, the interactional order informs the institution regarding ways in which professionals might work together to try to resolve such complex issues. Also while mental health care professionals take a variety of footings, certain professionals may privilege specific footings rather than others (i.e., the psychologist may take on a counselor footing more often than the enforcer or manager footing).

Future directions

When analyzing the discourse of mental health care professionals in a Brazilian psychiatric institution, one realizes that it is difficult to talk about sex even for these professionals. Sexuality and correlated issues are cultural taboo themes that still trigger a range of feelings and emotions, which seems to be more intense in a psychiatric setting due to the historical background of these institutions as previously noted (Goffman 1961; Foucault 1988; Birman 1994). Despite the difficulty in discussing such topics, the participants of this focus group acknowledge that sex matters. These discussions in a multidisciplinary team seem to have had at least a twofold function: they facilitated a deliberate set of responses from professionals to the sexual activities of patients (particularly in the absence of institutional guidelines) and they worked as a locus for the exchange of professional experiences, grounded in different fields of knowledge and expertise. Given the limit of our discussion, we have not focused on the impact of multidisciplinary team works in the institute; rather, our analysis highlights a shared concern among professionals related to their lack of interactional competence in coping with patients and their sexual practices.

Professionals report to patients' specific requests regarding their right to have sexual practices in the institution: 'And the citizen's request was the following: to build a room, because he's been here for two months or two months and a half, and he didn't have any privacy to have sex, which he needed so much.' By acknowledging patients/citizens' requests, professionals seem to implicitly align themselves with such demands (Goffman 1981; Harré and van Langenhove 1991). These requests clearly reinforce the need for further discussion. This focus group, in the words of a participant, explored topics that have not been addressed by mental health care professionals. The discussion also points to research and training developed by applied linguists and sociolinguists in areas of practical relevance (Sarangi and Roberts 1999).

It is widely known that the analysis of institutional discourse has implications for the understanding of how social life is organized (Drew and Heritage 1992; Heritage and Clayman 2010). Although professionals share the ultimate goal of the institution, to treat and care for the patients, the analysis presented in this chapter points to different perceptions of whether treatment and care should include the open discussion of sexuality. The professionals' lack of interactional knowledge about how to cope with such a complex and multilayered topic gives rise to a common feeling of professional perplexity. If one conceives health care as a set of practices that aims at the integral care and assistance of human beings, sexuality should be included.[13] This leaves us with the challenging task of providing interactional skills to Brazilian mental health care professionals, a role that applied and sociolinguists interested in the interface between mental health and linguistics are eager to play.

Related topics

Professional discourse; role performance; positioning; footing; mental health; psychiatric institution; sexual practices.

Notes

1 The authors gratefully acknowledge the relevant contributions made to the Projeto Interdisciplinar em Sexualidade, Saúde Mental e AIDS (PRISSMA) from those receiving care at the Institute of Psychiatry of the Federal University of Rio de Janeiro and PINEL, and the mental health care providers and other staff at these two institutions. This project is a participatory research study where data, results, and writing of manuscripts are shared by authors from Brazil and the US, and research and non-research members of the PRISSMA project: http://www.abiaids.org.br/projetos/projetoView.aspx?lang=pt&seq=9842&mid=5&fg=Projetos. The authors would also like to thank Scott P. Studebaker for the edits and comments on prior drafts of this chapter.

2 http://www.ccs.saude.gov.br

3 http://www.who.int/reproductive-health/gender/sexualhealth.html

4 All names in this chapter have been changed to protect confidentiality of the participants. The focus group was conducted in Portuguese. The English translation is not a word-for-word translation. Rather, it portrays the sense of the talk that is taking place at that moment. Thus the English segments are as close as possible to natural English discourse.

5 First names are used in various professional settings in Brazil.

6 Under Dr. João Ferreira's administration, the unusual and debatable mixed gender wards practice was introduced grounded in similar institutional experiences in Italy, which has also guided the Brazilian Psychiatric Reform Movement.

7 See Appendix 24.2 for the transcription conventions.

8 It is worth adding that the institution has an outdoor space where the day-hospital and the outpatient clinic are located. Also, there are several physical spaces where both patients and staff gather or circulate regularly: the cafeteria, the garden, the parking lot, the entrances, and restrooms.

9 The translation does not provide the true sense of the meaning of the original text in Brazilian Portuguese '*empata foda*' which has a sexual connotation.

10 In Brazil psychiatric inpatients do not vote, and do not keep their documents with them while they are in the emergency unit. Voting is mandatory in Brazil. Thus, when unable to vote, inpatients are positioned as 'minors or deprived from their citizenship'.

11 As a psychologist Nadia had group supervisor functions at the institute at the time of this research.

12 Mental health professionals must subscribe to the Brazilian Ethical Code on Health which determines that a patient's HIV positive status should only be disclosed when someone else's life is at risk.

13 In Brazil, a few universities and technical schools have lately included sexuality as a topic in their curricula (https://uspdigital.usp.br/jupiterweb/obterDisciplina?sgldis=MSP0674&verdis=1).

Further reading

Holmes, J. (2006) 'Workplace narratives, professional identity and relational practice'. In Anna de Fina, Deborah Schiffrin, and Michael Bamberg (eds) *Discourse and Identity*, 166–187, New York: Cambridge University Press. (This article examines how individuals construct and negotiate a range of social identities through the telling of workplace narratives.)

Pinto, D. (2011) 'Discourse Analysis, the use of image and the health field: theoretical–methodological aspects'. RECIIS – R. *Eletr. de Com. Inf. Inov. Saúde*, 5(2): 8–15, Jun; Rio de Janeiro. (This article discusses Discourse Analysis from an Interactional Sociolinguistics perspective and its application to mental health.)

Ribeiro, B.T. (2006) 'Footing, positioning, voice. Are we talking about the same thing?' In Anna de Fina, Deborah Schiffrin, and Michael Bamberg (eds) *Discourse and Identity*, 48–82, New York: Cambridge University Press. (The author discusses the theoretical and methodological notions of footing, positioning, and voice by investigating contextualization processes in talk and interaction.)

Ribeiro, B.T. and Pinto, D.S. (2006) 'Medical discourse: psychiatric interviews'. In Keith Brown (Editor-in-chief) *Encyclopedia of Language and Linguistics*, vol. 7, 658–664, 2nd edn, Oxford: Elsevier. (This text provides a comprehensive understanding of the implications of the interactive model for communication studies to psychiatry and mental health.)

Sarangi, S. (2011) 'Role hybridity in professional practice'. In S. Sarangi, V. Polese, and G. Caliendo (eds) *Genre(s) on the Move: Hybridisation and Discourse Change in Specialized Communication*, 271–296, Napoli: Edizioni Scientifiche Italiane. (The author discusses hybridity in light of the complex concepts of role and role set and suggests a linkage between the latter and discourse types with particular reference to professional practices in various settings.)

References

Bastos, F.I. and Szwarcwald, C.L. (2007) 'AIDS and pauperization: principal concepts and empirical evidence'. *Cadernos de Saúde Pública*, 16(Sup. 1): 65–76.

Birman, J. (1994) 'Between evil and scorn'. In: M.A. Loyola (ed.) *AIDS and Sexuality: The Viewpoint of Human Sciences,* 109–115, Rio de Janeiro: Relume-Dumará: UERJ.

Candlin, C. and Sarangi, S. (2011) 'Professional and organizational practice'. In C. Candlin and S. Sarangi (eds) *Handbook of Communication in Organizations and Professions*, 4–56, New York: Mouton de Gruyter.

Cournos, F. (1996) 'Epidemiology of HIV'. In Francine Cournos and Nicholas Bakalar (eds) *AIDS and People with Severe Mental Illness: A Handbook for Mental Health Professionals,* New Haven, CT: Yale University Press.

Cournos, F., Empfield, M., Horwath, E., McKinnon, K., Meyer, I., Schrage, H., et al. (1991) 'HIV seroprevalence among patients admitted to two psychiatric hospitals'. *American Journal of Psychiatry*, 148: 9.

Drew, P. and Heritage, J. (1992) *Talk at Work*, Cambridge: Cambridge University Press.

Erickson, F. (1999) 'Appropriation of voice and presentation of self as a fellow physician: aspects of a discourse of apprenticeship in medicine'. In S. Sarangi and C. Roberts (eds) *Talk, Work and Institutional Order: Discourse in Medical, Mediation and Management Settings*, 109–143, New York: Mouton de Gruyter.

Erickson, F. and Shultz, J. (1982) *The Counselor as Gatekeeper: Social Interaction in Interviews*, New York: Academic Press.

Foucault, M. (1988) *Madness and Civilization: A History of Insanity in the Age of Reason*, London: Vintage Books.

Goffman, E. (1961) *Asylums: Essays on the Social Situation of Mental Patients and Other Inmates*, New York: First Anchor.

——(1974) *Frame Analysis*, New York: Harper and Row.

——(1981) 'Footing'. In *Forms of Talk*, 124–159, Philadelphia, PA: University of Pennsylvania Press.

Guimarães, M.D.C., Acúrcio, F., Campos, L., Freitas, M.I., Melo, A.P., Oliveira, S.B., and Oliveira, H.N. (2007) *Seroprevalence Study of HIV, Syphilis, Hepatitis B and C in Public Institutions of Mental Health Care: A Multicentric Study*, Final Technical Report, Brasília/DF.

Gumperz, J.J. (1982) *Discourse Strategies*, Cambridge: Cambridge University Press.

——(1992) 'Contextualization and understanding'. In: A. Duranti and C. Goodwin (eds) *Rethinking Context*, 229–252, Cambridge: Cambridge University Press.

Harré, R. and van Langenhove, L. (1991) 'Varieties of positioning'. *Journal for the Theory of Social Behavior*, 21(4): 393–407.

Heritage, D. and Claymann, S. (2010) *Talk in Action: Interaction, Identities and Institutions*, Oxford: Blackwell.

Hirdes, A. (2009) 'The psychiatric reform in Brazil: a (re)view'. *Ciência & Saúde Coletiva*, 14(1), Jan./Feb.: 297–305.

Hoyle, S. and Ribeiro, B.T. (2002) 'Scripts, frames, and schemas'. In J. William Frawley (ed.) *International Encyclopedia of Linguistics*, 516–17, New York: Oxford University Press.

Krumm, S., Kilian, R., and Becker, T. (2004) 'Psychiatric inpatient care and sexuality'. *Psychiatrische Praxis*, 31(4): 212–217.

McCann, E. (2010) 'The sexual and relationship needs of people who experience psychosis: quantitative findings of a UK study'. *Journal of Psychiatric and Mental Health Nursing*, 17(4): 295–303.

McKinnon, K., Cournos, F., Herman, R., and Le Melle, S. (2005) 'HIV and people with serious and persistent mental illness'. In Kenneth Citron (ed.) *HIV & Psychiatry: A Training and Resource Manual*, 138–152, Cambridge: Cambridge University Press.

Menon, A.S. (1994) 'The high prevalence of unsafe sexual behaviors among acute psychiatric inpatients: implications for AIDS prevention'. *Journal of Nervous and Mental Disease*, 182: 661–666.

Ministry of Health of Brazil, National Program for STD and AIDS (2012) *Epidemiologic newsletter – AIDS and STD*, Year VIII, no. 1–01ª–26ª epidemiological weeks, Jan./Jun., Brasilia, Brazil: Ministry of Health of Brazil.

Pinto, D.S., Ribeiro, B.M.T., and Dantas, M.T.L. (2005) '"Let the heart speak out": interviewing practices by psychiatrists from two different traditions'. *Communication and Medicine*, 2: 177–188.

Pinto, D.S., Mann, C.G., Wainberg, M., Mattos, P., and Oliveira, S.B. (2007) 'Vulnerability to HIV, and mental health: an ethnographic study of psychiatric institutions'. *Cadernos de Saúde Pública*, 23: 2224–2233.

Ribeiro, B.T. (1994) *Coherence in Psychotic Discourse*, Oxford: Oxford University Press.

Ribeiro, B.T. and Bastos, L.C. (2005) 'Telling stories in two psychiatric interviews: a discussion on frame and narrative'. In Kanavillil Rajagopalan (ed.) *Applied Linguistics in Latin America, AILA Review*, 18: 58–75.

Rosenberg, S.D., Goodman, L.A., Osher, F.C., Swartz, M.S., Essock, S.M., Butterfield, M.I., et al. (2001) 'Prevalence of HIV, Hepatitis B, and Hepatitis C in people with severe mental illness'. *American Journal of Public Health*, 91: 31–37.

Sánchez, A.I.M. and Bertolozzi, M.R. (2007) 'Can the vulnerability concept support the construction of knowledge in collective health care?' *Ciência & Saúde Coletiva*, 12(2): 319–324.

Sarangi, S. (2005) 'Social interaction, social theory and work-related activities'. *Revista Calidoscópio*, 3(3): 160–169.

——(2010) 'Reconfiguring self/identity/status/role: the case of professional role performance in healthcare encounters'. In J. Archibald and G. Garzone (eds) *Actors, Identities and Roles in Professional and Academic Settings: Discursive Perspectives*, 27–54, Berne: Peter Lang.

Sarangi, S. and Roberts, C. (1999) 'Introduction: discursive hybridity in medical work'. In S. Sarangi and C. Roberts (eds) *Talk, Work and Institutional Order: Discourse in Medical, Mediation and Management Settings*, 61–74, New York: Mouton de Gruyter.

Shorter, E. (1997) *A History of Psychiatry: From the Era of the Asylum to the Age of Prozac*, New York: John Wiley.

Tannen, D. (1989) *Talking Voices. Repetition, Dialogue, and Imagery in Conversational Discourse*, New York: Cambridge University Press.

Tannen, D. and Wallat, C. (1993) 'Interactive frames and knowledge schemas in interaction: examples from a medical examination/interview'. In D. Tannen (ed.) *Framing in Discourse*, 57–76, New York: Cambridge University Press.

Wainberg, M., Gonzalez, A., Mckinnon, K., Elkington, K., Pinto, D., Mann, C.G., and Mattos, P. (2007) 'Targeted ethnography as a critical step to inform cultural adaptations of HIV prevention interventions for adults with severe mental illness'. *Social Science & Medicine*, 65: 296–308.

Appendix 24.1: Participants' information

Pseudonymous	*Gender*	*Profession*	*Time at the institution*
Diana	female	Sociolinguist/PRISSMA Researcher	–
Pedro	male	Psychologist/PRISSMA Researcher	–
Manuela	female	Medical intern	3 years
Denis	male	Medical intern	4 years
Wilma	female	Nurse technician	10 years
Nádia	female	Psychologist	3 years
Nilma	female	Social worker	2 years
Silvana	female	Nurse technician	2 years
Gustavo	male	Music therapist	8 years
Bruno	male	Laboratory technician	15 years
Guida	female	Occupational therapist	9 years

Appendix 24.2: Transcription conventions

.	Sentence-final falling intonation
,	Sentence final rising and fall intonation; more to come
?	Brazilian Portuguese question pattern
...	Pause (length of time was not assigned)
(...)	Transcription impossible
.....	Short text omitted
(words)	Uncertain transcription
[ ]	Unclear referent
-	Glottal stop or abrupt cutting off of sound
{ }	Description of non-verbal behavior

25

Clinical incident reporting, incident investigation, and incident disclosure

Rick Iedema

Introduction

The advent of the new century has seen healthcare communication undergoing a range of dramatic developments. These developments are due to the progressive technologization in the areas of information technology and medical technology, and continuing expansion in the variety of medical services and therapeutic drugs. These developments place a significant burden on healthcare professionals. They require more coordination of the growing number of treatments, and ongoing communication to plan and monitor patients' progress through those treatments. With this, clinical handover of treatment plans between teams has grown into a critical and complex dynamic to create links through the overall process of care (Iedema and Merrick in press).

At the same time, there has been increasing regulation and surveillance of the clinical–medical work that is done in health services. This scrutiny targets clinical and medical products and interventions. This is because they are becoming more complex and powerful, and therefore more prone to accidents. Accidents and incidents are common also because the health care that patients receive is more likely to draw on multiple medical specialties, as well as involving nursing teams, allied health services (physiotherapy, dietetics, etc.), community carers, and general practitioners. This service complexity arises from the need to cater to growing numbers of 'old old' patients who arrive with multiple co-morbidities (mostly chronic illnesses) and high-level care demands.

In turn, this complexity leads to rising levels of staff turnover, burnout, and conflict. It negatively affects the quality and safety of healthcare professionals' work. It has been estimated that one in every ten patients experiences an avoidable accident or incident, and that between 1 and 2 percent of patients experience serious harm, including permanent disability and death (US Institute of Medicine 1999). Growing public concern about the quality and safety of care has led to policies seeking to reform clinical practice. These policies require that healthcare professionals reflect on the risks and mishaps that occur, and engage in learning and practice improvement to make their work safer for future patients. This chapter addresses the varieties of communication that undergird these activities. In doing so, the chapter lays claim to significantly expanding the perspectives that have defined healthcare communication analysis to date.

Historical perspectives

Historically, healthcare communication has been approached principally from the perspective that healthcare communication involves only doctors and patients. Studies in linguistics (Coulthard and Ashby 1976), conversation analysis (Heritage and Maynard 2006), and discourse analysis (Ainsworth-Vaughn 2003) have privileged the doctor–patient consult as the site par excellence where healthcare communication is produced. These analyses revealed critical insights into how doctors legitimate their authority for patients, with more recent studies tracing changes towards more deliberative or 'relational' forms of consultation (Roter 2000). But ultimately, and paradoxically, the concern of these studies with the doctor–patient consult has inadvertently served to confirm rather than question the notion that doctors represent health care. This focus has thereby contributed to the exclusion from our analyses of nurses and other healthcare workers (Gelb-Safran et al. 2006; Iedema 2007b).

A new strand of work has now begun to delve into the multidisciplinary dimensions of healthcare provision. This work takes account of the roles of nurses, allied health professionals (psychologists, dieticians, physiotherapists, and occupational therapists), and health service managers in the provision of care. With this, our healthcare communication focus has moved beyond primary care (the realm of the general practitioner) into secondary and tertiary care, or the more complex domains of healthcare provision found in community health and in hospitals (Iedema 2007a). Examples of this work are in the areas of clinical team communication (Lingard et al. 2004), inter-specialty diagnostic work (Maseide 2003), nursing (Crawford et al. 1998) and nurse–doctor relationships (Riley and Manias 2007; Riley et al. 2007), and mental health (Brown et al. 2008), among others.

This latter work remains rather specialty-specific, however. As health care develops, there are more complex treatments and more variegated trajectories for patients, and this means new ways of communicating need to be generated as well. With some notable exceptions (Engeström et al. 2003; Kerosuo 2007), little is as yet known about the forms of communication that orchestrate care as continuum for the patient. More attention therefore needs to be paid to communication that cuts across these disciplines and specialties in order to create continuity of treatment and care for patients. This is critically important because as we know from clinical incident research, treatments increasingly often go wrong when they are transferred from one clinician to another, from one team to another, from one specialty to another, or from one institution to another (US Institute of Medicine 1999). One way of capturing these kinds of communication is to analyse instances where care breaks down.

Looking across health care, there are very specific kinds of communication that are emerging therefore for all healthcare professionals. They impose significant new communication demands. These are to do with trying to understand and relay what happened when care goes wrong, and what should have happened instead. One difficulty is that many healthcare incidents occur in the 'in-betweens' of care: at handover, referral, discharge, and so on. These processes have received little attention to date, both from health services and from academic researchers. Indeed, they have been allowed to remain taken as given, with little training being provided to clinicians about forms of communication designed to straddle in-betweens, and with even less focus provided on learning from errors and failures resulting from ineffective management of those in-betweens.

Critical issues and topics

Generally when providing care, but specifically when needing to learn from errors and failures, healthcare professionals can no longer operate as autonomous professionals, contributing specialty interventions without much regard for the overall plan, structure, and continuum of care. Healthcare professionals increasingly have to participate in multidisciplinary teams, and this means they have to communicate across professional, specialty, and institutional boundaries. These communication demands stretch well beyond the conventional parameters of health professional identity formation (Benner et al. 1999; Erickson 1999). In addition to learning how to nurse or how to doctor, healthcare professionals are expected to put together care treatments and trajectories that involve numerous specialists and patients. They also have to make their care processes transparent and explicit, measure their clinical outcomes, improve those outcomes, and report outcomes to their managers and health departments (Iedema 2006).

What these new kinds of communication have in common is that they articulate not just the clinical and medical dimensions of care provided to individual patients, but also the organizational dimensions of care provided to cohorts of patients. Thus, healthcare professionals are now expected to reflect on the effectiveness of their shared practices and design improvement strategies (Brown and Crawford 2003). This means they have to account for how well care is structured along the whole pathway of treatment. Besides this organizational focus, there is also a service quality focus. Thus, professionals are increasingly expected to strengthen quality by making their care more 'patient-centred' or 'relationship-centred' (Roter 2000; van Dulmen 2003).

The communication processes discussed in the next section are the culmination of the last two decades of health reforms. These reforms demand from healthcare professionals more transparent and reflexive approaches to practice design, more service-oriented and patient-centred attitudes towards consumers, and a more reflexive attitude towards errors and failures. Contemporary healthcare places particular emphasis on communication practices that address care gone wrong. These practices are called incident reporting, incident investigation, and incident disclosure. They are gaining in prominence and frequency because health care is becoming increasingly complex, and therefore increasingly prone to errors and failures. They are at the heart of professionals' attempt and need to 'tame' health care's runaway complexity by investigating past errors and failures and learning from them.

Current contributions and research: an analysis of emerging processes in healthcare communication

The analysis presented here of incident reporting, incident investigation, and incident disclosure targets how these processes unfold *in situ*. Incident reporting involves a clinician submitting a report to their health organization about a mishap. For its part, incident investigation brings clinicians together from different parts of the hospital to join a team that investigates the causes behind such a mishap. Finally, incident disclosure requires that clinicians discuss the details of mishaps with patients who were harmed by their care. To provide insight into these emerging communication processes, each of these processes is considered along three axes (Figure 25.1): its linguistic manifestation (the transcript: 'text'), its ethnographic dimension ('*in situ* narrative'), and its institutional–contextual dimension (here: 'the policy background').

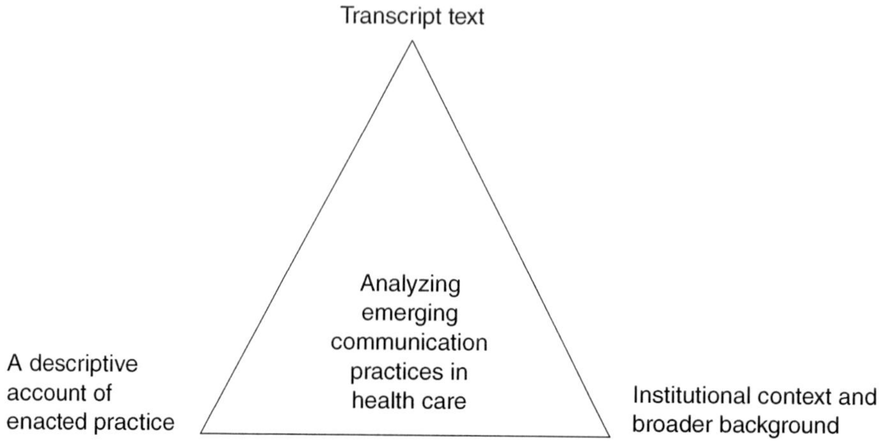

Figure 25.1 Analyzing emerging communication practices: three dimensions

In this chapter, I apply this analysis to three separate datasets. The first is a corpus of 124 incident reports. These incident reports were filed by retrieval clinicians – doctors and nurses who travel by plane or helicopter to rural and remote places in Australia where medical care is needed (Iedema et al. 2006a). As an emergency service, retrieval needs to happen quickly and efficiently, putting extra pressure on the clinicians and support staff involved. Every time there is a problem, clinicians are expected to write an incident report, and send this to their manager.

The second corpus contains notes about and transcripts of five 'root cause analysis' (RCA) meetings which we attended in 2005.[1] These meetings were arranged in response to different healthcare incidents, and all had the purpose of establishing what had gone wrong. The people attending the meetings were volunteers from around the hospital where the problem occurred, but not those originally involved in the incident. The error or failure was investigated until the root cause or root causes were clarified. Research has shown that RCA investigations give team members new responsibilities and powers, such as interviewing those involved in the incident, determining what should have happened, and outlining what those involved in the incident need to do to improve their practice (Iedema et al. 2006b; Iedema et al. 2006c). Indeed, RCA investigations involve delving into problems and harms that in the past were rarely if ever publicly addressed (Bosk 2003). Discourse analysis of this practice has shown that clinicians are faced with reasoning through the clinical and organizational dimensions of care practices, and such reasoning has made only tentative inroads into healthcare professional thinking to date (Iedema et al. 2006b).

The third corpus is a set of transcripts and notes collected from incident disclosure training sessions that we attended in 2008–2009. Incident disclosure is a practice that is becoming increasingly common for clinicians engaged in dangerous care situations. Health policymakers, clinicians, as well as consumers of health care are increasingly concerned to make sure unexpected clinical outcomes and hospital errors are communicated to patients who are harmed or to their families in the case of death (Australian Council for Safety and Quality in Health Care 2003; Canadian Medical Protective Association 2008; UK National Patient Safety Agency 2009). Termed *Open Disclosure* in Canada, New Zealand, the US, and Australia, and *Being Open* in the UK (UK National Patient Safety Agency 2009), these initiatives require clinicians and their colleagues to discuss incidents with patients and carers. Policymakers expect clinicians to be open and honest such that patients and their relatives need not file complaints, or, more importantly, take clinicians and services to court, incurring high costs and much loss of time. The incident disclosure training sessions that were observed were to induct clinicians into speaking openly and honestly about incidents. The sessions involved clinicians in role-playing disclosure communication with patient-actors on the basis of set 'incident' scenarios, in this case a delayed lung cancer diagnosis. In total, 28 hours of such training were observed (Iedema et al. 2009).

Incident reporting

Incident reporting is a genre that is rapidly gaining importance in health care. It is promoted for two reasons: to find out what recurrent errors occur in clinical practice, and to focus professionals on organizational causes rather than blame individuals (Runciman et al. 1993). This focus arose from analyses of organizational incidents showing that it is not individuals who are most often responsible for errors, but work process systems that are badly designed or allowed to deteriorate (Reason 1997). Hence, the emphasis in the incident reporting literature is on 'systems problems', not individuals' mistakes.

The following report is part of the first corpus referred to above: 124 incident reports filed by patient retrieval clinicians. The report reproduced below (Excerpt 1) describes a rather unfortunate event:

> *Excerpt 1*
> ***Story.***[2]
> No porter and wheelchair provided by commercial aircraft. Passenger had fractured left ankle, fractured right wrist, back pain.
> ***Outcome.***
> Increased pain and suffering for patient.
> ***Steps taken or treatment required.***
> Patient crawled to aircraft as she could not walk.
> ***Was this incident preventable?***
> Yes, by airline providing promised service of wheelchair and porter.

This first report describes not a major error but a relatively minor problem (Tucker and Edmondson 2003). The incident, in this case, consists in the airline failing to provide a porter and wheelchair causing a patient having to crawl to the retrieval aircraft. Discursively, the report positions the various parties in very different ways. The airline company is passivized ('by commercial aircraft'), and then buried in a circumstantial clause ('by airline providing [service]'). By contrast, the patient is mostly agent ('Patient had fractured left ankle', 'Patient crawled', 'she could not walk'), except in the 'Outcome' statement: 'Increased pain and suffering for the patient'.

Of course, these choices may have been motivated by the author wanting to maintain a voice of formality that avoids attributing blame: 'No porter or wheelchair provided', 'Increased pain and suffering for the patient'. These choices nevertheless give the impression of being emotionally charged. The patient is described as partaking in several actions despite her injuries, resulting in a very graphic image ('crawling'). At the same time, the airline is rendered grammatically invisible, as if to remind us of its absent service.

We can surmise that reporting an incident is a complex affair: authors can use language in ways that appear dispassionate while at the same time intimating tension and emotion. This tension evokes Sarangi and Roberts's distinction between the interactional and institutional orders of work (Sarangi and Roberts 1999): how people interact is constrained by institutional rules and resources. Here, the way bureaucratic formality dampens emotion about a wrong raises an interesting question: how do incident reporters' personal sentiments and work-related frustrations skew the formal bureaucratic objectives of systems and practice improvement that define incident reporting?

Before addressing this question, let us consider Excerpt 2. This second excerpt is about a rather more serious incident. A patient was intubated in order to stabilize his breathing, but the tube was put into his oesophagus instead of his airway, allowing him (if perhaps not actually causing him) to die.

> *Excerpt 2*
> ***Story.***
> Patient with severe intracerebral bleed. GCS 4 on admission. Intubated by doctor in Emergency Department. Left spontaneously breathing. Retrieval team arrived. Breath sounds heard within usual total assessment. Readied for transfer, paralysed for transport.
> Subsequent demise, presumed to be of neurological cause. Later review of CXR[3] (not looked at by retrieval team) showed ETT[4] in oesophagus.
> ***Outcome.***
> Cardiac arrest.
> ***Steps taken or treatment required.***
> As presumed to be neurological cause, patient already elderly and moribund, aggressive resuscitation not attempted.
> ***Was this incident preventable?***
> Yes – always check CXR when available, re-check airway if paralysing.

The two actors responsible for the death – 'doctor in Emergency' (who intubated incorrectly) and 'retrieval team' (who failed to check the intubation properly) – do not appear explicitly (grammatically) as agents in clauses. We are told that the retrieval team did not review the chest X-ray: 'CXR (not looked at by retrieval team'). As was the case in the first report seen above, in this second report cause is grammatically attenuated rather than foregrounded.

In contrast to the first report above, this second report was written by someone who was implicated in the incident (reporting clinician; personal communication). Pointing to the importance of ethnographic information revealing who on the team wrote this report, the reporting clinician was a member of the retrieval team that failed to check whether the tube was in the patient's airway ('Retrieval team arrived. Breath sounds heard …'). In this case, what is at issue is not the reporter's backgrounding the cause of the incident as a way of complying with bureaucratic standards of formality, but arguably avoiding specifying a causal relationship to limit their own contribution to the intubation not having been checked.

The above makes clear that incident reporting operates at the interstice between reporters' personal emotional responses to 'care gone wrong', inter-professional dynamics to do with status, reputation and fear of legal action, and formal policy demands centring on avoiding blame and promoting organizational learning and practice improvement. The formal nature of reporting an incident no doubt led reporters to avoid making explicit causal connections and instead to use implied and even attenuated attributions of cause. In the first report, the airline service was singled out, albeit very indirectly, for being absent. Blame was tangible in the graphic description of the consequences of the airline's absent service ('patient had to crawl'), amounting to what may be termed a 'token of judgment' (Martin 2000). In the second report, blame of the retrieval team who failed to check the GP's intubation is mitigated when the author grammatically attenuates the link between the team's actions and the patient's demise (cf. 'epistemic caution'; Heritage 1997). The final recommendation of this report ('always check the airway') clearly applies to the retrieval team itself as much as it applies to the hospital doctor who undertook the incident report.

Incident investigation

The spoken interaction shown below is one that involves clinicians in the task of investigating clinical errors as members of Root Cause Analysis or 'RCA' teams. As explained above, RCA investigations are initiated following incidents to enable clinicians to explore and understand what went wrong. In the case focused on here (Excerpt 3), the RCA team investigates a morphine overdose that was inadvertently administered to a motor vehicle accident patient. The clinician speaking below is a doctor:

> *Excerpt 3*
> The other thing was because he [the patient] was so gregarious and entertaining, they [the nurses] didn't – I don't know whether that may have contributed to them not, you know, figuring that that was an issue, because he was so alive and animated that even though he'd had that much morphine, it wasn't sort of affecting him when he arrived up into the theatre, so … as far as – they usually have a fairly sort of stringent checklist in theatre, but I think the gap, you know, in terms of relevant information – putting down the fact that he had that much morphine or the fact that they do crossover their responsibilities and not all the information – the relevant information is handed over, could contribute.
>
> *(RCA meeting #1 2005)*

There are multiple uncertainties for this RCA team member, confirmed by the several uncertainty markers in the talk ('I don't know', 'may have contributed', 'but I think', 'could contribute'). Uncertainty permeates team members' attempt to reconstruct how the incident happened. Team members have to grapple with how things are commonly done around the hospital, and posit causes for what happened and devise solutions from what they are discovering (Excerpt 4). The solution put forward by the same speaker heard above is that clinicians should be expected to fill out a form to clarify what they decided needed to be done and what was done.

> *Excerpt 4*
> It does make – I mean, I completely agree, I'm just not sure what the practical way of resolving it is because … the whole purpose of this is that there's a lot of verbal ordering going on and then the doctor [sighs? inaudible], but the problem is that it very rarely ends at a fixed point and often exactly this happens – that half way through the process, you sign it, but the process continues on for an hour beyond there. So, whether when you sign it, that's the end of that form and you move onto another form, but then you have the problem of keeping – the value of this is it's all in front of you of how much [medication] they've had.
>
> *(RCA meeting #1 2005)*

Expressions like 'I'm not sure', 'the problem of this is that …', and 'rarely' create space for alternative voices and contradictory meanings. This phenomenon has been referred to by Bakhtin (1981) as 'heteroglossia'. The speaker mobilizes heteroglossia to navigate the tension between getting the clinicians to sign off on a form, and yet being unable to minimize the complexity of diagnostic and treatment processes. Turning understanding of the incident into a solution ('get them to sign a form') thus harbours considerable uncertainty. Will filling out a form really prevent handover problems in future? Will such a solution be accepted by the clinical team that made the error of administering an overdose?

This latter question indicates that being a member of an RCA team, and investigating colleagues' incidents and proposing improvements are not straightforward, neutral activities. Indeed, RCA team members find themselves in a delicate position: besides having to appropriate the policy and procedural requirements according to which the RCA investigation is to formally unfold, team members find themselves having to ask probing questions, in order to be able to reconstruct complex events. Additionally, in asking these things they may become seen as 'the conscience' of the service, pursuing the clinicians who erred with questions, reasonings, and practice change recommendations (Iedema et al. 2006b; Iedema et al. 2006c).

The meeting talk above reveals that the team's questioning of practices and standards serves to bring into the open what normally remains taken-for-granted and therefore hidden: the existing 'negotiated order of the hospital' (Strauss et al. 1963). Seen in this light therefore, the investigation was much less straightforward than might have been apparent from its original, policy-defined aim: to identify incident causes and formulate process improvements.

Incident disclosure

As noted above, incident disclosure promotes openness about how incidents happened. Incident disclosure policy requires clinicians to explain what went wrong, and offer apologies to patients who are harmed. In doing so, clinicians are to avoid exposing themselves or their organization to undue legal risk. Apologies can avoid incurring the risk of legal liability by only expressing regret ('we are sorry *this happened*') and not acknowledging responsibility for what went wrong ('we're sorry *we did the wrong thing*') (Vines 2005). This makes doing disclosure hard for clinicians. Being limited to offering 'partial apologies' (*'I'm sorry this happened'*), clinicians may not be able to act with sincerity, and this may prevent them from 'connecting' with the harmed patient.

To appreciate how trainees in a disclosure workshop session tackle this challenge, let us consider the following role-play and discussion sequence. The data presented here were part of a larger study into incident disclosure training (see Iedema et al. 2009). As part of this training, clinicians were asked to role-play disclosing an incident to an actor/patient. In this role-play scenario, clinicians failed to follow-up with the patient about positive X-ray results a year previously. The X-ray showed the presence of lung cancer. Because this result was not communicated to the patient at the time and was only picked up one year later, this dramatically reduces his chances of survival.

In this first extract shown below, a person from the group steps up to the patient-actor and says:

> [name patient] what I would like to say to you is that though the information is still to be investigated, as senior clinicians we'd be offering you a sincere apology and say we'd go about finding out how it all happened.

In response to this, the patient-actor turns to the training facilitator and says, shaking his head, 'that makes no difference', indicating that this apology remains meaningless for him. Then another person assumes the role of discloser. This person says:

> [name patient] um this may not come out very well because we're shattered by what happened. We're very sorry this happened. We don't know how or why. But on behalf of the organization we're very sorry, and we'll make sure that we'll look after you from now on.

The patient-actor comments, again turning to the facilitator, 'this still feels like I've been thrown out of an airplane without a parachute'. The group ponders this for a while, and subsequently agrees that the patient-actor needs to be able to say what he himself feels. A third person from the group takes a seat next to the patient-actor and says:

> I certainly appreciate that that's how you might be feeling. [long pause]
> Perhaps there's some anger? [pause]

This draws a very different response from the patient-actor: he takes his glasses off, rubs his eyes, and says (to the person who addressed him, and 'in character'), 'I'll be bloody pissed off when I get out of here [the hospital].'

In exploring their inadequate attempts at communicating regret to the patient, the participants realize that they are not 'connecting' with the patient-actor. Their deliberations address why this might be so, and they agree that the patient-actor needs communicative space to express his emotions. He needs to be 'given the floor' (Edelsky 1981). Giving the other 'the floor' means that we show we are willing to listen to the other. This act of listening is what Egan (2006) termed 'active listening'.

Active listening is a technique that involves using silences and pauses to elicit input and responses from one's interlocutor. The effect of using these silences and pauses is quite marked in the scenario described above. In response to the third participant's silences and pauses, the actor assumes his 'patient' character for the first time: he draws breath, takes his glasses off (possibly signifying acceptance), and articulates in honest terms what he (as patient) will feel when he leaves the doctor's rooms. As this exchange unfolds, and no doubt realizing the power and significance of the pauses, everyone in the group remains silent and attentive. They know something important has happened: they have 'cracked' the problem: they got the actor-patient to engage with them.

The emotional dynamic just described is critical to incident disclosure. If those disclosing the incident fail to make room for the patient's thoughts and feelings, as occurred in much of the training seen above, the patient will leave without the full spectrum of his or her concerns, thoughts, and misgivings having seen the light. But through active listening, through creating pauses and silences that drew the patient-actor in, the clinicians were able to *connect* with him and get him to reveal his 'patient' feelings.

Active listening requires healthcare professionals to absorb patients' and relatives' emotional or dismissive responses without reacting negatively or defensively. They need to engage patients and relatives in 'riding out' the full momentum of their sentiments and misgivings about the harm (Charon 2001) and bring them back to communication that constructively addresses the question, 'where to from here?' By attuning themselves to patients' and relatives' emotions, clinicians shape a context such that those harmed will feel safe to articulate their feelings, concerns, and preferences for how to continue from here

(Hesson et al. 2012). This is critical to enabling those harmed to become reconciled to their sad circumstances, and, perhaps, to an imperfect future.

Framed thus, 'active listening' acts as risk containment strategy, as therapeutic tactic, and as humanizing gesture. Enabling the patient to reconnect with their clinicians may limit the risk that his or her harm will motivate them to remain angry and seek legal action. Equally, reconnecting with those in charge of the care is therapeutic: it means the patient's care and his care relationships can now resume. Third, active listening may draw everybody in, not merely the (actor-)patient. Seen thus, active listening may create a humanizing dynamic, with everyone – clinicians included – becoming entrained by it.

Recommendations for practice

The above analysis points to a significant expansion in the healthcare professional's communication repertoire. Above we considered communication practices that moved well beyond history-taking, breaking bad news, shared-decision making, and patient-centred care in the communication demands they place on clinicians. This communication repertoire expansion pertains principally to healthcare professionals relating to one another and how they constitute the work. Relating to colleagues and arranging tasks are no longer premised on the assumption that there is a strict professional hierarchy, with authority and decision-making power concentrated at the top of that hierarchy. Instead, communicating with immediate colleagues and devising decisions on-the-spot are now critical to resolving local issues and challenges. Such networked communication enables tasks to be dynamically arranged and rearranged in response to rising practice complexity.

Not surprisingly, in view of the above, teamwork relations are increasingly couched in terms like 'mindful interdependence' (Weick 2004) and 'distributed intelligence' (Iedema 2011). These terms highlight the importance of clinicians' negotiating local courses of action in a deliberative fashion, and they de-emphasize traditional kinds of work relationships premised on strict rules, predefined tasks, and rigid boundaries. The complexity of care limits the applicability of hierarchical knowledge relying on rules and boundaries, because complexity tends to require creative solutions or 'workarounds'.

Workarounds place very specific demands on the contemporary healthcare professional. This is because workarounds veer off into what Amalberti terms the 'illegal–normal' space of practice: the space where practice departs in sometimes dangerous ways from what is laid down in guidelines and protocols (Amalberti et al. 2006). Operating in and through this risky space, clinicians need to rely on communicative access and speed such that they can quickly negotiate any issues and problems arising. For this reason too, team simulations are now used to test and strengthen clinicians' ability to negotiate complex events quickly and locally, even if they have limited knowledge of each other as team members (Jeffs 2010).

In parallel with the above, relationships with patients have begun to shift from being patriarchal towards being deliberative (Roter 2000). Deliberation with colleagues is demanding, but deliberating professional and technical issues with patients can be even more demanding. This is because patients do not always command the health literacy level required for negotiating complex care issues, and neither do they always share clinicians' priorities and norms. This imposes a special burden on clinicians, needing to bring patients up to speed with the available options, the likely implications, normative issues, and their enhanced responsibility for final decisions.

Critical here too are communication training programs that involve healthcare professionals in simulated scenarios with patient-actors (Hall et al. 2009). These scenario role-plays enable clinicians to experience and learn from the difficulties of speaking to people who may not appreciate technical–clinical details, or have expectations that diverge from those assumed to be natural and necessary by the clinician.

Future directions

In the past, healthcare professional expertise was acted out according to relatively insulated, stable, and time-honoured knowledges and practices. The doctor–patient consult used to be considered to be the apotheosis of care. Now, healthcare professionals have to communicate with increasing numbers of stakeholders about the experiences, structures, policies, guidelines, reforms, and risks, failures and improvements that affect them and their work. Where before healthcare professional communication centred principally on mobilizing and applying formal medical knowledge, it now has expanded towards harnessing numerous professional and lay expertises, including reflexive and relational expertises oriented to realizing learning, listening, and openness (Gelb-Safran et al. 2006).

These developments have led to a considerable shift in the communication demands faced by healthcare professionals. Healthcare professionalization used to centre on adopting values and behaviours that were determined primarily by the clinicians' own fraternity (Erickson 1999). Now, these professionals are expected to identify with several values and discourses that run counter to their profession's interests (Freidson 1994): health reform, service culture, and patient-centredness. Professionals are expected to show enhanced sensitivity to complex circumstances and impending or existing risks, awareness of others' feelings, experiences, opinions and sentiments, and willingness to change in how things can be done and said. All these developments require new ways of communicating on the part of the healthcare professional, some of the more prominent and recent of which this chapter has exemplified and analyzed.

With this, healthcare communication analysis needs to shift from the classic sites that have predominated to date (e.g., the general practitioner's surgery), to sites where care complexity is acute, and where communication analysis is critical to assist professionals. Such sites include intensive care departments, acute surgery, community carer networks, family (end-of-life) conferencing, incident investigation, and incident disclosure. Here, however, established kinds of communication research come up against their own methodological limits (Iedema 2007a). Needing to come to terms with the analytical and methodological demands of these new sites and their peculiar complexity, communication analysis is in need of new approaches and different kinds of outcomes. This is critical if such analysis is to function in sites where professionals are in dire need of support with negotiating the rising complexity of their work.

Related topics

Professional practice; health policy reform; incident reporting; incident investigation; incident disclosure; affect.

Notes

1 'Root cause analysis' (RCA) is now applied in many post-industrial countries, including the US, UK, Canada, and Australia. RCA involves a team of clinician volunteers meeting to study what might have led to the error in question, and this usually encompasses doing interviews with clinicians involved in the incident, studying medical notes, and inviting experts to explain complicated issues to the team (Iedema et al. 2006c).
2 The bold headings are part of the form used to report the incident.
3 CXR stands for chest X-ray.
4 ETT stands for endotracheal tube, a tube used for intubation.

Further reading

Iedema, R., J. Mesman, and K. Carroll. (2013) *Visualising Healthcare Improvement: Innovation from Within*. Oxford: Radcliffe Medical Press.
Jones, L. and B.M. Watson. (2012) 'Developments in health communication in the 21st century.' *Journal of Language and Social Psychology* 20(10): 1–22.
Jones, R. (2013) *Health and Risk Communication*. London: Routledge.

References

Ainsworth-Vaughn, N. (2003) 'The discourse of medical encounters.' In D. Schiffrin, D. Tannen, and H.E. Hamilton (eds) *The Handbook of Discourse Analysis*, Oxford: Blackwell.
Amalberti, R., C. Vincent, Y. Auroy, and G. de Saint-Maurice. (2006) 'Violations and migrations in health care: a framework for understanding and management.' *Quality & Safety in Health Care* 15(Suppl 1): i66–i77.
Australian Council for Safety and Quality in Health Care. (2003) 'Open Disclosure Standard: a national standard for open communication in public and private hospitals following an adverse event in health care.' Commonwealth of Australia, Canberra.
Bakhtin, M.M. (1981) *The Dialogic Imagination*. Austin, TX: University of Texas Press.
Benner, P., P. Hooper-Kyriakidis, and D. Stannard. (1999) *Clinical Wisdom and Interventions in Critical Care: A Thinking-in-Action Approach*. Philadelphia, PA: W.B. Saunders.
Bosk, C. (2003) *Forgive and Remember: Managing Medical Failure*. Chicago, IL: University of Chicago Press.
Brown, B. and P. Crawford. (2003) 'The clinical governance of the soul: "deep management" and the self-regulating subject in integrated community mental teams.' *Social Science & Medicine* 56: 67–81.
Brown, B., P. Crawford, and L. Mullany. (2008) 'Clinical governmentality: a critical linguistic perspective on clinical governance in health care organizations.' *Journal of Applied Linguistics* 2(3): 273–298.
Canadian Medical Protective Association. (2008) 'Communicating with your patient about harm: disclosure of adverse events.' Canadian Medical Protective Association, Ottawa.
Charon, R. (2001) 'Narrative medicine: a model for empathy, reflection, profession, and trust.' *Journal of the American Medical Association* 286: 1897–1902.
Coulthard, R.M. and M.C. Ashby. (1976) 'A linguistic description of doctor–patient interviews.' In M. Wadsworth and D. Robinson (eds) *Studies in Everyday Medical Life*, London: Martin Robertson.
Crawford, P., B. Brown, and P. Nolan. (1998) *Communicating Care: The Language of Nursing*. Cheltenham: Stanley Thornes.
Edelsky, C. (1981) 'Who's got the floor?' *Language in Society* 10: 383–421.
Egan, Gerard. (2006) *The Skilled Helper: A Problem-Management and Opportunity-Development Approach to Helping*. New York: Brooks/Cole.
Engeström, Y., R. Engeström, and H. Kerosuo. (2003) 'The discursive construction of collaborative care.' *Applied Linguistics* 24: 286–315.
Erickson, F. (1999) 'Appropriation of voice and presentation of self as a fellow physician: aspects of a discourse of apprenticeship in medicine.' In S. Sarangi and C. Roberts (eds) *Talk, Work and the*

Institutional Order: Discourse in Medical, Mediation and Management Settings, New York: Mouton de Gruyter.

Freidson, E. (1994) *Professionalism Reborn: Theory, Prophesy and Policy*. Cambridge: Polity Press.

Gelb-Safran, D., W.L. Miller, and H.B. Beckman. (2006) 'Organizational dimensions of relationship-centred care.' *Journal of General Internal Medicine* 21: S9–S15.

Hall, J.A., D.L. Roter, D.C. Blanch, and R.M. Frankel. (2009) 'Nonverbal sensitivity in medical students: implications for clinical interactions.' *Journal of General Internal Medicine* 24: 1217–1222.

Heritage, J. (1997) 'Conversation analysis and institutional talk: analyzing data.' In D. Silverman (ed.) *Qualitative Research: Theory, Method and Practice*, London: Sage.

Heritage, J. and D.W. Maynard. (2006) 'Introduction: analyzing interaction between doctors and patients in primary care encounters.' In J. Heritage and D.W. Maynard (eds) *Communication in Medical Care: Interaction between Primary Physicians and Patients*, Cambridge: Cambridge University Press.

Hesson, A.M., I. Sarinopoulos, R.M. Frankel, and R.C. Smith. (2012) 'A linguistic study of patient-centered interviewing: emergent interactional effects.' *Patient Education and Counseling* 88(3): 373–380.

Iedema, R. (2006) '(Post-)bureaucratizing medicine: health reform and the reconfiguration of contemporary clinical work.' In F. Meyer and M. Gotti (eds) *Advances in Medical Discourse Analysis: Oral and Written Contexts*, Gottingen: Peter Lang.

——(2007a) 'Communicating hospital work.' In R. Iedema (ed.) *Discourses of Hospital Communication: Tracing Complexities in Contemporary Health Organizations*, Basingstoke: Palgrave-Macmillan.

——(ed.) (2007b) *Discourses of Hospital Communication: Tracing Complexities in Contemporary Health Organizations*. Basingstoke: Palgrave-Macmillan.

——(2011) 'Creating safety by strengthening clinicians' capacity for reflexivity.' *BMJ Quality and Safety* 20: S83–S86.

Iedema, R. and E. Merrick. (in press) 'Team work in health care: how clinicians negotiate the continuity of clinical tasks and care responsibilities.' In S. Sarangi and P. Linell (eds) *Team Talk: Decision-Making Across Boundaries in Health and Social Care*, London: Equinox.

Iedema, R., A. Flabouris, S. Grant, and C.M. Jorm. (2006a) 'Narrativizing errors of care: critical incident reporting in clinical practice.' *Social Science & Medicine* 62: 134–144.

Iedema, R., C.M. Jorm, J. Braithwaite, J. Travaglia, and M. Lum. (2006b) 'A root cause analysis of clinical errors: confronting the disjunction between formal rules and situated clinical activity.' *Social Science & Medicine* 63: 1201–1212.

Iedema, R., C.M. Jorm, D. Long, J. Braithwaite, J. Travaglia, and M. Westbrook. (2006c) 'Turning the medical gaze in upon itself: root cause analysis and the investigation of clinical error.' *Social Science & Medicine* 62: 1605–1615.

Iedema, R., C. Jorm, J. Wakefield, C. Ryan, and S. Dunn. (2009) 'Practising open disclosure: clinical incident communication and systems improvement.' *Sociology of Health & Illness* 31: 262–277.

Jeffs, L., S. Epsin, S.E. Shannon, W. Levinson, M. Kazman Kohn, and L. Lingard. (2010) 'A new way of relating: perceptions associated with a team-based error disclosure simulation intervention.' *Quality and Safety in Health Care* 19: 56–60.

Kerosuo, H. (2007) 'Renegotiating disjunctions in interorganizationally provided care.' In R. Iedema (ed.) *The Discourses of Hospital Communication*, Basingstoke: Palgrave.

Lingard, L., S. Espin, W.F. Whyte, G. Regher, G.R. Baker, R. Reznick, et al. (2004) 'Communication failures in the operating room: an observational classification of recurrent types and effects.' *Quality and Safety in Health Care* 13: 330–334.

Martin, J.R. (2000) 'Beyond exchange: appraisal systems in English.' In S. Hunston and G. Thompson (eds) *Evaluation in Text: Authorial Stance and the Construction of Discourse*, Oxford: Oxford University Press.

Maseide, P. (2003) 'Medical talk and moral order: social interaction and collaborative clinical work.' *Text* 23: 369–403.

Reason, J.T. (1997) *Managing the Risks of Organizational Accidents*. Aldershot: Ashgate.

Riley, R. and E. Manias. (2007) 'Governing the operating room list.' In R. Iedema (ed.) *The Discourse of Hospital Communication: Tracing Complexities in Contemporary Health Care Services*, Basingstoke: Palgrave-Macmillan.

Riley, R., E. Manias, R. Forsyth, and R. Iedema. (2007) 'Whiteboards: a mechanism of communication and social control in clinical practice.' *Communication & Medicine* 4: 165–175.
Roter, D. (2000) 'The enduring and evolving nature of the patient–physician relationship.' *Patient Education & Counseling* 39: 5–15.
Runciman, W.B., R.K. Webb, R. Lee, and R. Holland. (1993) 'The Australian Incident Monitoring study: system failure – an analysis of 2000 incident reports.' *Anaesthetic Intensive Care* 21: 684–695.
Sarangi, S. and C. Roberts. (1999) 'The dynamics of interactional and institutional orders in work-related settings.' In S. Sarangi and C. Roberts (eds) *Talk, Work and Institutional Order*, New York: Mouton de Gruyter.
Strauss, A., L. Schatzman, D. Ehrlich, R. Bucher, and M. Sabshin. (1963) 'The hospital and its negotiated order.' In E. Freidson (ed.) *The Hospital in Modern Society*, New York: Free Press of Glencoe.
Tucker, A.L. and A.C. Edmondson. (2003) 'Why hospitals don't learn from failures: organisational and psychological dynamics that inhibit system change.' *California Management Review* 45: 55–72.
UK National Patient Safety Agency. (2009) 'Being open: communicating patient safety incidents with patients, families and carers.' National Patient Safety Agency, London.
US Institute of Medicine. (1999) *To Err is Human: Building a Safer Health System*. Washington, DC: National Academy Press.
van Dulmen, S. (2003) 'Patient-centredness.' *Patient Education and Counseling* 51: 195–196.
Vines, P. (2005) 'Apologising to avoid liability: cynical civility or practical morality?' *Sydney Law Review* 27: 483–505.
Weick, K. (2004) 'Reduction of medical errors through mindful interdependence.' In K. Sutcliffe and M. Rosenthal (eds) *Medical Error*, San Francisco, CA: Jossey-Bass.

Part III

Patient–provider communication in interaction

26

Before the 'official diagnosis'

A focus on prediagnostic statements

Thomas Spranz-Fogasy

Introduction

Before pronouncing their diagnosis, doctors often comment on patients' utterances, verbalize their observations, announce test findings, explain relations, or draw preliminary conclusions during a verbal and/or physical examination. These utterances contain diagnostic elements which are set up for subsequent interactive use and which lead into the next stage of the examination. This all happens *before* the 'official diagnosis' (Stivers 1998: 241) and *with respect* to it. Utterances of this type will therefore be called *prediagnostic statements*.

While questions in the context of the examination as well as diagnostic statements and directives within the treatment phase of doctor–patient interaction have all been looked at in great detail by conversation analysts and researchers from other fields in the social sciences, prediagnostic statements have rarely been investigated as an independent topic (but see Stivers 1998; Heritage and Stivers 1999; Mangione-Smith et al. 2003; Heritage et al. 2010); rather they were included in the general context of diagnosis (Heath 1992; Maynard 2003 and elsewhere; Peräkylä 1997 and elsewhere). The reason for this lies in their characteristic oscillation between examination and diagnosis. However, this in-between quality and, consequently, their inconspicuous appearance in medical interaction provide invaluable insights not only into medical interaction itself but also into a variety of linguistic features, cognitive phenomena, and interactional processes contained therein (Heritage and Stivers 1999).

This chapter combines a review of recent research on prediagnostic statements with some initial findings from my current work on this issue in the context of conversation analysis. I will first sketch the broader context of the research and then present an example of a medical examination which I will use as the central database for an analysis of important phenomena and functions of this particular utterance type.

Phase models and sequential analysis

Nearly all publications analyzing doctor–patient interaction in the English-speaking world refer to the idealized logical sequence model by Byrne and Long (1976: 21); more recent publications also do this, but place a much greater emphasis on the role of the patient

(Heritage and Maynard 2006; Heritage and Clayman 2010). The model characterizes diagnosis as a stage of its own, i.e., stage IV: 'The doctor, or the doctor and the patient, or the patient (in that order of probability) consider the condition' (Byrne and Long 1976: 21). This premise – diagnosis as a discrete event (Stivers 1998) or a distinct action (Heath 1992) – is also dominant in all publications dealing with diagnosis or prediagnostic statements (e.g., Heritage and Stivers 1999; Maynard 2003; Peräkylä 1998). In a similar way, models of doctor–patient interaction that have been developed in other countries define diagnosis as a separate event, e.g., as a 'Pragmem' in German 'Functional Pragmatics' (Meyer 2004), or as a component of the action scheme in the German theory of Interaction Constitution (Kallmeyer 2005; Nowak and Spranz-Fogasy 2009). In all models, the core elements of doctor–patient interactions in primary care are threefold: (verbal and physical) examination, diagnosis, and treatment. Additionally, these core elements are mainly characterized by three complementary utterance types: examining questions, diagnostic statements, and treatment directives. Accordingly, many of the doctors' statements are categorized as being part of the diagnostic phase but are actually uttered prediagnostically *within* the examination. Only online commentaries during physical examination are clearly differentiated from diagnosis because of their function within the examination phase (see Stivers 1998).

One reason for the paucity of information on prediagnostic statements as a phenomenon in their own right is based on the conceptual conflict between Byrne and Long's (1976) phase model and the sequential orientation of conversation analysis (Schegloff 2007). Maynard's *news delivery sequence* (Maynard 2003) focuses on the sequential context of the diagnosis, i.e., 'turns in which the doctor names the patient's disease', an activity type which Peräkylä considers to be the 'core of the overall activity of diagnostic information giving' (Peräkylä 1998: 304). The *news delivery sequence* contains four steps: (1) announcement of news, (2) announcement response, (3) elaboration of news, (4) assessment of news (Maynard 2003: 95). In the case of bad news doctors often insert a perspective-display sequence where they remind patients of test results and other findings. As such, prediagnostic statements in this sequence are not seen as being elements of the examination phase.

Peräkylä also deals with prediagnostic statements when distinguishing between *straight factual assertion* and the *evidence formulating pattern* (Peräkylä 1997). The latter is prediagnostic per se and many examples of the first type in Peräkylä's articles are prediagnostic as well, e.g., the announcement of findings or a diagnosis of exclusion (Peräkylä 1997, 1998, 2002, 2006). However, Peräkylä's research does not aim to identify divergent types of utterances for breaking medical news but to analyze their function within the relation between authority and accountability. He convincingly demonstrates that doctors present themselves as 'accountable for the evidential basis' of their diagnoses by coordinating their 'design and placement' instead of just claiming *unconditional authority*, as Parsons or Freidson argue (Peräkylä 1998: 301). Peräkylä's main concern is to show the relevance and strength of conversation analysis in analyzing social phenomena such as authority, for example.

At first sight, divergent modeling and divergent intentions concerning inquiry into diagnosis are not that problematic, but they sometimes hide important interactional phenomena connected with processing knowledge and understanding during examination. In this regard, analyses of prediagnostic commentaries and online commentaries during physical examination turn out to be more instructive.

Explicit inquiries into prediagnostic utterances have been undertaken by Stivers (1998), Heritage and Stivers (1999), Mangione-Smith et al. (2003), and Heritage et al. (2010). As Heritage and Stivers point out, there was no previous research on this topic worth mentioning. They found only one reference in Byrne and Long, who wrote that 'few doctors actually explain what they are doing when they examine (1976: 24) and cited only one example for this utterance type: 'Now I'm listening to your lungs. *They sound clear*' (ibid. 25). Roter and Hall subsumed only one prediagnostic utterance under the coding category of 'positive talk': 'Your blood pressure is great' (Roter and Hall 1992: 83f.).

To underline this point again, each of these four articles on prediagnostic/online commentaries reveals a particular research interest connected with that kind of utterance. Whereas Heritage and Stivers (1999) state that online commentary during the physical examination is a 'method to shape patient expectation', Mangione-Smith et al. (2003) and Heritage et al. (2010) take it as 'a communication tool for avoiding inappropriate antibiotic prescribing' according to the respective titles. Stivers deals with prediagnostic commentaries in a veterinarian clinic focusing on all 'diagnostically relevant statements that describe what the physician is seeing or feeling, anticipate or speculate on diagnosis' (1998: 241). Similarly, Heritage and Stivers (1999), Mangione-Smith et al. (2003), and Heritage et al. (2010) define online commentary but with explicit reference to physical examination, while Stivers (1998) and Heritage and Stivers (1999: 1503) cover prediagnostic utterances at 'any point prior to the delivery of the diagnosis'. All of the studies actually dealing with prediagnostic statements (i.e., including Maynard and Peräkylä) claim that there are differences with regards to content, design, production, placement or positioning, and receipt as relevant criteria to dissociate them from an 'official diagnosis' or 'explicit diagnostic evaluations' (Stivers 1998; Peräkylä 1998; Heritage and Stivers 1999; Mangione-Smith et al. 2003; Maynard 2003; Heritage et al. 2010).

In order to gain comprehensive insights into the phenomenology and interactive function of this utterance type we will take all prediagnostic statements during the – verbal *and* physical – examination into consideration and include doctoral utterances focusing on *diagnostically relevant elements* in a *declarative mode* and mentioned *before* the official diagnosis in our working definition of prediagnostic statements.[1]

This definition of prediagnostic statements also includes *online explanations* during physical examination which Heritage and Stivers explicitly exclude (Heritage and Stivers 1999: 1501), as well as *diagnostic explanations* during the verbal part of the examination (see Example 1, line 55). Peräkylä explicitly excludes 'preliminary diagnostic statements ... before the final diagnosis' (Peräkylä 1998: 304) but analyzes, for example, diagnoses of exclusion which are, by definition, not final diagnoses and are therefore classified as prediagnostic statements in the present chapter.

Finally, using the term 'statement' instead of 'commentary' enables us to apply a more neutral term; generally, prediagnostic statements do not include a kind of assessment, and the presentation of previously recorded findings is not an online reference as it is necessary for online commentaries.

The following chapter presents the context of inquiry and a description of data at first and proceeds with the sample analysis with subsections of linguistic, cognitive, and interactive dimension. Further sections deal with combinations of prediagnostic statements and interactive consequences. A summary reviews the results of this chapter.

Context of inquiry and data

This contribution should be seen in the context of a larger research project at the Institute for the German Language (Mannheim) which is concerned with 'verbal and communicative displays of understanding in interaction' (http://www.ids-mannheim.de/prag/verstehen/home_eng.html). The project deals with linguistic resources, often grammaticalized, which function specifically as displays of understanding, including the sequential practices of claiming and demonstrating, negotiating and repairing understanding, and covers the relationship between tasks and displays of understanding, genre, participation framework, and social structure (Deppermann and Schmitt 2009). We study these questions by drawing on audio and video recordings of interactions from different fields of practice, medical interaction being one of them. The findings in this chapter are based on 30 medical interactions by four doctors from different medical fields (general practitioner, internist, or urologist). The encounters lasted a total of 4h55min, ranging from 1min13sec to 35min12sec per interaction. The doctors produced a total of 138 prediagnostic statements. First, I will present a single case study and refer to other interactions later on.

Sample Analysis

The following transcript contains a complete medical examination in a general practice from the opening question in line 1 (Robinson and Heritage 2006; Heritage and Robinson 2006) to the final, albeit rather vague, diagnosis in line 70. During this examination, the doctor asks questions, carries out a physical examination, and occasionally formulates in a paradigmatic way seven prediagnostic statements (marked by bold). The transcription follows GAT2 (Selting et al. 2009), the standard transcribing conventions used in Germany (conventions are explained in Appendix 26.1 at the end of this chapter). The example is long due to the necessity of translating into English.

Example 1 AA_BI_03 (00:00–01:40)

D: NA weswegen kommen sie denn HER?
well why are you here
P: ja ich habe seit drei tagen einen ä:h (0.2) FINger
wo ich nicht weiß:-
well for three days I have a uh finger where I don't know
(0.1) was ich damit MAchen soll;
what I should do with it
(0.8) also ich' wenn ich' (0.2)
well I when I
gestern abend hab ich n BRIEF geschrieben;=
yesterday evening I wrote a letter
=da is er also ganz DICK gewo:rden, (0.5)
then it got really swollen
D: hm::?=
hm
P: =und das is als ob hier ein (0.1) ne NAdel
oder irgendwas> DRIN wär; (1.0)
and that is as though here a a needle
or something would be inside
D: ham se n unfall gehabt?
did you have an accident
P: n 'überHAU:PT nichts passiert;
n nothing happened at all
P: [(in letzter zeit)]
lately

13 D: **[nich erINNERlich;]**
not rememberable
(0.1) was is n das hier für n kleines LOCH- (0.2)
what is this little hole here
P: ja das heiß:t (0.3)
yes that means
da hat mich glaub ich eine KATze:,
(1.0) gehakt-
there I think a cat hooked me
D: wann WARN [das?]
when was it
P: [das is-]
that is
20 o:ch-
och
(0.1) des is- (1.3)
that is
moment ich bin (0.2) ich KOMM nämlich jetzt
von auSTRA:lien; und ä:h-
(1.2)
wait a second I am I that is to say I have just got back
from australia right now and uh
25 meine güte des müsste vielleicht am- (0.7)
oh my goodness that must have been perhaps
letzte woche (0.2) DONnerstag gewesen sein.
(0.8)
last week on thursday
28 D: **ja:: aber hoffentlich hängt das nicht damit zuSAMmen**
yes but hopefully it is not related to that
[nich, (.) die hat] ZWEImal hier reingehackt;
TAG it has hooked me twice here
30 P: [ja also sie hat-]
yes so it had
D: [nich]
TAG
P: [nein]
no
das (0.2) das bin ICH gewesen;
that that was me
das is [also] [die-]
that is so the
35 D: [ja:] [und] HIER hat ne katze gekratzt; (0.4)
yes and here a cat scratched
und DA tuts auch we:h? (.) an der stelle?
and that's where it also hurts at this point
P: nein also HIE:R; (0.4) sticht es; (0.4)
no well here it pricks

D: da:- (0.4)
there
P: ja-
yes
40 (0.2) da-
there
(0.2) ziemlich; (0.7)
quite a lot
42 D: das is wohl der grund; (1.6)
that must probably be the reason
an den ANdern fingern ist nichts;
there is nothing on the other fingers
P: ÜBERhaupt nichts nein-
absolutely nothing no
D: und die wird das wird ganz DICK hier;
and the is here it is swelling
P: zum beispiel gestern abend hab ich n BRIEF geschrieben=
=also da hab ich n gar nich mehr grA:de gekriegt;
for example yesterday evening I wrote a letter
well I wasn't able to straighten it at all
D: ja ja:,
yes yes
(0.5) und über NACHT klingt das dann wieder AB;
and overnight it wears off again
50 P: ja also DA is:-
yes well there is
D: an 'andern geLEN[ken oder so haben sie GAR nichts;
you have nothing on other joints or so
P: [nein überHAUPT nichts; (.) ÜBER
no nothing at all
P: haupt nichts;]
nothing at all
D: nichts,]
nothing
(0.5) 'hmhm->
hmhm
55 (3.9) katzen haben manchmal (0.3) allerhand DRECK unter den
cats sometimes have quite a lot of dirt under the
P: ja:, (0.3) [ja-] [hmhm-]
yes yes hmhm
D: [fin]gern; nich [unter den] krallen;
fingers TAG under the claws
P: ja-
yes
D: nich wahr?
don't they
60 da KANN schon mal was passIEr[n;]
indeed something may happen then

P: [ja;]
yes
also TOLLwütig is sie nich weil des is ene:;
well it is not rabid because that is a

63 **D: ne- (.)**
no
das [GLAUB ich-]
I believe that

P: [ne Eigene] katze gewesen nich-
pet cat nich

D: [ja:, das das GLAUB ich auch nich;]
yes I don't believe that that either

P: [und (...);]
and

68 **D: das hat mit TOLLwut nix zu [tUN;]**
that doesn't have anything to do with rabies

P: [ja-]
yes

70 D: das is 'ein 'ein: sicher ein: WEICHteilinfekt-
that s a a surely a soft tissue infection

P: 'hmhm,
hmhm

D: den se da HAben; [ne,]
that you have here TAG

P: ['hmhm]
hmhm

D: sONST sind sie immer gesund gewesen- (0.4)
otherwise you have always been healthy

The examination presented here reveals many aspects relevant for an analysis of prediagnostic statements which can be roughly characterized as follows; they

- come up during the examination phase and are placed before the final diagnosis;
- are mostly self-initiated by the doctor;
- are barely discussed by patients;
- function as summaries, often as shortcuts, and appear as staging posts (Heritage and Stivers 1999: 1510) within the examination process with a tendency towards increased density as they get closer to the point of diagnosis;
- cannot be differentiated clearly from declarative questions (as the patient's response onset in line 30 suggests);
- have some linguistic features in common: they are of the same declarative syntactic type but with different pragmatic functions, and they reveal fine-grained modifications via modal and epistemic verbs, particles, and other lexical resources;
- display cognitions via cognitive categories (e.g., *rabies*), cognitive concepts (e.g., *reason*), and cognitive operations (e.g., inference procedures, as in line 28);
- display the local state of understanding and certainty;
- are characterized as preliminary and partial in nature and, as a result, provide a starting point for further examination.

Even just a quick first glance reveals how many interactional phenomena and functions prediagnostic statements contain. In the following sections we will look at them more systematically with respect to three fundamental analytical dimensions: linguistic, cognitive, and interactive. If necessary, occasionally I include references to other interactions of my data sample.

The linguistic dimension

During a medical examination, the patient's presentation of his/her complaints, signs, and symptoms are at the focus of talk (Hamilton 2004). The doctor's questions and the patient's answers are dominant utterance types when eliciting relevant information for diagnosis and treatment. Iteratively, prediagnostic statements appear as declarative utterances mentioning elements of the patient's condition (such as findings, reviews, causes, diagnoses of exclusion, or preliminary diagnoses) but not explicitly (diagnostically) labeling that condition as a whole. Thus the first linguistic feature of prediagnostic statements is their declarative, predicating quality. But this feature can be ambiguous for both participants and analysts. Declarative questions share the same syntactical structure but are, for the most part, clearly identifiable as questions via the context or their prosody (Heritage and Claymann 2010; Spranz-Fogasy 2010).

Example 1 contains such an ambiguous utterance. In line 28 the doctor assumes a connection between the patient's complaints and her being injured by a cat: *but hopefully it is not related to that*. The doctor continues her examination with her next question, treating her declarative utterance as a statement, while the patient begins with an answer, having identified the same utterance as a declarative question. Here, the boundaries between declarative and interrogative utterances become indistinct – but that also reveals an important resource for interlocutors to deal with complex and sometimes unclear topics in a very flexible way.

Prediagnostic statements are also afforded flexibility with the help of other linguistic features, namely lexical and pragmatic features. From a lexical perspective, alongside medical terms, prediagnostic statements often characteristically contain modal verbs, epistemic verbs, or assessment terms. By doing so, the doctor adapts his/her utterances to his/her state of knowledge and understanding. The same is the case with the number of other modifiers such as modal particles, other adverbs, or connectors regularly found in prediagnostic statements. Such modifiers either 'downgrade epistemic certainty' (Stivers 1998: 251) or upgrade it. In Example 1 in line 42 the doctor downgrades her certainty with the adverb *probably* and later upgrades it in her diagnosis of exclusion in line 68 with the generalizing adverb *anything*.

Additionally, the pragmatic function of prediagnostic statements is very flexible, ranging from certain assertion, report, comment, explanation, definition, demonstration, and assessment to assumption, etc. (Stivers 1998: 251). Obviously, flexibility is the main linguistic trademark of prediagnostic statements but not uniquely so: other utterance types in an examination also involve caution as an examination is, per se, an interactional state of uncertainty for the participants.

The cognitive dimension

As already indicated in the descriptions of the linguistic features, many of them also refer to cognitive aspects of prediagnostic statements. Medical terms, epistemic verbs, evaluative expressions, conclusive particles and conjunctions display the doctor's cognitive access to the patient's presentation or to his/her own observations. It seems as though the doctor's online thinking is revealed in this way. (But remember that some topics remain unspoken as investigations into diagnoses suggest, e.g., bad news is often concealed, shrouded, or just alluded to (Maynard 2003). As Heritage and Stivers (1999: 1503) state, online commentaries are most often used to report on signs that are absent or mild or non-serious; conversely unfavorable information is often obviously withheld by doctors.)

Example 1 documents the doctor's development from knowing nothing (*well why are you here*, line 1) to stating a specific diagnosis (*that s a a surely a soft tissue infection*, line 70) via

1 assuming a relation between the cat's 'hooking' the patient and her complaints (*but hopefully it is not related to that,* line 28),
2 identifying an assumed reason (*that must probably be the reason,* line 42),
3 explaining the connection (*cats sometimes have quite a lot of dirt under the ... claws ... indeed something can happen,* line 55), and
4 definitely excluding a particular diagnosis (*that doesn't have anything to do with rabies,* line 68).

Here, the doctor focuses on cognitive elements like relation, reason, connection, or exclusion. Cognitive elements as part of prediagnostic statements are of two types: (medical and other, more general) cognitive categories or concepts and (general) cognitive operations. In the following, I refer to the database of all 30 interactions.

Cognitive categories and concepts in prediagnostic statements allow categorical access to medically relevant aspects of a disease. They contain aspects like figures (e.g., as set point values), space (e.g., body parts or organs), time (e.g., the frequency of complaints), vital signs (e.g., blood pressure), excretion (e.g., urine or stool), and findings (e.g., bacteria, fracture). More abstractly, conceptual categories mentioned in prediagnostic statements may include symptoms (vertigo) or symptom complexes, bodily reactions (inflammation), diagnoses (preliminary, exclusional), syndromes, disease theory, quality (enlarged, scarred) or probability (see Example 1, line 42). All these categories and concepts prediagnostically organize the cognitive space where the later diagnosis should then be found (Cicourel 1987). They do that in the manner of jigsaw pieces or mosaic tiles which are part of a whole but are not to be placed in position in advance but within a process of constricting diagnostic plausibility which can only be dealt with sequentially.

The organizing elements of this process are the cognitive operations doctors deal with in their prediagnostic and diagnostic statements. These operations are generally in use in human interaction but are specified for medical purposes in doctor–patient interaction. Examples of such operations are

- attribution (*towards the anus it is not that enlarged the prostate*; the examples given in this list are from other examinations of our corpus),
- comparison and contrast (*here (-) it is different (-) definitely a difference*),
- inference (*urine from yesterday (--) leukocyte so an infection so far(.) urine culture (-) (so) no bacteria it might be something like (.) chlamydia (myco)plasma*),
- or abduction (*if there were symptoms of paralysis sometimes it can even be nerval disorders of the bladder*).

These operations always relate two or more phenomena or categories in a particular manner and thus create the basis for the summarizing conclusion expressed in the form of an official diagnosis. Whereas the official diagnosis is clearly a medical concept, even when expressed in everyday terminology, prediagnostic statements oscillate between the professional medical world of the doctor and the lay world of the patient and they more or less mediate between both worlds.

The interactive dimension

Within the interactive dimension, we first look at general features of occurrence of prediagnostic statements and after that we focus on aspects of their local positioning.

Occurrence

Prediagnostic statements are, by definition, utterances that are made before the final diagnosis during the medical examination. Heritage and Stivers (1999: 1503) characterize them as 'an intermission in and subordinate to the activity of examination which is underway', thus suspending the current examination for a short time. Realized in this way, prediagnostic statements are 'rarely overtly addressed to patients or directly acknowledged by them' (1504), and are sometimes even a 'type of thinking out loud' (Stivers 1998: 246); thus they do 'not require response but allows for it' (Stivers 1998: 249). In Example 1 the first three cases of prediagnostic statements display that kind of unclear addressing (lines 13, 28, 42) while the last four cases are directly and overtly addressed to the patient as they are semantically marked as direct responses (lines 55, 60, 63, 68).

In most cases, prediagnostic statements emerge in a sequential position not made conditionally relevant by a previous utterance. Rather they are self-initiated utterance types in response to the patient's presentation or observations by the doctor him- or herself. Depending on organizational premises, prediagnostic statements can sometimes be realized before the examination begins. Prediagnostic statements such as the announcement of findings like blood pressure, blood levels, or urine status, etc., refer to preliminary examinations performed by nurses or referrals by colleagues which the doctor notices before meeting the patient. This is the default case in the United States where practices and clinics are organized with preliminary examinations; in Germany such a set-up is mostly found in specialized practices and much less frequently in general practices.

In the course of the medical examinations the frequency of prediagnostic statements increases depending on the doctor's state of diagnostic certainty. Obvious and plain symptoms are often accompanied by early and more firm realizations of prediagnostic statements as compared to diffuse and complex clinical syndromes where prediagnostic statements start hesitantly. In our data sample, doctors with a psychosomatic background often refrain from making prediagnostic statements for a long time during the examination, trying to provide as much time as the patient needs. In contrast, biomedically oriented doctors try to identify symptoms and signs of a disease as soon as possible and organize the diagnostic process in stages that way; often early anchoring via firm findings may be observed, e.g., obvious symptoms, test results, or machine-aided findings. So they organize their diagnostic proceedings from firm elements via the less firm ones to more general firm findings or a final diagnosis right at the end.

Local positioning

As mentioned before, prediagnostic statements are, for the most part, initial utterances that follow a patient's presentation, the doctor's own observations, or longer stretches of the examining interaction. In most cases, they stand turn-initially if they do not occupy the entire turn. This also sets them apart from other typical activities within the examination such as questions, for example.

There are several types of prediagnostic statements connected with different sequential positions. Prediagnostic statements may occur as:

- *statements in advance*, like the announcement of results of previously run tests;
- *direct response* to a patient's utterance; e.g., in Example 1, the patient rejects a *rabies* diagnosis which she thought had been insinuated by the doctor's explanation (line 63–68); the doctor then responds affirmatively *I don't believe that either* and strengthens her opinion with an explicit statement: *that doesn't have anything to do with rabies*;
- *online commentaries* on a running physical examination (many examples are given in Heritage and Stivers 1999; Mangione-Smith et al. 2003; and Heritage et al. 2010);
- a *result* of a sequence of topically specified questions; in Example 1, the doctor's statement, *that must probably be the reason* in line 42, matches the patient's answer to several questions concerned with identifying the frequency, exact location, and quality of the pain;
- a *summary* of longer phases of verbal and physical examination, e.g., after a long, extended presentation of different complaints about the patient's nose and throat, supplemented by information about treatment in the past and after a short physical examination, the doctor states:

  Example 2 IA_03 (02:49–02:54)
  D: sie sind EIgentlich so mit ihrem GANzen
  hals Nasen bereich nicht zuFRIEden.=
  [=hab ich] den EINdruck-
  actually you are kind of not satisfied with
  your entire nose throat area is my impression

  with this summary of the whole examination to date, the doctor focuses on the patient's experiences rather than on the physical aspects of the complaints;
- an *explanation* for the aetiology or other diagnostic aspects of the complaints under discussion; after clarifying all the relevant diagnostic aspects in a question-and-answer mode with an accompanying physical examination, the doctor in Example 1 starts an explanation in two steps (line 55–60): first, she describes the frequent fact that *cats sometimes have quite a lot of dirt under the ... claws* before drawing a general conclusion that *indeed something may happen*.

All these different types of prediagnostic statements indicate that doctors have some conversational rights at their disposal and that they use these rights to interrupt the current examination for an intermittent fixation of an interim result for the diagnostic findings, their evaluation, or explanation. The examples given show free choice of action and placement for such a statement. But on very rare occasions, prediagnostic statements are sometimes also reactive, in the sense of an affirming or negating response to an explicit request by the patient. In my data there was only one such case:

Example 3 AA_HD_01(05:44–05:51)
P: (-) oder was kann es sonst sEIn?
or what else can it be
(2.7) ((Schreibgeräusche))
((writing noises))
D: .hh (-) für mich hört sich das so
for me it sounds
wie so ne strESSsymptomatik an-
like a stress symptom

Before this segment, the patient assumed that she had a circulation problem, but the doctor obviously reacted skeptically to that theory. So the patient decides to ask the doctor directly about an alternative diagnosis. Note that the doctor does not present a diagnosis but an assumption and by doing so withdraws from the requested obligation and makes use of his interactional rights.

Combinations and interactive consequences of prediagnostic statements

Prediagnostic statements are no stand-alone units of talk within doctor–patient interactions. They are often connected with other prediagnostic statements in a row contributing to the diagnostic process as a whole, and engendering consequences in a systematic way.

Combinations of prediagnostic statements

Prediagnostic statements are not necessarily realized as single utterances. Sometimes the doctor makes two or more prediagnostic statements in a row, either in order to give more than one piece of information or to display associations, assumed connections, or inferences. Such a combination is often merely additional, but occasionally the doctors present an explanation, abstract from bare facts, or build up inferences from different findings as in the following example:

Example 4 UR_13 (00:28–01:41)
D: (.) IM ejakulat (.) sind zu viele WEIße blutkörperchen drin–
in the ejaculate (.) there are too many white blood cells
(.) [das heißt] also (--) auch
[that means] consequently also
P: [mhm]
[uhum]
D: die zeichen der entzÜNdung;
the signs of inflammation
(-)
P: ja
yes
D: das heißt
that means
(-) Eine beteiligung der prostataSAmenblasen (.) is sO anzunehmen–
(-) an involvement of the seminal vesicles of the prostate (.) is to be assumed

P: mhm
uhum
(--)
D: .h äh der strAHl (.) is AUch (.) für=n (.) JUNgen
uh the stream (.) is even (.) for a (.) young
(.) patienten (-) zu schlecht–
patient (-) too bad
[...]
D: bei ihnen also
to you well
(.) kann ich nur sagen
i can only say
(.) eingeschränkter harnstrAHl,
reduced urinary stream
(.) das kann SOwohl .h entzündungsbedingt sein–
that can be both (-) inflammation-related
(.) und die entzündung is ja wieder DA,
and the inflammation is back again
P: mhm
uhum
D: äh (.) das macht natürlich auch noch die entzündung ne gewisse
uh of course the inflammation causes (a) certain
schwellung der schleimhAUt;
swelling of the mucous membrane too
(-)
P: mhm
uhum
[...]
D: gut–
well
(---) JA (-) jetzt–
yes now
(--) gestrige urIn (--) LEUkocyten,
yesterday's urine leukocytes
also insofern ne infekTION,
well in this respect an inflammation
(.) urinkulTUR (-) (also) keine bakterien NAchzuweisen;
urine culture (-) (well) no bacteria to be detected
P: mhm
uhum
D: es dÜrfte wieder so was sein;
that might be again something like this
(.) chlaMYdien (myko)plasmen;
chlamydia (myko)plasmas

Here the doctor successively informs the patient about three different findings concerning the *ejaculate* (line 1), the *urinary stream* (line 10), and *urine leukocytes* (line 23). Each of these findings is discussed individually but also in relation to the other two findings. Single discussions result in a relevant conclusion or assessment. The combined discussion finally leads to a working diagnosis: *that might be again something like this chlamydia (myko) plasmas* which operates as an official diagnosis in the following interaction and treatment. This example also illustrates the complexity of the 'diagnostic overview', which involves putting different aspects together and adjusting them in a total judgment.

Interactive consequences

The main emphasis of conversation analytic research related to the present topic is on interactive consequences and functions of prediagnostic statements. Heath (1992) states that patients respond minimally to diagnoses, only in terms of acknowledgment or agreement markers, or do not react recognizably at all. Peräkylä (1998, 2002) affirms these findings by and large for his Finnish data. Nonetheless, he also states that extended responses sometimes occur in reaction to 'instructed seeing of evidence' which is a prediagnostic statement according to our definition here. In Example 1, a similar reaction can be observed when the doctor explains the probable aetiology of the patient's complaints by *dirt* under the cat's claws and the patient denies the presumably insinuated *rabies* (line 62ff.).

Nevertheless, the weak response to diagnosis and prediagnostic statements is overwhelming and requires (further) discussion. Peräkylä explains that 'by explicating the evidence the doctors make a part of their medical reasoning available' (Peräkylä 1998: 307; see also Stivers 1998). This is not meant to be taken as an invitation to discussion for the patient but, instead, as an offer for passive participation. Heritage and Stivers characterize online commentaries as staging posts on the way to a conclusion, building up evidence incrementally, and this step-by-step quality makes it 'extremely difficult for the patient to contradict' (Heritage and Stivers 1999: 1511).

Heritage supports Peräkylä's views on reasoning availability when stating that '"online commentary" is "evidence formulating" and reveal a process of diagnostic reasoning to the patient' (Heritage 2005: 99) while for Maynard citing the evidence 'bring[s] the recipient to a state of realization jointly and collaboratively' as 'a predecessor account to asserting the condition' (Maynard 2004: 71). In his view, this interactional work 'seeks to achieve a sense of mutuality, understanding, and agreement' and these 'practices of talk-in-interaction establish objectivity' for speakers, recipients, and anyone else (ibid.). In their research on diagnosis, Maynard and also Peräkylä focus on the relation between prediagnostic statements and the official diagnosis and state that preliminary statements and their positioning within the examination index a diagnosis which is still to come.

In her study of veterinarian examinations, Stivers (1998) analyzes the more immediate consequences of prediagnostic statements and distinguishes between two primary uses: forecasting the next steps and allowing for negotiation. Prediagnostic statements are a resource for exploring the client's willingness to agree to diagnostic tests that are liable to pay off and as such they are a means of tacit negotiation of the final treatment and diagnosis – in her opinion, this makes decision-making highly flexible. In later studies, Stivers and others identify online commentaries as a powerful resource to resist patient pressure for inappropriate antibiotic medication (Heritage and Stivers 1999; Mangione-Smith et al. 2003; Heritage et al. 2010).

In our own German data, the patients' responses to prediagnostic statements are overwhelmingly absent or minimal, too (Schöffler and Spranz-Fogasy 2012). In addition to the reasons discussed above, this seems to be due to the preliminary quality of prediagnostic statements, which makes additional considerations or examinations necessary. In this respect, the subsequent activities of doctors turn out to be more informative. Prediagnostic statements are almost always followed on by further examining activities, be it questions on other aspects of the complaints or a request for a physical examination or for other kinds of diagnosis. The first three statements in Example 1 (lines 13, 28, 42) demonstrate this.

In a few cases, doctors directly move onto a concluding diagnosis as is the case in Example 1 when the doctor changes from the diagnosis of exclusion (*that doesn't have to do with rabies*) to the final diagnosis *that's a a surely a soft tissue infection* (line 70); or the doctor proceeds to preliminary proposals for treatment. In this manner, prediagnostic statements turn out to be an organizational link between topical, pragmatic, and empractic activities accomplishing topic and agenda setting (Manning and Ray 2002; Boyd and Heritage 2006). The basis for that is their quality as sum-ups or the notionalization of stages of the examination (see Deppermann 2011), often in combination with a reduction in the complexity of the local issue (Spranz-Fogasy and Deppermann 1998).

Summary

At first glance, prediagnostic statements seem to be an inconspicuous utterance type which for a long time were not considered to be worth mentioning in analyses of the examination phase of doctor–patient interactions or were otherwise subsumed in research on communicating the diagnosis as just 'a predecessor account to asserting the condition' (Maynard 2004: 71). In the context of analyses of physical examinations, prediagnostic statements were inevitably conspicuous because of their obvious placement *before* the diagnosis, following the interaction, and this is also true for verbal examinations.

As can be seen in Example 1, the path from knowing nothing about the patient's complaints, expressed in the opening question *well why are you here* (line 1, for discussion on opening questions see Heritage and Clayman 2010; Robinson 2006; Robinson and Heritage 2006; Heritage and Robinson 2006) to the certain diagnosis *that s a a surely a soft tissue infection* (line 70) is iteratively marked by prediagnostic statements displaying increasing certainty on the part of the doctor. This example shows an idealized default course of such interactions because it is not the case in every doctor–patient interaction due to remaining unclear or over-complex symptoms and signs (Maynard and Frankel 2003).

Every prediagnostic statement in Example 1 closes one brief discussion phase and sets new topics and agenda (Heritage 2010). It is a feature set by doctors to regularly organize their state of knowledge and understanding and at the same time to display that state to their patients by letting them participate, step by step, in the course of medical action and interaction.

In that way, doctors organize mutuality and intersubjectivity between the lay world of the patient and the world of medical expertise they represent themselves. As the picture of a disease is built up piece by piece, the interaction is aligned with that, and prediagnostic statements express one relevant diagnostic mosaic tile at a time. The wide variety of cognitive categories, concepts, and operations mentioned in prediagnostic statements reveals the amount of professional and everyday knowledge that is necessary for a proper examination and diagnosis. Furthermore, the flexibility of linguistic resources displays the local state of provisionality related with that via the pragmatic mode, calibrating the content or modifying certainty.

The general fluency of the activity types used in verbal examinations is also useful for that purpose: they occur as interrogatives, comments or assertives, or change their status from a more decisive to a vaguer one by means of placement, content, prosody, or modification.

More so than other utterance types within the examination phase, prediagnostic statements operate in both ways locally and broadly. When summing up different utterances or observations, giving explanations or denying patients' assumptions, they refer to a later diagnosis by indicating their fragmental and preliminary quality in relation to that.

Analyses of prediagnostic statements reveal not only linguistic, cognitive, and interactional relevancies but are instructive regarding applications for practice. Stivers (1998) already noted that they are an important resource, not only for informing clients but also for tacit negotiation of further and occasionally expensive diagnostics. Heritage and Stivers (1999) characterize prediagnostic statements as a method of shaping patient expectations concerning prescriptions while Mangione-Smith et al. (2003) demonstrate how 'no problem' prediagnostic statements build up an effective and time-neutral method for resisting patients' prescription demands. Consequently, Heritage et al. (2010) explicitly propose avoiding such 'no problem' commentaries.

These analyses of prediagnostic statements, supplemented by the conversation analytic research on diagnosis which also deals with prediagnostic statements but in their sequential role as part of the 'official' diagnostic statement itself (Heath 1992; Maynard 2003 and elsewhere; Peräkylä 1998 and elsewhere), suggest that the doctor's display of knowledge and understanding is also a powerful resource in establishing and maintaining patients' trust via participation and this leads to increased compliance (Peräkylä 2006).

Future directions

Research on prediagnostic statements is still in its infancy although it has given us important insights as described above. Further directions can be derived from the limitations of the given analyses but also from their results.

Heritage et al. (2010) state limitations due to the small sample of records with respect to differentiation between participants, their gender, interaction types, or geographic distribution. By incorporating appropriate parts of studies on diagnosis, its announcement and its sequencing, as has been done in this context, this database may be extended, but not sufficiently, of course. More visits from other medical areas have to be included in addition to pediatric and primary care visits.

Furthermore different degrees of gravity in relation to upcoming diagnoses play an important role for the realization or withholding of prediagnostic statements. Maynard's dictum of more complex and more hesitant pre-announcements being associated with cases of bad news (Maynard 2003) indicates that doctors may not make problematic statements that are open or transparent if they suspect a serious disease. Here, new research methods are needed, such as video stimulated comments or video recall (Pomerantz 2005).

Concerning linguistic desiderata, prediagnostic statements indicate, more than many other utterance types, the fluidity of linguistic categories. Transitions from declarative sentences to questions are obviously fluent, as it is the display of epistemic stance and certainty via verb use, modification, content, placement, or receipt. In this respect, prediagnostic statements are a paradigmatic and instructive research object.

The sheer number of cognitive categories, concepts, and operations turns prediagnostic statements into an outstanding issue for research on the interplay of interaction and cognition. An exhaustive record of cognitive elements may help to reconstruct professional organization of thinking and their influence on interactional acting and vice versa. More so than questions (Spranz-Fogasy 2010), prediagnostic statements display understanding explicitly; in relation to medical interaction this includes understanding the complaints and the disease as well as understanding the patients, their presentation, and their behavior. Prediagnostic statements reveal what has already been understood and what still needs to be understood, including their partiality and provisional nature, and as a result they open the window to processes of interactive understanding.

The analysis of prediagnostic statements as part of the news delivery sequence draws attention to the function of prediagnostic statements within the examination as a whole. Different utterance and action types, such as questions, answers, physical examinations, or prediagnostic statements, interreact and guide the examination process. Different question types, such as wh-questions, syntactic questions with subject-auxiliary inversion (in German the verb in first position), or declarative questions, reveal different states of knowledge and understanding (Heritage and Clayman 2010; Spranz-Fogasy 2010) while prediagnostic statements often mark an interim result established by a particular succession of the utterance and action types at issue. Analyzing the interplay of actions and their relation to the examination process will deepen our knowledge of the interactive organization of knowledge and understanding and its necessary stages.

Related topics

Doctor–patient interaction; diagnosis; cognition; understanding.

Note

1 Postdiagnostic statements, which deal with diagnostic elements in the same way as prediagnostic statements, are excluded here, although they often aim to establish acceptance of and the patient's trust in and compliance for subsequent treatment – a function which prediagnostic statements also fulfill in preparation for the final diagnosis and treatment proposals (Maynard 2003; Stivers 1998; Heritage and Stivers 1999; Peräkylä 2006).

Further reading

Deppermann, A., Reitemeier, U., Schmitt, R., and Spranz-Fogasy, T. (2010) *Verstehen in professionellen Handlungsfeldern*, Tübingen: Narr.

Edwards, D. and Potter, J. (2005) 'Discursive psychology, mental states and descriptions', in H. te Molder and J. Potter (eds) *Conversation and Cognition*, Cambridge: Cambridge University Press, 241–259.

Gill, V., Pomerantz, A., and Denvir, P. (2010) 'Pre-emptive resistance: patients' participation in diagnostic sense-making activities', *Sociology of Health & Illness*, 31(1): 1–20.

Heritage, J. and Raymond, G. (2005) 'The terms of agreement: indexing epistemic authority and subordination in assessment sequences', *Social Psychology Quarterly*, 68: 15–38.

Maynard, D. (2006) 'Cognition on the ground', *Discourse Studies*, 8: 105–115.

References

Boyd, E. and Heritage, J. (2006) 'Taking the history: questioning during comprehensive history-taking', in J. Heritage and D.W. Maynard (eds) *Communication in Medical Care: Interaction between Primary Care Physicians and Patients*, Cambridge: Cambridge University Press, 151–184.

Byrne, P.S. and Long, B.E.L. (1976) *Doctors Talking to Patients: A Study of the Verbal Behaviour of General Practitioners Consulting in their Surgeries*, London: HSMO, Royal College of General Practitioners.

Cicourel, A. (1987) 'Cognitive and organizational aspects of medical diagnostic reasoning', *Discourse Processes,* 10: 346–367.

Deppermann, A. (2011) 'Notionalizations: the transformation of descriptions into categorizations', *Human Studies*, 34(2): 155–181.

Deppermann, A. and Schmitt, R. (2009) 'Verstehensdokumentation: Zur Phänomenologie von Verstehen in der Interaktion' [Understanding displays: the phenomenology of understanding in interaction], *Deutsche Sprache*, 3(08): 220–245.

Hamilton, H.E. (2004) 'Symptoms and signs in particular: the influence of the medical concern on the shape of physician–patient talk', *Communication & Medicine*, 1(1): 59–70.

Heath, C. (1992) 'The delivery and reception of diagnosis in the general-practice consultation', in P. Drew and J. Heritage (eds) *Talk at Work: Interaction in Institutional Settings*, Cambridge: Cambridge University Press, 235–267.

Heritage, J. (2005) 'Revisiting authority in physician–patient interaction', in J. Duchan and D. Kovarsky (eds) *Diagnosis as Cultural Practice*, New York: Mouton de Gruyter, 83–102.

——(2010) 'Questioning in medicine', in A. Freed and S. Ehrlich (eds) *'Why Do You Ask?': The Function of Questions in Institutional Discourse*, New York: Oxford University Press, 42–68.

Heritage, J. and Stivers, T. (1999) 'Online commentary in acute medical visits: a method of shaping patient expectations', *Social Science & Medicine*, 49(11): 1501–1517.

Heritage, J. and Maynard, D.W. (eds) (2006) *Communication in Medical Care: Interaction between Primary Care Physicians and Patients*, Cambridge: Cambridge University Press.

Heritage, J. and Robinson, J.D. (2006) 'The structure of patients' presenting concerns: physicians' opening questions', *Health Communication*, 19(2): 89–102.

Heritage, J. and Clayman, S. (2010) *Talk in Action: Interactions, Identities, and Institutions*, Oxford: Wiley-Blackwell.

Heritage, J., Elliott, M.N., Stivers, T., Richardson, A., and Mangione-Smith, R. (2010) 'Reducing inappropriate antibiotics prescribing: the role of online commentary on physical examination findings', *Patient Education and Counseling*, 81(1): 119–125.

Kallmeyer, W. (2005) 'Konversationsanalytische Beschreibung' [Conversation analytical description], in U. Ammon, N. Dittmar, K.J. Mattheier, and P. Trudgill (eds) *Sociolinguistics/Soziolinguistik. An International Handbook of the Science of Language and Society/Ein internationales Handbuch zur Wissenschaft von Sprache und Gesellschaft*, vol. 1, revised edn, New York: de Gruyter, 1212–1225.

Mangione-Smith, R., Stivers, T., Elliott, M., McDonald, L., and Heritage, J. (2003) 'Online commentary on physical exam findings: a communication tool for avoiding inappropriate antibiotic prescribing?', *Social Science & Medicine*, 56(2): 313–320.

Manning, P. and Ray, G. (2002) 'Setting the agenda: an analysis of negotiation strategies in clinical talk', *Health Communication*, 14(4): 451–473.

Maynard, D.W. (2003) *Bad News, Good News. Conversational Order in Everyday Talk and Clinical Settings*, Chicago, IL: University of Chicago Press.

——(2004) 'On predicating a diagnosis as an attribute of a person', *Discourse Studies*, 6(1): 53–76.

Maynard, D.W. and Frankel, R.M. (2003) 'Indeterminacy and uncertainty in the delivery of diagnostic news in internal medicine: a single case analysis', in P.J. Glenn (ed.) *Studies in Language and Social Interaction: In Honour of Robert Hopper*, Mahwah, NJ: Erlbaum, 393–410.

Meyer, B. (2004) *Dolmetschen im medizinischen Aufklärungsgespräch. Eine diskursanalytische Untersuchung zur Wissensvermittlung im mehrsprachigen Krankenhaus* [*Interpretation in medical briefings. A discourse analytic analysis of transfer of knowledge in multilingual hospital*], Münster: Waxmann.

Nowak, P. and Spranz-Fogasy, T. (2009) 'Medizinische Kommunikation – Arzt und Patient im Gespräch' [Medical communication – doctor and patient in discussion], in A. Bogner et al. (eds) *Jahrbuch Deutsch als Fremdsprache [Yearbook German as a foreign language]. Intercultural German Studies*, vol. 34, München: Iudicium, 80–96.

Peräkylä, A. (1997) 'Conversation analysis: a new model of research on doctor–patient communication', *Journal of the Royal Society of Medicine*, 90(4): 205–208.

——(1998) 'Authority and accountability: the delivery of diagnosis in primary health care', *Social Psychology Quarterly*, 61(4): 301–320.

——(2002) 'Agency and authority: extended responses to diagnostic statements in primary care encounters', *Research on Language and Social Interaction*, 35(2): 219–247.

——(2006) 'Communicating and responding to diagnosis', in J. Heritage and D.W. Douglas (eds) *Communication in Medical Care: Interaction between Primary Care Physicians and Patients*, Cambridge: Cambridge University Press, 214–247.

Pomerantz, A. (2005) 'Using participants' video stimulated comments to complement analyses of interactional practices', in H. te Molder and J. Potter (eds) *Talk and Cognition: Discourse, Mind and Social Interaction*, Cambridge: Cambridge University Press, 93–113.

Robinson, J.D. (2006) 'Soliciting patients' presenting concerns', in J. Heritage and D.W. Maynard (eds) *Communication in Medical Care: Interaction between Primary Care Physicians and Patients*, Cambridge: Cambridge University Press, 22–47.

Robinson, J.D. and Heritage, J. (2006) 'Physicians' opening questions and patients' satisfaction', *Patient Education and Counseling*, 60(3): 279–285.

Roter, D. and Hall, J. (1992) *Doctors Talking with Patients, Patients Talking with Doctors: Improving Communication in Medical Visits*, Westport, CT: Auburn House.

Schegloff, E. (2007) *Sequence Organization in Interaction. A Primer in Conversation Analysis*, Cambridge: Cambridge University Press.

Schöffler, M. and Spranz-Fogasy, T. (2012) "ja m–hm' – Patientenreaktionen auf prädiagnostische Mitteilungen' ['yes uhm' – Patients' reactions and prediagnostic statements], *Zeitschrift für Angewandte Linguistik*, 57(1): 1–32.

Selting, M. et al. (2009) 'Gesprächsanalytisches Transkriptionssystem 2 (GAT 2)', trans. E. Couper-Kuhlen and D. Barth-Weingarten (2011) 'A system for transcribing talk-in-interaction: Gat 2', *Gesprächsforschung – Online Zeitschrift zur verbalen Interaktion* [*Conversation and Discourse Analysis*], 12: 1–51. Online. Available HTTP: <http://www.gespraechsforschung-ozs.de/heft2011/px-gat2-englisch.pdf> (accessed 8 November 2012).

Spranz-Fogasy, T. (2010) 'Verstehensdokumentation in der medizinischen Kommunikation: Fragen und Antworten im Arzt-Patient-Gespräch' [Understanding displays in medical communication: questions and answers in doctor–patient interaction], in A. Deppermann, U. Reitemeier, R. Schmitt, and T. Spranz-Fogasy (eds) *Verstehen in professionellen Handlungsfeldern* [*Understanding in professional fields of activity*], Tübingen: Narr, 27–116.

Spranz-Fogasy, T. and Deppermann, A. (1998) 'Kommunikationsstörungen durch den Gesprächsprozeß. Zur Entstehung von Interaktionsdilemmata durch zeitliche Komplexierung' [Communication problems in the conversational process. The development of interactional dilemmas based on temporal complexity], in R. Fiehler (ed.) *Verständigungsprobleme und gestörte Kommunikation* [*Comprehension problems and disturbed communication*], Opladen: Westdeutscher Verlag, 44–62.

Stivers, T. (1998) 'Pre-diagnostic commentary in veterinarian–client interaction', *Research on Language and Social Interaction*, 31(2): 241–277.

Appendix 26.1: Transcription conventions GAT (Selting et al. 2009)

[ ] *[ ]*	overlap and simultaneous talk
=	fast, immediate continuation with a new turn or segment (latching)
(.)	micro pause, estimated, up to 0.2 sec. duration appr.
(-), (--), (---)	short, intermediary, longer estimated pause of appr. 0.2–0.5, 0.5–0.8, 0.8–1.0 sec. duration
(2.8)	measured pause of appr. 2.8 sec. duration (to tenth of a second)
s_geht	cliticizations within units
:, ::, :::	lengthening, by about 0.2–0.5, 0.5–0.8, 0.8–1.0 sec.
äh, öh, etc. *(uh, uhm, etc.)*	hesitation markers, so-called 'filled pauses'
'	cut-off by glottal closure
haha hehe hihi	syllabic laughter
((lacht))	description of laughter
akZENT	focus accent
ak!ZENT!	extra strong accent
?	rising to high
,	rising to mid

-	level
;	falling to mid
.	falling to low
.h, .hh, .hhh	inbreaths of appr. 0.2–0.5, 0.5–0.8, 0.8–1.0 sec. duration
h, hh, hhh	outbreaths of appr. 0.2–0.5, 0.5–0.8, 0.8–1.0 sec. duration
((coughs))	non-verbal vocal actions and events
( )	unintelligible passage
(solche)	assumed wording
(solche/welche)	possible alternatives
((...))	omission in transcript

27

After the diagnosis

News disclosures in long-term cancer care

Karen S. Schaepe and Douglas W. Maynard

Introduction

Prospective cancer patients hear the diagnosis in one of three ways: following an acute episode in the emergency room; during a clinic visit after presentation with sub-acute symptoms (fatigue or a rash); or asymptomatically, as when cancer is discovered by routine blood work as part of a physical exam or in the course of treatment for an unrelated condition (an infection or broken bone). Whatever the circumstances, patients often recall a specific moment when the news hits home – what Maynard (2003: 19) calls a 'noetic crisis' in which the world of everyday life, including one's taken-for-granted healthy body, is utterly called into question. For some, the 'realization' (Maynard 1996) is experienced as a sudden visceral shock:

> 'We've discovered there is a malignancy.' A flush went through my body and out of my mouth came a sound like a guttural animal cry.
>
> *(Cripe 2008)*

For many patients there is a period of denial:

> [The doctor said,] 'I'm going to refer you right away today to an expert ... but I really believe it is [cancer].' But I was thinking it can't be, you know, it just can't be.
>
> *(Patient interview by Schaepe, February 2008)*

Accordingly, realization of the news can take time and occur when the patient is well into treatment:

> I was down there [at the clinic] probably halfway through the first week of chemo before I even realized – well, you know, before it really sunk in. Like holy man, I'm sick! And oh, I can't change my mind on anything now because they're already pumping drugs in me!
>
> *(Patient interview by Schaepe, March 2008)*

Whether realization comes quickly or takes time, the diagnostic episode is only one frame of a larger picture. In this chapter, we address the larger picture of what happens in the delivery and reception of news concerning treatment, side effects, remission, recurrence, palliation, and other matters as cancer patients move beyond diagnosis and enter the treatment phase of the disease.

Currently, the literature on delivery of bad news in cancer care is skewed toward the initial disclosures of the diagnosis, and guidelines for delivering news to cancer patients focus primarily on minimizing the shock and the disbelief associated with the initial diagnosis. Strategies to reduce shock include using a 'perspective display sequence' (Maynard 1992) – i.e., asking before telling, firing a 'warning shot' (Buckman 1984) or 'forecasting' (Maynard 1996), 'dosing' information, and responding to patient emotion with empathy (Frankel 2000). Strategies used to contain disbelief and insure understanding include clarifying information frequently and summarizing plans for future treatment at the end of the encounter (Baile et al. 2000; Buckman 1992; Girgis and Sanson-Fisher 1998). The crux is that, while these techniques may be helpful for delivering an initial diagnosis, they are less useful for the multiple other occasions of news delivery occurring in the context of week-to-week or month-to-month and even more widely spaced follow-up encounters.

Schaepe (2011) offers an example of problems that news deliveries later in an illness trajectory can encompass, in this case due to miscommunication and a lack of coordination between medical clinics. A 24-year-old patient had developed leukemia as a result of the chemotherapy used to treat her sarcoma. Three months following a stem cell transplant to treat the leukemia, interpretation of an X-ray suggested that the patient's original sarcoma had returned. In fact, the cancer had not recurred and a mistake had been made in reading the X-ray. The mother of the patient recalled:

> We were actually celebrating her '100 days,' and two days before, Sarah called Dr. Y and said, 'I've got this pain in my hip and I don't know if I pulled something or what.' He said, 'Well, you know, to play it safe, why don't you get an X-ray?' ... So she did that [at a clinic local to the family's celebration], and then the doctor that read it was actually a nurse practitioner and had told us that the radiologist had read it. But long story short, *she* read it. She read it backwards. And even though Sarah and I both explained that on her one hip it's going to look like she's got a tumor, but it's a dead tumor. And the pain was actually on the other side. Anyway, she read it wrong and called us the next day at the resort we were at and told Sarah right there on the phone that, you know, 'Sorry. Your cancer's back.'
>
> *(Schaepe 2011: 917)*

Not surprisingly, the family cut short their celebration, returned home that day, and Sarah had another X-ray at the home clinic where the mistake was subsequently revealed. Afterward, the dominant feeling expressed by the patient and her family was a sense of betrayal. As the mother noted:

> I actually had talked to the nurse practitioner. I just grabbed the phone from Sarah because she was screaming and crying and saying, 'No, not again! Not again! Not again!' When I talked to her [the nurse practitioner] I said, 'Are you sure? Are you absolutely sure?' 'Yes, I'm sure.' And, you know, you trust them.
>
> *(Schaepe 2011: 917)*

This may be an extreme case, but it points to the multiple occasions to disclose and receive news and illustrates the troubles that can, and often do, accompany the long treatment process after diagnosis. For Sarah and her family an ambiguous pain may be nothing or could signal relapse; in either case, choosing to have the X-ray also meant taking the errant news about its results at face value, picking up, and going home. Then, the family learned that the film had been read 'backwards', which should have been good news, except that it left them bereft of their former trust in the medical community.

Communication and long-term care

Three issues emerge in the small literature concerning news deliveries in the long-term context of treatment for cancer care. First are suggestions that disclosures are often either indirect or entirely absent (Bensing et al. 2003; Christakis 1999; Helft 2005; Lutfey and Maynard 1998). Recent observations by Schaepe (2013) confirms earlier research (Lutfey and Maynard 1998) that doctors and patients, especially in the transition from curative to palliative care, allude to rather than directly announce the news that this transition is happening and that a terminal phase is proximate. We show an example later in the chapter, and it raises an issue of whether and how there can be more transparent communications regarding stages of cancer treatment, including end-of-life transitions.

Second, guidelines often frame best practice strategies assuming that news will be disclosed in the context of a doctor–patient dyad (Bensing and Verheul 2009; Eggly et al. 1997) rather than a doctor–patient–family member(s) grouping. Sarah's case (above) illustrates how a whole family, outside of the clinic, was involved. In fact, of the 44 oncology follow-up visits in Schaepe's study (2013), 33 involved one or more family members or friends. This finding is consistent with other research in oncology suggesting that the majority of patients bring a companion to some or all of their clinic visits (Beisecker and Moore 1994; Ellingson 2002). Although older patients are most likely to bring a companion for support and help in processing information, younger patients also bring friends and family with regularity (Labrecque et al. 1991). What is less conclusive in the literature is the actual role of companions in clinic interactions. That is, they are sometimes characterized as forceful advocates and/or antagonists (Adelman et al. 1987, 2000), interpreters and neutral mediators between the doctor and patient, medication managers, or caretakers (Coe and Prendergast 1985). Alternatively, companions are sometimes characterized as occupying a relatively passive role (Hasselkus 1992).

Third, widely used guidelines such as the SPIKES protocol (Baile et al. 2000) assume that oncologists can improve the interaction by preparing mentally for the delivery of bad news. The guidelines encourage clinicians to rehearse the way they intend to convey bad news to cancer patients and thereby avoid poorly worded and anxiety-producing hesitations. While this may be useful for getting through initial, discrete disclosures of diagnostic news, subsequent disclosures during routine clinic visits, especially when these encounters included a companion, rarely provide physicians with sufficient control of the conversation (Eggly et al. 2006; Mei-Hui 2007). That is, patients and companions may produce multiple interruptions and spontaneous shifts to secondary issues (Hasselkus 1992; Labrecque et al. 1991). In one clinic visit (Schaepe 2013), the doctor's announcement about 'concerning' changes in a patient's blood work was met with questions about how this might affect vacation plans. The patient and caregiver engaged in a side conversation for several minutes before the doctor closed discussion of the topic by suggesting they come back to it again the following week.

Related to the problem of mental rehearsal are situations where doctors and patients engage in deliberate indirect communication. Vague language and the absence of explicit questioning may not always reflect ineptitude so much as reveal a context operating by a different logic based on distinct social goals. Schaepe (2013) documents a case in which a doctor told a patient and his wife that the blood counts were 'off'. The doctor did not elaborate, however, and the patient and his wife did not ask for clarification although they sensed this information was significant. In a post hoc interview, the couple admitted they did not inquire further because they worried that their failure to comply with the doctor's orders from an earlier visit may have caused the abnormal lab results. The patient said, 'I thought maybe I screwed something up,' with his wife adding, 'We were afraid to tell the doc about it.' This illustrates how concerns about maintaining the therapeutic relationship and worries about their own caretaking skills may have actually led both parties to prefer indirect over explicit communication.

These three matters – problems of indirectness, assumptions about the dyadic nature of doctor–patient interaction, and suggestions that, by mental rehearsal, physicians can control the disclosure process – may affect initial diagnostic news deliveries, but they are particularly salient for understanding disclosures about health status occurring over the long term, with family and other caretakers present. We return to these issues and the sparse research on them at the end of the chapter. First, we set a context for further discussion by providing background about cancer disclosures generally and the implications for long-term care. We also address different methodologies that research employs and report findings from associated studies. Then we engage in 'taking stock', by addressing three prominent issues for future research, and conclude the chapter.

Research on disclosures in oncology

Using a variety of search terms such as 'cancer', 'communication', 'bad news', 'prognosis', 'truth-telling', 'disclosure', and 'decision-making', an initial query of social science databases yielded approximately 550 articles falling into five categories: (1) systematic and literature reviews, (2) normative/best practice articles, (3) opinion/editorial pieces, (4) empirical studies, and (5) intervention-based research. We first review what has been written about the doctor's position in news deliveries including initial as well as subsequent disclosures, and then examine facets of the patient's perspective over time.

Physician dread and lack of preparation

Empirical research accounts for about a quarter of the articles on news delivery overall (Walsh et al. 1998). These studies cluster into investigations based on self-report data and those drawing from observation or recordings of actual clinic encounters. Of the two, the self-report literature is larger, and uses surveys, structured and semi-structured interviews, and focus group data collected from doctors, patients, and (to a lesser degree) other clinical staff and patient companions. Although a comprehensive assessment of this literature falls beyond the scope of this chapter, two recurring findings are worth mentioning. One is that physicians often characterize delivering bad news as the most dreaded part of their work. Indeed, the dread may be enough to turn doctors away from clinical medicine toward professions such as radiology, forensic pathology, or others (Maynard 2003: 23). Another finding is that few doctors indicate having had formal training and instead most have learned to deliver news through a process of trial and error (Friedrichsen and Milberg 2006; Ptacek et al. 1999; Schildmann et al. 2005).

Routinized behavior

Taken together, physician dread and a lack of preparation raise the possibility that physicians may adopt forms of routinized behavior in order to manage the news delivery. Such a strategy is documented in a Canadian study (Taylor 1988) that analyzes the delivery of positive breast biopsy results to 118 female patients. Because physicians perceive telling bad news as stressful, Taylor (1988: 129) reports that physicians find 'predictable ways to routinize this task'. She observed 17 surgeons with no previous contact with their patients delivering the biopsy news to the women. All disclosures included three phases: the preamble (where the surgeon sets the stage with somber tone and phrases like 'serious illness' and 'difficult decision'), confrontation (the actual disclosure of the diagnosis), and diffusion (softening the blow through reassuring language). As Taylor (1988: 116) says, 'During each of the three phases of disclosure, each clinic physician adopted a favorite technique and used it routinely.' Of the 188 cases, 10 percent of surgeons favored 'truth-telling', revealing just what they knew about the cancer prognosis; 15 percent admitted uncertainty; and 30 percent engaged in 'dissimulation', offering a diagnosis/prognosis that could not be substantiated clinically. Notably, the largest group, 45 percent of surgeons, used techniques of evasion to suppress discussion of information about long-term survival. Taylor (1988) concludes that the tendency to develop one stance for news delivery – independent of context and patient – helped the surgeons control the length of the encounter, the range of topics discussed, and the likelihood of an emotional outburst from the patient.

Patient contributions to routinized disclosures

Of course, routinized exchanges regarding diagnosis may be more collaborative than unilateral. Leydon (2008) examines first-time interactions involving three oncologists and 27 patients with head, neck, breast, or colon cancer diagnoses and uncertain outcomes. Doctors engage in 'proximate pairing', a stylization by which good news is paired with bad or uncertain information about the patient's cancer and its treatment. Stylized behavior is initiated by the doctor but patients readily take up optimistic talk such that both parties contribute to routinized exchanges.

The collaborative nature of routinization has also been documented in long-term care. Drawing on a corpus of audiotaped visits between three doctors and 21 male patients after surgery for testicular cancer, a Swedish study (Sanden et al. 2001) outlines organizational features contributing to routinization. Because these are 'non-urgent' appointments, many of the same activities occur at each visit. Time constraints play a central role in the agenda of the doctor and as these constraints become familiar, patients increasingly orient to this agenda. Routinization also takes hold because of the ever-present specter of possible bad news from post-operative evaluations and tests. Sanden et al. (2001) argue that although the discussion of sensitive issues and new bad news might be expected to disrupt established routines, in fact, patients are aware of adverse possibilities, and this awareness may actually foster superficial discussions that preserve a sense that things are still 'okay'. Patients may help to intensify routinized forms of interaction by their own contributions. As the relationship between the doctor and the patient develops, either party may introduce more non-medical topics and 'small talk' that has the effect of lightening the overall conversation and making it difficult to address more serious health issues when necessary (Maynard and Hudak 2008).

Patients' experiences

When we shift from the physician's perspective to that of the patient, investigators have considered two contrasting features: persistence and change. In terms of persistence, Thorne et al. (2009) interviewed 200 cancer patients over a two-year period, finding that a sense of 'being known' emerged as critically important to patients as part of the context of hearing both good and bad news. In characterizing whether or how doctors 'know' them (which contributes to trust), patients cited being talked to as a person independent of their disease, eye contact, the ease with which the doctor comported themselves physically in the exam room, and remembering the patient's name as well as medical history. Patients also noted the importance of not being rushed and physician acknowledgment of the socio-emotional challenges of the disease.

Just as there are features that persist across time, Gray et al. (2000) point to changes in disclosure patterns. In this study, 34 men with prostate cancer and their wives were interviewed separately on three occasions: prior to prostatectomy, 8–10 weeks after surgery, and 11–13 months post-surgery. The men's need for support, fear of stigmatization, exigencies of the workplace, and desires to avoid burdening others all affected their decisions to share or not share information about progress or regress of the disease over time. In the beginning both the men and their wives engaged in disclosure to others, but, by the end of a year, disclosures had tapered off considerably to brief updates to just one or two people. Among the men, the reduction in disclosures over time reflected a desire to 'return to normal'. Their wives, however, were more likely to disclose more information throughout treatment and follow-up and to view this activity positively. Gray et al. (2000) also note that during the time disclosures to family and friends were diminishing, discussions increased between husband and wife about treatment news and with whom to share it.

Methods for studying disclosures in long-term cancer care

In comparison to the number of clinical accounts about initial disclosures, the research on news deliveries in long-term cancer care is relatively small. Most focus on the prognosis but there are studies that address news pertaining to current health status as well.

Quantitative analysis

Much longitudinal research on cancer draws on survey research or coding systems. Survey-based studies often measure changes in awareness, changes in emotional status and related variables across two or more points in time. Burns et al. (2007), for example, conducted interviews with 163 terminal cancer patients and their caregivers at diagnosis and again at 12 weeks to assess changes in awareness of the intent of palliative treatment. Initially, only about one-third of subjects understood that the treatment goal was non-curative, but in the months before death, in nearly 90 percent of cases at least one member of the pair understood that the process was palliative only. Using a similar comparative design, Keogh et al. (1998) employed psychometric anxiety scales to assess stress and depression in 28 bone marrow transplant patients and their caregivers at intervals to find that post-transplant anxiety was highest around three months after the procedure. Likewise, Weisman and Worden (1976) interviewed 120 newly diagnosed cancer patients at four intervals during the first 100 days to assess changes in coping strategies and found that for all patients, vulnerability to psychosocial distress increases with a worsening prognosis. However, variations in the level of distress during the terminal phase could often be predicted by a baseline assessment during the first 100 days.

Unlike survey research but still quantitatively oriented, coding studies of long-term care focus on classifying face-to-face behavior using various indices. Most frameworks build in one way or another on Bales' (1950) Interaction Process Analysis (IPA), originally developed to study small groups by organizing interactional activities into 12 complementary-paired categories of affective and task-oriented behaviors. IPA has been used to classify behavior act-by-act and then record the number and duration of specific acts occurring during an encounter between doctor and patient (Connor et al. 2009). The Roter Interaction Assessment System (Roter and Hall 1989; Smith et al. 2009) or RIAS is the most widely used coding tool and has been called the 'gold standard' for studying doctor–patient interaction (Groopman 2004). Modeled on Bales', this system expands the number of task and affective behavior categories from 12 to 29. Researchers code directly from the recorded observations (Roter and Hall 2006) and organize items in line with Lazare et al.'s (1995) three functions model of medical interviewing, an approach that involves: (1) developing rapport, (2) gathering data on the patient's problem, and (3) educating and treating the patient. Studies in oncology that draw on the RIAS approach often generate 'communicator profiles' and frequencies of specific behaviors within a clinic visit to develop correlations with patient satisfaction (Eide et al. 2004; Ford et al. 1996; Ong et al. 2000; Timmermans et al. 2005). Quantitative coding approaches are often viewed as the most systematic, efficient, and reliable way to assess doctor–patient interactions, however, critics point out that researchers are not actually assessing interaction but rather static behavioral states that are counted, categorized, and compared over time (Heritage and Maynard 2006; Peräkylä 2004).

Qualitative analysis

The qualitative approaches used to study doctor–patient interaction include ethnography, discourse analysis, and conversation analysis. As a rule, qualitative longitudinal research differs from quantitative analyses in terms of the depth of attention to how and why events unfold as they do – change understood as interactive, multifaceted, and incremental.

Ethnography is the approach traditionally used to study longitudinal interactions in various institutional contexts. Several early projects in medical settings deserve mention due to their influence on the study of oncology interactions. Among these are Julius Roth's *Timetables* (1963), which drew on his personal experience with tuberculosis as well as extensive field observations in three hospitals to highlight discrepancies in the way patients and doctors characterize the passage of time. The disparity between how physicians and patients conceptualized time proved critical to ongoing communication problems. Based on fieldwork with 14 pediatric polio sufferers and their parents, Fred Davis's *Passage through Crisis* (1963) revealed the role of families in management of polio, laying blame for communication breakdowns on the medical staff. Davis observed that physicians frequently engaged in evasive communication tactics and used technical language out of impatience dealing with family units. Erving Goffman's *Stigma* (1963) and work on 'impression management' (1959) has aided understanding of the psychosocial challenges faced by patients coping with chronic illness and how these pressures can lead sufferers to retreat from social contact.

The most comprehensive ethnographic investigations on chronic illnesses are those of Strauss and colleagues (Strauss 1975; Strauss et al. 1984) who attend to the patient's subjective and temporal experience of stigma as well as the structural constraints associated with hospital schedules and various medical technologies. Strauss's notion of an 'illness trajectory' has been influential on the work of many qualitative sociologists and researchers studying illnesses such as cancer longitudinally. Charmaz's (1993) *Good Days, Bad Days: The Self in Chronic Illness and Time* draws on interviews and informal conversations with patients coping with a range of chronic illnesses including cancer. Charmaz considers how people with chronic illness experience a transformation in identity and focuses on the news disclosure process in particular. Telling the news to family and friends includes announcing and recounting what the physician has reported to the patient about the illness and its prognosis. Two specific postures associated with news sharing are 'protective disclosing' (planning what to tell, to whom, and when) and 'spontaneous disclosing' (minimal planning and sometimes impulsive telling). Charmaz (1993: 121–133) also explores 'strategic' announcing, by which ill persons work to control information as well as their recipient's response, and 'selective' informing or acknowledging aspects of illness while minimizing others, in an effort to protect their friends as well as themselves. Overall, this work explores the meaning of illness in terms of the affected person's self and identity, disclosure and identity being deeply intertwined.

Discourse analytic studies identify themes and patterns within doctor–patient encounters. For example, Fagerlind et al. (2008) studied clinic conversations involving patients with gastrointestinal cancer and generated six categories of conversation. The study found that physicians concentrated on responses to treatment and the severity of side effects and tended to avoid quality of life, coping, and psychosocial concerns raised by patients. In another study, The et al. (2000) identified themes in lung cancer patient information-seeking strategies that can lead to false optimism about prognosis. In a third, Rodriguez et al. (2007, 2008), researching first-time encounters between oncologists and patients referred with previously diagnosed and incurable cancer, summarized patterns in language use (analogies, metaphors, etc.) when referring to death. Discourse analysis is also used to reveal patterned absences in doctor–patient interactions. Audrey et al. (2008), for example, followed patients with advanced colorectal, pancreatic, and non-small cell lung cancers who were moving from curative to palliative care to see how much information oncologists include about the survival benefits of palliative chemotherapy. Curtis et al. (2005), examine tape recordings of 15 family conferences in which the topic was about withdrawing life support or other bad news. The analysis focused specifically on missed opportunities – defined as places to listen and respond to family members, to acknowledge and address emotions, or to elicit patient preferences about palliative care and address concerns about clinical abandonment. The most common missed opportunities involved those where the physician could have listened more carefully and thereby responded better to family concerns.

Conversation Analysis (CA) is the third approach used to study doctor–patient interaction. CA stands apart from other qualitative methods in its use of recorded interaction to identify the practices used to accomplish communication actions and create a locally meaningful level of social organization. CA holds that the delivery of diagnostic news is not a unilateral achievement by a physician but is a co-constructed and collaborative activity between doctor and patient (Heath 1992; Maynard 1997; Peräkylä 1998). To date, the CA literature has only rarely focused on cancer specifically, despite its advantages in going beyond 'contributions of individuals' to fully appreciate the institutional and 'interactional environment' in which complex communications about cancer occur.

Delivering and receiving news of a change of disease state is a feature of cancer disclosures that Lutfey and Maynard (1998) have addressed. The focus is an oncologist with three of his male patients and their partners, and how the doctor, the patient, and the family member in each case cautiously – through stepwise perspective displays and allusive talk – discuss the transition to terminal status.

One example involved a patient, 'John', who had been under treatment for melanoma and brain metastases for a number of years, and whose recent severe symptoms resulted in a hospital stay, when it was determined that the tumor had become untreatable. In the patient's hospital room, with the man's wife also present, 'Dr. T' (the oncologist) discusses John's impending release and the difficulties it would entail, and only vaguely referred to 'what's happening' with the cancer. Over the course of the interview, through a variety of invitations and questions soliciting John's own perspective, Dr. T moved from inexplicit reference to forthcoming declines, to ask how the 'melanoma' was 'affecting' John. In reply to this question, John said, 'Yeah I have a sense of it for sure. Absolutely. Uh doesn't make it any easier, but it gives me a sense of knowing what's going on, which is very important to me.' The 'what's going on' reference was followed by Dr. T, in the segment below, working to inform John that it was no longer possible to treat the cancer, and that the clinicians could only treat his symptoms (transcript is normalized, but silences are indicated in parentheses in tenths of seconds, and emphasis is shown by underlining):

Lutfey and Maynard (1998: 337)

Dr T: Um but it seems now that (0.3) we might have to switch
gears (0.2) and (0.4) work on treatments (0.4) that (0.3)
help relieve (0.4) or (0.6) improve the complications of the
cancer like pain or any other symptoms that it might cause
because it's very hard for me or Doctor Terrie to identify
any treatment in particular to attack the cancer directly.=
John: =Mm hm.
(1.3)
Dr T: That may be something that you were a- aware of before.
((nodding))=
John: =Mm hm.
(1.4)
Dr T: Um (0.3) and I think we can do a good job of (0.3) keeping
you pretty pain free or if there are any other symptoms that
the melanoma causes or relieving- relieving that make you feel
better.
John: Mm
Dr T: But (0.7) tchh uhmm (0.6) we have after a lot of thought
we haven't come up with any (.) treatment for the melanoma
itself.
John: Right (2.4) I unfortunately am quite aware of that myself.
(0.6)
Dr T: Mm hm.

Dr. T metaphorically proposes to 'switch gears' (lines 1–2) and treat pain rather than the cancer, and implicates another oncologist in the decision to stop treatment (lines 5–6). In response, John provides a minimal acknowledgment (line 7). After a silence (line 8), Dr. T (line 9) offers an interpretation of this acknowledgment, suggesting that it might indicate a prior awareness, which John confirms (line 11). Next, following another silence (line 12), Dr. T reformulates his delivery of the news (lines 13–16), suggesting that they 'can do a good job' of pain control. After John's quiet acknowledgment (line 17), Dr. T produces another version of the message that they cannot treat the 'melanoma itself' (lines 18–20). Now, John displays agreement and states his 'unfortunate' awareness 'of that' (lines 21–22). The overall message here is one about stopping the cancer treatment and starting pain treatment as a patient is, to put it in stark terms, being sent home from the hospital to die.

Along with other cases that Lutfey and Maynard (1998) examine, this one shows how cautious a physician may be in approaching the topic of transition from treatable to untreatable cancer and from dealing with the cancer itself to now helping the patient cope with its painful effects and his inevitable decline. The patient responds to the oncologist's message with rather terse utterances that permit the doctor to forge ahead with his news. The caution in this case fits a general pattern in which physicians, to use Jefferson's (1985) terminology, may 'gloss' more concrete versions of what they have to say about disease and death; patients, in the interaction, fundamentally affect how much such glosses (including euphemisms and other vague or indirect references) can become 'unpackaged' or explicated in transparent terms.

Pilnick (1998) examines multiple clinic visits between pharmacists and leukemia patients and addresses the issue of asymmetry in clinical discourse (Maynard 1991; ten Have 1991). The research draws on 43 audiotaped follow-up consultations between pharmacists, patients, and their companions in a leukemia pediatric outpatient clinic over a two-month period. Pilnick challenges existing literature that simplistically interprets asymmetry in provider–patient communication during one encounter as evidence of an enduring power imbalance, noting that, when considering successive encounters, asymmetries between provider and patient change. With a condition such as leukemia, patients gradually come to assume a greater sense of 'ownership' of the disease, in part through adoption of medical terminology. Thus, Pilnick (1998) argues that the patient's experience with the disease has a long-term leveling effect on the distribution of expertise between doctor and patient.

One of the most remarkable studies in relation to CA and cancer is that of Beach (2009), who does not focus on the clinical experience of cancer per se, but on conversations between family members and a variety of non-clinical others. The case focuses on one female patient who is a wife and mother in the family. Her son happened to record the phone call when he first heard the diagnostic bad news about Mom from his father. After that, he decided to record all of his conversations, which covered a 13-month period before his mother died and involved the son talking to her, his father, his ex-wife, additional family members, airline employees (as he made arrangements to visit his mother), and other agencies and people. Among the topics Beach (2009) explores are how Dad initially tells Son about Mom's cancer, and how Son receives this news; how Mom and Son come to display intense forms of affect as the prognosis worsens; and how family members relate to one another and to doctors in light of differing states of knowledge about the cancer. Also analyzed is how family members employ 'figurative expressions' to act with resolve, stick together in the face of extreme circumstances, and use humor to manage their own and each other's emotions as they confront finality.

Future directions

Taking stock

In this chapter, we have suggested that the cancer literature on delivering news overemphasizes the initial diagnosis and underemphasizes the challenges associated with disclosures in the months and years following diagnosis. As such, this literature neglects a number of features salient to long-term care such as transparency in communication regarding the patient's illness, the presence of family when news is disclosed, and the highly charged and unpredictable multi-party social context. We note that physicians often approach the task of delivering bad news with both dread and little training for how to convey such news, which can result in development of routinized disclosure strategies that are ill-fitted to the unique circumstances of patients and family members. For their part, patients who emphasize the importance of 'being known' by their doctor may inadvertently reinforce development of these routines by seeking reassurance in small talk that avoids sensitive topics. Adding to the complexities with which practitioners must deal are the evolving needs of patients and family members over time.

Despite a paucity of research on disclosures in long-term cancer care, a number of investigations, representing different methodological traditions, exist. In the quantitative tradition, survey research documents changes in awareness, stress, and depression as well as patient satisfaction with care; however, this research has been unable to establish causal links between specific physician behaviors and patient outcomes. Coding studies have attempted to add precision to analysis of the relationship between clinician behavior and patient satisfaction, but so far this research has also been inconclusive – and even contradictory – especially when exploring the 'value-added' by affective talk at different phases of the doctor–patient relationship.

The shortcomings of quantitative research in documenting concrete features of clinical relationships are well known. Qualitative research provides a more fine-grained understanding of these relationships through interviewing and observation (ethnography), study of the patterns and themes as well as patterned absences in discussions about the cancer trajectory (discourse analysis), and systematic examination of the sequences and structures of naturally occurring interaction (conversation analysis).

For clinicians, what about long-term cancer communication remains elusive and vitally in need of better understanding? Which topics require research initiatives? We highlight just three topics: the significance of multi-party interactions, how patients share health news with family and friends, and problems associated with realism and hope. Our approach to these questions stresses ethnographic and conversation analytic investigation.

Three issues for further research

Multi-party research

As noted in the introduction to this chapter, studies of the oncology outpatient setting that consider the effect of a family caregiver on the conversation with the doctor are few, despite increasing recognition that many cancer patients do bring a companion to some or all of their clinic visits. The research is mixed on whether physicians prefer the presence of a third party, but some self-report literature suggests that they do (Coe and Prendergast 1985). However, other research finds that while family members often viewed themselves as ad hoc clinicians, doctors were more likely to view them as 'surrogate patients' (Hasselkus 1992). More to our concerns, few studies provide grounded analyses of multi-party encounters involving cancer patients, family members, and physicians. How does the turn-by-turn unfolding of interaction differ in multi-party as opposed to two-party clinic encounters? Are there important differences in the way that doctors, patients, and family members show their mutual understanding and retention of the information disclosed?

Sharing health status news with others

From the physician's perspective, naming the disorder and disclosing the news are the primary events that must take place before treatment can commence. From the patient's perspective, however, learning the diagnosis launches a social journey requiring repeated episodes of self-disclosure of health-related news to family, friends, and co-workers. How does sharing what patients learn about the course of their own illness influence therapeutic outcomes? Research suggests that patients with fewer confidants often have lower survival rates (Burns et al. 2005), and that those who conceal news from loved ones are more prone to obsess in isolation and experience mood disturbances (Roemer and Borkovec 1994). Also, handling the disease alone may not only be stress-inducing but also suppress immune responsiveness, which causes susceptibility to other illnesses besides their cancer (Larson and Chastain 1990). Sharing the diagnosis with family and friends, therefore, is not a tangential activity occurring between important disease-related events, but an important social dimension of the illness experience in its own right (Charmaz 1993; Schaepe 2013). Further research on disclosure of clinically related news in the context of long-term illness needs to explore whether and how patients share the news with others.

Optimism

Editorials and opinion pieces in medical journals on cancer communications often focus on the moral acceptability of withholding information to protect the hope of patients and their families. Implicitly, these writings point to the importance of understanding the strategic relationship between bad news and good news. Leydon (2008), for example, examines 27 consultations between oncologists and patients just prior to treatment, and observes a tendency to pair good news with bad news. Although this practice may smooth rough spots in what otherwise would be a very difficult conversation, Leydon finds that it may have unintended and undesirable consequences as well. Specifically, it can confuse patients and families about the state of a disease and foster unrealistic expectations about what further treatment can accomplish. Likewise, in a study of nurses and patients in four inpatient and outpatient chemotherapy units, Jarrett and Payne (2000: 83) suggest an institutional discourse of optimism essentially 'permeate[s] all levels of the hospital communication process' with dubious clinical implications. Maynard (2003: 160) suggests the phenomenon is more general than this, in that participants in settings beyond the hospital or other institutions also display an orientation to a 'benign order of everyday life' through the asymmetric ways in which they handle bad news and good news.

Given the tendency to offset bad news with good news, physicians often err on the side of providing hope in ways that distort the realistic picture for patients. In the case of 'prognostic disclosure practices', Campbell et al. (2010: 461) observe, patients often 'have a serious misunderstanding of their disease and may believe they are being treated with curative intent despite having incurable, metastatic cancer'. Recommendations for better disclosure practices focus on oncologists and what they can do unilaterally, although their practices are only one side of the transaction. We still know very little about the actual detailed interactional contingencies and outcomes involved in balancing bad news and good news, realism and hope, and related features embedded in talk and social interaction over the course of treatment for cancer.

Conclusion

Drawing on and expanding Corbin and Straus's (1985, 1988) concept of the 'work' associated with managing a chronic type of illness such as cancer, Donovan-Kicken et al. (2012) suggest that communication is a type of this 'work' and, for both theoretical and practical reasons, needs appreciation in terms of the effort it entails. Often communication is conceived in terms of the 'conduit metaphor' (Reddy 1979), which implies that the matter is a straightforward one of sending information down a pipeline for unproblematic removal at the other end, whereas the concept of 'work' points to situational demands and sensitivities, divisions of responsibility among practitioners, patients, and family members, needs for preparation and planning, and 'message design' (Donovan-Kicken et al. 2012). The concept of work is a rich one in terms of pointing to particulars of sites, persons, anticipations, and actual talk that characterize the environments of cancer care conversations. As Schaepe (2013, 2011) has shown with regard to the long-term disclosure process, communication work occurs in many different contexts after the initial diagnosis, and therefore involves an immense variety of messages regarding treatment outcomes, recurrences, prognostications, and the like. Moreover, disclosure is indelibly an interactional phenomenon, which requires methodologies suited to analyze the delivery of news, its reception, its avoidance, the contributions by various clinical as well as family personnel, and the contingencies that mental or other types of preparation can only partly anticipate. From such research, it may be possible to develop guidelines for disclosure events occurring past the initial diagnosis and involving many different healthcare and social contexts.

Related topics

Doctor–patient interaction; bad news; cancer disclosures; family caregivers; ethnography; conversation analysis.

Further reading

Beach, Wayne A. (2009) *A Natural History of Family Cancer: Interactional Resources for Managing Illness*. Cresskill, NJ: Hampton Press.

Epstein, Ronald M. and Street, Jr., Richard L. (2007) *Patient-Centered Communication in Cancer Care: Promoting Healing and Reducing Suffering*. NIH Publication No. 07-6225. Bethesda, MD: National Cancer Institute.

Lutfey, Karen and Maynard, Douglas W. (1998) 'Bad news in oncology: how physician and patient talk about death and dying without using those words', *Social Psychology Quarterly*, 61: 321–341.

Maynard, Douglas W. (2003) *Bad News, Good News: Conversational Order in Everyday Talk and Clinical Settings*. Chicago, IL: University of Chicago Press.

Schaepe, Karen S. (2011) 'Bad news and first impressions: patient and family caregiver accounts of learning the cancer diagnosis', *Social Science & Medicine*, 73: 912–921.

References

Adelman, R.D., Greene, M.G., and Charon, R. (1987) 'The physician–elderly patient–companion triad in the medical encounter: the development of a conceptual-framework and research agenda', *Gerontologist*, 27: 729–734.

Adelman, R.D., Greene, M.G., and Ory, M. (2000) 'Communication between older patients and their physicians', *Clinics in Geriatric Medicine*, 16(1): 1.

Audrey, S., Abel, J., Blazeby, J.M., Falk, S., and Campbell, R. (2008) 'What oncologists tell patients about survival benefits of palliative chemotherapy and implications for informed consent: qualitative study', *British Medical Journal*, 337: a752.

Baile, W.F., Buckman, R., Lenzi, R., Glober, G., Beale, E.A., and Kudelka, A.P. (2000) 'SPIKES – A six-step protocol for delivering bad news: application to the patient with cancer', *Oncologist*, 5: 302–311.

Bales, R.F. (1950) *Interaction Process Analysis: A Method for the Study of Small Groups*. Reading, MA: Addison-Wesley.

Beach, W.A. (2009) *A Natural History of Family Cancer: Interactional Resources for Managing Illness*. Cresskill, NJ: Hampton Press.
Beisecker, A.E. and Moore, W.P. (1994) 'Oncologists' perceptions of the effects of cancer patients' companions on physician–patient interactions', *Journal of Psychosocial Oncology*, 12: 23–39.
Bensing, J. and Verheul, W. (2009) 'Towards a better understanding of the dynamics of patient–provider interaction: the use of sequence analysis', *Patient Education and Counseling*, 75: 145–146.
Bensing, J., Van Dulmen, S., and Tates, K. (2003) 'Communication in context: new directions in communication research', *Patient Education and Counseling*, 50: 27–32.
Buckman, R. (1984) 'For Debate ... Breaking Bad News – Why Is It Still So Difficult?', *British Medical Journal*, 288(6430): 1597–1599.
——(1992) *How to Break Bad News: A Guide for Health Care Professionals*. Baltimore, MD: Johns Hopkins University Press.
Burns, C.M., Craft, P.S., and Roder, D.M. (2005) 'Does emotional support influence survival? Findings from a longitudinal study of patients with advanced cancer', *Supportive Care in Cancer*, 13: 295–302.
Burns, C.M., Broom, D.H., Smith, W.T., Dear, K., and Craft, P.S. (2007) 'Fluctuating awareness of treatment goals among patients and their caregivers: a longitudinal study of a dynamic process', *Supportive Care in Cancer*, 15: 187–196.
Campbell, T.C., Carey, E.C., Jackson, V.A., Saraiya, B., Yang, H.B., Back, A.L., and Arnold, R. (2010) 'Discussing prognosis: balancing hope and realism', *Cancer Journal*, 16: 461–466.
Charmaz, K. (1993) *Good Days, Bad Days: The Self in Chronic Illness and Time*. New Brunswick, NJ: Rutgers University Press.
Christakis, N.A. (1999) *Death Foretold: Prophecy and Prognosis in Medical Care*. Chicago, IL: University of Chicago Press.
Coe, R.M. and Prendergast, C.G. (1985) 'The formation of coalitions – interaction strategies in triads', *Sociology of Health & Illness*, 7: 236–247.
Connor, M., Fletcher, I., and Salmon, P. (2009) 'The analysis of verbal interaction sequences in dyadic clinical communication: a review of methods', *Patient Education and Counseling*, 75: 169–177.
Corbin, J.M. and Strauss, A. (1985) 'Three lines of work', *Qualitative Sociology*, 8: 224–227.
——(1988) *Unending Work and Care: Managing Chronic Illness at Home*. San Francisco, CA: Jossey-Bass.
Cripe, L. (2008) 'Closing the gap', presentation at Cancer Stories Conference, November 8, Indianapolis, IN.
Curtis, J.R., Engelberg, R.A., Wenrich, M.D., Shannon, S.E., Treece, P.D., and Rubenfeld, G.D. (2005) 'Missed opportunities during family conferences about end-of-life care in the intensive care unit', *American Journal of Respiratory and Critical Care Medicine*, 171: 844–849.
Davis, Fred. (1963) *Passage through Crisis: Polio Victims and Their Families*. Indianapolis, IN: Bobbs-Merrill.
Donovan-Kicken, Tollison, A., and Goins, E. (2012) 'The nature of communication work during cancer: advancing the theory of illness trajectories', *Health Communication*, 27(7): 641–652.
Eggly, S., Afonso, N., Rojas, G., Baker, M., Cardozo, L., and Robertson, R.S. (1997) 'An assessment of residents' competence in the delivery of bad news to patients', *Academic Medicine*, 72: 397–399.
Eggly, S., Penner, L., Albrecht, T.L., Cline, R.J., Foster, T., Naughton, M., et al. (2006) 'Discussing bad news in the outpatient oncology clinic: rethinking current communication guidelines', *Journal of Clinical Oncology*, 24: 716–719.
Eide, H., Frankel, R., Haaversen, A.C.B., Vaupel, K.A., Graudaard, P.K., and Finset, A. (2004) 'Listening for feelings: identifying and coding empathic and potential empathic opportunities in medical dialogues', *Patient Education and Counseling*, 54(3): 291–297.
Ellingson, L.L. (2002) 'The roles of companions in geriatric patient–interdisciplinary oncology team interactions', *Journal of Aging Studies*, 16: 361–382.
Fagerlind, H., Lindblad, A.K., Berstrom, I., Nilsson, M., Naucler, G., Glimelius, B., and Ring, L. (2008) 'Patient–physician communication during oncology consultations', *Psycho-Oncology*, 17: 975–985.
Ford, S., Fallowfield, L., and Lewis, S. (1996) 'Doctor–patient interactions in oncology', *Social Science and Medicine*, 42: 1511–1519.
Frankel, R.M. (2000) 'Challenges and opportunities in delivering bad news', *Physician's Quarterly*, 25: 1–6.

Friedrichsen, M. and Milberg, A. (2006) 'Concerns about losing control when breaking bad news to terminally ill patients with cancer: physicians' perspective', *Journal of Palliative Medicine*, 9: 673–682.

Girgis, A. and Sanson-Fisher, R.W. (1998) 'Breaking bad news 1: current best advice for clinicians', *Behavioral Medicine*, 24(2): 53–59.

Goffman, E. (1959) *Presentation of Self in Everyday Life*. New York: Anchor.

——(1963) *Stigma: Notes on the Management of Spoiled Identity*. Englewood Cliffs, NJ: Prentice-Hall.

Gray, R.E., Fitch, M., Phillips, C., Labrecque, M., and Fergus, K. (2000) 'To tell or not to tell: patterns of disclosure among men with prostate cancer', *Psycho-Oncology*, 9: 273–282.

Groopman, J.E. (2004) *The Anatomy of Hope: How People Prevail in the Face of Illness*. New York: Random House.

Hasselkus, B.R. (1992) 'Physician and family caregiver in the medical setting: negotiation of care', *Journal of Aging Studies*, 6: 67–80.

Heath, C. (1992) 'Diagnosis and assessment in the medical consultation', in P. Drew and J. Heritage (eds) *Talk at Work*. Cambridge: Cambridge University Press.

Helft, P.R. (2005) 'Necessary collusion: prognostic communication with advanced cancer patients', *Journal of Clinical Oncology*, 23: 3146–3150.

Heritage, J. and Maynard, D.W. (2006) 'Introduction: analyzing interaction between doctors and patients in primary care encounters', in J. Heritage and D.W. Maynard (eds) *Communication in Medical Care: Interaction between Primary Care Physicians and Patients*. Cambridge: Cambridge University Press.

Jarrett, N.J. and Payne, S.A. (2000) 'Creating and maintaining "optimism" in cancer care communication', *International Journal of Nursing Studies*, 37(1): 81–90.

Jefferson, G. (1985) 'On the interactional unpackaging of a "gloss"', *Language in Society*, 14: 435–466.

Keogh, F., O'Riordan, J., McNamara, C., Duggan, C., and McCann, S.R. (1998) 'Psychosocial adaptation of patients and families following bone marrow transplantation: a prospective, longitudinal study', *Bone Marrow Transplantation*, 22: 905–911.

Labrecque, M.S., Blanchard, C.G., Ruckdeschel, J.C., and Blanchard, E.B. (1991) 'The impact of family presence on the physician–cancer-patient interaction', *Social Science and Medicine*, 33: 1253–1261.

Larson, D.G. and Chastain, R.L. (1990) 'Self-concealment: conceptualization, measurement, and health implications', *Journal of Social and Clinical Psychology*, 9: 439–455.

Lazare, A., Putnam, S.M., and Lipkin, M. (1995) 'Three functions of the medical interview', in M. Lipkin, S.M. Putnam, and A. Lazare (eds) *The Medical Interview: Clinical Care, Education, and Research*. New York: Springer-Verlag.

Leydon, G.M. (2008) '"Yours is potentially serious but most of these are cured": optimistic communication in UK outpatient oncology consultations', *Psycho-Oncology*, 17: 1081–1088.

Lutfey, K. and Maynard, D.W. (1998) 'Bad news in oncology: how physician and patient talk about death and dying without using those words', *Social Psychology Quarterly*, 61: 321–341.

Maynard, D.W. (1991) 'On the interactional and institutional basis of asymmetry in clinical discourse', *American Journal of Sociology*, 97: 448–495.

——(1992) 'On clinicians' co-implicating recipients in the delivery of diagnostic news', in P. Drew and J. Heritage (eds) *Talk at Work: Interaction in Institutional Settings*, Cambridge: Cambridge University Press.

——(1996) 'On "realization" in everyday life: the forecasting of bad news as a social relation', *American Sociological Review*, 61(1): 109–131.

——(1997) 'The news delivery sequence: bad news and good news in conversational interaction', *Research on Language and Social Interaction*, 30: 93–130.

——(2003) *Bad News, Good News: Conversational Order in Everyday Talk and Clinical Settings*. Chicago, IL: University of Chicago Press.

Maynard, D.W. and Hudak, P.L. (2008) 'Small talk, high stakes: interactional disattentiveness in the context of prosocial doctor–patient interaction', *Language in Society*, 37(5): 661–688.

Mei-Hui, T. (2007) 'Who gets to talk? An alternative framework evaluating companion effects in geriatric triads', *Communication & Medicine*, 4: 37–49.

Ong, L.M.L., Visser, M.R.M., Lammes, F.B., and De Haes, J. (2000) 'Doctor–patient communication and cancer patients' quality of life and satisfaction', *Patient Education and Counseling*, 41: 145–156.
Peräkylä, A. (1998) 'Authority and accountability: the delivery of diagnosis in primary health care', *Social Psychology Quarterly*, 61: 301–320.
——(2004) 'Two traditions of interaction research', *British Psychological Society*, 43: 1–20.
Pilnick, A. (1998) '"Why didn't you say just that?" Dealing with issues of asymmetry, knowledge and competence in the pharmacist/client encounter', *Sociology of Health & Illness*, 20: 29–51.
Ptacek, J.T., Fries, E.A., Eberhardt, T.T.L., and Ptacek, J.J. (1999) 'Breaking bad news to patients: physicians' perceptions of the process', *Supportive Care in Cancer*, 7: 113–120.
Reddy, M.J. (1979) 'The conduit metaphor', in A. Ortony (ed.) *Metaphor and Thought*. Cambridge: Cambridge University Press.
Rodriguez, K.L., Gambino, F.J., Butow, P., Hagerty, R., and Arnold, R.M. (2007) 'Pushing up daisies: implicit and explicit language in oncologist–patient communication about death', *Supportive Care in Cancer*, 15: 153–161.
——(2008) '"It's going to shorten your life": framing of oncologist–patient communication about prognosis', *Psycho-Oncology*, 17: 219–225.
Roemer, E. and Borkovec, T.D. (1994) 'Effects of suppressing thoughts about emotional material', *Journal of Abnormal Psychology*, 103: 467–474.
Roter, D. and Hall, J.A. (1989) 'Studies of doctor–patient interaction', *Annual Review of Public Health*, 10: 163–180.
——(2006) *Doctors Talking with Patients/Patients Talking with Doctors: Improving Communication in Medical Visits*. Westport, CT: Praeger.
Roth, J. (1963) *Timetables: Structuring the Passage of Time in Tuberculosis Treatment and Other Careers*. New York: Bobbs Merrill.
Sanden, I., Linell, P., Starkhammar, H., and Larsson, U.S. (2001) 'Routinization and sensitivity: interaction in oncological follow-up consultations', *Health*, 5: 139–163.
Schaepe, K.S. (2011) 'Bad news and first impressions: patient and family caregiver accounts of learning the cancer diagnosis', *Social Science & Medicine*, 73: 912–921.
——(2013) 'Affective communication: management of bad news following cancer diagnosis and stem cell transplant'. Unpublished PhD dissertation, Department of Sociology, University of Wisconsin: Madison, WI.
Schildmann, J., Cushing, A., Doyal, L., and Vollmann, J. (2005) 'Breaking bad news: experiences, views and difficulties of pre-registration house officers', *Palliative Medicine*, 19: 93–98.
Smith, S.W., Atkin, C., Skubisz, C.M., Nazione, S., and Stohl, C. (2009) 'The impact of personal and/or close relationship experience on memorable messages about breast cancer and the perceived speech acts of the sender', *Journal of Cancer Education*, 24: 129–134.
Strauss, A. (1975) *Chronic Illness and the Quality of Life*. St. Louis, MO: Mosby.
Strauss, A., Corbin, J., Faberhaugh, S., Glaser, B., Maines, B., Suczek, B., and Wiener, C. (1984) *Chronic Illness and the Quality of Life*. St. Louis, MO: Mosby.
Taylor, K.M. (1988) 'Telling bad news: physicians and the disclosure of undesirable information', *Sociology of Health & Illness*, 10: 109–132.
ten, Have, P. (1991) 'Talk and institution: a reconsideration of the "asymmetry" of doctor–patient interaction', in D. Boden and D.H. Zimmerman (eds) *Talk and Social Structure*. Cambridge: Polity Press.
The, A.M., Hak, T., Koeter, G., and Van Der Wal, G. (2000) 'Collusion in doctor–patient communication about imminent death: an ethnographic study', *British Medical Journal*, 321: 1376–1381.
Thorne, S., Armstrong, E.A., Harris, S.R., Hislop, T.G., Kim-Sing, C., Oglov, V., et al. (2009) 'Patient real-time and 12-month retrospective perceptions of difficult communications in the cancer diagnostic period', *Qualitative Health Research*, 19: 1383–1394.
Timmermans, L.M., Van Der Maazen, R.W.M., Verhaak, C.M., Van Roosmalen, M.S., Van Daal, W.A.J., and Kraaimaat, F.W. (2005) 'Patient participation in discussing palliative radiotherapy', *Patient Education and Counseling*, 57: 53–61.
Walsh, R.A., Girgis, A., and Sanson-Fisher, R.W. (1998) 'Breaking bad news 2: What evidence is available to guide clinicians?', *Behavioral Medicine*, 24: 61–72.
Weisman, A.D. and Worden, J.W. (1976) 'The existential plight in cancer: significance of the first 100 days', *International Journal of Psychiatry in Medicine*, 7: 1–15.

28

Managing hopeful moments

Initiating and responding to delicate concerns about illness and health

Wayne A. Beach

Introduction

Communication between patients and their doctors involves many social activities. With diseases such as cancer, one prominent research agenda focuses on how *bad* news gets raised, delivered, and responded to (e.g., Maguire and Faulkner 1988; Fallowfield 1993; Lutfey and Maynard 1998; Baile et al. 2000; Beach 2002; Maynard 1996, 1997, 2003, 2006, 2007; Fallowfield and Jenkins 2004; Maynard and Frankel 2006; Barclay et al. 2007; Cleary et al. 2009; Del Vento et al. 2009). Oncology interviews are often described as preoccupied with managing possibilities of dying as well as other challenging, delicate, and highly emotional moments. Societal attitudes also associate cancer with bad news and terminal illness. While numerous popular and mediated campaigns emphasize that cancer is not a 'death sentence' (e.g., MSNBC 2007; NY Times 2008), but a chronic disease managed by over ten million American survivors, misconceptions abound that 'c'ancer (the 'c' word) inevitably leads to dying. A simple Internet search on 'Why is cancer the 'c' word?' yields thousands of articles, personal interviews, anecdotal testimonies, and videos – most of which describe cancer as a distinct and stigmatizing disease triggering anxiety, trepidation, and even horror.

Given the predominance of dark and foreboding conceptions about cancer and cancer clinics, it may seem incongruous and even ironic to suggest that few other medical settings are more 'benign' than interactions designed to manage 'malignancies' during oncology encounters. However, from repeated and close inspections of a large collection of video recorded and transcribed oncology interviews, we are discovering the existence of an alternative social order: Patients and doctors systematically work together to counter hopeful solutions to potentially despairing circumstances. Bad news is countered with good news, and health and well-being are treated as more desirable than sickness. Talk about death and dying are minimized and relatively infrequent. These practices mobilize patients and doctors to seek relief from troubling symptoms, reassurance about inherently ambiguous futures, comfort and strength in the face of fearful reactions to seemingly countless challenges associated with cancer and other health threats. In these ways clinical orientations mirror everyday, ordinary conversations as participants routinely display resistance to troubles, and exit troubling matters by introducing remedial or good topics, optimistic projections, or 'bright side sequences' (Jefferson 1980a, 1980b, 1988; Holt 1993, 1996; Maynard 2003; Beach 2009). For example, outside of clinics in home environments, family members talking through cancer on the telephone have been shown to enact hopeful behaviors when managing uncertain circumstances and working together to support, commiserate, fight illness battles, and construct positive futures (Beach 2009).

Despite the significance of these social actions, little is known about the communicative work of hopeful conduct in the cancer clinic or during primary care. Collaborative and interactionally organized communicative processes have been overlooked in favor of individuals' perceptual experiences assessed through self-report scales, interviews, surveys, diaries, and anecdotal reports (Peräkylä 1991; Beach and Andersen 2003, 2004). This chapter begins with a brief chronology of research findings identifying moments where hopeful actions are raised and responded to in ordinary (e.g., family) interactions as well as primary and cancer medical encounters. Doctors' responses to patients' hopeful concerns are also examined to reveal that what patients nominate, and treat as important, can be redirected to accommodate biomedical agendas and priorities. Next, analysis turns to selected instances of how doctors work to edify patients' health circumstances. A case study is provided of how an oncologist delivers and manages hopeful news to a lung cancer patient by initiating, delivering, and summarizing good news evidencing treatment effectiveness. Discussion raises implications for ongoing studies of hopeful conduct, relationships between justifying wellness and offering reassurance, and how close examinations of hopeful moments can promote improved clinical care.

Data and method

Data excerpts selected for this chapter are drawn from video recordings and transcriptions of 25 primary care, 150 oncology interviews, as well as 61 phone calls involving family members talking about and through cancer over a 13-month period. Encounters between cancer patients and their doctors were collected at an institution designated by the National Cancer Institute (NCI) as a Comprehensive Cancer Center. Conversation analytic (CA) methods (Atkinson and Heritage 1984; Drew and Heritage 1992; Sacks 1992; Sidnell and Stivers 2013), anchored in repeated listenings of recordings in unison with systematic inspections of carefully produced transcriptions (for transcription symbols see Appendix 28.1 at the end of this chapter), have been employed to generate an empirical foundation for understanding hopeful conduct during oncology interviews.

Sample analysis: exemplars of hopeful conduct-in-interaction

Hopeful social actions demonstrate a minimum of three general qualities: (1) any communicative orientation displaying expectation, anticipation, and/or desire of positive outcomes enhancing signs of life, wellness, and well-being; (2) may be stated explicitly (i.e., lexical as with hope, hoping, hopeful) or implicitly; and (3) emerge in the course of pursuing a displayed preference for good rather than bad news.

To exemplify the sequential environments within which hopeful moments get initiated and responded to during interaction, analysis begins with an excerpt from a phone call between a mother and a son during their first opportunity to discuss mom's recent cancer diagnosis. Attention is then given to a series of examples from both primary and cancer care. To understand how doctors can be purveyors of hope, instances are drawn from post-encounter interviews with patients, field notes, and moments from a single video recorded oncology interview.

Family cancer phone calls

When beginning to examine a corpus of phone calls involving family members talking about and through cancer (Beach 2009), initial observations identified how a series of bad or difficult topics got punctuated with good or hopeful possibilities. The excerpt below occurred only minutes into the second of 61 phone calls. Mom had just informed son that her cancer diagnosis was very serious, perhaps the 'worst' news that she could have received:

Excerpt 1: SDCL: NH2: 2–3

Mom:	→	So. (0.4) It's r(h)e::al °b(h)a:d°.
		(0.8)
Mom:		((coughs))
Son:		pt .hh I guess.
		(0.4)
Mom:		And uh: >I don't know what else to tell you.<
		(1.0)
Son:		.hh hhh Yeah. (0.2) um- ((hhhh)). Yeah, I don't know what to
		say either.
Mom:	→	No there's nothing to say. >You just-< .hh I'll I'll wait to talk
		to Doctor (name) today. = He's the cancer man and =
Son:		= Um hmm.
Mom:	→	See what he has to say, and (0.4) just keep goin' forward. I
		mean- (.) I might be real lucky in five years. It might just be
		six months.
		(0.4)
Son:		Yeah.
Mom:		°Who knows.°
Son:		Phew::.
Mom:		Yeah.
Son:		.hh hhh (.) Whadda you do: with this kind of thing. I mean-
Mom:		>Radiation chemotherapy.<
		(1.2)
Son:		Oh bo:y?
Mom:		Yeah.
		(0.5)
Mom:	→	My only hope- I mean (.) my only choice.
Son:		Yeah.
Mom:	→	It's either that or just lay here and let it kill me.
		(1.0)
Mom:	→	And that's not the human condition.
Son:		No. (1.0) I guess [not.]

Following mom's 'r(h)e::al °b(h)a:d°.' (line 1) summary of her diagnosis, both mom and son state there is little or nothing more to say. Yet mom continues by describing that she is waiting to see what the doctor, 'the cancer man', might have to say (lines 10–13). Relying on a doctor specializing in cancer care, as an authoritative medical source, provides one hopeful option to 'just keep goin' forward' (line 13). Mom does not explicitly invoke 'hope', though her actions indirectly imply that the doctor is a valued and potential source for news updates (both good and bad) as her cancer journey unfolds. A 'lucky' scenario is then depicted (line 14): 'five years' of remaining life amounts to good news, especially when compared with the next and possible duration of 'six months'. Moments later, mom responds to son's question (line 21) by referring to radiation and chemotherapy as 'My only <u>ho</u>pe- I mean (.) my only <u>cho</u>ice.' (line 27). This is a curious display of hopefulness and a restriction with dire consequences: if mom chooses to avoid treatments, it could kill her (line 29), and that is not an outcome she prefers.

From this excerpt it is seen that hopeful actions can be indirect (lines 10–14) or explicit (line 27). The close proximity of good/hopeful and bad news is also apparent: mom could live for 'five years' or 'six months'. Treatment options are mom's primary hope, but her choices are both restricted and (if avoided) could lead to death. Such ambiguities are routine when managing cancer and a wide variety of other potentially threatening illnesses. In everyday living, it is also a recurring tendency for good/hopeful topics to premonitor and be in close proximity to subsequent troubles (e.g., see Jefferson 1980a, 1980b; 1984a, 1984b; 1988; Maynard 2003). For mom and son, managing the outset of a serious cancer diagnosis involves investing hope in her doctor and prescribed treatments, yet being realistic about a serious cancer threat that may (and eventually did) take mom's life earlier than hoped for. In short, good and bad news function as intricate balancing mechanisms that are not artificially separated in ordinary interactional circumstances.

Initiating and responding to hopeful actions in primary care and cancer clinics

During medical interviews, patients initiate a wide variety of *patient-initiated actions* (PIAs) extending beyond yes/no answers to doctors' questions (Stivers and Heritage 2001; Boyd and Heritage 2006; Stivers 2007; Beach 2012). For example, PIAs may be evident in any combination of the following: asking questions about their illness and care, making requests for what they want and need, bidding for acknowledgment or reassurance, resisting and/or challenging doctors' recommendations, describing symptoms and impacts on daily living (e.g., pain, discomfort, diet, sleep, exercise), and initiating stories or narratives about how life-world experiences (e.g., work, relationships, finances, faith) are connected with illness. In turn, physicians can be responsive to what patients have raised and nominated as primal concerns, or avoid patient's concerns by shifting toward their own biomedical agendas. These are *doctor-responsive actions* (DRAs) that occur following patients' attempts to initiate actions.

Invoking hopeful concerns

A series of moments have been identified where primary care patients initiate hopeful concerns about their health condition. The patient below is a mechanic who scheduled a visit to address his injured back:

Excerpt 2: Street: 2:6:5, p. 277

1 Doctor: You kept thinking it'd get better.
2 Patient: Yeah.
3 Doctor: [[Then it didn't.]

Patient: → [[Hoping it would] get better, because you know I have to work.
→ (1.2)
Doctor: → Ka:y. I don't know too much about cars. Tell me, how heavy
is an intake manifold.

In response to doctor's 'You kept thinking it'd get better.' (line 1), patient extends his initial 'Yeah.' to produce two key actions. First, 'Hoping it would get better' (line 4) is an upgrade to doctor's prior 'thinking'. With 'Hoping' patient displays an expectation or desire for healing, and also next provides a viable reason for his hope: He has to work but cannot do so with a hurt back. While the consequences of his not working (e.g., paying bills or providing for family) are not specified, the importance of his working is made available to the doctor. In response, followed by a marked (1.2) pause, doctor's ' Ka:y' minimally acknowledges patient's concern (line 6) before shifting topic to 'intake manifold' (Beach 1995). What is not addressed is the importance of patient's hopefulness (i.e., a need to work). Further, no reassurance or offer is made to form a partnership to better insure patient's healing and getting back to work as soon as possible.

A similar instance involves a cancer patient previously diagnosed with melanoma/skin cancer (Beach et al. 2005). She now seeks referral to a cancer clinic to insure that no new cancer sites have developed. This excerpt begins as patient completes a story about a friend also diagnosed with cancer. But her friend is facing serious metastasis, requiring that she travel long distance to a major cancer center for advanced treatment:

Excerpt 3: OC#1: 17–18

Patient: (Now we have)- ah a friend of mine- (.) a friend- (.) it wrapped
around the stem <of his bra::in.> .hhh [° Like] oh my God.°=
Doctor 1: [Mm hm.]
Patient: =It metastasized in his le:g (.) °Ya know.° But he's down at Anderson.=
Doctor 1: =Mm hm.
Patient: → So: hope::fully I caught mine early enough.
Doctor 1: → Well that's the thing. If you had a ah seven millimeter=
Patient: =Mm hm.=
Doctor 1: → =ah (.) melanoma (.) the: (.) ah (.) survival is much better (.) if yo:u
do a resection early on, and I had mentioned to you about the
(sentinel) lymph node biopsy ((continues))

Patient brings her story to a close by stating 'So: hope::fully I caught mine early enough.' (line 6). Even though her friend's condition is much more serious than her own, patient does not unequivocally claim such good news. Instead, she makes her hope available to doctor and provides a window of opportunity for receiving confirmation and reassurance (Suchman et al. 1997). Both are withheld, however, as doctor's 'Well'-prefaced response does not disagree nor strongly affiliate with patient's hopeful summary of her condition. Doctor does acknowledge patient having had an early resection, but also provides a 'textbook' or biomedical response that describes '(sentinel) lymph node biopsy' (line 11) as a technical procedure somehow related to patient's history with melanoma. What is left unaddressed, then, is a much more basic and hopeful concern initiated by patient: whether her cancer was caught 'early enough' or not.

A third and final primary care example involves what many doctors find troubling at the outset of an interview: a patient treated as wanting to know what is wrong before undergoing medical history-taking and physical examination (Jones and Beach 2005). This patient does not make a specific request, but says '=Well I hope you can find out what's wrong with me.' (line 8):

Excerpt 4: S14: 1

Doctor: H'lo Mister Steen.=
Patient: =Good morning.
(2.0)
Doctor: I'm Physician Krone.
(0.2)
Patient: Pleased to meet sir.
Doctor: Nice to meet you.=
Patient: → =Well I hope you can find out what's wrong with me.
Doctor: → We(h)ll I hadn't even seen you yet.
Patient: → (At's whuh) I say I still say I hope you can find
[out what's wrong with me.]
Doctor: → [O:h, okay. (0.4) Well we will.]
Patient: → Whatever you think whatever yo: (0.5) u:h (0.3) whatever
it is tell me: so I can (0.7) eh- (0.7) (keepn gih) get somethin
done about it. Cause (.) ma:n (0.4) it's worrying me.

In stating 'I hope', patient does not seek a specific answer about his illness condition. As with previously examined moments, what patient does seek is some acknowledgment and recognition that the doctor shares a hope to discover and resolve patient's problem(s). Patient's action is met with some resistance, however, as doctor states he hasn't even interviewed the patient yet (line 9). Doctor makes this obvious assertion rather than simply acknowledging that patient's stated 'hope' is also doctor's priority. In response (lines 10–11), patient again informs doctor that his point is not to request that this doctor tell him what only a medical history and diagnosis will reveal. Instead, patient is persistent with 'I still say I hope you can find out what's wrong with me.'. Marked by 'Oh.', displaying awareness of new information (Heritage 1984), doctor now claims to understand that patient's fundamental concern is about hope, not definitive answers. Yet doctor's 'O:h, okay. (0.4) Well we will.' (line 12) remains somewhat resistant. And by invoking the institutional 'We.' (Heritage and Drew 1992), doctor deflects a stronger and more personal commitment to insure patient that he too shares patient's hopeful orientation. With persistence, patient's next turn (lines 13–15) –marked with anxious hesitation, dysfluency, and stuttering – demonstrates his need to hear whatever the doctor might say, and do, to relieve patient's 'worrying'. It is now apparent that this 'worrying' underlies patient's pursuit and displayed need for confirmation of shared hopeful orientations – hopeful worrying that the doctor did not discern, or even if so, did not actively attend to.

Across the three instances (above) patients' are not passive (e.g., see Robinson 2003; Street et al. 2003, 2005) but design their hopes to assuage worry (and fear): a mechanic is not able and needs to work (Excerpt 2), a cancer patient treats 'early enough' as less threatening than a late detection (Excerpt 3), and a patient twice solicits a doctor's shared hopeful orientation to identify and solve health problems 'Cause (.) ma:n (0.4) it's worrying me.' (Excerpt 4). At least for these cases, doctors' responses are tailored less to what patients treat as important, and more to agendas that tend to avoid, gloss, or even dismiss what patients have put forth as primary concerns. Drawn from a considerably larger collection, these instances provide preliminary and compelling evidence that what patients are hopeful about may not be acknowledged, directly addressed, nor affirmed by doctors. This is not to say that doctors, without exception, give more priority to their agendas rather than patients' hopes. This chapter concludes with an extended instance where a doctor works diligently to deliver good news to a lung cancer patient, information allowing for anticipation of a hopeful and healthy future.

Justifying wellness in a comprehensive cancer clinic

We are increasingly discovering that patients devise innovative ways to raise and pursue their hopeful concerns (Beach 2013; Beach and Dozier 2012). The following instances reveal alternative practices used by cancer patients to substantiate being well, rather than predisposed to or actually being sick. In the face of structural (e.g., question–answer) constraints, and even when doctors take actions to limit patients' contributions, patients initiate and continue to pursue diverse courses of hopeful actions. In response to 'no problem' questions, designed by oncologists to constrain both length and topics addressed by patients' answers, patients expand yes/no answers to achieve actions such as managing vulnerability, taking resilient stances toward healthy living, and countering sick-role symptoms indicative of cancer.

In Excerpt 5, patient uses extreme language (Pomerantz 1986) to assert and legitimate the absence of family cancer history:

Excerpt 5: ND14: P1: 4

1 Doctor: And you said that there's no family history of cancer whatsoever?
2 No breast, ovary, colon, or whatever?
3 Patient: → No. Nothing. Absolutely nothing.

While a 'No.' response to doctor's no-preference question could suffice, patient expands his answer to include 'Nothing. Absolutely nothing.'. This response is not just overly redundant; it is built progressively to unequivocally provide stronger evidence for wellness.

The cancer patient in Excerpt 6, diagnosed with chronic lymphocytic leukemia (CLL), could have also provided a 'No.' response to doctor's prior question – a question which presumes no change in bowel habits:

Excerpt 6: OC6: 6

1 Doctor: You haven't noticed any change in your bowel habits at all?
2 Patient: → pt I have regular u:h bowel movements eve[ry morning.]
3 Doctor: [°Mm hm.°] °Mm hm.°
4 Patient: → It hasn't changed for years and years and years.
5 Doctor: Mm hm.
6 Patient: → No- <u>no</u> difference.
7 Doctor: pt .hh Not taking any medicines right now?
8 Patient: ↑No.
9 Doctor: A:nd don't have any allergies of any sort?
10 Patient: No.

Instead, patient makes a point that bowel movements occur 'every morning.' (line 2), i.e., without exception. He then bolsters his argument by stating that no change had occurred for 'years and years and years' before concluding with 'No- <u>no</u> difference.' (lines 4 and 6).

Taken together, patient invests considerable efforts to justify regularity, a position patient treats as not symptomatic of increased problems with CLL. It is also worth noting, and a routine occurrence across our data, that despite patients' repeated wellness efforts doctors tend to withhold acknowledgment, and move quickly forward to next items advancing their biomedical agenda (as with the two no-preferenced questions in lines 7 and 9, above).

This kind of turn and position expansion, designed by patients to optimize wellness and minimize potential cancer problems, also occur in each of the two moments drawn from two additional and different oncology interviews. In Excerpt 7, by not simply stating 'Yes', patient first reports that her pap smear was not just okay but 'Perfect.' (line 2):

Excerpt 7: ND10P5: 10

((Patient had just reported having a mammogram 2–3 weeks ago.))

1	Doctor:	And was it okay?
2	Patient: →	Perfect.
3	Doctor:	Okay. Have you ever had an ab[normal one.]
4	Patient: →	[No, always]perfect.
5	Doctor:	Okay. [And when-].
6	Patient: →	[Mammogr]ams were always perfect.

She then and twice (lines 4 and 6) reasserts this good news announcement with 'always perfect.'. With extreme and repeated language, patient works diligently to pronounce that recent and prior breast images revealed no visible problems (indeed, were 'Perfect.').

Similarly, as doctor in Excerpt 8 assumes no problems with patient's arm movements, the patient's next 'No no no!' takes an exclaimed stance that all is well:

Excerpt 8: ND3 P3: 11

1	Doctor:	And can you go like so? No problem moving your arms
2		[at all]?
3	Patient: →	[No] no <u>no</u>! And I am doing all different exercises =
4	Doctor:	= Mm hm.=
5	Patient: →	= and dressing and everything.
6	Doctor:	Mm hm.

Further, patient explains he cannot just move his arms well, but is 'doing all different exercises' including 'dressing and everything' (lines 3 and 5). With 'all' and 'everything', and by visually moving his arms freely (apparent in the video recording), patient cumulatively substantiates his claim for wellness.

Doctors as purveyors of hope

Attention thus far has been given to how doctors pay minimal attention to patient's efforts to initiate hopeful concerns and justify wellness. Some doctors do not respond directly to what patients raise as hopeful concerns, pursuing instead to ask next history-taking questions, provide biomedical information, or even resist patient's psychosocial issues (e.g., 'worrying'). But it is important to emphasize that doctors are also purveyors of good news, and invest considerable efforts to create a foundation for building hope to advance health and healing (e.g., see Groopman 2004). While systematic research efforts to explicate doctors' good news/hopeful actions are minimal, some attention has been given to how doctors edify patients. Relying on individual interviews with patients following visits with their doctor, Fallowfield (1991) provides the following example:

> *Excerpt 9: Fallowfield 1991: 44 (see also Maynard 2003: 42–43); italics mine*
> I can't speak highly enough of Mr. C. He was very gentle and kind and
> didn't hurry me even though it was a busy clinic with lots waiting. He
> let me get dressed, then he sat me down, held my hand, and asked
> me what I thought was wrong. *When I said 'cancer', he said that*
> *I was right but that I shouldn't feel too worried as the lump was very*
> *small and there wasn't any lumpiness under my arms, which is a good sign.*

Patient provides an endearing description of this doctor and the care provided in the clinic. Two observations are important for the present analysis. First, the doctor delicately asked the patient what she thought was wrong, and only following patient's 'cancer' guess, did the doctor confirm her suspicion. Maynard (1992, 2003), describes this sequence as a 'perspective display series' (p. 42), a cautious way for doctors to initially solicit a patient's opinion or perspective, receive patient's reply or assessment, and only then confirm or provide an alternative assessment. (This basic sequence is also apparent in the final Excerpt 12, examined below.) Second, doctor's response to patient's 'cancer' reply was reported by patient to be both reassuring and hopeful: The patient should not be too worried, as the lump was small and seemingly had not spread – a 'good sign'.

Two related examples below are drawn from Peräkylä's (1991) field notes, in a Finnish leukemia ward, and illustrate how positive and optimistic attention was given to patients' conditions:

> *Excerpt 10: Peräkylä (1991: 413)*
> The patient [a 30-year-old woman who had recently contracted leukemia] is
> talking about her job and at one point says, '*if I get better*.' The doctor intervenes
> and says, '*No, listen, it's always going to be when you get better*.'

> *Excerpt 11: Peräkylä (1991: 413)*
> (The consultant explains that the cell count of Mr. K, in his sixties, may allow
> him to leave the hospital – if results from his bone marrow sample are good.)
>
> Patient: *So things are looking good?*
> Consultant: *As far as the cell count is concerned. Let's hope that*
> *the results of the bone marrow examination are just as good.*

In Excerpt 10, patient's 'if I get better' is corrected by doctor's 'when you get better'. And in Excerpt 11, patient's inquiry about possible good news is confirmed in terms of 'cell count'. Doctor next states a 'hope' that such good news will be extended to bone marrow results.

These examples from interviews and field notes provide a useful backdrop for examining a real-time interview between a cancer patient and oncologist.

The serial ordering of minimizing efforts

This analysis concludes with a more detailed case study of practices employed by an oncologist to inform a lung cancer patient about his cat scan (or CT imaging) results. The CT images (see Figure 28.1) provide cross-sectional views of tissue, including organs, allowing doctors to determine the presence or absence of tumors, their precise size and location, and how (or if) a tumor might be involved with connecting tissue and/or organs. These findings are also numerically summarized in the medical record for doctor's inspection.

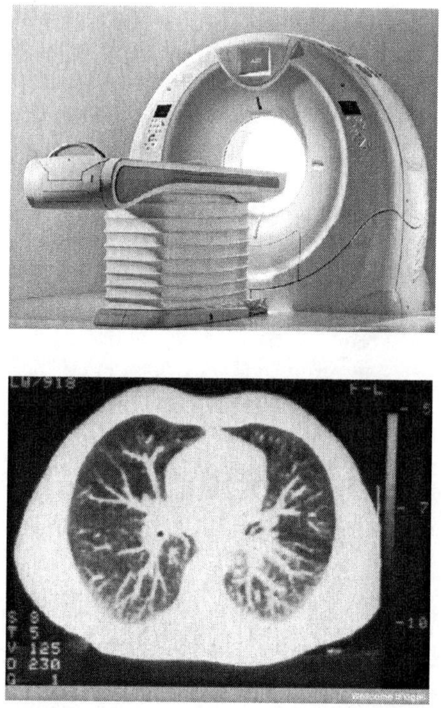

Figure 28.1 Cat scanner and image of the chest showing both lungs

Particular attention will be given to how the doctor initiates, elaborates, and bodily demonstrates good cancer news to both the patient and his co-present wife. Through the serial ordering of talk and local gestures (e.g., pinched fingers), the doctor offers both clarification and reassurance when calibrating that, and how, problem tumors have gotten smaller. The series of moments examined below focus not on single, isolated activities but on how a doctor's talk and embodied actions, especially his pinched fingers, get fluidly transformed from one task to another in the course of describing the size of 'nodes', how that size has changed, and (in the end) what counts as 'normal' (e.g., see Gutzmer and Beach 2012). These actions reveal the fluidity, precision, and critical importance involved as potential cancer threats get explained and minimized.

'It still measures one point six.'

This lung cancer patient had recent cat scans and a bone marrow transplant. The primary purpose for his visitation was to receive news about whether treatments and transplant had reduced sizes of tumors (or not):

Excerpt 12: OC D1 P7: 7–8 (1:46)

1 Doctor: So you know the results of your cat scans?
2 (0.2)
3 Patient: pt U::h, Patty said they were r:eally good. =She [was really] happy.=
4 Doctor: [°Uh huh.°]
5 Doctor: =Yeah.=
6 Patient: =Uh she said that there was a little sca:rring. And u:h, she called it-

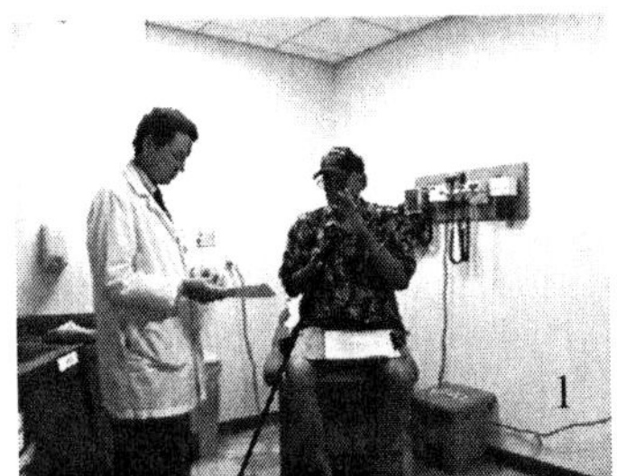

7 u::h the name of the- part of the lung. = I don't- [(.) don't kno]w exactly.
8 Doctor: [° Mm hm. °]
9 Ri::ght. Well a- any- any place we saw enla:rged nodes before
10 they're sma↓ller. = So that's the first important thing. A:nd u:h (0.2)
11 there's- the biggest node that's left is sorta deep down in he:re. It
12 still measures one point six, which is about like tha:t. (1.2)

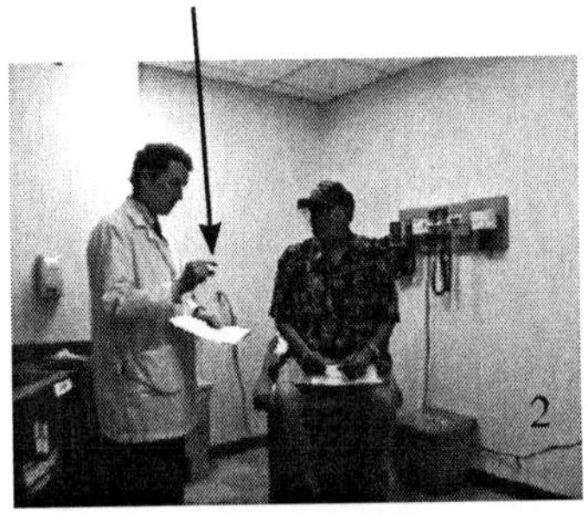

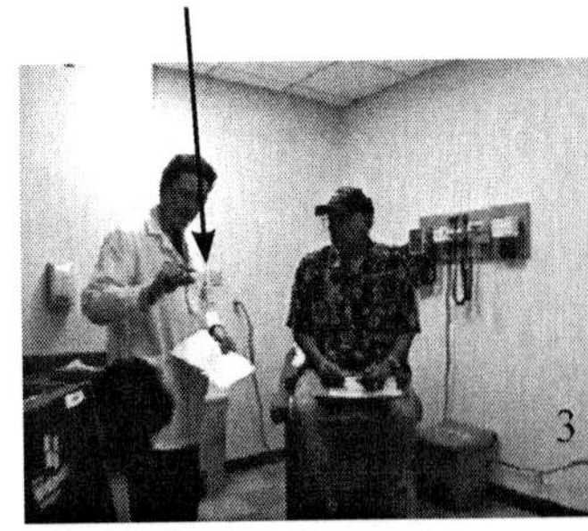

((shows fingers to patient's wife))

13 And previously it had been like tha:t? So- um but- but- a- anything a

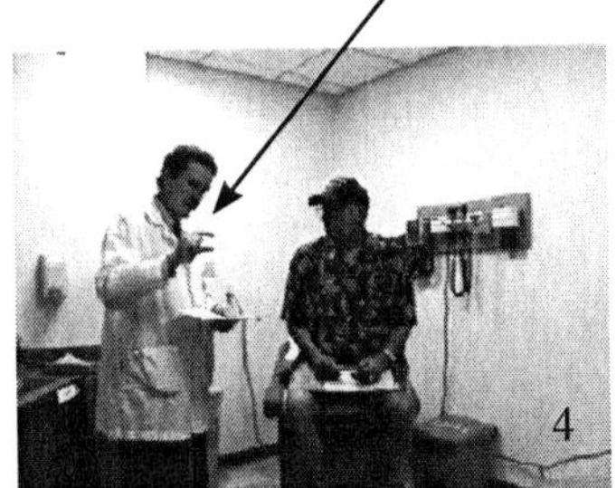

((depicts larger size))

< ce:ntimeter (.) or so (0.2) and le:ss is considered no:rmal. >

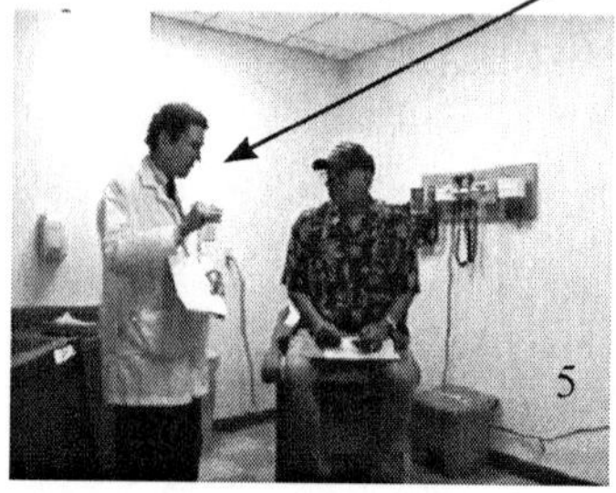

((pinched fingers reduced in size while hand lowers))

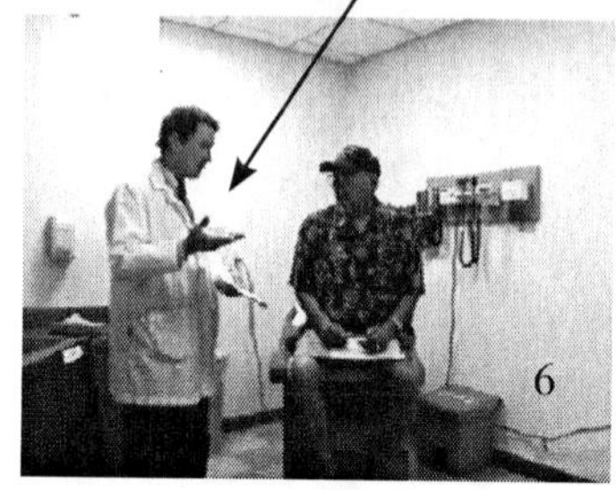

((opens hand to depict normal))

>So what we'll do we'll just follow this particular lymph node. <
Now d-did you have a pe:t sca:n before your transplant.
Patient: No. [((° I don't think so.°]))
Doctor: [Never had a pet] scan? Okay. So this was your one month
roughly um (.) cat scan. An' we'll repeat these again in thr:ee
months and continue to look at any places that use to ha:ve
increased no:des and just keep an eye on them.=
Patient: =Y-you know ac-according to- when I first was uh first came to
no:w.
Doctor: °Mm hm°.
Patient: I feel like I breath a lot better.
Doctor: °Mm hm°.

In line 1, doctor begins by soliciting patient's knowledge about his cat scans. Rather than directly announcing the news, asking for patient's information is a cautious way for doctor to proceed. Hearing the patient's perspective allows doctor to assess both patient's knowledge and general orientation to good or bad news about the cat scans (Maynard 1992, 2003). In this case, patient reports that 'Patty' (perhaps a clinical staff member) 'said they were r:eally good. =She was really happy.=' (line 3). Rather than claiming entitlement to know about these good results, and take a personal stance toward them, patient relies on a third party to authoritatively report these findings (see Bergmann 1992; Holt 1996; Holt and Clift 2006). Yet with 'really', twice emphasizing how good/happy Patty was with the results, patient does upgrade the news as more than simply 'good'.

This obvious good news is next countered with possible bad news of 'scarring' (line 6). As the patient proceeds to describe what Patty had stated about such scarring, in Frame 1 he opens both hands to represent the shape of the lung he is envisioning. But he cannot name the 'part of the lung' Patty had portrayed. With the disclaimer 'I don't know' (line 7), he claims insufficient knowledge as a non-medical expert (see Beach and Metzger 1997; Gill 1998; Gill et al. 2001). The patient is tentative, and downgrades his ability to know or definitively report on either the details of his lungs or the exact nature of the cat scan findings. In this way, patient makes available the limits of his knowledge to doctor, useful information which doctor's initial question (line 1) was designed to elicit.

Without hesitation doctor then confirms an important fact: that 'enlarged' nodes are now 'smaller'. Stated in plain, non-technical language doctor provides a preview and bottom-line, positive assessment of cat scan results (lines 9–10). This up-front forecast of good news offers a lens for patient and his wife to make sense of forthcoming details. To depict that the 'biggest' node remains and is embedded in the lung, doctor points to and taps his left chest to indicate 'sorta deep down in he:re' (line 11, video frame not included).

Building a metric: calibrating reduction in tumor size as evidence of treatment effectiveness

In Frame 2, doctor illustrates the 'one point six' size of this deeper node with pinched fingers. Here and throughout Frames 2–6, patient's gaze is directly focused on doctor's gestural depictions, an extended gaze revealing the fundamental importance of what doctor is demonstrating: reduction in tumor size.

During a (1.2) pause in Frame 3, patient's wife orients to the importance of this moment by leaning forward to better see what doctor was portraying. In response doctor rotates his body, and moves his pinched fingers to the right to accommodate the wife's visual access and thus understanding. Transferred across the talk comprising these moments, doctor's spatial gesture remains steady and becomes a focal resource signifying tumor size. Doctor retains a bodily position visually available to both patient and wife (Frame 4), and enlarges the space between his fingers when stating 'it had been like that' (line 13). This slight separation of his fingers represents how the size of the node was larger prior to treatment. He then draws his fingers together and moves his hand downward (Frame 5) when uttering 'a centimeter or so and less' (line 14). This lowered hand movement is lexically tied with 'less' to emphasize an actual reduction in size. With these actions, evident in Frame 6, doctor exhibits the shrinking importance of 'less'. He then opens and raises his hand when stating 'normal'.

Doctor makes clear that most nodes have gotten smaller, but the single remaining mode – at 'one point six' – is only slightly larger than normal. While the ultimate goal of cancer care is to eliminate malignant tumors altogether, and prevent them from recurring, the doctor here works diligently to characterize that this patient's condition nevertheless qualifies as good news and thus hopeful. Vocal and embodied evidence is recruited to illustrate that shrinking nodes, calibrated through increasing and decreasing pinched fingers, were the result of effective treatments. And by comparing the remaining 'biggest' node as nearing 'normal', doctor provides patient and his wife welcome news that, at least for the foreseeable future, cancer is being managed well as they embark on a hopeful path toward wellness.

Future directions

In his book *The Anatomy of Hope*, Groopman (2004) asserts that hope is less delusional than optimism and is 'the very heart of healing.' (p. xvi). The moments analyzed in this chapter begin to anchor our understandings of hopeful conduct in ordinary, frequently delicate, at times all-too-real circumstances. When real or potential illness needs to be managed, and the pursuit of health and healing are not just individual ambitions but collaboratively produced and inherently social activities, hopeful speakers produce distinct actions: They take (often affective) stances, make bids for acknowledgment and reassurance, justify their wellness to minimize cancer (and other health) threats, and overall work diligently to emphasize the importance of good rather than bad news. We have also seen, however, that raising hopeful concerns does not guarantee that doctors or patients will fully acknowledge or align with actions such as hopeful bids for reassurance.

When bad news arises, or health threats loom, being hopeful can be a steadfast resource for simply moving forward and managing health circumstances as best possible. The excerpts examined herein serve as humble reminders that hope gets practically and at times explicitly/lexically recruited to manage diverse circumstances. We have seen how a mother, dealing with the outset of a serious cancer diagnosis, informs her son that her only hope and choice is to seek cancer treatments because it's 'not the human condition' to just lay there and let it kill her. Other key moments, each in their own way, have been shown to be equally compelling: When a mechanic hopes to work, a melanoma patient hopes she 'caught mine early enough', and at the very beginning of a primary care interview, a worried patient hopes the doctor can share a hopeful commitment to find out what's wrong. Yet references to 'hope' need not be explicitly invoked for speakers to advance hopeful cases for wellness. Attention has also been given to efforts invested by patients to emphasize no family history of cancer, regular bowel movements, perfect mammograms, and an ability to move arms freely. These are often reasonable and well-justified sets of actions, significant because they can be used to avoid or minimize symptoms that could be indicative of cancer diagnosis or recurrence.

Summary

In closing, the materials included in this chapter are drawn from considerably larger collections of instances involving direct and indirect displays of hopeful conduct. Ongoing research draws similar attention to circumstances surrounding 'uncertainty' and 'fear' as interactional achievements, as well as inevitable relationships between hope, uncertainty, and fear as new cancer patients raise concerns and pursue responses from doctors. We are also comparing interactional conduct with patients' pre-post-assessments of hope, fear, uncertainty, and post-evaluations of communication satisfaction (Beach and Dozier 2012). From these efforts a more comprehensive analysis will reveal how patients' predispositions to care influence, and are influenced by, actual communication during oncology interviews. Such findings will also yield specific educational and clinical recommendations for better understanding patient-initiated actions (PIAs), more effectively responding to patients' primal concerns, and the fundamental importance of relying on digitized video recordings (and transcriptions) to produce innovative curricula designed to improve communication skills throughout cancer care. For example, when patients explicitly express their hopes, it could be highly effective for doctors to simply respond 'I hope so too.'. So doing not only acknowledges and reassures patients that their hopes were heard, but provides doctors an opportunity to offer realistic assessments of those hopes and demonstrate how they might work together as partners to achieve hoped-for outcomes.

Acknowledgment

This project was supported by the National Cancer Institute (NCI) of the National Institutes of Health (NIH) through Grant #CA122472-2.

Related topics

Communication and cancer; conversation analysis; death and dying; good and bad news; hope and optimism; patient-initiated actions; patient–provider interactions.

Further reading

Balint, M. (1957/1972) *The doctor, his patient, and the illness*. Madison, CT: International University Press. (One of the earliest descriptions of how patients offer and doctors respond (or not) to patients' primary concerns.)

Beach, W.A. (ed.) (2012) *Handbook of patient–provider interactions: Raising and responding to concerns about life, illness, and disease*. Mahwah, NJ: Hampton Press. (This handbook includes 52 chapters and chronicles 50 years (1957–2007) of efforts by clinicians, medical scientists, and social science researchers to closely examine communication during medical interviews.)

Beach, W.A. and Mandelbaum, J. (2005) 'My mom had a stroke': Understanding how patients raise and providers respond to psychosocial concerns. In L.H. Harter, P.M. Japp, and C.M. Beck (eds) *Constructing our health: The implications of narrative for enacting illness and wellness* (343–364). Mahwah, NJ: Lawrence Erlbaum. (A case study of how root issues of illness (caregiving stress) are raised indirectly by patient and thus not addressed by medical interviewer.)

Engel, G.F. (1977) The need for a new biomedical model: A challenge for biomedicine. *Science* 196, 129–136. (A foundational examination and critique of the limits of biomedicine for addressing patients' psychosocial experiences of illness.)

Heath, C. (2002) Demonstrative suffering: The gestural (re)embodiment of symptoms. *Journal of Communication* 52, 597–616. (Analysis of how patients use their bodies (e.g., hands and facial expressions) to dramatize their illness experiences, re-enacting for the doctor the very sensations associated with their symptoms.)

References

Atkinson, J.M. and Heritage, J. (eds) (1984) *Structures of social action: Studies in conversation analysis*. Cambridge: Cambridge University Press.

Baile, W.F., Buckman, R., Lenzi, R., et al (2000) SPIKES – A six-step protocol for delivering bad news: Application to the patient with cancer. *Oncologist* 5, 302–311.

Barclay, J. S., Blackhall, L.J., and Tulsky, J.A. (2007) Communication strategies and cultural issues in the delivery of bad news. *Journal of Palliative Medicine* 10, 958–977.

Beach, W.A. (1995) Conversation analysis: 'Okay' as a clue for understanding consequentiality. In S.J. Sigman (ed.) *The consequentiality of communication* (121–162). Hillsdale, NJ: Lawrence Erlbaum.

——(2002) Between dad and son: Initiating, delivering, and assimilating bad cancer news. *Health Communication* 14, 271–299.

——(2009) *A natural history of family cancer: Interactional resources for managing illness*. Cresskill, NJ: Hampton Press.

——(2013) Patients' efforts to justify wellness in a comprehensive cancer clinic. *Health Communication* 28, 577–591.

Beach, W.A. and Metzger, T.R. (1997) Claiming insufficient knowledge. *Human Communication Research* 23, 562–588.

Beach, W.A. and Andersen, J. (2003) Communication and cancer? Part I: The noticeable absence of interactional research. *Journal of Psychosocial Oncology* 21, 1–23.

——(2004) Communication and cancer? Part II: Conversation analysis. *Journal of Psychosocial Oncology* 21, 1–22.

Beach, W.A. and Dozier, D. (2012) Fears, uncertainties, and hopes: Patient-initiated actions (PIAs) and doctors' responses during oncology interviews. Manuscript.

Beach, W.A., Easter, D.W., Good, J.S., and Pigeron, E. (2005) Disclosing and responding to cancer *fears* during oncology interviews. *Social Science & Medicine* 60, 893–910.

Bergmann, J. (1992) Veiled morality: Notes on discretion in psychiatry. In P. Drew and J. Heritage (eds) *Talk at work: Interaction in institutional settings* (137–162). Cambridge: Cambridge University Press.

Boyd, E. and Heritage, J. (2006) Taking the patient's medical history: Questioning during comprehensive history taking. In J. Heritage and D. Maynard (eds) *Communication in medical care: Interactions between primary care physicians and patients* (151–184). Cambridge: Cambridge University Press.

Cleary, M., Hunt G.E., and Horsfall J. (2009) Delivering difficult news in psychiatric settings. *Harvard Review of Psychiatry* 17, 315–321.

Del Vento, A., Bavelas J., Healing S., MacLean G., and Kirk, P. (2009) An experimental investigation of the dilemma of delivering bad news. *Patient Education & Counseling* 77, 443–449.
Drew, P., and Heritage, J. (eds) (1992) *Talk at work: Interaction in institutional settings*. Cambridge: Cambridge University Press.
Fallowfield, L. (1991) *Breast cancer*. London: Routledge.
——(1993) Giving bad news. *Lancet* 341, 476–478.
Fallowfield, L. and Jenkins, V. (2004) Communicating sad, bad, and difficult news in medicine. *Lancet* 363, 312–319.
Gill, V.T. (1998) Doing attributions in medical interaction: Patients' explanations for illness and doctors' responses. *Social Psychology Quarterly* 61, 342–360.
Gill, V.T., Halkowski, T., and Roberts, F. (2001) Accomplishing a request without making one: A single case analysis of a primary care visit. *Text* 21, 55–82.
Groopman, J. (2004) *The anatomy of hope: How people prevail in the face of illness*. New York: Random House.
Gutzmer, K. and Beach, W.A. (2012) 'Having an ovary this big is not normal': How doctors negotiate patients' sickness or wellness during oncology interviews. Manuscript.
Heritage, J. (1984) A change-of-state token and aspects of its sequential placement. In J.M. Atkinson and J. Heritage (eds) *Structures of social action: Studies in conversation analysis* (229–345). Cambridge: Cambridge University Press.
Heritage, J. and Drew, P. (1992) Analyzing talk at work: An introduction. In P. Drew and J. Heritage (eds) *Talk at work: Interaction in institutional settings* (3–65). Cambridge: Cambridge University Press.
Holt, E. (1993) The structure of death announcements: Looking on the bright side of death. *Text* 3, 189–212.
——(1996) Reporting on talk: The use of direct reported speech in conversation. *Research on Language and Social Interaction* 29, 219–245.
Holt, E. and Clift, R. (2006) *Reporting talk: Reported speech in interaction*. Cambridge: Cambridge University Press.
Jefferson, G. (1980a) The analysis of conversations in which 'troubles' and 'anxieties' are expressed. Final report for the (British) Social Science Research Council: Report nos. HR 4805/1–2.
——(1980b) On 'trouble premonitory' response to inquiry. *Sociological Inquiry* 50, 153–185.
——(1984a) On stepwise transition from talk about a trouble to inappropriately next-positioned matters. In J.M. Atkinson and J. Heritage (eds) *Structures of social action: Studies in conversation analysis* (191–222). Cambridge: Cambridge University Press.
——(1984b) On the organization of laughter in talk about troubles. In J.M. Atkinson and J. Heritage (eds) *Structures of social action: Studies in conversation analysis* (347–369). Cambridge: Cambridge University Press.
——(1988) On the sequential organization of troubles talk in ordinary conversation. *Social Problems* 35, 418–444.
Jones, C.M. and Beach, W.A. (2005) 'I just wanna know why': Patient's attempts and doctors' responses to premature solicitation of diagnostic information. In Judith F. Duchan and D.Kovarsky (eds) *Diagnosis as cultural practice* (103–136). New York: Mouton de Gruyter.
Lutfey, K. and Maynard, D.W. (1998) Bad news in oncology: How physician and patient talk about death and dying without using those words. *Social Psychology Quarterly* 61, 321–341.
Maguire, P. and Faulkner, A. (1988) Communicate with cancer patients: 1. Handling bad news and difficult questions. *British Medical Journal* 297, 907–909.
Maynard, D.W. (1992) On co-implicating recipients in the delivery of diagnostic news. In P. Drew and J. Heritage (eds) *Talk at work: Interactions in institutional settings* (331–358). Cambridge: Cambridge University Press.
——(1996) On 'realization' in everyday life: The forecasting of bad news as a social relation. *American Sociological Review* 61, 109–131.
——(1997) The news delivery sequence: Bad news and good news in conversational interaction. *Research on Language and Social Interaction*, 30, 93–130.
——(2003) *Good news, bad news: Conversational order in everyday talk and clinical settings*. Chicago, IL: University of Chicago Press.
——(2006): 'Does it mean I´m gonna die?': On meaning assessment in the delivery of diagnostic news. *Social Science & Medicine* 62, 1902–1916.

——(2007) The news delivery sequence: Bad news and good news in conversational interaction. *Research on Language and Social Interaction* 30, 93–130.
Maynard, D.W. and Frankel, R.M. (2006) On diagnostic rationality: Bad news, good news, and the symptom residue. In J. Heritage and D.W. Maynard (eds) *Communication in medical care: Interaction between primary care physicians and patients* (248–278). Cambridge: Cambridge University Press.
MSNBC (2007) Cancer is no longer a death sentence. www.msnbc.msn.com/id/17760785/ns/nbcnightlynews/t/cancer-no-longer-death-sentence
NY Times (2008) Cancer as a disease, not a death sentence. http://www.nytimes.com/2008/06/17/health/17brody.html
Peräkylä, A. (1991) Hope work in the care of seriously ill patients. *Qualitative Health Research* 1, 407–433.
Pomerantz, A. (1986) Extreme case formulations: A way of legitimizing claims. *Human Studies* 9, 219–229.
Robinson, J.D. (2003) An interactional structure of medical activities during acute visits and its implications for patients' participation. *Health Communication* 15, 27–59.
Sacks, H. (1992) *Lectures on conversation: Volumes I and II*. Jefferson, G. (ed.). Oxford: Blackwell.
Sidnell, J. and Stivers, T. (eds) (2013) *Handbook of conversation analysis*. Cambridge: Blackwell-Riley.
Stivers, T. (2007) *Prescribing under pressure: Parent–physician conversations and antibiotics*. Cambridge: Cambridge University Press.
Stivers, T. and Heritage, J. (2001) Breaking the sequential mold: Answering 'more than the question' during comprehensive history taking. *Text* 21, 151–186.
Street, R.L., Krupat, E., Bell, R.A., Kravitz, R.L., and Haidet, P. (2003) Beliefs about control in the physician–patient relationship: Effect on communication in medical encounters. *Journal of General Internal Medicine* 18, 609–616.
Street, R.L. Jr., Gordon, H.S., Ward, H.M., Krupat, E., and Kravitz, R.L. (2005) Patient participation in medical consultations: Why some patients are more involved than others. *Medical Care* 43, 960–969.
Suchman, A., Markakis, K., Beckman, H.B., and Frankel, R. (1997) A model of empathic communication in the medical interview. *Journal of the American Medical Association* 27, 678–682.

Appendix 28.1: Transcription symbols

In data headings such as 'OC# D1P1: 6–7', 'OC' stands for 'Oncology', D1 P1 is Doctor 1 Patient 1, and 6–7 are the pages of the transcription for that interview. The transcription notation system employed for data segments is an adaptation of Gail Jefferson's work (e.g., see Atkinson and Heritage 1984: ix–xvi). The symbols may be described as follows:

:	Colon(s): Extended or stretched sound, syllable, or word.
_	Underlining: Vocalic emphasis.
(.)	Micropause: Brief pause of less than (0.2).
(1.2)	Timed Pause: Intervals occurring within and between same or different speaker's utterance.
(( ))	Double Parentheses: Scenic details.
( )	Single Parentheses: Transcriptionist doubt.
.	Period: Falling vocal pitch.
?	Question Marks: Rising vocal pitch.
↑↓	Arrows: Pitch resets; marked rising and falling shifts in intonation.
° °	Degree Signs: A passage of talk noticeably softer than surrounding talk.
=	Equal Signs: Latching of contiguous utterances, with no interval or overlap.
[ ]	Brackets: Speech overlap.
[[	Double Brackets: Simultaneous speech orientations to prior turn.
!	Exclamation Points: Animated speech tone.

- Hyphens: Halting, abrupt cut off of sound or word.

> < Less Than/Greater Than Signs: Portions of an utterance delivered at a pace noticeably quicker than surrounding talk.

OKAY CAPS: Extreme loudness compared with surrounding talk.

hhh .hhh H's: Audible outbreaths, possibly laughter. The more h's, the longer the aspiration. Aspirations with periods indicate audible inbreaths (e.g., .hhh). H's within (e.g., ye(hh)s) parentheses mark within-speech aspirations, possible laughter.

pt Lip Smack: Often preceding an inbreath.

hah Laugh Syllable: Relative closed or open position of laughter.
heh
hoh

29

Medication and morality

Analysis of medical visits to address chronic pain

Felicia Roberts and Jennifer S. Kramer

Introduction

Research about language and health in the context of chronic pain is international in scope (Alamo et al. 2002 (Spain); Bieber et al. 2006 (Germany); Haugli et al. 2004; Laerum et al. 2006; Eggly and Tzelpis 2001 (USA); Werner and Malterud 2004 (Norway); Kenny 2004 (Australia)), but surprisingly sparse. Considering that pain-related complaints are among the top 20 reasons for visits to the doctor (similar in frequency to well baby exams, complaints of fever, and skin rash (NAMCS 2008)) and that the medical use of opioids has increased by a factor of 10 since 1990 (Okie 2010), there is clearly a need for analysis of the language practices that constitute medical visits where pain and pain medications are discussed. Research has addressed how patients describe their pain (see Salovey et al. 1992 for a review), but the interactional dynamics of primary care encounters for pain management are as yet underspecified. In this chapter we address this gap in knowledge by focusing on the moral dimension of these visits, specifically examining stances regarding pain medication as embodied in patients' and physicians' language practices.

But why focus on the moral dimension of these interactions? We introduce here, and explain further below, two key reasons: (1) morality inheres at all levels of interaction and is therefore foundational to the study of any language event (Bergmann 1998; Linell and Rommetveit 1998), and (2) until we take seriously the study of the moral landscape in health care, as produced in participants' interactions, we will not be able to fully grasp how best to devise interventions and training for improving health communication (Maynard 2003; Churchill 1997).

To date, the focus of the research on chronic pain in medical encounters has examined decision-making styles as they relate to both patient satisfaction and health outcomes (Alamo et al. 2002; Bieber et al. 2006; Laerum et al. 2006). Using message-coding methods (Eggly and Tzelpis 2001), focus groups (Haugli et al. 2004), and interviews (Werner and Malterud 2004; Kenny 2004), this international effort has been concerned primarily with understanding the therapeutic relationship in the pain management context. However, what is left unexamined is the normative and evaluative work within these healthcare visits. Understanding this interactional work, using actual medical encounters as the empirical basis for knowledge building, is where language scholars can contribute to the development of communication strategies appropriate for pain patients. Potentially, there is room to develop more sensitive and holistic practices for assessing pain and for discussing pain management.[1]

This study, which draws on audiotaped interactions between primary care physicians and persons with chronic pain, will focus on the issue of medication use and addiction. This choice is made because of the tendency to perceive those complaining of chronic pain as potentially merely drug seeking (Elder et al. 2006) or as having underlying psychological rather than biological conditions (Chibnall et al. 1995; Holloway et al. 2007). As this analysis demonstrates, patients orient to these concerns by deflecting the 'addict' characterization, by cooperatively constructing and therefore displaying an understanding of addiction, and by representing themselves as responsible users of medication.

Morality in discourse

Two kinds of morality must first be distinguished before embarking on the current analysis. As identified by Bergmann (1998) and Linell and Rommetveit (1998), there is a 'proto' or 'elemental' morality which is present in *any* dialogic activity; it is the reciprocal ascription of responsibility for behavior in a world held in common (Bergmann 1998: 284). This proto-morality or 'discourse internal ethics' transcends cultural and historical contexts; Maynard (2003) refers to this as the *morality of discourse.*

Built upon this fundamental moral structure is the more commonly understood, second-order morality which refers to topics 'as they are coped with' in interaction and to which evaluative or normative attitudes are explicitly or implicitly addressed (Linell and Rommetveit 1998: 466). This second form, *morality in discourse* (Maynard 2003), tends to be culturally and historically specific and is the form of morality explored in this chapter. It is also the form scholars refer to when calling for better mapping of the moral landscape in medicine (Churchill 1997). However, because medical interactions are primarily service encounters (Jefferson and Lee 1981), moral issues are generally subordinate to the practical exigencies of providing healthcare services (Heritage and Lindstrom 1998). Thus, while patients may display an orientation to health behaviors such as smoking, drinking, or weight loss as morally laden (as good or bad), (Halkowski 2012; Webb 2009) medical professionals tend to treat these behaviors in a more neutral or bureaucratic manner (Linell and Rommetveit 1998: 470); for example, by refraining from commenting on patients' self-assessments (Webb 2009). Some medical domains, such as psychiatric intake interviews (Bergmann 1992) and midwifery (Linell and Bredmar 1996) are treated by both provider and patient as morally sensitive, but morality is not a topic of conversation. Thus, to get a glimpse of the moral landscape in medical interaction we attend to what is enacted through language and embodied action, through implicit or explicit claims, judgments, ascription of obligations, and so on. Attention to this more subtle interactional work can help reveal the normative and evaluative contours of the pain context.

Materials and methods

The materials for this analysis are based on close transcription and analysis of 21 audio recorded clinic visits in which chronic pain was the patient's chief concern. The visits were in the same primary care clinic and were collected over approximately four months in 2004 and 2005 (Kramer 2008). The 12 physicians included in the study were family practice specialists.

The analytic framework and technical toolkit for the analysis are grounded in conversation analysis which privileges co-participants' displayed orientations to producing and making sense of social actions through their vocal and embodied practices (Sacks et al. 1974; see also Heritage 1984; Pomerantz and Fehr 1997). This chapter presents three exemplars to support the theoretical proposition concerning the interconnectedness of language practices and moral order. The goal is not to generalize to the population of chronic pain sufferers, but to open the door to consideration of the features of the pain context that are constituted through talk-in-interaction.

Analysis

Of the 21 visits recorded, 12 involve a routine return visit of chronic pain patients. We take three of those cases to serve as exemplars of patients' orientation to medication use and addiction as moral issues. In the first case a patient works to retrospectively account for her non-prescription ibuprofen use as responsible, not addictive. In the second, a patient and physician co-construct the dangers of dependence on opiate medication. Finally, having established patients' overt orientation to the moral dimension of medication use, we turn to an extended analysis of a patient's request for the refill of opiate medications, unpacking the more subtle interactional work that constructs such a request as morally laden.

Explicit orientation to medication use as a moral issue

Two cases are presented in this section to exemplify patients' explicit orientation to the moral dimensions of medication use, even the use of non-opiates, and the ostensibly related issue of addiction.

Patient A is a 40-year-old woman who has experienced chronic back pain for 12 years. The current visit is a routine follow-up to review her pain status and medications, but she also raises a new concern: recurrent, severe headaches over the past two weeks. As part of a series of questions to diagnose possible causes of the headaches, the doctor asks the patient what alleviates the pain. The patient reports taking 'Advil' which is one of many brand names for non-prescription ibuprofen, a non-steroidal anti-inflammatory. Although the amount of ibuprofen the patient reports taking is not unusual (600 mg) she engages, nonetheless, in extended interactional work to back off of the self-disclosure as though it were an indicator of improper use. The larger than recommended dosage can indicate that she is experiencing severe pain and therefore pushing the limits of proper use, but she moves to construct a portrait of herself as someone who would not knowingly go over such a limit. The moral implication is that she is favoring rational action over pain relief, thus embodying a cultural or moral value of self-restraint.

Excerpt 1: I read the labels (Patient A; 20:00)

DR: What makes it better.
PT: Laying down. Taking, taking three- ya know I take- almost six hundred
milligrams of ibuprofen.
(0.2)
PT: An I mean I'm not takin it till where I:'m ya know addicted to it

DR: [mm
PT: [I'm spa:cing it out.
DR: mhm,
PT: Ya know cuz I know:: I read the labels °and everything° so I'm not taking it one right after the other.=
DR: =Sure.
PT: Ya know an overdosing on the advil.=
DR: =Right.
PT: Cuz I'm just not that way.
DR: mhm.

In line 2, the patient first reports 'laying down' and then taking ibuprofen, initiating a self-repair on the dosage information. She moves from the presumably less medically precise number of pills ('three') to a more technically accurate, though not entirely clear-cut measure of 'almost six hundred milligrams' (lines 2–3). Although over-the-counter ibuprofen is generally dosed in 200 mg pills, there can be some variation by brand, thus the repair on the metric (from pills to milligrams) indexes a move toward both precision and self-awareness of consumption. In contrast to research on patient alcohol reports, which finds that patients have a tendency to use 'nonstandard metrics' to resist physicians' efforts to generate specific alcohol usage rates (Halkowski 2012), this patient offers a nearly precise, and technically relevant, measure of ibuprofen usage. Since the recommended over-the-counter dosage for adults is 200–400 mg, the hedge 'almost' (line 2) on the 600 mg indicates that she is approaching a threshold of 'too much' (i.e., indexing serious pain) but, as yet, not quite over an acceptable limit.

From a structural and pragmatic standpoint, the sequence initiated by the physician's question could now accountably be complete. The information provided by the patient addresses the conditional relevance (Schegloff 1968) set up by the initial question; she has reported both laying down and taking medication to address her pain. However, exploiting the brief gap at line 4, the patient self-selects, adding additional, unsolicited information about *how* she takes the ibuprofen, treating her prior report as requiring something further.

Indeed, the ensuing talk (lines 5–7) deflects any implication about addiction or irresponsible behavior. At line 5, the 'An I mean' preface, indicates a correction on her prior talk, recasting the description ('six hundred milligrams') as in need of clarification. This seems an implicit recognition that 600 mg could be misunderstood as indicating a larger than recommended single dosage, something possibly indicative of irresponsible behavior. The utterance develops into a claim that she is not 'taking it till where [she's] addicted' (line 5), thus explicitly invoking a morally laden term and simultaneously deflecting it.

The patient's use (at line 5) of 'till where' (similar to 'almost' at line 2) implies someone on the verge of, or at the boundary of, some acceptable line between responsible and irresponsible behavior. The physician doesn't assess any of the talk so far; although there is an opportunity at the transition relevance place at the end of line 7, where the utterance is grammatically and prosodically complete (Sacks et al. 1974; Ford and Thompson 1996). Rather, at line 8, the physician passes the floor back to the patient who, perhaps in pursuit of some recognition of the appropriateness of her behavior, produces a characterization of herself as someone who regularly reads and follows label instructions (note the present tense and plural noun 'labels' at line 9).

The physician acknowledges the report with a confirming 'sure' (line 11) which could be the end of this now expanded sequence (i.e., expanded beyond the initial response to 'what makes it better'). However, at line 12, the patient moves to further deflect any implication she is improperly using 'advil' or, by extension, any other medication (line 14). In line 12, she deploys the term 'overdose' which is both technical and moral; overdosing can indicate anything from accidental to irresponsible to willfully negligent use of medication. While it can project all of those meanings, here the patient is confronting a meaning of negligence or moral weakness: she builds her utterance at line 12 as a continuation, linked through its parallel grammatical structure (present progressive) to the prior negation 'so I'm not taking it one right after the other ... and overdosing on the advil' (lines 9–12), causally connecting (with turn-initial 'cuz') that claim with the further self-characterization that she is 'just not that way'.

In sum, by invoking then deflecting any implication of addiction, the patient displays an overt orientation to use of this relatively benign, over-the-counter medication as a moral issue; moral in the sense that evaluative/normative attitudes are explicitly or implicitly addressed (Linell and Rommetveit 1998). While the doctor displays uptake of the patient's talk (lines 6, 8, 11, 13, 15), she never assesses or pursues it either positively or negatively; the interactional space is simply left open. It may well be that the physician's neutral stance is actually contributing to what we might gloss here as the patient's defensive posture. Possibly in pursuit of an assessment or some form of reassurance from the physician, the patient extends her initial report to account for her ibuprofen use as responsible.

In the next example (Excerpt 2, below) it is the physician who introduces the topic of medication ('the problem with narcotics'). He treats it in a technical manner, while the patient displays an arguably moral stance.

Patient B is a 33-year-old male who has been experiencing ongoing pain from screws in his knee which were placed there during surgery following an accident. This is a routine follow-up visit in which he reports increasing sleeplessness. The physician implicitly suggests it may be connected to increased pain, given an apparent effort to reduce the patient's opiate medication. The talk then turns to 'the problem with narcotics.'

Excerpt 2: Weaning down (Patient B; 1:55)

1 PT: It's jus gettin to the point where I hh I'm not sleepin at night, uh::m
2 (0.6) .tch (0.2) jus gettin, (0.6) it's gettin, it's gettin ba::d.
3 (2.0)
4 DR: .hh An (0.2) we've been tryin ta wea::n down the
5 narcotic[s
6 PT: [yea::[h
7 DR: [Are you noticing a difference:?
8 PT: Yeah. Pain [wise,]
9 DR: [Pain is] worse?
10 PT: Up.
11 DR: The problem ya know with narcotics are that
12 PT: They're- you can get uh:m
13 DR: You get tolerant.
14 PT: Tolerant and uhm (.) possibly addictive.
15 DR: Yeah. There's w- there's a wert- your body can become dependent on it,
16 PT: mm=
17 DR: =you can become addicted, and your body can become tolerant.
18 PT: uh huh.
19 DR: What happens with the tolerance is that your- you end with more

[receptors,
PT: [you need more. Need more [and more]
DR: [so you need] more and more narcotic ta
PT: keep goin.
DR: right.

In lines 1–2, the patient reports ongoing, worsening pain. The general framing is similar to Patient A, above, in that he also describes a situation that is approaching some invisible line of reasonable acceptance ('it's jus gettin to the point' at line 1). The deployment of the present progressive along with the physical difficulty he has in producing the utterance formulate both immediacy and discomfort.

The physician responds to this description by offering a reminder about a prior decision to 'wean down the narcotics' (lines 4–5), lexically linking back, with the conjunction 'An' (line 4), the launch of his own utterance to the patient's report of things 'getting bad'. To gloss this, the physician artfully connects the patient's discomfort with the change in opiate medication, introducing 'the problem with narcotics' (line 11) as a general informing. At line 12, the patient attempts to complete the physician's utterance, displaying an understanding of where the informing may be going.

Their collaborative interactional work embodies a shared perspective and, for the moment, the 'puzzle' introduced by the doctor (about the problem with narcotics) is effectively resolved at line 13 where the physician produces the relevant technical term ('tolerant'). However, the patient does not treat the term as sufficient. He repeats it, but extends the utterance to include 'possibly addictive' (line 14) displaying recognition that the problem can be larger than mere tolerance. It is thus the patient, as in Excerpt 1, who introduces the more socially charged term, pre-emptively addressing himself to addiction as the essential 'problem' potentially indicated initially by the physician.

Although the patient has opened the door to a discussion of addiction in the context of his particular circumstances, the physician first introduces the generalized term 'dependence' and then acknowledges the pathway through to addiction and drug tolerance (lines 15–20). The second person possessive ('your body can become dependent') is an ambiguous formulation, allowing that the patient may be included in those who are dependent/addicted, but it is the more socially neutral term 'tolerance' that is topicalized (line 19).

In overlap (line 21), the patient again moves to collaboratively contribute, not in the direction of 'more receptors' which would constitute a physiological explanation of tolerance, but in the direction of an understanding that the person who is tolerant would 'need more and more' [medication] to address his/her pain. The patient's formulation is thus focused on human behavior, and moves the conversation toward human action and away from biology. Through repetition of the patient's words, extension of the utterance to include the term 'narcotic' (line 22) and a token of receipt (line 24), the physician confirms the patient's generic characterization of patients' (not yet this particular patient's) ever increasing need for medication just to 'keep going'.

In this oblique discussion of the patient's use of opiates, we catch a glimpse of the differing stances of the participants as they construct this stretch of talk. The physician's essentially technical stance embodies an institutional responsibility to help the patient understand what might be causing his increasing discomfort, but in a non-judgmental (non-moralistic) manner. This is evidenced by his focus on 'tolerance' and the biological explanation related to receptors. The patient's stance, in contrast, tends toward the evaluative and the behavioral: first, he introduces the term 'addictive' characterizing 'the problem with narcotics' as uncontrolled or unlimited need for medication ('more and more') and concomitant dependence just to maintain life ('[to] keep goin'). These are potentially socially and culturally deviant activities that therefore pose not just a physical but also a moral challenge.

Implicit orientation to medication as moral issue

The previous examples demonstrated how patients display an explicit orientation to medication use and related addiction risks as culturally/morally suspect, presenting themselves as both responsible and aware. The final example presents a case where the interactional work is perhaps more subtle, but the moral work is similar. In this case, the patient is framing, through a series of neutral reports about his remaining medication, an implicit request for an opiate prescription refill. The physician resists the implied request, putting the patient in the position of moving toward an ever explicit formulation. The patient does so, but in a manner that simultaneously suggests the extent of his pain and his reasonable approach to the medication.

Patient C is a 40-year-old male who was surgically treated for back pain and who found out, on the same day as the visit transcribed here, he will need another surgical procedure. Just prior to the excerpt transcribed below (Excerpt 3), the patient had asked if he could get the required pre-surgery physical during the current visit, but the doctor responds she is too busy that day. Line 1 of Excerpt 3 thus refers to scheduling that pre-surgery visit. Once that business has been attended to, the main reason for the visit is raised by the patient: refilling his prescriptions for Oxycontin (the brand name for generic oxycodone, a federally controlled opiate analgesic) and Endocet (a combination of the opiate oxycodone and acetaminophen, a nonsteroidal anti-inflammatory). The patient refers to these medicines as 'oxycotten' and 'ambiset' and they are transcribed as such, below. The patient also refers to 'breakthrough pain' which is the medical term for pain that occurs between scheduled administrations of analgesics and which is handled by other medications, in this case with Endocet.

Excerpt 3: Request for oxycontin & endocet refills (Patient C; 1:25)

PT: So you'll just hafta:: schedule me,
DR: Okay.
PT: For that=But^h [basically I'm I'm- (0.6) I'm outta
DR: [(wha-)
PT: the oxycottens that ya gave me,
DR: Okay.
PT: But I still have like thirty of the ambiset?
(0.6)
DR: [°mmm°]
PT: [And uh-] the surgery's gonna be au:gust fifth,
DR: [mkay.
PT: [So what is it uh :: (.) so: actually the thirty day period (.) I won't
see ya next month. Because #I'll be havin surgery I'll be in the
hospital.#
DR: You mean you're not gonna: s[neak $aw]ay and come see me?$
PT: [°°hh°°]
PT: heh heh.=
DR: =$Just kidding.$=

PT: =Yeah maybe in a wheelchair. [Ha ha ha ha ha ha .hh]
DR: [Okay. (0.2) Alright.]
PT: .hh Uhm ((clears throat)) So I guess I just (1.0) you know basically
need (.) some more oxycotten, and maybe[thirty]
DR: [m h m]
PT: ambiset because I [probably] got (0.4) fifteen to twenty of the
DR: [mhm::]
PT: ambisets left out of the sixty you gave me.
DR: Mhm.
PT: .hh And I been (0.2) pretty much eatin a lotta them for breakthrough
pain. ya know.
DR: [Hm
PT: [Stickin to the (.) ya know stickin to the thirty, (1.0) uh milligrams
a oxycotten?
DR: [Mhm.
PT: [Ya know up in the mornin and at night. But eatin a lotta the ambiset
for breakthrough pain.
DR: Mh[m
PT: [ya know. So.
DR: Okay. How's <u>is</u> your p[ain?
PT: [And ahhhh Bad. hhhh
DR: How is it compared to last time I saw you?
PT: Ehh bout the same.= I'm (.) bout a nine.

In lines 3–5, the patient completes his utterance about scheduling the physical and then rushes through the transition space (Schegloff 1987) to produce a report that he is out of oxycontin. At this point in the sequence, the launch of the utterance with the contrastive conjunction 'but' is hearable as transitional to a now official 'first topic' of this service encounter (Robinson 2006; Schegloff and Sacks 1973; Zimmerman 1992). Note, however, that the utterance is simply a report, not a grammatically formulated request for a medication refill. In everyday settings the report/description format serves (at least) two functions simultaneously: (1) as a vehicle for an implicit request (Drew 1984; Schegloff 1988, 1995), and (2) as a means to avoid an official stance on some matter at hand (e.g., see Drew 1984 on the use of reports for rejecting invitations). This same potentiality provides a resource in medical settings for patients to make requests without actually asking (Gill et al. 2001; Robinson 2001). In the current instance, however, the physician never engages with the patient's report as a request; she co-constructs this as the patient's multi-unit turn in progress, providing tokens of uptake or continuers (lines 6, 9, 11), but never actually addressing the implicit request.

The moral work getting done to this point can be analyzed from several vantage points. Through this series of reports, the patient avoids 'intruding on the doctor's medical judgment' (Robinson 2001: 33), simultaneously indexing the delicacy of the implicit request for opiates and the delicacy of making a request of one's physician. Further, by not setting up conditional relevance of a response (i.e., a request has not actually been articulated) the patient leaves open the possibility of refusal. Thus, in terms of rights, responsibilities, normative and evaluative attitudes (i.e., *morality in discourse*), the talk so far embodies the patient's orientation to the issue of the medication refill as (a) potentially problematic, (b) potentially indelicate, and, therefore, (c) potentially refusable.

For her part, the physician is not making it obvious that she is sympathetic to the implication of the patient's reports. While his description of using up the medication might be an indication of the patient's pain level, the physician does not assess or seek clarification in that direction (see Robinson 2001 for a contrasting case). Indeed, her resistance to the patient's request becomes more salient as the interaction continues. The patient offers new information: because of the surgery date, he will miss his next opportunity to get his prescription refilled ('won't see ya next month' lines 12–14). Here the physician accountably avoids the implication by simply fitting her response to the surface content of the utterance: she makes light of it through a non-serious, arguably ironic or even flirtatious question (line 15, 'You mean you're not gonna sneak away and come see me?'). The patient laughs briefly (line 17), but the apparent failure of the doctor's joke (as evidenced by the physician's recourse to the explanation 'just kidding' at line 18) is underscored by the patient's troubles-resistant laughter (Jefferson 1985; Glenn 2003) at line 19.

Exiting this joking episode in a distinctly non-jocular tone, the patient now expresses an explicit and specific 'need' for more medication (lines 21–26), which he accounts for by his (revised) estimate of the number of Endocet he has remaining. Interestingly, the number of pills he now claims to have (15 to 20) is actually far less than the 30 he originally mentioned (line 7). If the physician is listening carefully, this could cast aspersions on the patient's reliability; however, the fact that he describes himself as 'eatin a lotta them' (line 28) for breakthrough pain could also account for any impression of imprecision: the formulation indexes breakthrough pain that is frequent and serious enough that he may not actually have a concrete idea of how many pills remain. Whether the patient knows or not, whether the physician is listening carefully or not, neither of these questions can be answered here. What is clear, however, is that the smaller amount of remaining medication can work to upgrade the urgency of the need for the refill.

Paradoxically, such unobserved and possibly uncontrolled use could be construed as irresponsible; however, to briefly characterize what ensues, the patient then presents a more clinical description of the oxycodone use: taking them twice a day as directed at the dosage directed (lines 31–34). Thus, the patient's re-mention of 'eatin a lotta the ambiset' (line 34) is now in a context of responsible (i.e., prescribed) oxycodone use. The implication to be drawn is that the underlying pain is severe enough for him that the oxycodone is not sufficiently handling it, since he often resorts to breakthrough medications.

The moral landscape is thus similar to the previous cases: patients are managing responsibly in the face of pain, but they present themselves as being at the brink. The fact that they are at the doctor's office is evidence of rationality in that they are 'appropriately' (morally, correctly) seeking medical intervention (see Halkowski 2006 on 'the patient's problem'), but the interventions they seek are potentially suspect. Thus, these patients embody, through talk-in-interaction, an awareness of the social and cultural values that inhere in the practice of using pain medications, even when those substances are medically indicated.

Future directions

Understanding the moral dimension of medical encounters in the chronic pain context provides a basis for connecting micro-linguistic practices with public health issues. This study is among projects aiming toward such trans-disciplinary knowledge, as described in Kreps and Maibach (2008), and effectively realized in applied conversation analytic research (e.g., Heritage et al. 2010; Mangione-Smith et al. 2006; Stivers 2007). Studying the language practices that lead to prescription of pain medication is admittedly only one piece of a highly complex public health puzzle concerning over-prescription and diversion of opiates (Okie 2010), but since there is so little empirical research based on actual interactions in the pain context, the field is wide open for investigation, innovation, and theorizing. Indeed, pain education is generally lacking in medical curricula (Lippe et al. 2010); for example, only five of the 133 medical schools in the United States require courses on pain (Committee on Advancing Pain Research 2011: 366). The time is ripe, therefore, for studies of the pain context which take into account participant orientations as expressed through language and embodied action. This kind of research will afford scholars foundational material for developing empirically grounded and interactionally relevant training and education programs.

Three observations made in this chapter could be pursued. First, there may be a contrast in orientation toward pain medication use and alcohol consumption, and specifically how we talk about those substances with physicians. It seems that precision about medication use is favored, in contrast to patients' resistance to precision in the alcohol reporting context (Halkowski 2012). A second and related observation is the possibility of a preference by patients to display stoicism by reporting attempts to manage pain with physical interventions before reporting use of medication (e.g., Patient A). And third, that pain patients present themselves as managing in the face of their difficulties, but just barely. These last two observations point to tensions in the health context that could be further examined in light of Halkowski (2006) and the concept of 'the patient's problem' or the fine line between involvement and detachment. Importantly, researchers might explore patient–physician communication in the realm of cancer pain, where patients clearly have etiology, yet may still struggle with receiving sufficient pain medication (NIH 1997), even within the hospice setting (Kimberlin et al. 2004). Likewise, it would be enlightening to explore the context of complementary/alternative medicine, as there is currently no research that examines interactions between chronic pain patients and their complementary or alternative care providers.[2]

Summary

This chapter started with the premise that morality inheres at all levels of discourse and is therefore a relevant target for linguistic analysis. In the health context, only a few studies have developed this approach; thus, the current analysis attempted to fill that gap by sketching how patients treat the issue of addiction and their own medication use as morally laden. We found that they did this by explicitly raising and deflecting these related concerns or by collaboratively constructing, and thereby displaying, their understanding of the issues. The work patients do through language reveals they are alert to the moral implications of medicine as palliative: all three patients project restraint, awareness, and responsibility, indicating they view these moral qualities as relevant dimensions to be addressed. In other words, patients reveal through the content of what they say, when and how they say it, and by the collaborative interactional activities they engage in with physicians that moral character is at stake and must be defended.

We have also seen that, in line with prior research, physicians tend to take a bureaucratic or neutral stance within these pain-related interactions, treating these encounters as having no particular moral content. Interestingly, it is the patients themselves that display sensitivity, through their own language behavior, to the issue of addiction. Although the physician in Excerpt 3 does take a more resistant stance to the patient's implicit request, potentially treating it as inapposite, that implication recedes under cover of favoring scientific (chart-relevant) measures of the pain experience. Admittedly, these initial findings require further elaboration, confirmation, and refutation as we continue to refine our understanding of this important domain in personal and public health.

Related topics

Pain medication; morality in discourse; addiction; physician–patient interaction; prescribing.

Notes

1 The Joint Commission on Accreditation of Healthcare Organizations (JCAHO) requires its accredited organizations to include pain as a vital sign to be collected from all patients on initial intake (Rosenfeld 2003). However, there is no systematic means to assess pain (Lippe et al. 2010); many organizations, including the US Veterans Affairs, simply use a 0 to 10 scale for patient pain severity self-report (Mularski et al. 2006).

2 However, one study comparing physicians and chiropractors generally found that patients suffering from low back pain who saw chiropractors were more 'satisfied' than those who saw physicians (Hertzman-Miller et al. 2002). The higher satisfaction ratings were based on communication factors such as information giving and advice.

Further reading

Drew, P. and Wootton, T. (eds) 1988, *Erving Goffman: Exploring the Interaction Order*, Cambridge: Polity Press. (A collection of essays that contemplate and critique Goffman's concept of the interaction order, examining morality among other key constructs.)

Hilbert, R.A. (1984) 'The acultural dimensions of chronic pain: flawed reality construction and the problem of meaning', *Social Problems,* 31(4): 365–378. (This is foundational for understanding how language and culture prohibit pain sufferers from relating their subjective experience.)

Shorter, E. (1997) 'Somatization and chronic pain in historic perspective', *Clinical Orthopaedics and Related Research*, 336: 52–60. (This is a comprehensive overview by a prominent historian of medicine about the emergence of chronic pain as a cultural phenomenon.)

References

Alamo, M.M., Moral, R.R., and de Torees, L.A.P. (2002) 'Evaluation of a patient centered approach in generalized musculoskeletal chronic pain/fibromyalgia patients in primary care', *Patient Education and Counseling,* 48: 22–31.

Bergmann, J.R. (1992) 'Veiled morality: notes on discretion in psychiatry', in P. Drew and J. Heritage (eds) *Talk at Work: Interaction in Institutional Settings,* Cambridge: Cambridge University Press.

Bergmann, J. (1998) 'Introduction: morality in discourse', *Research on Language and Social Interaction,* 31: 279–294.

Bieber, C., Müller, K.G., Blumenstiel, K., Schneider, A., Richter, A., Wilke, S., et al. (2006) 'Long-term effects of shared decision-making intervention on physician–patient interaction and outcome in fibromyalgia: a qualitative and quantitative 1 year follow-up of a randomized control trial', *Patient Education and Counseling,* 63: 357–366.

Chibnall, J.T., Duckro, P.N., and Richardson, W.D. (1995) 'Physician frustration with chronic pain patients can and should be avoided', *Headache Quarterly,* 6: 123–125.

Churchill, L.R. (1997) 'Bioethics in a social context', in R.A. Carson and C.R. Burns (eds) *Philosophy of Medicine and Bioethics: A Twenty-year Retrospective and Critical Appraisal,* Dordrecht, the Netherlands: Kluwer Academic Publishers.

Committee on Advancing Pain Research, Care, and Education, Board of Health Sciences Policies, and Institute of Medicine (2011) 'A call for cultural transformation of attitudes toward pain and its prevention and management', *Journal of Pain & Palliative Care Pharmacotherapy*, 25: 385–369.

Drew, P. (1984) 'Speakers' reportings in invitation sequences', in J.M. Atkinson and J. Heritage (eds) *Structures of Social Action: Studies in Conversation Analysis*, Cambridge: Cambridge University Press.

Eggly, S. and Tzelpis, A. (2001) 'Relational control in difficult physician–patient encounters: negotiating treatment for pain', *Journal of Health Communication*, 6: 323–333.

Elder, N., Ricer, R., and Tobias, B. (2006) 'How respected family physicians manage difficult patient encounters', *Journal of the American Board of Family Practice*, 19: 533–541.

Ford, C. and Thompson, S. (1996) 'Interactional units in conversation: syntactic, intonational and pragmatic resources for the management of turns', in E. Ochs, E.A. Schegloff, and S. Thompson (eds) *Interaction and Grammar*, Cambridge: Cambridge University Press.

Gill, V.T., Halkowski, T., and Roberts, F. (2001) 'Accomplishing a request without making one: a single case analysis of a primary care visit', *Text*, 21: 55–81.

Glenn, P.J. (2003) *Laughter in Interaction*, Cambridge: Cambridge University Press.

Halkowski, T. (2006) 'Realizing the illness: patients' narratives of symptom discovery', in J. Heritage and D. Maynard (eds) *Communication in Medical Care: Interaction between Primary Care Physicians and Patients*, Cambridge: Cambridge University Press.

——(2012) '"Occasional" drinking: some uses of a nonstandard temporal metric in primary care assessment of alcohol use', in W.A. Beach (ed.) *Handbook of Patient–Provider Interactions: Raising and Responding to Concerns about Life, Illness, and Disease*, Cresskill, NJ: Hampton Press.

Haugli, L., Strand, E., and Finset, A. (2004) 'How do patients with rheumatic disease experience their relationship with their doctors? A qualitative study of experiences of stress and support in the doctor–patient relationship', *Patient Education & Counseling*, 52: 169–174.

Heritage, J. (1984) *Garfinkel and Ethnomethodology*, Cambridge: Blackwell.

Heritage, J. and Lindstrom, A. (1998) 'Motherhood, medicine, and morality: scenes from a medical encounter', *Research on Language and Social Interaction*, 31: 397–438.

Heritage, J., Elliott, M.N., Stivers, T., Richardson, A., and Mangione-Smith, R. (2010) 'Reducing inappropriate antibiotics prescribing: the role of online commentary on physical examination findings', *Patient Education and Counseling*, 81: 119–125.

Hertzman-Miller, R.P., Morgenstern, H., Hurwitz, E.L., Yu, F., Adams, A.H., Harber, P., and Kominski, G.F. (2002) 'Comparing the satisfaction of low back patients randomized to receive medical or chiropractic care: results from the UCLA low-back pain study', *American Journal of Public Health*, 92: 1628–1633.

Holloway, I., Sofaer-Bennett, B., and Walker, J. (2007) 'The stigmatization of people with chronic back pain', *Disability and Rehabilitation*, 29: 1456–1464.

Jefferson, G. (1985) 'On the organization of laughter in talk about troubles' in J.M. Atkinson (ed.) *Structures in Social Action*, Cambridge: Cambridge University Press.

Jefferson, G. and Lee, J.R.E. (1981) 'The rejection of advice: managing the problematic convergence of a "troubles teller" and a "service encounter"', *Journal of Pragmatics*, 5: 399–422.

Kenny, D.T. (2004) 'Constructions of chronic pain in doctor–patient relationship: bridging the communication chasm', *Patient Education and Counseling*, 52: 297–305.

Kimberlin, C., Brushwood, D., Allen, W., Radson, E., and Wilson, D., (2004) 'Cancer patient and caregiver experiences: communication and pain management issues', *Journal of Pain and Symptom Management*, 28: 566–578.

Kramer, J.S. (2008) 'Analyzing physician/patient chronic pain communication through primary goals, secondary goals, stages of change and processes of change', unpublished dissertation, Purdue University, Indiana.

Kreps, G.L. and Maibach, E.W. (2008) 'Transdisciplinary science: the nexus between communication and public health', *Journal of Communication*, 58: 732–748.

Laerum, E., Indahl, A., and Skouen, J.S. (2006) 'What is "the good back consultation"? A combined qualitative and quantitative study of chronic low back pain patients' interaction with and perceptions of consultations with specialists', *Journal of Rehabilitative Medicine*, 38: 255–262.

Linell, P. and Bredmar, M. (1996) 'Reconstructing topical sensitivity: aspects of face-work in talks between midwives and expectant mothers', *Research on Language and Social Interaction*, 29: 347–379.

Linell, P. and Rommetveit, R. (1998) 'The many forms and facets of morality in dialogue: epilogue for the special issue', *Research on Language and Social Interaction*, 31: 465–473.

Lippe, P.M., Brock, J.D., Crossno, R., and Gitlow, S. (2010) 'The first national pain medicine summit: final summary report', *Pain Medicine*, 11: 1447–1468.

Mangione-Smith, R., Elliott, M.N., Stivers, T., McDonald, L.L., and Heritage, J. (2006) 'Ruling out the need for antibiotics: are we sending the right message?', *Archives of Pediatrics and Adolescent Medicine*, 160: 945–952.

Maynard, D.W. (2003) *Bad News, Good News: Conversational Order in Everyday Talk and Clinical Settings*, Chicago, IL: University of Chicago Press.

Mularski, R.A., White-Chu, F., Overbay, D., Miller, L., Asch, S.M., and Ganzini, L. (2006) 'Measuring pain as the 5th vital sign does not improve quality of pain management', *Journal of General Internal Medicine*, 21: 607–612.

NAMCS (2008) *National Ambulatory Medical Care Survey: 2008 summary tables (p. 9, Table 9)*, Bethesda, MD: National Centers for Health Statistics. Online. Available HTTP: <http://www.cdc.gov/nchs/fastats/docvisit.htm> (accessed 3 May 2012).

NIH (1997) 'Symptoms in terminal illness: a research workshop', Rockville, MD: National Institutes of Health.

Okie, S. (2010) 'A flood of opiods, a rising tide of deaths', *New England Journal of Medicine*, 363: 1981–1985.

Pomerantz, A. and Fehr, B.J. (1997) 'Conversation analysis: an approach to the study of social action as sense making practices', in T.A. van Dijk (ed.) *Discourse as Social Interaction*, London: Sage.

Robinson, J.D. (2001) 'Asymmetry in action: sequential resources in the negotiation of a prescription request', *Text*, 21:19–54.

——(2006) 'Soliciting patients' presenting concerns', in J. Heritage and D. Maynard (eds) *Communication in Medical Care: Interaction between Primary Care Physicians and Patients*, Cambridge: Cambridge University Press.

Rosenfeld, A. (2003) *The Truth about Chronic Pain: Patients and Professionals on How to Face It, Understand It, Overcome It*, New York: Basic Books.

Sacks, H., Schegloff, E.A., and Jefferson, G. (1974) 'A simplest systematic for the organization of turn-taking for conversation', *Language*, 50: 696–735.

Salovey, P., Seiber, W.J., Smith, A.F., Turk, D.C., Jobe, J.B., and Willis, G.B. (1992) 'Reporting chronic pain episodes on health surveys', *Vital and Health Statistics*, 6: 1–71.

Schegloff, E.A. (1968) 'Sequencing in conversational opening', *American Anthropologist*, 70: 1075–1095.

——(1987) 'Recycled turn beginnings: a precise repair mechanism in conversation's turn-taking organization', in G. Button and J.R.E. Lee (eds) *Talk and Social Organization*, Clevedon, UK: Multilingual Matters.

——(1988) 'Goffman and the analysis of conversation', in P. Drew and A. Wooten (eds) *Erving Goffmann: Exploring the Interaction Order*, Cambridge: Polity Press.

——(1995) 'Discourse as an interactional achievement III: the omnirelevance of action', *Research on Language and Social Interaction*, 28: 185–211.

Schegloff, E.A. and Sacks, H. (1973) 'Opening up closing', *Semiotica*, 7: 289–327.

Stivers, T. (2007) *Prescribing Under Pressure: Parent–Physician Conversations and Antibiotics*, New York: Oxford University Press.

Webb, H. (2009) '"I've put weight on cos I've bin inactive, cos I've ad me knee done": moral work in the obesity clinic', *Sociology of Health & Illness*, 31: 854–871.

Werner, A. and Malterud, K. (2004), 'It is hard work behaving like a credible patient: encounters between women with chronic pain and their doctors', *Social Science & Medicine*, 57: 1409–1419.

Zimmerman, D.H. (1992) 'The interactional organization of calls for emergency assistance', in P. Drew and J. Heritage (eds) *Talk at Work: Interaction in Institutional Settings*, Cambridge: Cambridge University Press.

30

The role of the electronic patient record in the clinical consultation

Deborah Swinglehurst and Celia Roberts

Introduction

One of the most significant recent influences on the clinical consultation in UK general practice is the almost universal adoption of electronic patient records (EPRs) in place of paper medical records. Although often taken for granted by clinicians, managers, administrators, and patients, there is limited understanding of how, and to what extent, EPRs shape communication and care processes. The EPR places new demands on the clinician and presents fresh challenges to the researcher of interaction.

Good communication skills are regarded as a core defining feature of the profession of general practice. Assessment of these skills forms a key component of licensing examinations required for entry into UK general practice, but the EPR is absent from these examinations and the consultation continues to be conceptualized as a communication dyad occurring between clinician and patient. In general, professional training aspires to equip the clinician with predefined skills and focuses on the evaluation of task-oriented doctor behaviours with minimal attention to the unfolding consultation as a *co-constructed* interaction. The EPR tends to be regarded as little more than a neutral 'data container', somewhat irrelevant to the ongoing process of talk and meaning-making. In this chapter we will show that this may be an important misconception.

We will begin by describing the historical context in which the widespread use of the EPR has emerged. We will then review some of the literature reporting on the role of the computer in the consultation. Against this backdrop we will introduce a novel methodological approach to examining the 'EPR-in-use', an orientation which embraces the complexities of the EPR in its social context. This approach brings together discourse analysis – a 'micro' analysis of the unfolding interaction – and attention to the wider ethnographic context (Swinglehurst et al. 2011; Greenhalgh and Swinglehurst 2011). This dual orientation is important, since the influence of the EPR extends both within and beyond the consultation. Drawing on the work of Goffman and Bakhtin we suggest that the EPR can be usefully conceptualized as a collection of voices which are multilayered. Conceptualizing the EPR in this way sensitizes us to the many semiotic planes to which clinicians orient as they incorporate new technologies such as the EPR.

Using a short data extract which illustrates our approach to transcription and analysis, we will demonstrate that the EPR contributes in profound ways to shaping how the interaction unfolds. Our research leads us to conclude that far from being a simple data-container, or a peripheral 'add-on' to the clinical consultation, the EPR is integral to the contemporary consultation and deserves greater prominence in the analysis of healthcare interactions.

Historical perspectives on the computer in the consulting room

The EPR has not evolved in a vacuum but from previous iterations of paper medical records and in response to wider social influences, which we will mention briefly here. The broad structure of modern-day electronic clinical systems can be traced to Weed's proposals for *problem-oriented medical records* (POMRs) which have informed record-keeping practices since the 1960s (Weed 1968). Computers started to appear in consulting rooms in the 1980s and 1990s, but were initially used primarily for appointment scheduling and prescribing. More recently, in response to wider socio-political pressure for technological development, it has become the norm for record keeping to be done electronically.

In 2000, the UK government removed the legal obligation for paper record systems – and with it the requirement for dual recording which had thwarted general practitioners' (GPs') early aspirations for 'paperless' practice. This was soon followed by the establishment of the National Programme for Information Technology (NPfIT), encompassing a vision for a fully networked electronic record, accessible from all points of care. Although this programme folded in 2010, the political zeal for data capture at the point of care remains strong, with an emphasis on the need for increasingly structured electronic records (Department of Health 2010).

Another important development in the UK context was the introduction of a new GP contract in 2004, incorporating the 'Quality and Outcomes Framework' (QOF) – an incentive scheme which rewards GPs financially for demonstrating performance against pre-specified clinical and organizational indicators (General Practitioners Committee 2009). Crucially, this depends on gathering data for institutional audit. The emergence of QOF, alongside the rise of evidence-based medicine (EBM), and an increasing emphasis on accountability in the public sector contribute to what Foucault (1970) would refer to as the *conditions of possibility* for the almost universal uptake of the EPR in recent years.

Previous research on the computer in the consultation

Most previous studies of healthcare interaction either ignore the EPR or 'contain' it by focusing on the computer rather than on the EPR in its full complexity. The EPR has both a *material* dimension (e.g., the screen, keyboard, mouse – what most people would call the 'computer') and a *textual* dimension (medical information, prompts, alerts, and structured fields for completion as displayed in the EPR). We believe that our research is unique in the extent to which it engages with both of these (interrelated) dimensions. By grappling with this complexity we can gain new insights into *what is actually going on* in the consultation, and how this relates to the wider institutional context.

Much of the existing research sits within the tradition of medical informatics and assumes a positivist ontological stance towards computers and technologies (asking questions such as *What is the effect of technology A on health outcome B?*). Even within communications research this positivist orientation is common, researchers seeking out the 'impact' of the computer as if it is quite separate from the communication. The computer is often assumed to be the *cause* of various communication problems, and yet the solutions proposed invariably (and rather confusingly) lie with the *doctor*. For example, a recent review of such studies concludes that the computer has a:

> positive impact on information exchange, but exerts a negative influence on patient centredness ... The negative impact on communication can be partially overcome by spatial organization of the doctor's office and by physician computer skills and behavioural style.
>
> *(Shachak and Reis 2009)*

Early studies suggested that doctors spend a significant amount of time gazing at the computer (Margalit et al. 2006; Warshawsky et al. 1994; Herzmark et al. 1984). Als described the computer as a 'veracious character' or 'magic box' – something to which the doctor might nod or point whilst presenting facts derived not from the computer itself, but from the doctor's own abstractions (Als 1997). She suggested that patients synchronized their talk with pauses in the GP's computer work. The nature of this synchrony was a particular interest of Greatbatch et al., who made an important contribution to the field in the 1990s, when computer use was gathering momentum (Greatbatch et al. 1995; Greatbatch et al. 1993; Greatbatch 1992).

Greatbatch analyzed video recordings of doctor–patient consultations occurring in a practice before and after the introduction of computers for prescribing. His ground-breaking work highlighted the interaction of clinician, patient, and computer as a collaborative one, in which computer use and communicative conduct are coordinated and shaped by reference to each other (Greatbatch et al. 1995; Greatbatch et al. 1993; Luff et al. 1992; Greatbatch 1992). He found that the initiation and extension of patients' unsolicited turns at talk (i.e., those utterances that were not solicited by the doctor) were recurrently synchronized with the doctor's computer use (Greatbatch et al. 1993; Greatbatch 1992). The findings suggested that patients monitor doctors' bodily conduct, to identify upcoming boundaries in keyboard use, hence avoiding interrupting an activity in progress. Furthermore, patients are able to anticipate these boundaries *in advance of their occurrence*. His identification of computer use as embedded within work practices and interactions as a collaborative activity (rather than a single-user activity) is especially important. He suggested that the more a doctor 'backgrounded' computer use, the less the patient was constrained by it in his own interactional moves (Greatbatch et al. 1995). However, recent commentators argue that now the EPR is used exclusively, it may require a level of attention that is impossible to 'background' (Booth et al. 2004).

Increasingly, research interest is focusing on the computer as a 'third party' in what is called the 'triadic' consultation (Pearce et al. 2009; Pearce 2007; Booth et al. 2002; Scott and Purves 1996). For example, Scott and Purves described a 'three way interactive DCP model' with each 'component' (Doctor, Computer, Patient) regarded as having an effect on relationships between the other two and arguing that it is insufficient to analyse the consultation without attending to the third ubiquitous component (Scott and Purves 1996). Others have drawn attention to the 'intrusive' nature of the computer (Booth et al. 2004; Sullivan 1995). Booth et al. developed a classification system based on different doctor behaviours at 'moments of transition', when doctors' attention switched between patient and screen (Booth et al. 2002). Others have attempted to consider the relationship between doctors' consulting styles and their EPR use, with Frankel suggesting that clinicians' baseline communication skills are carried forward *and amplified* with a computer record (Ventres et al. 2006; Ventres et al. 2005; Frankel et al. 2005).

In a recent study, Pearce sought to describe the nature of relationships within the triadic consultation (which he calls the 'new' consultation) using tagging software to facilitate analysis of videos of 141 consultations (Pearce et al. 2009; Pearce et al. 2008; Pearce 2007). Critical of previous work for being primarily doctor-centric and for continuing to frame a triadic relationship as a series of dyadic relationships, he brought Goffman's dramaturgical theories to his analysis (Goffman 1974), considering the consultation as a 'play' and regarding the computer as a non-human actant. He described the openings of consultations as doctor-openings, patient-openings, or computer-openings and identified the computer as exhibiting agency within a three-way relationship in which information, power, and authority shifted in 'ever-revolving circles' between the three actants (Pearce et al. 2008; Pearce 2007).

Notwithstanding these recent re-framings of the consultation as 'triadic', most research on the computer in the consultation pre-dates the almost universal uptake of EPRs. It establishes that the computer has a significant influence within the consultation, but leaves open the question of what is *actually being accomplished* as clinicians interact with the computer, and what this might *mean* for patients. A striking observation is the focus of most interactional research on the 'computer' and not, in fact, on the EPR. The computer remains something of a 'black box'. The consultation also tends to be studied in isolation with little attempt to situate it within a wider social, organizational, or institutional context. In the remainder of this chapter we will describe a novel approach which seeks to overcome these objections and which embraces the complexity of actual social practices. This offers a new way of looking at and reflecting upon professional practice with potential to bring new understandings of what the EPR *is* and what is being accomplished through its integration in primary care.

The potential of novel methodologies to extend our understanding of the EPR

Technological advances not only influence record keeping practices but also change what is possible for the researcher of interaction. Our work has involved ethnographic observation in two GP practices over an eight-month period, in both clinical and non-clinical spaces. This included video-recording consultations with parallel screen capture of what we have called the 'EPR-in-use' – namely the dynamic display on the computer monitor of the patient's electronic record as the consultation progresses.

The ethnographic work served the practical purpose of getting to know participants and familiarization with practice procedures. It was also an opportunity to experience what Gumperz calls the 'communicative ecology' of the practices – an understanding of communicative practices and wider organizational discourses within which particular interactions are situated – for example, what gets talked about, by whom, and in what ways (Gumperz 1999). It also helped us to understand the tools and technologies that people use; the occasions for using them; the jargon that is routinely exchanged between practice members; the documents and artefacts that are written and referred to in day-to-day work. These are all aspects that Heath identifies as crucial to understanding complex organizational environments (Heath and Hindmarsh 2002). They are particularly important to an understanding of the EPR, since the EPR is not constrained by the spatial boundaries of the consulting room, but has what Iedema calls a wide 'organizational reach' (Iedema 2003). It is difficult to appreciate the influence of the EPR in the interaction without at least some appreciation of this wider organizational landscape.

We collected consultation data from 54 consultations, including 19 clinicians (doctors and nurses) across the two research sites. A digital camcorder (Sony Handycam DCR-SR72) with wide angle lens and remote control was used alongside a commercially available screen capture tool, generating two separate video files which were synchronized and merged using video editing software (Adobe® Premiere® Elements 4) (see Figure 30.1).

Our work is a contribution to an emerging field called linguistic ethnography (Rampton et al. 2004). Linguistic ethnography has evolved from an appreciation of both the strengths and pitfalls of different ways of studying language and communication in the social sciences. For example, micro-analytic approaches such as conversation analysis pay detailed attention to the interaction as emerging context but with little regard to the wider socio-political context. Approaches such as critical discourse analysis focus on the wider socio-political context but pay limited attention to the detail of local interaction and the meanings that emerge for participants. Linguistic ethnographers investigate both the detail of interactions as they occur and the wider social, historical, and political context within which social interaction occurs. The implicit assumption is that whilst each consultation is unique, it is nevertheless shaped by the constraints and opportunities that the wider institutional context presents. This is pertinent to a study of the EPR, not only because of the distributed nature of the EPR, but also because of the way in which the EPR comes to constitute this context. We will discuss this further in our data analysis.

A linguistic ethnographic approach offers an orientation to data gathering and analysis which is explicitly social constructionist in perspective. That is, it assumes that reality is socially constructed, and that language does not just *reflect* or express intentions or decisions (the representational role of language) but it *makes* them (the constitutive role of language) (Roberts and Sarangi 2005). It also assumes that persons, encounters, and institutions are profoundly interlinked and that the linkages between these are worthy of study. What it does not provide is a set of clearly defined methods for analysis, rather a range of 'sensitizing concepts' (Blumer 1969: 148).

Methodology: our approach to transcription and analysis

DS familiarized herself with the dataset through repeated viewings of the video data. Twelve consultations were selected for full transcription, using Jefferson conventions for the spoken

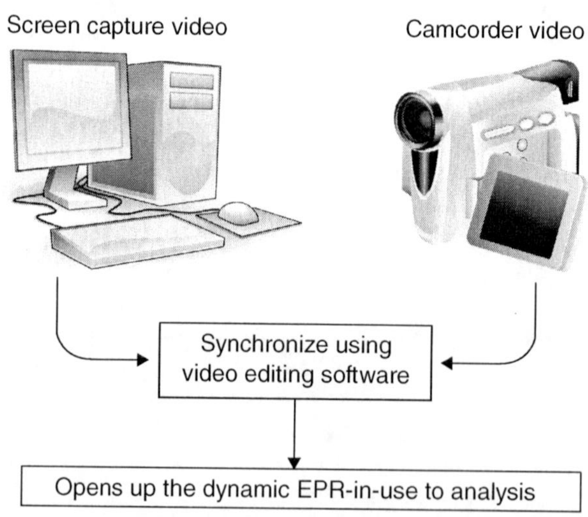

Figure 30.1 Capturing video of the EPR and the interpersonal interaction

word (Atkinson and Heritage 1984) (see Appendix 30.1 at the end of this chapter) to which we added the use of a horizontal arrow (→ or ↔) to indicate direction of gaze between clinician/patient/EPR screen. Table 30.1 shows an extract of data from one consultation. We adapted an approach suggested by Jewitt for transcription of multimodal data, with different modes presented in adjacent columns, and time as an anchor (Jewitt 2006) (see Table 30.1).

We mapped consultations, adding two columns ('material' and 'textual') for observations, analytic notes, and reflections. This approach kept us alert to the relationship between computer and EPR and to the interrelationship between different modalities. We identified what have been called *focal* and *analytic* themes (Roberts and Sarangi 2005), linking analytic themes from linguistics and sociology to focal themes relevant to professional concerns. For example, analytic themes included 'face-work' (Goffman 1967; Goffman 1955) and changes in 'footing' (Goffman 1981). Focal themes included the extent to which the EPR is shared, notions of asymmetry in the consultation, and agenda setting (e.g., how and to what extent the EPR opens up certain agendas and closes down others). This cyclical approach (see Figure 30.2) contributed to a growing understanding of the role of the EPR, and to a parallel evolution of a conceptual framework for analysis of the consultation.

Developing a conceptual framework for analysing the triadic consultation

We do not intend to describe our conceptual framework in detail here, but will outline some of the principles informing its development and highlight two particularly useful analytic concepts. This is a novel area of study and we did not set out with a set of specific (and potentially limiting) analytic questions in mind. Our conceptual framework evolved through

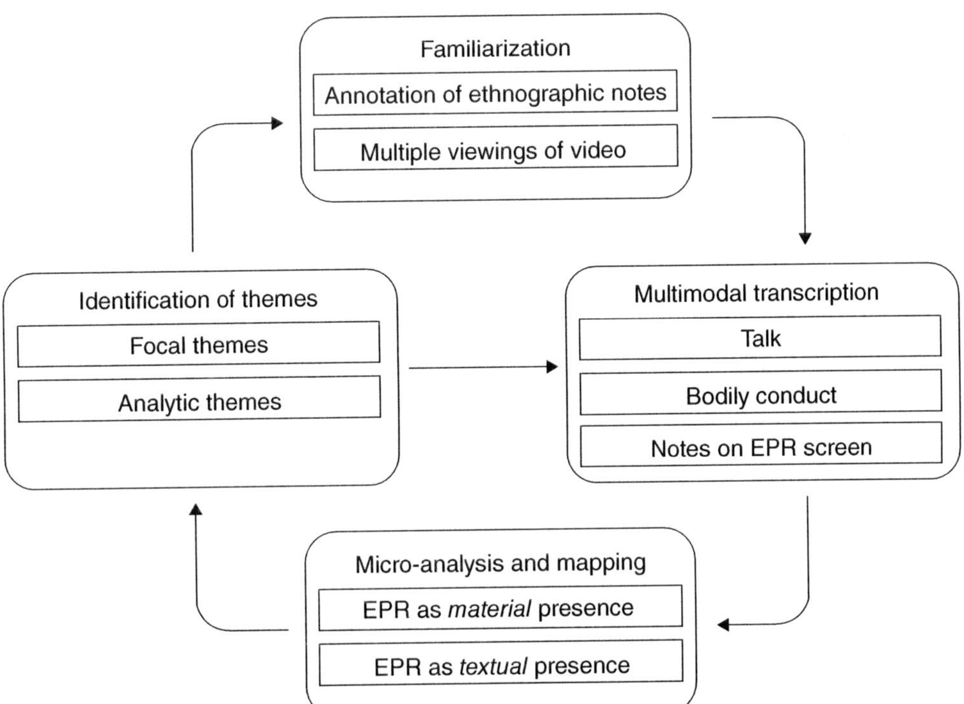

Figure 30.2 Approach to transcription and analysis

repeated viewing of video data, and a combination of fine-grained micro-analysis of evolving interactions with broader analysis of ethnographic field notes as described above. This allowed us to shift constantly between what Erickson has called the 'social microscope' and the 'social telescope' (Erickson 2004: 16), drawing on an eclectic range of discourse analysis approaches. This eclectic approach is not unusual in discourse analysis and allows some flexibility; different analytical tools may be used to a greater or lesser extent at different stages in the analysis.

We found the work of Goffman and Bakhtin very valuable in the analysis of the triadic consultation. Two concepts that formed part of the overall analytic framework were 'engagement/involvement' (Goffman 1966b) and the 'dialogic voice' (Bakhtin 1981b; Vološinov 1973). We will describe these briefly.

Goffman: engagement and involvement

Goffman defines engagement and involvement as follows:

> To be engaged in an occasioned activity means to sustain some kind of cognitive and affective engrossment in it, some mobilization of one's psychobiological resources; in short it means to be involved in it.
>
> *(Goffman 1966b: 36)*

> A demand regarding engrossment is a demand on the inner spirit of the engrossed person.
>
> *(Goffman 1966b: 38)*

A consultation is an example of what Goffman called a 'focused interaction' (Goffman 1966a) and one where we might expect both clinician and patient to display such involvement. Crucial to Goffman's definition is the combination of the cognitive and the affective, and he draws attention to the role of bodily conduct (or 'body idiom' to use Goffman's terminology) in this respect. Although the involvement an individual sustains is a matter of inward feeling, Goffman argues that the assessment of involvement relies on outward expression, on how involvement is 'allocated'. Therefore, actual involvement is not only inaccessible (to interactants and analysts alike) but may be of little significance (Goffman 1966b: 38). What matters – and what is consequential to the unfolding of interactions in social life – is this outward expression (or display) of involvement, since this is all that interactants (and analysts!) have to go on in their evaluation of a social situation.

Introducing the EPR into the consulting room places new pressures on the social interaction which clinicians and patients must manage. A particular challenge for the clinician is the requirement to make 'on-the-spot' judgements about the allocation of involvement, and how to avoid the possibility that involvement in the interpersonal interaction is disrupted.

Bakhtin/Vološinov: the dialogic voice

Bakhtin/Vološinov[1] described the *dialogic* nature of communication – the idea that meaning is only possible at the point at which speaker and listener (or writer and reader) connect, and that the specific meaning will vary depending on this immediate social context, and is therefore never neutral (Bakhtin 1981b). Spoken utterances and written texts must be understood in terms of how they are responding to and anticipating other utterances or texts (including spoken or written texts). Vološinov states that the word is a 'two-sided act … the product of the reciprocal relationship between speaker and listener' (Vološinov 1973: 86).

He also emphasized the importance of both the immediate and wider social context of this interactional exchange:

> the forms of signs are conditioned above all by the social organization of the participants involved and also by the immediate conditions of their interaction.
>
> *(Vološinov 1973: 21)*

One consequence of the dialogic nature of communication is that any single utterance contains a response to what has preceded the utterance (a 'hearing') as well as anticipation of what may follow (a 'speaking').

The fundamental question for Bakhtin is 'Who is doing the talking?' and his dialogic orientation entails a constant reflection on how meaning is constructed through chains of representation, each speaker 'populating' language with his own intention. Words are appropriated, and reproduced voices are transformed and given a new evaluative accent, bringing to bear a particular semantic and expressive intention in the quest to make oneself understood in a particular social context (Bakhtin 1981a). This depends on what Bakhtin calls a 'responsive understanding', which is itself also dialogic and evaluative (Bakhtin 1986).

The integration of the EPR into the consultation complicates the matter of 'who is doing the talking'. A close study of the interaction reveals ways in which 'voices' emerge as being distributed between people and technologies, and the EPR becomes recognizable as a source of silent (but often consequential) voices, many originating beyond the 'here and now' of the immediate interaction and constituting important context for the unfolding interaction.

We will now consider a short case study.

Case study: tracing 'involvement' and 'voice' in the triadic consultation

These data (Table 30.1) are from a consultation between a male GP (D) and a female patient (P) who has been recently diagnosed with hypertension (high blood pressure). Six days before this consultation the practice nurse took a blood sample from the patient to measure her cholesterol level. The computer screen is visible to the patient but she is unable to read the details.

Just before this exchange, the GP advises that the patient's cholesterol is high. Both parties express some surprise at the result:

GP: *'they turn out you've got quite ↑high cholesterol'*
P: *'which seems really bizarre…cos I can't think of anything that I have'*

The patient explains that she eats '*loads of fruit, loads of veg'*, then the GP takes a family history (there is nothing relevant) before they interact as shown in Table 30.1.

A detailed line-by-line analysis of this transcript is published elsewhere and will not be repeated here, but may be of interest to some readers (see Further reading) (Swinglehurst et al. 2011). Here we will use the data to illustrate the value of our novel methodological approach to understanding the EPR's influence, highlighting some broad principles which should be considered by researchers interested in exploring the role of new technologies in the interaction.

Table 30.1 Transcript of data (D = doctor; P = patient)

Time	*D/P*	*Spoken word*	*Bodily conduct*	*EPR Screen*
3.30	D	uh well yo:ur l:ow density cholesterol	D-> EPR; P-> D	Consultation screen showing two entries dated 6 days ago:
		is is quite high um::(.) over seven so::	D sits back in chair -> EPR	
3.36	D	((sniff))	D scratches nose, raises eyebrows	1) (nurse): *Blood sample taken. Biochemical screening test (Fasting cholesterol).* Text note: *will make app in a week to see Dr X*
		(0.8)		
3.37	D	<al:tho:ugh ju:st because> you've got high blood pressure you don't necessarily	D->EPR	
		need anything to lower cholesterol (.)	D turns slightly - > P	2)(path lab): displays blood test results incl. *Cholesterol 10, Serum LDL cholesterol >7 see doc please.*
		.hh >even though you've got hypertension<	D returns gaze - > EPR	QOF alert (remains throughout consultation). Shows P is on "QOF register" for hypertension and has two QOF items outstanding: "*notes summarised*" and "*recent medication review*"
3.45	D	I think you'll probably be well advised to have something t- to lower it↑=	D frowns	
3.49	P	=°°yeah°° mean as a child I couldn't take (.) milk and I still don't like milk	P - > forwards; D -> EPR	
3.53	D	no↓		
		(1.0)		
3.54	P	ehm (.) I can take (0.4) >sort of< hot milk in custard (0.4) but someone gave me a glass of hot milk and I would really be ill.		
4.01	P	ha	P-> D; D - > EPR	
4.02	D	right (.) yeah		
4.03	P	so maybe there was an intolerance right from a baby		
		ha	P smiles	
		(0.2)		
4.07	D	we↑↓ll		
4.08	P	who kno↑ws °°ha ha°°	P shakes head slightly, smiling	
4.09	D	°°ha°°	D smiles -> EPR and leans forward -> EPR, placing R hand on keys	
		((C))	Key stroke	Returns to today's consultation screen "Problem title" is automatically highlighted
		(1)		
4.10	D	°u::::hm°		
4.12		((typing for 4.5 seconds))	D -> EPR, typing P looking ahead	"Problem title" selected, then enters keystrokes "Framing" – EPR displays a pick list of 9 choices about cardiovascular risk (Framingham risk scores codes)
		(0.5)	P - > keyboard	
4.16	P	I noticed when I was having my blood test	P - > forwards; D typing	D selects first choice, "*10 yr CHD risk (Estimate, Fram)*"

Time	*D/P*	*Spoken word*	*Bodily conduct*	*EPR Screen*
		(1.0)	D -> EPR, P-> forwards, raises finger in air	A box displays: *"Estimated 10 year CHD risk is 15% The system has calculated that: Average of last 2 systolic BPs is 145 The Total/HDL cholesterol ratio is 6.10 Stopped smoking for over a year, no ECG LVH, No diabetes is the above information correct? (Y/N):*
4.20	P	mm Nurse B***	D -> EPR, P-> forwards and points with finger	
		was showing me (0.4) .hhh on the screen cos she was trying to work out what you wanted it said a fasting blood test (.)	P-> forwards P points again on *fasting*	
		but I didn't (.) ↑ neither of mine (.) were fasting blood tests	P shaking head; D turns to gaze at P	
4.29	D	oh weren't they?	D < - > P	
	P	no		
4.31	D	oh right↓		
		(1)	D looks back to screen; P - > D	
4.33	D	((cough))		Consultation screen displays: *"Additional: Est 10 yr CHD 15%"* indicating that GP responded "Y"
		o::kay. well we'll do it again: (0.5) [then] in that case [((C))	D -> EPR; types keystroke	
		[before] panicking or worrying too much about it ↑ [((C))	D sits upright, keystroke, then rotates chair away from P, reaching for something on desk	

Inspection of the fourth column (bodily conduct) shows that during this minute of interaction, there is only one complete utterance (4:29 '*oh weren't they*?') during which the doctor and patient are focusing their visual attention on each other. The GP is gazing at the EPR the rest of the time. It is oversimplistic to conclude that the GP is not 'focusing' on the patient. Indeed Robinson suggests that patients have a distributed existence (he refers to the *patient embodied* and the *patient inscribed*) observing that patients may remain the focus of the wider activity (consulting) even if not the focus of the GP's gaze (Robinson 1998). Scanning the fifth column suggests that the GP is reading (initially) and then interacting with the patient's EPR, but there is a stark difference between the nature of the unfolding events of column 5 (EPR screen) when compared to the spoken interpersonal interaction (column 3).

Goffman's notion of involvement is a more helpful orientation here than the consideration of gaze alone. As the interaction progresses from 3.30 to 4.16 we observe a widening gap between the patient's concerns (she constructs a narrative to explore whether her raised cholesterol may result from milk intolerance) and the GP's concerns (he begins to calculate the patient's cardiovascular risk at 4:12). The patient begins her narrative at 3:49, but does so as she withdraws her gaze from the GP, looking forwards to tell her story. In doing so the patient mirrors the GP's failure to secure eye contact. The result gives the appearance of parallel 'interactions'.

The patient uses escalating, increasingly medical language, progressing from a *dislike* of milk (3:49), to being *really ill* (3:54) to possible *intolerance* (4:03) – an example of what Pomerantz calls 'extreme case formulation' (Pomerantz 1986). This may be an attempt to secure involvement of the GP (who is occupied with the EPR) and is a good illustration of the importance of the *dialogic* nature of communication – the notion that meaning is only possible at the point at which speaker and listener connect (Bakhtin 1981b). In their work on interviews between careers counsellors and students, Erickson and Shultz found that the failure of students to provide an anticipated 'listening response' led to counsellors engaging in 'hyperexplanation' – either giving successive reasons or 'talking down' (lowering the level of abstraction from one repetition to the next) (Erickson and Shultz 1982). Interestingly, in this sequence the patient makes the GP accountable to the absence of an active listening response by 'talking up' her explanation, fitting her 'lay' explanation into a medical framework. But her short narrative ends definitively when the GP leans forward towards the EPR, and intensifies his attention towards it (and away from the patient) to start typing.

Who (or what) is the focus of the GP's involvement in this extract? At one level we might suggest that the GP is focused on the 'computer' but we have already suggested that this may be oversimplistic. The screen capture gives us clearer insight into what is actually going on and highlights the importance of the EPR in constituting the ongoing context for interaction. The GP is dealing with a concern which is never explicitly articulated in this consultation, but which he anticipates from 3.37. At 3:37 he says: '*<al:though just because> you've got high blood pressure you don't necessarily need anything to lower cholesterol(.) .hh even >even though you've got hypertension<*'. Here he is indexing a specific body of expert medical knowledge – Bakhtin would call this the 'superaddressee' (Bakhtin 1986) – the multifactorial nature of cardiovascular risk. He deals with this concern from 4:12 onwards as he interacts with the EPR to calculate the patient's Framingham cardiovascular risk score.

As analysts we gain a privileged view of this consultation, and one which (it turns out) is not fully shared with the patient. The GP is divided between attending to the 'here and now' of the interpersonal interaction and the 'there and then' of negotiating the discourse of cardiovascular risk – a more institutional framing of the patient, and one that the EPR readily facilitates. In terms of Bakhtin's notion of 'voice' the EPR brings a voice which represents the patient as one of a population, or a series of numerical variables, and contributes to making sense of her cholesterol within a biomedical frame. We have coined the phrase 'dilemma of attention' to describe the way in which the EPR sharpens the tension between different ways of framing the patient – the patient as 'individual' and the patient as 'one of a population' (Swinglehurst et al. 2011). In this example, this 'silent' voice sits uncomfortably alongside the patient's attempts at sense-making in terms of dietary habits and possible milk intolerance.

The EPR has revolutionized the generation of certain *kinds* of knowledge. Risk calculation is an example of the kind of data that can be readily gathered and put to powerful institutional uses: audit, generation of epidemiological data, assessment of GP 'performance'. But it also fosters an orientation to a particular version of patienthood – or a different order of indexicality – one that may compete with the demands of the 'here and now' in the consultation. By anticipating this framing of the patient as early as 3:37, the GP's display of involvement is not only with the 'computer' but with the EPR *and the particular version of patienthood that it privileges*. This ultimately contributes to a closing down of the patient's narrative at 4:09 and to difficulty for the patient in voicing her own concerns. Goffman's involvement is difficult to maintain when attending to the EPR incorporates both physical realignments and orientations to different semiotic planes (different 'voices').

We should point out that the EPR is not necessarily prescriptive in its demands for attention. The clinician and the EPR exist in a recursive relationship, in that the EPR shapes the doctor's actions and the doctor in turn shapes the EPR. To this end the *agency* of the EPR may be regarded as partial and highly contingent on the immediate social context of its use. In this example, the EPR displays QOF alerts throughout the consultation, reminding the GP of institutional objectives (e.g., medication review, notes summarization) but the GP does not attend to them. Indeed our ethnographic observation revealed 'notes summarization' as a labour-intensive task, usually delegated to 'back office' administrators. Regarding the risk calculation, the EPR is not prescriptive in insisting this be done. However, once the GP begins the calculation, the EPR contributes significantly to its unfolding – the calculation cannot be progressed (or abandoned) unless the doctor continues interacting with the EPR. The question it displays at 4:20 demands an answer.

The patient's utterance at 4:20 is an important crux of this consultation – her revelation that she had not fasted before the blood test on which this cholesterol result rests. It is perhaps not surprising that this is the one comment that draws the GP's attention away from the EPR and secures his gaze. Not only does this remark conflict with the nurse's records (3:30, entry 1) but it is immediately relevant to the activity of risk calculation in which the GP is engaged. The patient's utterance here gives us a glimpse of the way in which the EPR conveys voices beyond the consulting room. She treats her 'noticing' of the entry in the EPR as a delicate matter – it reveals the possibility that an error has occurred, and draws attention to different practices between doctor and nurse around screen-sharing (the screen is not shared in this consultation). She invokes the screen (i.e., the EPR) as agent of the 'misunderstanding', politely reframing a human error as a technical one.

In his final utterance the GP says (at 4:33) '*o::kay we'll do it again (0.5) then in that case.*' Not only does he speak as an institutional representative ('*we'*) but he exercises some authority by referring only to the institutional side of this proposal; that the patient will attend (again) for another blood test is taken for granted. Precisely as he speaks, his keystroke accepts the cardiovascular risk calculation (15 percent) as a searchable coded entry in the patient's EPR, constructing an enduring and particular definition of reality. Although from a medical perspective a non-fasting sample may indeed be adequate in a risk calculation, his spoken utterance orients to the patient's display of doubt in her result. We see the EPR contributing to two parallel chains of representation, and the construction of two different realities occurring in tandem. The first results from the clinician's engagement with the EPR, culminating in his documentation of the cardiovascular risk as a coded entry. The second is more subtle and complex. It involves the GP, the nurse, the patient, and the EPR – and culminates with the doctor exercising his authority by ordering a repeat test.

To recap, this analysis shows the importance of the EPR in constituting the ongoing context for interaction, especially by delivering institutional voices into the 'here and now' and tending to privilege particular versions of reality. This places complex challenges upon clinician and patient especially with respect to achieving involvement in the consultation.

Summary and implications for research practice

In this chapter we have briefly charted the historical context for the study of the EPR in the consultation, and have reviewed the state of research in this area. We have introduced a novel methodological approach which illustrates both the complexity of the EPR and the challenges faced by researchers wishing to study it. What the EPR *is* or *can be* depends to some extent on one's epistemological stance towards it and towards the interaction of which it is a part. It is important to contemplate this question before embarking on any study of the role of technologies in communication. Whether and how one chooses to 'contain' a technology informs methods of data collection, transcription, and the range of possible analytical approaches. We have argued our case for 'opening up' the EPR and grappling with its complexity, but in doing so one must accept that the EPR is indeed a highly complex entity.

An approach like ours brings a richness of understanding but it is a researcher-intensive process – one minute of interaction takes many hours to transcribe and analyze. However we hope we have demonstrated the potential limitations of studying the contemporary consultation *without* reference to the EPR, since this is nowadays an integral part of general practice and makes an important contribution to the unfolding context for consulting.

We have drawn attention to the recursive relationship between clinician and EPR. That is, the EPR cannot be understood in isolation; its influence is highly contingent on the immediate social context of its use (Swinglehurst et al. 2011). Furthermore, because its 'presence' extends beyond the 'here and now' into different spaces and different times, the EPR simultaneously makes new things possible (which paper records support less readily) whilst also posing big challenges for the immediate interaction. In particular, the EPR contributes to what we have called a 'dilemma of attention' by sharpening the tension between different ways of framing the patient – the patient as 'individual' and the patient as 'one of a population', the latter being a more institutional framing of the patient (Swinglehurst et al. 2011). Although the EPR is not prescriptive of particular practices, we suggest that it encourages a privileging of this 'institutional' framing of the patient. This tendency to sharpen the asymmetry between 'individual' and 'institutional' framings of the patient may sit uncomfortably alongside the identity of general practice as a discipline that is committed to the 'patient-centred' ideal.

Related topics

Electronic patient records; ethnography; linguistic ethnography; triadic consultation; involvement; dialogism; multimodality.

Note

1 The authorship of some of the Bakhtin/Vološinov writings is controversial, with some critics believing that work attributed to Vološinov may actually have been written by Bakhtin.

Further reading

Bakhtin, M. (1981a) 'Discourse in the novel', in *The Dialogic Imagination: Four Essays by M.M. Bakhtin*, M. Holquist, ed., Austin, TX: University of Texas Press, pp. 259–422. (This essay, a translation of Bakhtin's original work of the early 1930s, includes a more detailed description of Bakhtin's radical notion of dialogism and introduces the reader to several key Bakhtinian concepts.)

Goffman, E. (1966b) 'Involvement', in *Behavior in Public Places*, New York: Free Press, pp. 33–42. (A short, easy-to-read introduction to 'involvement' illustrated with examples from everyday social life.)

Greenhalgh, T. and Swinglehurst, D. (2011) 'Studying technology use as social practice: the untapped potential of ethnography', *BMC Medicine*, 9: 45. (This paper highlights the philosophical underpinnings of different study designs, building a case for ethnography as the preferred methodological approach for studying technologies in complex social systems such as health care.)

Rampton, B., Tusting, K., Maybin, J., Barwell, R., Creese, A., and Lytra, V. (2004) *UK Linguistic Ethnography: A Discussion Paper.* Downloadable from: http://www.uklef.net/documents/papers/ramptonetal2004.pdf (This discussion paper introduces linguistic ethnography as a new area of scholarship highlighting the methodological potential and challenges of combining ethnography and linguistics.)

Swinglehurst, D., Roberts, C., and Greenhalgh, T. (2011) 'Opening up the "black box" of the electronic patient record: a linguistic ethnographic study in general practice', *Communication and Medicine*, 8(1): 3–15. (This paper, on which many of the ideas in this book chapter are based, incorporates a more detailed line-by-line analysis of the transcript and might be usefully read alongside this chapter to broaden general understanding of the methods and methodology employed.)

References

Als, A.B. (1997) 'The desk-top computer as a magic box: patterns of behaviour connected with the desk-top computer: GPs' and patients' perceptions', *Family Practice*, 14: 17–23.

Atkinson, J.M. and Heritage, J. (1984) 'Transcript notation', in *Structures of Social Action: Studies in Conversation Analysis*, J.M. Atkinson and J. Heritage, eds, Cambridge: Cambridge University Press, pp. ix–xvi.

Bakhtin, M. (1981a) 'Discourse in the Novel', in *The Dialogic Imagination: Four Essays by M.M.Bakhtin*, M. Holquist, ed., Austin, TX: University of Texas Press, pp. 259–422.

Bakhtin, M. (1981b) *The Dialogic Imagination: Four Essays*, Austin, TX: University of Texas Press.

——(1986) *Speech Genres and Other Late Essays*, Austin, TX: University of Texas Press.

Blumer, H. (1969) *Symbolic Interactionism*, Berkeley, CA: University of California Press.

Booth, N., Kohannejad, J., and Robinson, P. (2002) *Information in the Consulting Room (iiCR). Final Project Report*, University of Newcastle upon Tyne, Department of Health, SCHIN.

Booth, N., Robinson, P., and Kohannejad, J. (2004) 'Identification of high-quality consultation practice in primary care: the effects of computer use on doctor–patient rapport', *Informatics in Primary Care*, 12: 75–83.

Department of Health (2010) *Liberating the NHS: An Information Revolution.* Available HTTP: < http://www.gov.uk/government/uploads/system/uploads/attachment_data/file/216664/dh_129580.pdf> (accessed 16 October 2013).

Erickson, F. (2004) *Talk and Social Theory*, Cambridge: Polity.

Erickson, F. and Shultz, J. (1982) *The Counselor as Gatekeeper*, New York: Academic Press.

Foucault, M. (1970) *The Order of Things*, London: Tavistock/Routledge.

Frankel, R., Altschuler, A., George, S., Kinsman, J., Jimison, H., Robertson, N., and Hsu, J. (2005) 'Effects of exam-room computing on clinician–patient communication', *Journal of General Internal Medicine*, 20: 677–682.

General Practitioners Committee (2009) *Quality and Outcomes Framework. Guidance* – Updated August 2004. Available HTTP: <http://www.nhsemployers.org/payandcontracts/GeneralMedicalServicesContract/QOF/pages/QualityOutcomesFramework.aspx> (accessed 4 November 2012).

Goffman, E. (1955) 'On face-work: an analysis of ritual elements in social interaction', *Psychiatry: Journal of Interpersonal Relations*, 18: 213–231.

——(1966a) 'Introductory definitions', in *Behavior in Public Places*, New York: Free Press, pp. 13–30.

——(1966b) 'Involvement', in *Behavior in Public Places*, New York: Free Press, pp. 33–42.

——(1967) 'On face-work', in *Interaction Ritual: Essays On Face-to-Face Behaviour*, New York: Pantheon Books, pp. 5–45.

——(1974) *Frame Analysis: An Essay on the Organization of Experience*, York, PA: Northeastern University Press.

——(1981) 'Footing', in *Forms of Talk*, Philadelphia: University of Pennsylvania Press, pp. 124–159.

Greatbatch, D. (1992) *System Use and Interpersonal Communication in the General Practice Consultation: Preliminary Observations*, Cambridge: Rank Xerox Research Centre.

Greatbatch, D., Luff, P., Heath, C., and Campion, P. (1993) 'Interpersonal communication and human–computer interaction: an examination of the use of computers in medical consultations', *Interacting with Computers*, 5: 193–216.

Greatbatch, D., Heath, C., Campion, P., and Luff, P. (1995) 'How do desk-top computers affect the doctor–patient interaction?', *Family Practice*, 12: 32–36.

Greenhalgh, T. and Swinglehurst, D. (2011) 'Studying technology use as social practice: the untapped potential of ethnography', *BMC Medicine*, 9: 45.

Gumperz, J.J. (1999) 'On interactional sociolinguistic method', in *Talk, Work and Institutional Order*, S. Sarangi and C. Roberts, eds, Berlin: Mouton de Gruyter, pp. 453–471.

Heath, C. and Hindmarsh, J. (2002) 'Analysing interaction: video, ethnography and situated conduct', in *Qualitative Research in Action*, T. May, ed., London: Sage, pp. 99–121.

Herzmark, G., Brownbridge, G., Fitter, M., and Evans, A. (1984) 'Consultation use of a computer by general practitioners', *Journal of the Royal College of General Practitioners*, 34: 649–654.

Iedema, R. (2003) 'The medical record as organizing discourse', *Document Design*, 4: 64–84.

Jewitt, C. (2006) 'Towards a multimodal analysis', in *Technology, Literacy and Learning: A Multimodal Approach*, Abingdon: Routledge, pp. 32–52.

Luff, P., Heath, C., and Greatbatch, D. (1992) 'Tasks-in-interaction: paper and screen based documentation in collaborative activity', CSCW 92 Proceedings of the ACM conference on Computer-supported Cooperative Work, pp. 163–170.

Margalit, R.S., Roter, D., Dunevant, M.A., Larson, S., and Reis, S. (2006) 'Electronic medical record use and physician–patient communication: an observational study of Israeli primary care encounters', *Patient Education and Counseling*, 61: 134–141.

Pearce, C. (2007) 'Doctors, patients and computers, the new consultation', PhD Thesis, Department of General Practice, University of Melbourne.

Pearce, C., Trumble, S., Arnold, M., Dwan, K., and Phillips, C. (2008) 'Computers in the new consultation: within the first minute', *Family Practice*, 25: 202–208.

Pearce, C., Dwan, K., Arnold, M., Phillips, C., and Trumble, S. (2009) 'Doctor, patient and computer – a framework for the new consultation', *International Journal of Medical Informatics*, 78: 32–38.

Pomerantz, A. (1986) 'Extreme case formulations: a new way of legitimating claims', *Human Studies (Interaction and Language Use Special Issue)*, 9: 219–230.

Rampton, B., Tusting, K., Maybin, J., Barwell, R., Creese, A., and Lytra, V. (2004) UK Linguistic Ethnography: A Discussion Paper. Available HTTP: <http://www.uklef.net/documents/papers/ramptonetal2004.pdf>

Roberts, C. and Sarangi, S. (2005) 'Theme-oriented discourse analysis of medical encounters', *Medical Education*, 39: 632–640.

Robinson, J.D. (1998) 'Getting down to business: talk, gaze and body orientation during openings of doctor–patient consultations', *Human Communication Research*, 25: 97–123.

Scott, D. and Purves, I. (1996) 'Triadic relationship between doctor, computer and patient', *Interacting with Computers*, 8: 347–363.

Shachak, A. and Reis, S. (2009) 'The impact of electronic medical records on patient–doctor communication during consultation: a narrative literature review', *Journal of Evaluation in Clinical Practice*, 15: 641–649.

Sullivan, F. (1995) 'Intruders in the consultation', *Family Practice*, 12: 66–69.

Swinglehurst, D., Roberts, C., and Greenhalgh, T. (2011) 'Opening up the "black box" of the electronic patient record: a linguistic ethnographic study in general practice', *Communication and Medicine*, 8: 3–15.

Ventres, W., Kooienga, S., Marlin, R., Vuckovic, N., and Stewart, V. (2005) 'Clinician style and examination room computers: a video ethnography', *Family Medicine*, 37: 276–281.

Ventres, W., Kooienga, S., Vuckovic, N., Marlin, R., Nygren, P., and Stewart, V. (2006) 'Physicians, patients, and the electronic health record: an ethnographic analysis', *Annals of Family Medicine*, 4(2): 124–131.

Vološinov, V. (1973) *Marxism and the Philosophy of Language,* Cambridge, MA: Harvard University Press.

Warshawsky, S.S., Pliskin, J.S., Urkin, J., Cohen, N., Sharon, A., Binztok, M., and Margolis, C.Z. (1994) 'Physician use of a computerized medical record system during the patient encounter: a descriptive study', *Computer Methods and Programs in Biomedicine*, 43: 269–273.

Weed, L. (1968) 'Medical records that guide and teach', *New England Journal of Medicine*, 278: 593–600.

Appendix 30.1

| onset of overlapping speech

| end of spate of overlapping talk

|| speakers start a turn simultaneously

: preceding sound is lengthened or drawn out

(more : means greater prolongation)

<u>Underlining</u> emphasis

.hhh inbreath

Hhh outbreath

= no pause between speakers; contiguous utterances

((   )) a non verbal activity (e.g. C = keystroke in this work)

(text) unclear fragment of text

(.) pause of less than 0.2 seconds

(0.4) pause, in tenths of a second

↑↓ marked rising / falling intonation

>text< the talk they surround is quicker than surrounding talk

°° the talk they surround is quieter than surrounding talk

. falling tone (not necessarily end of sentence)

? rising inflection (not necessarily a question)

CAPITALS louder than surrounding talk

<text> the talk they surround is slower than surrounding talk

31 Provider–patient communication about complementary and alternative medicine

Evelyn Y. Ho and Christopher J. Koenig

Introduction

In a landmark study in the *New England Journal of Medicine,* Eisenberg et al. (1993) reported higher than expected complementary and alternative medicine (CAM) use in the US and precipitated a flood of research about CAM. The study concluded that physicians should ask patients about CAM use. Since then, researchers have been studying not only CAM use but also whether and how often patients and physicians communicate about CAM. As research in this area flourished, more complex concerns regarding CAM communication developed, including examining barriers to CAM communication that raised questions about provider training, patient and provider knowledge about CAM, and the possibilities for patient-centered care, shared decision-making, and culturally competent health care.

In the two decades since Eisenberg et al. (1993), other national studies estimate that up to 38.3 percent of US adults use some form of CAM treatment (Barnes et al. 2008). In 2006, the National Center for Complementary and Alternative Medicine (NCCAM) and the American Association of Retired Persons (AARP) conducted a joint study of CAM users over 50. Findings indicated that only 31 percent of CAM users discussed CAM with their physicians (NCCAM 2007). In response to these findings, NCCAM launched the *Time to Talk* campaign in 2008 to encourage healthcare providers to ask patients about CAM and to teach patients how to ask providers about CAM. A follow-up study in 2010 found that 58 percent of CAM users had discussed CAM with their provider (NCCAM 2011). Some studies have used *Time to Talk* to develop patient education materials that teach patients how to talk to their providers about CAM (Ho et al. 2012).

While extensive self-report research has been conducted on CAM communication, cutting-edge research employs audio-visual recordings that document actual conversations between providers and patients about CAM. Studies using discourse and conversation analysis examine how CAM communication is interactionally negotiated by considering the communicative context of the medical visit. These innovative methods have the potential to elucidate CAM communication through detailed examination of the communication process to promote positive health outcomes.

Current research and critical issues

In the following sections, we review research about CAM communication. However, many of these studies are difficult to compare not only because their population samples are so different, but also because of variation in research design. There are two significant methodological points of interest related to defining, measuring, and reporting what data are being presented.

First, while some studies report percentages of *all* participants who discussed CAM, others report percentages of *current CAM users*. Depending on what is measured and reported, these numbers can imply drastically different conclusions. For example, in a 2010 study of US adults over 50, only 33 percent of *all* respondents had ever discussed CAM with their providers while 58 percent of *CAM users* had ever discussed CAM (NCCAM 2011). Compare these findings to four years previously when only 31 percent of *CAM users* had ever discussed CAM with their providers and 22 percent of *all* respondents had discussed CAM (NCCAM 2007). By comparing equivalent data, CAM communication with biomedical providers appears to be rising.

Second, most studies operationalize communication using the dichotomous variables of *disclosure/non-disclosure* or *discussion/non-discussion*. This creates problems for comparison across studies because CAM disclosure may not be the same as CAM discussion. For example, if a patient lists CAM use on an intake form, CAM use may be considered disclosed, but unless a provider subsequently asks about that patient's CAM use, it may not actually be discussed during a medical visit. Additionally, if a patient mentions CAM and the provider ignores or does not respond, it is not clear if this would be considered disclosure or discussion. This interactional issue will be discussed later in this chapter.

Self-reported CAM discussion rates

A large body of research reports rates of CAM communication, especially around CAM use and disclosure and discussion rates. Across these studies, CAM discussion rates vary tremendously depending on a number of factors, including the population sampled, whether disclosure or discussion was measured, and the research methods used. Most studies report between 23 and 72 percent disclosure rates (Robinson and McGrail 2004). Research outside the US mirrors these CAM disclosure rates. On the low end, only 18.75 percent of cancer patients in Norway disclosed using herbal preparations (Engdal et al. 2008) and on the high end, 60 percent of a national sample of older Australians reported that they always discuss their CAM use with their physicians (Zhang et al. 2007). Compare these relatively low numbers to discussion of biomedical treatments in CAM settings. In a study of breast cancer patients who were simultaneously seeing CAM providers, only 50 percent of them disclosed their CAM use to their biomedical provider whereas 90 percent discussed biomedical diagnoses and treatments with their CAM providers (Adler et al. 2009).

Reviews of CAM communication generally conclude that patient demographics are not reliable predictors of CAM disclosure (Robinson and McGrail 2004). However, individual studies are mixed. Some research finds that patients with higher incomes and education (Liu et al. 2009; NCCAM 2011) and those with better access to care are more likely to disclose CAM use (Chao et al. 2008). Most studies, including those based on US national samples, find that ethnic minorities disclose CAM use less often than non-Latino Whites (Kennedy et al. 2008; Young et al. 2009) and that women typically disclose CAM use more often than men (Busse et al. 2005; NCCAM 2011). From the provider's side, female physicians (Corbin

Winslow and Shapiro 2002), those who are younger in the profession (Sleath et al. 2001), and those who have had more training about CAM (Staples et al. 2007) tend to recommend CAM more. Providers who use CAM themselves also recommend CAM more (Corbin Winslow and Shapiro 2002; Mak et al. 2009). Physicians report that they are more likely to recommend CAM if it is available at their current clinic (Wahner-Roedler et al. 2006) and if there is more evidence-based research about CAM (Janamian et al. 2011). In fact, most providers want more education and information about CAM (Janamian et al. 2011). Finally, some studies find that patients were more likely to disclose CAM use if their primary care providers employed a more participatory style of decision-making (Sleath et al. 2005).

Barriers to CAM talk

Overwhelmingly, US studies conclude that, first, patients initiate conversations about CAM more often than providers and, second, the main reason patients neither disclose nor discuss CAM is because providers do not routinely ask about it during medical visits (NCCAM 2011; Robinson and McGrail 2004). However, studies outside the US often report other reasons for non-disclosure, including that CAM is perceived as safe (Chang et al. 2011), that disclosure is unnecessary, or that patients just did not think about it (Zhang et al. 2007).

Barriers to CAM communication can be understood in three ways. First, communication about CAM is a problem of initiation: neither provider nor patient thinks to raise the topic of CAM. In fact, the most commonly reported barrier to CAM communication is that the provider did not ask (Engdal et al. 2008; NCCAM 2011). However, research also finds that both providers (Corbin Winslow and Shapiro 2002) and patients (Busse et al. 2005) are uncomfortable discussing CAM. Second, CAM communication is a problem of information: neither provider nor patient has – or believes the other to have – enough information to usefully discuss CAM (Busse et al. 2005; Chang et al. 2011). Third, communication about CAM is a problem of context or situation: neither patient nor provider perceives the medical visit as an appropriate place to talk about CAM. Research in this area finds both patients (Young et al. 2009) and providers may avoid discussing CAM because they do not feel it is relevant to the visit (Roberts et al. 2005). In addition, some patients report that they do not expect their medical provider to integrate their CAM and biomedicine; instead, patients preferred to self-manage their overall health care, including CAM use (Adler et al. 2009).

CAM talk by CAM modality

While early research in CAM communication generally grouped all CAM together, later research separates CAM communication by modality. There are few similarities across studies that analyze communication by CAM modality. For example, based on a US national sample, practitioner-based CAM such as biofeedback (72 percent) and chelation therapy (75 percent) is disclosed more than self-care CAM such as folk medicine (33 percent) or homeopathy (35 percent) (Chao et al. 2008). However, another study found that patients were most comfortable discussing biofeedback, massage, chiropractic, and relaxation as opposed to energy healing, naturopathy, magnetic therapy, and aromatherapy (Wahner-Roedler et al. 2006).

Herb and supplement disclosure has received more attention than other CAM modalities because they have the highest likelihood of contraindications with pharmaceutical medications. In one national study, although 18.9 percent of the US population reported using herbs and supplements, only one-third of study participants disclosed herbs or supplement use with their physicians (Kennedy et al. 2008). There are a variety of reasons a patient might not disclose herb or supplement use. Some commonly used herbs are also everyday foods and may or may not be considered CAM. For example, many Hispanic patients use herbs such as cinnamon, cloves, cumin, chamomile, and garlic as part of traditional folk medicine, but physicians may not be aware of the therapeutic use of these herbs (Howell et al. 2006).

CAM communication in clinical settings

Recent research examining CAM communication has begun to focus more specifically on particular medical settings and clinical conditions. While research on CAM in clinical settings covers the spectrum from HIV/AIDS (Liu et al. 2009) to pediatrics (O'Keefe and Coat 2010), the most developed area of CAM communication research is in oncology.

Research in cancer settings has found not only that CAM use may be higher with this population (Roberts et al. 2005) but also that CAM disclosure may be higher especially with oncologists (Humpel and Jones 2006) compared to primary care providers (Mao et al. 2011; Yates et al. 2005). Studies of cancer patients typically show higher CAM disclosure than national averages with as many as 65.6 percent of cancer patients in Hawaii (Tasaki et al. 2002). One explanation for these differences is based on the extremely high usage rates of CAM – 91 percent in a study of those receiving cancer treatment (Yates et al. 2005). Another explanation is that cancer may be one area in which CAM and biomedicine are more consciously integrated (Mao et al. 2011). In addition, it is also important to note that despite talking about CAM more, patients are still wary about having these conversations because of previous negative or indifferent reactions from providers and a fear or further rejection of their CAM use (Humpel and Jones 2006).

Outcomes of CAM conversations

The assumption underlying research is that increased communication about CAM should lead to benefits including avoidance of adverse events between CAM and prescription medication, increased satisfaction, and shared decision-making (Perlman et al. 1999). However, research focused on outcomes is not well developed and no studies have empirically tested the relationship between communication and clinical health outcomes concerning CAM. Some studies report that both providers and patients believe that communication about CAM enhances the therapeutic relationship (Richardson et al. 2004). Other studies find correlations between disclosure and patient satisfaction (Liu et al. 2009). However, research also reports that patients are unsatisfied with CAM communication because they perceived physicians to have negative or indifferent attitudes toward CAM in general (Tasaki et al. 2002). While almost all studies about CAM communication conclude that communication may lead to clinically significant outcomes, more extensive research can be done in this area to better understand how the actual conversations work and their relationship to outcomes. We will address this in more depth later in the chapter.

Interactional approaches to studying CAM communication

Most studies reviewed thus far primarily use surveys or questionnaires to determine the knowledge, attitudes, beliefs, and conversation-initiation behaviors of providers and patients. Very few studies problematize CAM communication. Studies that analyze actual communicative dynamics surrounding CAM can be divided into two types: (1) semi-structured interviews, which enables reports of knowledge, attitudes, and beliefs about CAM; and (2) audio-visual recordings of actual interaction between physicians and patients, which we suggest is the gold standard for future research about CAM communication. In the following sections, we discuss three different bodies of research focused on CAM communication as interactionally negotiated.

Interview studies

Several previous studies used interviews to ask patients and providers about the interactional process of CAM communication. In contrast to survey-based research, these studies reveal that barriers to talking about CAM depend on the longitudinal relationship between patient and provider across medical visits. For example, Tasaki et al. (2002) used open-ended qualitative interviews with cancer patients to investigate CAM communication with oncologists. They found that nearly 70 percent of patients reported not disclosing CAM use or continuing CAM conversations due to anticipated negative provider responses (Tasaki et al. 2002). This study expands understandings of barriers to communication because it reveals that reasons for initial disclosure may differ from barriers to continued conversations about CAM use over time.

In another study, Shelley et al. (2009) used sequenced semi-structured interviews and focus groups with healthcare providers and staff at several primary care clinics with Hispanic and Native American patients to investigate communication about CAM use. They found that patients' perceptions of provider attitudes influenced whether they disclosed and discussed CAM use. Patients did not expect providers to be experts, but they wanted providers to know that they were proactively supporting their health in other ways that were culturally relevant and meaningful. These findings indicate that provider initiation is key to having discussions, but only if that initiation is done in a non-judgmental way.

Interview studies are a significant departure from survey research in at least three ways. First, disclosure is an interactive process in which multiple barriers may affect conversation about CAM. Second, this research shows that CAM communication can move beyond discussion about safety and efficacy, which requires providers to be knowledgeable about CAM. Finally, CAM communication is one way in which providers can explicitly build a therapeutic alliance because CAM communication facilitates a window into patient preferences and values more generally (Shelley et al. 2009).

Content analysis of recorded interaction

A few studies move beyond asking participants to self-report about CAM communication by using audio- or video-recorded interaction from actual patient visits to empirically investigate CAM communication. Sleath et al. (2001) used audio-recordings to count CAM modalities mentioned and patient disclosure rates. They also documented the number of physician and patient questions about CAM during the actual visits as 3.4 percent and 2 percent respectively (Sleath et al. 2001). While this study begins to examine the interactive nature of CAM communication, it does not fully take advantage of the recordings to explore the communication process.

Two additional studies use audio- or video-recordings of consultations between cancer patients and oncologists to investigate and expand our understandings of CAM communication (Juraskova et al. 2010; Schofield et al. 2003). While patients (or family members) were found to primarily initiate CAM discussions, these studies recognize that physicians play an important role through how they respond. Providers primarily encouraged patient use of CAM modalities, but providers also discouraged, were neutral towards, or even ignored patient mentions of CAM use (Juraskova et al. 2010; Schofield et al. 2003).

What distinguishes these studies from previous CAM research is that these articles recognize that CAM talk is not simply about who initiates the talk or which CAM modalities are mentioned. Instead, participants' orientations to CAM occur as an interactive negotiation between provider and patient. However, one of the limitations of these studies is their use of content analysis which treats communication as a dichotomous variable that either does or does not happen and therefore treats physician's behavior in isolation from the larger communicative context which these orientations are achieved in and through talk.

Discourse analysis of recorded interaction

Only one previous study using audio-recordings shows that disclosure of and discussion about CAM are interactionally negotiated. Koenig et al. (2012) use discourse analysis to contextualize providers' responses to patient-initiated CAM talk within the larger communicative situation. By focusing on the turn-by-turn interactional processes, Koenig et al. show how providers' responses help shape patient participation in negotiating treatment decisions about CAM use as an interactional outcome. Building on previous studies (Juraskova et al. 2010; Schofield et al. 2003), this study conceptualizes physicians' responses as a continuum. At one end, physicians encouraged CAM use when it was perceived to be primarily helpful and not harmful. In the middle, providers could stay neutral about their recommendations by claiming not to have knowledge of CAM modalities or by disattending CAM mentions altogether. For example, when a patient disclosed using CAM, his physician adopted a neutral stance by saying, 'You can use (CAM) if you want to.' The analysis suggests that while the physician's turn may appear to vaguely encourage CAM use, in context the patient may hear the physician's turn as mitigated disapproval. At the other end of the continuum, physicians discouraged CAM use when it was perceived to be harmful or could interfere with biomedical treatments. This study is a significant departure from previous research because it shows the interactionally dynamic process through which physicians' responses can lead to differential outcomes within the medical visit.

Two discourse analytic case studies

In this section, we present two case studies to illustrate how discourse analytic research can provide insight into CAM communication. The following data were collected as part of a study examining how patients communicate with their primary care physicians about acute and chronic problems. Five primary care physicians in Northern California were video-recorded with 10 patients each. The UCLA institutional review board approved this study. Transcription conventions (see Appendix 31.1 at the end of this chapter) are a subset of the full conversation analytic symbols (Jefferson 2004).

Case study 1: Oregano oil

In the following extract, the physician and patient are meeting for the first time in a private, fee-for-service internal medicine clinic. At the beginning of the visit, the patient presents allergy-like symptoms that have persisted over one week. She reports trying an over-the-counter allergy medicine. Because this remedy did not alleviate her symptoms, she decided to make an appointment with this physician who has an office near her residence. After presenting her problem, the physician asks a general history-taking question in line 01.

Extract 1: 'I take oregano oil'

01 MD: And uhm, do you take any medications?
02 (.)
03 PT: Mm [mm.
04 MD: [herbs, vitamins, supplements?
05 (0.2)
06 PT: Uh::m, no.=Sometimes I take vitamins:,
07 (0.8) ((MD types into electronic medical record))
08 PT: uh: if I'm sick, occasionally, I take like
09 <u>o</u>regano oil?=
10 MD: =M[m, ((MD types into electronic medical record))
11 PT [but I haven't been taking that this time.
12 MD: °o[kay. ((MD types into electronic medical record))
13 PT: [<just because my stomach has felt kinda
14 upset and that-
15 (0.4) ((MD looks up from computer))
16 MD: Yeah.
17 PT: Yeah, I don't like the taste of oregano
18 [(either.)
19 MD: [<u>Oh</u>(heh heh)ka(heh)y.=.hh
20 (0.2)
21 MD: And how did you find <u>me</u>?

After a micropause (line 02) the patient provides a preferred negative response, 'mm mm' (line 03). From the patient's perspective, the physician's question asks if she regularly takes any *pharmaceutical* medications, which she declines. Rather than moving on to a next question, the physician adds a grammatical increment in the next turn position to elicit whether the patient uses any CAM treatments, such as 'herbs, vitamins, supplements?' (line 04). Previous literature has shown that physicians do not typically ask patients if they use CAM because physicians assume patients would volunteer CAM use (Robinson and McGrail 2004). While the three-part list does not repeat the original question syntax, its placement in the turn after the patient's answer is hearable as a re-specification of the 'any medications' question. This extension implies that when the physician asked about 'any medications', the physician is soliciting all treatment the patient routinely takes, including CAM.

The patient delays her answer with two forms of mitigation, a 0.2 second gap (line 05) and a stretched 'uh::m' (line 06) before finally producing a <u>no</u> (line 06). However, what initially seems to be a 'no' answer turns out to be reversed, 'sometimes I take vitamins:,' (line 06). During the 0.8 second pause, the physician types into the patient's electronic medical record, and the patient continues, 'if I'm sick, occasionally I take like oregano oil?' (lines 08–09), a CAM remedy derived from the culinary herb. The initial mitigation may address the physician's first question, namely, that he is asking about treatment the patient may *regularly* take rather than treatments she takes 'sometimes' (line 06) or 'occasionally' (lines 08–09). However, in qualifying her CAM use, the patient constructs herself to be an occasional, rather than a regular, CAM user. As her answer comes to an end, the upward-intonation on 'oregano oil?' (line 09) projects more talk, which the physician receipts (line 10) as he types into the electronic medical record.

After discussing her historical CAM use, the patient notes that she did not use CAM for the current illness episode (line 11) by citing two specific reasons: (1) her stomach has been upset (lines 13–14) and (2) she doesn't like the taste of oregano (line 17–18). These reasons are significant because they provide insight into the patient's decision-making process about CAM use. While she may use oregano oil when she is sick, it may not be a regular part of her health behavior because it has unwanted side effects, such as upset stomach and bad taste. Balancing side effects may play a role in deciding what treatment forms to use. In response to the patient's expanded answer, the physician acknowledges the elaborated answer (line 19) before moving to a next question (line 21), thereby closing this part of the interview.

This case provides three insights into CAM communication as an interactional process. First, physicians' behaviors can help shape interactional outcomes with respect to disclosure about CAM. During the history-taking phase of the acute medical visit, physicians routinely ask patients about the medications they use. However, questions about medication use may often fail to elicit a full spectrum of treatments that patients use beyond prescription or over-the-counter medication. In this extract after asking specifically about 'medicine', the physician follows-up with a three-part list that specifically solicits disclosure about possible CAM use. As a result, the patient discloses occasional CAM use. This implies that the design features of a question about CAM use, the activity within which the question is asked, and the placement within the overall context of the medical visit, may shape the interactional trajectory of CAM disclosure.

Second, in disclosing her CAM use, the patient also reveals some clues about her treatment decision-making. CAM treatment is one option out of several other treatment options, including over-the-counter and prescription medication. By disclosing *any* CAM use, she provides insight into the range of possible treatment options she might consider during an illness episode, including over-the-counter and CAM treatments. In this sense, any disclosure about CAM use helps inform providers about patient treatment preferences and values that may not otherwise be brought to light. Further, the patient specifically mentions avoiding a particular CAM treatment due to undesirable side effects. This implies that while the patient may consider using a CAM treatment *in general*, the decision to use or not use CAM is weighed against a range of perceived risks and benefits vis-à-vis other treatment options.

Finally, once the patient discloses occasional CAM use, rather than inquiring more, the physician moves on to a next history-taking question. This suggests that further discussion does not always follow from disclosure about CAM use. The physician moves onto a new question without discussing the safety, efficacy, or possible contraindications of the CAM treatment and without acknowledging the patient's occasional preference for CAM treatment. Thus, through his immediately next behavior, the physician treats the patient's mention of CAM as disclosure and passes on the opportunity to discuss CAM use in more depth.

Case study 2: Eat yogurt

In this visit, the patient presents flu-like symptoms and coughing consistent with a bacterial upper respiratory infection. As the initial treatment recommendation, the physician recommends a 5-day course of antibiotics. After an extended sequence of instruction giving, the physician asks the patient if she has experienced yeast infections after taking antibiotics. When she affirms that she has, the physician recommends a complementary form of treatment, 'Eat yogurt.' (line 79).

Extract 2. 'Eat yogurt'

79 MD: Eat yogurt.
80 PT: Eat yogurt?
81 MD: Yo:gurt with uh live cultures, which most
82 yogurt does have because the antibiotics
83 would give you yeast infectio=<well, some
84 women will get yeast infections so-
85 PT: Okay.
86 MD: Uhm, (0.2) and just to prevent it, you can eat
87 uh yogurt.=and if you do end up getting a
88 yeast infection, call me and we can get you
89 a medication and so-
90 PT: ((nods)) <I also wanted to ask you,
91 ((continues presenting a second problem))

Following an extended discussion about antibiotics, the physician attends to one side effect of the proposed biomedical treatment: antibiotics kill the bacteria responsible for illness as well as the intestinal flora that may contribute to good gastrointestinal health. Some CAM and integrative providers recommend taking probiotics through either dietary supplements or food, such as yogurt, to counter these side effects.

In response, the patient repeats the recommendation with question intonation, 'Eat yogurt?' (line 80), simultaneously displaying surprise and inviting elaboration. The physician confirms the recommendation, complying with her invitation through specifying the type of yogurt she should eat with finer granularity, 'yo:gurt with uh live cultures, which most yogurt does have' (lines 81–82). The physician continues his speaking turn, 'because the antibiotics would give you yeast infectio=<well, some women will get yeast infections so-' (lines 82–84), explaining the reason for the complementary recommendation after completing the course of antibiotics.

Apparently hearing the physician's second recommendation as potentially complete, the patient accepts it (line 85), bringing the sequence to possible completion. However, rather than moving onto the next activity in the visit, the physician continues his explanation: 'Uhm, (0.2) and just to prevent it, you can eat uh yogurt.' (lines 86–87). Once fully produced, the physician's full recommendation becomes clear retrospectively: while antibiotics will help to rid the patient of symptoms related to the bacterial infection that brought her to the physician's office in the first place, the antibiotics also have possible associated symptoms, namely, yeast infections, which the yogurt may help prevent as a complementary treatment by re-populating the 'good' bacteria in the patient's body after the course of antibiotics.

Before the patient responds to the completed explanation, the physician continues his speaking turn a second time, addressing the contingency that the complementary treatment may either not work or that the patient may choose not to follow (lines 87–89). He suggests that if the patient does end up getting a yeast infection, 'call me and we can get you a medication and so-' (lines 88–89). The patient nods her head, presumably acknowledging this contingency and shifts to a new activity, an inquiry about an unrelated medical problem that ends the discussion.

This case provides further insight into CAM communication in primary care visits. Most previous research has shown that patients typically initiate CAM discussion, however in this case the physician volunteers a complementary treatment for a possible future medical problem. This is notable in at least two ways. First, the physician demonstrates his understanding of the strengths and limitations for both biomedical and complementary forms of treatment. While the antibiotics will help treat the patient's upper respiratory infection, antibiotics also have the potential to put the patient at risk for another medical problem, a yeast infection. Second, this physician uses a sophisticated treatment strategy that employs both biomedical and CAM modalities. He first suggests the complementary treatment, yogurt, as an easy, 'do it yourself' treatment to help prevent a future yeast infection. However, while yogurt may help to prevent yeast infections after antibiotics, as a complementary therapy, it also may not work, for which he offers future biomedical treatment options. Sequencing complementary then biomedical treatment options shows the physician to be attentive to the patient's possible treatment preferences, which may help bolster his relationship with the patient through a balanced, integrative approach to treatment that includes multiple treatment modalities.

Second, this case shows that discussion about CAM treatment can take place within the treatment recommendation phase of acute medical visits. Previous research that uses content analytic methods do not typically consider the context of when CAM is discussed. When coding for 'CAM discussion', content analyses typically only notice the presence vs. absence of discussion throughout the entirety of a medical visit, regardless of the activity, such as problem presentation, history taking, or treatment recommendation. Discourse analysis, however, examines the language used by participants to understand their orientations to the activity as constitutive of the activity at hand. While CAM disclosure may be typical during a history-taking activity, CAM conversation may be more typical during treatment recommendation activities. However, this is an empirical matter that future research should address more fully.

These two case studies demonstrate the utility of a discourse analytic approach to the study of CAM communication. In contrast to survey-based and content analytic studies, discourse analytic studies can examine the antecedents for analytic constructs, such as disclosure and discussion, to better understand how CAM communication occurs in naturally occurring conversation. Discourse analysis provides fine-grained attention to the local activities, relationship between patient and provider, and overall communicative context that all contribute to differential outcomes for CAM communication within acute medical visits. As research into the efficacy and safety of CAM continues, healthcare providers will have the opportunity to learn more about CAM treatment modalities.

Future directions

Communication about CAM in biomedical settings is an area that is ripe for future investigation. Continued discourse analytic research that analyzes actual interaction between patient and provider will expand knowledge about CAM communication and may have important effects on health outcomes and delivery.

Future research needs to examine the current purpose of CAM communication in health care and determine when and how CAM talk is relevant. Disclosure of current CAM use has been suggested as a way for providers to uncover patient preferences and to address issues of safety and efficacy related to CAM use itself and in combination with biomedical treatment. However, these conversational goals are situationally specific, and both provider and patient goals may not necessarily match in all conversations. As this review and case studies demonstrate, CAM use may not always be immediately relevant to the particular illness experience being discussed at a patient visit. For example, a patient's use of breathing exercises for overall well-being may not seem relevant in an appointment to refill cholesterol medication. However, a holistic approach might elicit why the patient does the exercises, what she hopes to gain from the exercises, and how the exercises play a role in the patient's overall perceptions of health and wellness.

Second, providers and patients may be trained more specifically about how to approach CAM communication to achieve particular goals. Future research could continue to usefully examine chronic illnesses, such as cancer in which CAM is often used, and focus on how patients use CAM alongside biomedical treatments. Additionally, future research can examine where in clinical encounters physicians should ask about CAM use, such as immediately after asking about regularly used medications, and how to best word those questions so patients understand the question as asking about CAM separate from – and in addition to – pharmaceutical treatment modalities. Asking about CAM immediately after other medications may help to reinforce the idea that CAM is treatment. As a corollary, patients may also be trained about how to communicate about CAM in a way that helps them use CAM communication to explain their health beliefs and preferences for treatment decision-making. While providers may try to engage the conversation as one about safety, patients can also affect those conversations to remind providers about why they are using other treatment modalities.

Third, scant research has examined CAM communication outside the context of physicians and patients. Future research should investigate CAM interaction with allied health professionals such as pharmacists, nurses, social workers, nutritionists, or health educators. While pharmacists may participate the most actively with patients about issues of drug/CAM safety, nurses, social workers, and health educators may be better trained to discuss CAM as a matter of patient health beliefs and preferences.

While research on CAM communication has been prolific, most has focused on measuring how often patients disclose CAM use and the barriers to that disclosure. To this extent, the notion of communication in these studies is primitive and focused mainly on disclosure rather than discussion. Most research treats patient CAM disclosure as a discrete event that occurs only one time, such as when a physician asks, 'Have you ever used CAM?' In this way, communication is deemed 'successful' merely because it occurred.

Providers often underestimate the numbers of their patients who use CAM, and both patients and providers have reasons not to talk about CAM: patients may anticipate a negative provider reaction; providers may not feel they have the knowledge or evidence to have a useful conversation about CAM as evidence-based; or one or both parties may view CAM talk as irrelevant to the biomedical visit. However, studies analyzing the actual conversations of patients and providers around CAM show that the communicative event is complex and both providers and patients play different roles and have different goals in discussing CAM. With more people integrating CAM and biomedicine, interactionally sensitive examinations of these conversations can provide empirically based suggestions for how these conversations can best occur to strengthen the therapeutic alliance between providers and patients. With better knowledge about when CAM talk occurs, how it is interactionally negotiated, and what role it serves within the clinical visit, researchers can then provide specific suggestions for how to improve CAM talk with the ultimate goal to improve global health outcomes.

Related topics

Complementary medicine; alternative medicine; holistic medicine; integrative medicine; provider–patient interaction; treatment decision-making; discourse analysis.

Further reading

Ho, E.Y., D'Agostino, T.A., Yadegar, V., Burke, A., and Bylund, C.L. (2012) 'Teaching patients how to talk with biomedical providers about their complementary and alternative medicine use', *Patient Education and Counseling,* 89(3): 405–410.

Juraskova, I., Hegedus, L., Butow, P., Smith, A., and Schofield, P. (2010) 'Discussing complementary therapy use with early-stage breast cancer patients: exploring the communication gap', *Integrative Cancer Therapies,* 9: 168–176.

Koenig, C.J., Ho, E.Y., Yadegar, V., and Tarn, D.M. (2012) 'Negotiating complementary and alternative medicine use in primary care visits with older patients', *Patient Education and Counseling,* 89(3): 368–373.

Schofield, P.E., Juraskova, I., and Butow, P.N. (2003) 'How oncologists discuss complementary therapy use with their patients: an audio-tape audit', *Supportive Care in Cancer,* 11: 348–355.

Shelley, B.M., Sussman, A.L., Williams, R.L., Segal, A.R., and Crabtree, B.F. (2009) '"They don't ask me so I don't tell them": patient–clinician communication about traditional, complementary, and alternative medicine', *Annals of Family Medicine,* 7: 139–147.

References

Adler, S.R., Wrubel, J., Hughes, E., and Beinfield, H. (2009) 'Patients' interactions with physicians and complementary and alternative medicine practitioners: older women with breast cancer and self-managed health care', *Integrative Cancer Therapies,* 8: 63–70.

Barnes, P.M., Bloom, B., and Nahin, R.L. (2008) 'Complementary and alternative medicine use among adults and children: United States, 2007', CDC National Health Statistics Report no. 12. Hyattsville, MD: National Center for Health Statistics.

Busse, J.W., Heaton, G., Wu, P., Wilson, K.R., and Mills, E.J. (2005) 'Disclosure of natural product use to primary care physicians: a cross-sectional survey of naturopathic clinic attendees', *Mayo Clinical Proceedings,* 80: 616–623.

Chang, H.Y., Wallis, M., and Tiralongo, E. (2011) 'Use of complementary and alternative medicine among people with type 2 diabetes in Taiwan: a cross-sectional survey', *Evidence-based Complementary and Alternative Medicine*, Article ID 983792.

Chao, M.T., Wade, C., and Kronenberg, F. (2008) 'Disclosure of complementary and alternative medicine to conventional medical providers: variation by race/ethnicity and type of CAM', *Journal of the National Medical Association,* 100: 1341–1349.

Corbin Winslow, L. and Shapiro, H. (2002) 'Physicians want education about complementary and alternative medicine to enhance communication with their patients', *Archives of Internal Medicine,* 162: 1176–1181.

Eisenberg, D.M., Kessler, R.C., Foster, C., Norlock, F.E., Calkins, D.R., and Delbanco, T.L. (1993) 'Unconventional medicine in the United States – prevalence, costs, and patterns of use', *New England Journal of Medicine,* 328: 246–252.

Engdal, S., Steinsbekk, A., Klepp, O., and Nilsen, O.G. (2008) 'Herbal use among cancer patients during palliative or curative chemotherapy treatment in Norway', *Supportive Care in Cancer,* 16: 763–769.

Ho, E.Y., D'Agostino, T.A., Yadegar, V., Burke, A., and Bylund, C.L. (2012) 'Teaching patients how to talk with biomedical providers about their complementary and alternative medicine use', *Patient Education and Counseling,* 89(3): 405–410.

Howell, L., Kochhar, K., Saywell, R., Zollinger, T., Koehler, J., Mandzuk, C., et al. (2006) 'Use of herbal remedies by Hispanic patients: Do they inform their physician?', *Journal of the American Board of Family Medicine,* 19: 566–578.

Humpel, N. and Jones, S.C. (2006) 'Gaining insight into the what, why and where of complementary and alternative medicine use by cancer patients and survivors', *European Journal of Cancer Care,* 15: 362–368.

Janamian, T., O'Rourke, P., Myers, S.P., and Eastwood, H. (2011) 'Information resource needs and preference of Queensland general practitioners on complementary medicines: result of a needs assessment', *Evidence-Based Complementary and Alternative Medicine,* Article ID 810908.

Jefferson, G. (2004) 'Glossary of transcript symbols with an introduction', in G.H. Lerner (ed.) *Conversation Analysis: Studies from the First Generation*, Philadelphia, PA: John Benjamins.

Juraskova, I., Hegedus, L., Butow, P., Smith, A., and Schofield, P. (2010) 'Discussing complementary therapy use with early-stage breast cancer patients: exploring the communication gap', *Integrative Cancer Therapies*, 9: 168–176.

Kennedy, J., Wang, C.C., and Wu, C.H. (2008) 'Patient disclosure about herb and supplement use among adults in the US', *Evidence-Based Complementary and Alternative Medicine*, 5: 451–456.

Koenig, C.J., Ho, E.Y., Yadegar, V., and Tarn, D.M. (2012) 'Negotiating complementary and alternative medicine use in primary care visits with older patients', *Patient Education and Counseling*, 89(3): 368–373.

Liu, C., Yang, Y., Gange, S.J., Weber, K., Sharp, G.B., Wilson, T.E., et al. (2009) 'Disclosure of complementary and alternative medicine use to health care providers among HIV-infected women', *AIDS Patient Care STDS*, 23: 965–971.

Mak, J.C.S., Mak, L.Y.H., Shen, Q., and Faux, S. (2009) 'Perceptions and attitudes of rehabilitation medicine physicians on complementary and alternative medicine in Australia', *Internal Medicine Journal*, 39: 164–169.

Mao, J.J., Palmer, C.S., Healy, K.E., Desai, K., and Amsterdam, J. (2011) 'Complementary and alternative medicine use among cancer survivors: a population-based study', *Journal of Cancer Survivorship*, 5: 8–17.

NCCAM, AARP. (2007) 'Complementary and alternative medicine: what people 50 and older are using and discussing with their physicians', National Center for Complementary and Alternative Medicine and American Association of Retired Persons.

——(2011) 'Complementary and alternative medicine: what people aged 50 and older discuss with their health care providers', National Center for Complementary and Alternative Medicine and American Association of Retired Persons.

O'Keefe, M. and Coat, S. (2010) 'Increasing health-care options: the perspectives of parents who use complementary and alternative medicines', *Journal of Paediatrics and Child Health*, 46: 296–300.

Perlman, A.I., Eisenberg, D.M., and Panush, R.S. (1999) 'Talking with patients about alternative and complementary medicine', *Rheumatic Disease Clinics of North America*, 25: 815–822.

Richardson, M.A., Masse, L.C., Nanny, K., and Sanders, C. (2004) 'Discrepant views of oncologists and cancer patients on complementary/alternative medicine', *Support Care Cancer*, 12: 797–804.

Roberts, C.S., Baker, F., Hann, D., Runfola, J., Witt, C., Mcdonald, J., et al. (2005) 'Patient–physician communication regarding use of complementary therapies during cancer treatment', *Journal of Psychosocial Oncology*, 23: 35–60.

Robinson, A. and McGrail, M.R. (2004) 'Disclosure of CAM use to medical practitioners: a review of qualitative and quantitative studies', *Complementary Therapies in Medicine*, 12: 90–98.

Schofield, P.E., Juraskova, I., and Butow, P.N. (2003) 'How oncologists discuss complementary therapy use with their patients: an audio-tape audit', *Supportive Care in Cancer*, 11: 348–355.

Shelley, B.M., Sussman, A.L., Williams, R.L., Segal, A.R., and Crabtree, B.F. (2009) '"They don't ask me so I don't tell them": patient–clinician communication about traditional, complementary, and alternative medicine', *Annals of Family Medicine*, 7: 139–147.

Sleath, B., Rubin, R.H., Campbell, W., Gwyther, L., and Clark, T. (2001) 'Ethnicity and physician–older patient communication about alternative therapies', *Journal of Alternative and Complementary Medicine*, 7: 329–335.

Sleath, B., Callahan, L., Devellis, R.F., and Sloane, P.D. (2005) 'Patients' perceptions of primary care physicians' participatory decision-making style and communication about complementary and alternative medicine for arthritis', *Journal of Alternative and Complementary Medicine*, 11: 449–453.

Staples, J.K., Wilson, A.T., Pierce, B., and Gordon, J.S. (2007) 'Effectiveness of CancerGuides®: a study of an integrative cancer care training program for health professionals', *Integrative Cancer Therapies*, 6: 14–24.

Tasaki, K., Maskarinec, G., Shumay, D.M., Tatsumura, Y., and Kakai, H. (2002) 'Communication between physicians and cancer patients about complementary and alternative medicine: exploring patients' perspectives', *Psycho-Oncology*, 11: 212–220.

Wahner-Roedler, D.L., Vincent, A., Elkin, P.L., Loehrer, L.L., Cha, S.S., and Bauer, B.A. (2006) 'Physicians' attitudes toward complementary and alternative medicine and their knowledge of specific therapies: a survey at an academic medical center', *eCAM*, 3: 495–501.

Yates, J.S., Mustian, K., Morrow, G.R., Gillies, L.J., Padmanaban, D., Atkins, J.N., et al. (2005) 'Prevalence of complementary and alternative medicine use in cancer patients during treatment', *Supportive Care in Cancer,* 13: 806–811.

Young, L.A., Faurot, K.R., and Gaylord, S.A. (2009) 'Use of and communication about dietary supplements among hospitalized patients', *Journal of General Internal Medicine,* 24: 366–369.

Zhang, A.L., Xue, C.C.L., Lin, V., and Story, D.F. (2007) 'Complementary and alternative medicine use by older Australians', *Annals of the New York Academy of Sciences*, 1114: 204–215.

Appendix 31.1: Transcription symbols

DOC:/PAT:	Speaker identifications are for physician (DOC) and patient (PAT).
[overlap]	Square brackets indicate onset and offset of overlapping talk.
=	Equal signs indicate utterances are run together with no gap of silence.
-	Hyphens indicate a preceding sound is cut off or self-interrupted.
°word°	Degree signs indicate decreased volume relative to surrounding talk.
(0.8)	Numbers in parentheses measure silences in seconds, tenths of a second.
(.)	Parenthesis with period indicates a micropause, less than 2/10s of a second.
wo:rd	Colons represent prolongation or stretching of the preceding sound.
word.	Periods represent falling or turn-final intonation contours.
word,	Commas represent continuing or turn-continuative intonation contours.
word¿	Inverted question marks represent intonation rising higher than comma.
word?	Question marks represent rising intonation contours.
word	Underlining represents emphasis relative to surrounding talk.
<slow>	Less than–greater than symbols indicate decreased pace.
>fast<	Greater than–less than symbols indicate increased pace.
.hh	Period followed by h's indicate in-breaths; the more h's, the longer.
hh	H's alone indicate out-breaths or laughter; the more h's, the longer.
wo(h)rd	Single parenthesis filled with h's indicate breathy delivery of talk.
(word)	Single parenthesis filled indicates transcriptionist doubt.
((word))	Double parenthesis filled indicates transcriber's description or characterization of some event.

32

Negotiation of health, illness, and treatment in Korean Oriental medical discourse[1]

Ki-tae Kim

Introduction

Sociolinguistic studies of medical discourse have explored what is negotiated in the interaction between medical professionals or healthcare providers and their patients. The majority of these insightful studies have focused on interactions in what medical anthropologists identify as biomedicine, with only minimal attention being paid to other medical systems such as complementary and alternative medicine (CAM; see Chapter 31) and enthnomedicines. Such a modernistic take on medicine has unfortunately resulted in uncritically assuming the purported biomedical notions of health and causes of illness, and has not ventured beyond such notions as germs, genes, and lifestyles. They, in turn, have ended up neglecting interactions in systems other than those between the orthodox professional physicians and their patients in biomedicine.

According to Singer and Baer's (2007: 108) evolutionary view of illness theories and healing systems, however, such a take is disproportionately limiting even in modern industrial societies, let alone in medically postmodern societies. For excluded from consideration are the interactions of 'heterodox professional physicians' from 'professionalized heterodox medical systems' (e.g., Ayurvedic medicine in South Asia and traditional Chinese medicine such as herbal medicine and acupuncture in the People's Republic of China) (Baer et al. 2003: 10) with their patients (as well as those of religious, folk, and other healers) and their notions of health and causes of illness.[2] In light of some medical anthropologists' view of biomedicine as 'the predominant ethnomedicine in modern societies' (Singer and Baer 2007: 114–120) and hence only one of many medical practices, then, research on biomedical interaction sheds inadequate light on the negotiations of medical beliefs and practices in other medical communities, where other medicines coexist with the orthodox biomedicine as heterodox or additional medicines, be they legitimate or illegitimate. Then, the biomedical notions of health and etiology implicitly assumed or explicitly negotiated in biomedical interaction cannot be so readily transferred to non-biomedical interactions under a plural medical system.

Such is the situation where medicines in the Republic of Korea currently stand. The medical system is legally dual, biomedicine and Korean Oriental medicine (hereafter, KOM) constituting two legitimate medical service providers.[3] As the notions of health and illness in the two, nonetheless, are fundamentally divergent and not unquestionably transferrable, those negotiated and explored in biomedical interaction shed little light on the parallels in Korean Oriental medical discourse (henceforth, KOM discourse) or those of any other medical systems.[4]

Noting this gap in previous studies, this chapter will examine the discursive construction of the basic notions of health and etiology in KOM discourse. To do so, the next section will introduce KOM as the professionalized heterodox medicine vis-à-vis the orthodox biomedicine. The subsequent section will describe the data for this study: naturally occurring consultations between two KOM doctors and their patients. Sample analysis will investigate how the participants in KOM discourse, specifically the doctors, negotiate their medical beliefs and practices in KOM pathology and recuperation under the principle of moderation based on the other three foundational principles. The final section will summarize the findings and discuss the implications for future studies.

Historical background: KOM as the heterodox medicine

Oriental medicine in Korea was 'the dominant discourse' (Gee 1992) or 'the standard language' (Fairclough 1989: 56–58) of medicine in Korea from antiquity and, in fact, the only legitimate medical authority in the country until the arrival of Western biomedicine in the late eighteenth century (Baker 2003; KNKOMA 2009; Na 2012). Firmly based on the naturalistic Taoistic Traditional Chinese Medicine (TCM) (*han.uyhak*, 漢醫學), yet integrating Indian and Arabic Oriental medicines, KOM gradually developed its own identity (KNKOMA 2009), however. In particular, Ceyma I (1837–1900) integrated the neo-Confucian humanism into medicine and proposed the *Sasang* Constitutional or Four-Constitution Medicine when he published *Longevity and Life Preservation in Eastern Medicine* (東醫壽世保元) in 1894 (Baker 2003; Chae 2003; Kim, C. 2001: 153).[5] This new type of Oriental medicine, which has since characterized (if not been equated with) KOM, differentiates itself from others not only because of the four congenital, biophysical, psychosocial, and reactional constitutions that it posits, but also because of its emphasis on the human management and control over them according to one's own constitution.[6] In short, Oriental medicine in Korea has historical legitimacy over biomedicine because of its incomparably longer history.

Despite the fact that the advent of Western biomedicine and the Japanese occupation of Korea and subsequent oppression of Oriental medicine drove it to the brink of extinction in the early nineteenth century (KNKOMA 2009), KOM has bounced back and secured legal legitimacy comparable to that of biomedicine in Korea. For example, Oriental doctors must go through the same rigor of a six-year medical training as their biomedical counterparts do, and hence, are legally authorized *uylyoin*s 'medical specialists' under the Korean Medical Law, just as biomedical doctors and dentists are (Medical Law of Korea Ch. 1, Article 2).[7] The replacement of *han* (漢) 'Chinese' in *han.uyhak* (漢醫學) with the homophonous *han* (韓) 'Korean' in 1986 even further corroborated its legal legitimacy as *the Korean* Oriental medicine (Medical Law of Korea, Appendix 3825; Na 2012: 48).

As much as KOM is legally recognized as *one of the two* medical authorities in Korea, then, its legal status is fundamentally different from that of what is variously known as *herb medicine, irregular medical system,* or *unorthodox medicine* in other countries (the last two terms from Singer and Baer 2007: 128).[8] If biomedicine in Korea is the orthodox medicine in the aforementioned modernistic sense of medicine, the contemporary KOM, then, functions as the heterodox medicine. Nonetheless, little attention has been paid to how anatomy, physiology, and pathology in such heterodox medicines are negotiated and constructed, and that is what this study illuminates.

Description of KOM interactions examined

The particular consultations explored in the next section come from approximately 15 hours of naturally occurring conversations between Oriental doctors and their patients. The researcher, with the consent of the doctors and the patients, participant-observed and tape-recorded them over the summer of 2001 at two hospitals in one of the metropolitan areas in Korea.[9] One of them was a large general hospital that had a much more prominent and larger biomedical ward, which was lexically *un*marked, than the Oriental ward, which was lexically prefaced with *hanpang* (韓方) 'Korean Oriental Medicine'. Dr. Song, who alone participated in the study at the Oriental ward, appears in the analysis below.[10] The other institution was a medium-sized hospital that specialized in integrative (in)fertility and, hence, also had a biomedical ward. However, since the hospital itself was renowned for its Oriental approach, the Oriental ward, which nonetheless was lexically prefaced with *hanpang* (韓方), was more prominent than the biomedical ward, which was prefaced with *yangpang* (洋方) 'Western medicine'.[11] Out of a few doctors who participated in the study, Dr. Cho features in the analysis below. More details about these doctors and the patients who appear in this study are presented in Tables 32.1 and 32.2.[12]

Sample analysis: negotiation of pathology and recuperation in KOM interactions

This section explores the discursive manifestations of the pathology and recuperation in KOM.[13] More specifically, it focuses on the discursive construction of the principle of moderation among the four basic principles of KOM. To this end, however, it first lays a theoretical foundation by briefly highlighting the key anatomical and physiological notions

Table 32.1 Participating Oriental doctors

Code	*Dr's name*	*Dr's sex*	*Dr's age*	*Type of institution and specializations*
N	Dr. Song	Male	40s	Large general hospital, with both medicines; Dr. Song's official specialization is Oriental neuropsychiatry.
CE	Dr. Cho	Male	30s	Medium-sized hospital with both medicines that focuses on Oriental infertility and a few other Oriental specializations; Dr. Cho is an Oriental internist.

Table 32.2 Participating patients

Dr's name	*Pt's name*	*Pt's stated condition*
Dr. Song	Mr. Kim	Backache; diarrhea; eczema; chronic fatigue; cold sensation
	Ms. Kwen	Pain in the breasts
Dr. Cho	Ms. Hwang	Severe fatigue
	Ms. Lee	Fatigue; much less severe earache and eye strains than in the previous session
	Ms. Se	Fatigue; irregular menstruation; swelling (due to prescription medication)

in the other three principles (i.e., the affairs–mind–body–objects principle, the heaven–human–nature–order principle, and the principle of constitutionally different congenital formation of organs). It then turns to the principle of moderation to illustrate how illness and recovery are negotiated in KOM.[14]

Basic anatomy and physiology in anthropocultural and holistic KOM

First, KOM anatomy and physiology are humanistic and anthropocultural and stipulated by the heaven–human–nature–order principle, which places the basic anatomical units in close association with the psychological, ethical, sociological, and (meta)physical constructs. Such associations are formed according to the overarching affairs–mind–body–objects principle, which 'classifies all affairs and objects of humans, society, and the universe into four types' (AKOM 2000).[15] Accordingly, KOM places more emphasis on one's effort and practice on the psychosocial factors within each given constitution in maintaining one's health. Lee, U. (1997: 438) schematizes such anthropocultural harmonism as shown in Table 32.3.[16]

In reading Table 32.3 and the sample interactions later, one must remember that KOM sees the human body (and relevant biophysical and psychosocial factors) as consisting of the four main organ *groups*:[18] the lung, pancreas, liver, and kidney groups. As Table 32.4 demonstrates, each organ group, frequently referred to as the representative organs alone without the word 'group', is a unit of several closely associated individual organs from the anatomical perspective of contemporary biomedicine.[19]

The anatomical perspective of KOM leads us to the principle of constitutionally different congenital formation of organs. KOM sees people born with different functional strengths in the four main organ groups, according to which one falls into one of the four constitutions: a *Thayyangin*, a *Soyangin*, a *Thayumin*, or a *Soumin*, as Table 32.5 summarizes.

Table 32.3 Body parts from the anthropocultural perspective under the heaven–human–nature–order principle

Heaven[17]	Celestial Time	Society	Ethics	The Earth
	(Ears)	(Eyes)	(Nose)	(Mouth)
Human	Duty/Task	Social Life	Public Reliance	Residence
	(Lungs)	(Pancreas)	(Liver)	(Kidneys)
Nature (of Human)	Tactics	Management	Self-examination of one's behavior	Magnanimity
	(Chin/Jaw)	(Chest)	(Naval)	(Abdomen)
Order (of Human)	Discernment	Dignity	Skills/Talents	Method/ Scheme
	(Head)	(Shoulders)	(Waist)	(Hips/buttocks)

Source: Based on Lee, U. (1997: 440); my translations.

Table 32.4 Organ groups in *Sasang* Constitutional Medicine and the corresponding anatomical organs in biomedicine

	Lung Group (upper quarter)	**Pancreas Group** (upper middle quarter)	**Liver Group** (lower middle quarter)	**Kidney Group** (lower quarter)
Representative Organs	lungs	pancreas	liver	kidney
Other Organs in the Group	esophagus, tongue, ear, brain, skin	stomach, breast, eye, spine, muscle	small intestine, navel, nose, waist, subcutaneous tissue	large intestine, genitals, mouth, bladder, bones

Source: Based on Chong (2001).

Table 32.5 General features of the four *Sasang* constitutions and the functionality of each organ group

	Thayyangin	*Soyangin*	*Thayumin*	*Soumin*
Nature	Sorrow	Anger	Gladness (Joy)	Enjoyment (Pleasure)
Developed organ (Strong organ)	Lung	Spleen	Liver	Kidney
Underdeveloped organ (Weak organ)	Liver	Kidney	Lung	Spleen
Character (Psychosocial traits)*	Creative Positive Progressive Charismatic Heroic Rash mind	Unstable Easily get bored Sacrificing Righteous Easily acceptable Hot tempered Anxious mind	Gentle Commercial Endurable Humorous Look foolish Coward Fearful mind	Neat, mild Negative Intelligent Organized Selfish Jealous Persistent Nervous mind
Body shape (Physique)	Developed nape of the neck, Slender waist	Developed chest, Small hips	Thick waist, weak nape of the neck	Developed hip, weak chest
Healthy sign	Urination	Bowel movement	Perspiration	Digestion
Unhealthy sign	Bubbles in mouth, emesis	Constipation	No perspiration	Indigestion

Source: Chae et al. (2003: 521); parentheses indicate the terms used in this chapter.

* See Chae et al. (2004) for further information about personality types in *Sasang* Constitutional Medicine.

Note that the congenital strengths and weaknesses of each organ group in each constitution do not imply that one constitution is bound to be congenitally healthier or stronger than the others, but suggest that every constitution is imperfect and imbalanced in one way or another.

Since the principle basically states that all the constitutions are partially imperfect, it is essential in understanding KOM interactions; the issue, then, is how imbalanced a person of any constitution becomes and how one restores the constitutional equilibrium. The KOM anatomy and physiology introduced so far leads us to the principle of moderation, under which the discursive construction of KOM pathology and recuperation will be explored.

The principle of moderation to restore the broken constitutional equilibrium

This section explores how KOM views one's healthy state as a constitutionally stable equilibrium, an unhealthy state as a constitutionally unstable imbalance and recuperation as a return to the stable balance. After first introducing the notions of health in KOM, this section examines the participants' negotiation of how one becomes ill by going off the healthy equilibrium toward the Axis of Illness and, subsequently, how one recuperates from an unhealthy condition by healing and moving oneself toward the Axis of Health under the principle of moderation. For the notions of constitutional health, pathology, and recuperation, initial theoretical explorations are followed by sample analyses.

Notions of health in KOM: constitutionally stable equilibrium

Table 32.5 implicates that no one is perfect with optimally balanced organ groups and that such congenital imbalance is considered normal in KOM. Then aren't all of us doomed to be ill from the beginning?

This leads us to a brief introduction to pathology in KOM. The reason one gets ill is traced back to the degree of the imbalance at a given time, not to one's congenital constitutional strengths and weaknesses. Chong (2001) represents such a pathologic view through the diagram in Figure 32.1 and offers the following explanation:

> This organ imbalance is regarded as being completely normal because it is from birth and constitution. However, if a person somehow becomes ill, as shown in [Figure 32.1], the angle of the axis of imbalance is broken and becomes more acute. The more serious the illness, the more acute the angle becomes. But if adequate treatment is performed, the angle reverts to its original slope and the illness is cured. That is the so-called pathological viewpoint of constitution[al] medicine.

In other words, the congenital imbalance in the functionality of the organ groups itself (represented as the solid line in Figure 32.1) is not a health threat in any of the four constitutions

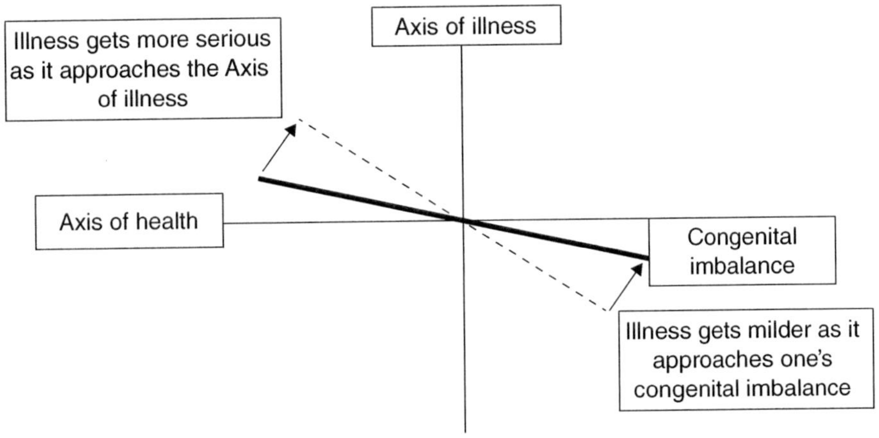

Figure 32.1 Organ imbalance

Source: Chong (2001: http://www.koreanmedicine.org/english/lecture-03.html); my translations in the illustration.

although each imbalance indicates that a person of the constitution is *prone* to certain constitutional symptoms (*Cheycil pyengcungs*). In a sense, therefore, the congenital imbalance itself is construed as a balance or at least a stable imbalance. Now that we have discussed the genotypic constitutional imbalance, let's examine an excerpt where it emerges in an unfolding interaction.

Excerpt 1 demonstrates that the congenital equilibrium of a female patient (Ms. Lee) is negotiated in an actual interaction. Dr. Cho states that the patient's body has the constitutional (im)balance (line 98) that consists of the cold interior and the hot exterior (lines 95 and 97):[20]

Excerpt 1

95 D: → Your interior is cold
96 P: Is it?/
97 D: → Yes your interior is cold your exterior is hot
98 → since you have such, such balance in your body
99 you should always warm your body [CE]

Now, the distribution of heat, warmth, cool, and cold in the interior and exterior of each constitution in relation to the functional strengths of the organ groups is beyond the scope of this chapter. What is important in this excerpt is that the doctor describes the thermal distribution as her congenital constitutional 'balance' (line 98), which is a stable imbalance to be precise.

Going off the healthy equilibrium toward the Axis of Illness: basic KOM pathology

If for some reason, one tips the balance off toward the Axis of Illness, one starts to develop warning signs or unhealthy signs (*Taypyeng*). If the imbalance gets more acutely away from the congenital imbalance, then one starts to show symptoms that raise red flags (*Cwungpyeng*) or develop grave illnesses. All of these scalar symptoms are constitution-specific, but the pathologic principle is the same across all the four constitutions.

Such a pathological approach to illness frequently emerges in two patterns in the data for the current study. In the first type, the doctor points out that the patient is out of balance (equilibrium) for one reason or another. In the second, the doctor discusses one or more of the scalar symptoms either as a current condition or as a prognosis. Let's examine these two types through Excerpts 2 and 3 respectively.

Excerpt 2 is a segment from one long interaction primarily because this is Ms. Hwang's first encounter with Dr. Cho, and consequently, prior to the excerpt, he was posing a full range of questions (including the patient's facial complexion and sweating pattern in the sauna) to identify her constitution and the source of her complaints. Based on them, he states that her body is out of balance (lines 366 and 367). Put more precisely, his diagnosis contends that the patient is out of her congenital constitutional (im)balance off toward the Axis of Illness. He then explicates the gradual and accumulative progress of her conditions (lines 370 through 373) and provides a couple of examples of the aggravating factors such as stress and overwork (lines 375 through 378), which he links to her current conditions (i.e., listlessness and vertigo in line 374). He argues that none of her organs is in an abnormally bad condition (lines 379 through 381),[21] but that the combination of all the damaging factors has accumulated to knock her overall equilibrium off (line 382) and disrupted her metabolic rhythm (line 390), resulting in the broken balance in her system (line 392):

Excerpt 2

366 D: → But your bodily condition itself now
367 → is way out of balance now
368 P: Right
369 (??) Probably due to overwork
370 D: Then now sort of the things that have piled up up to now,
371 In other words now your body is um slowly um
372 Now even though the symptom itself appears now
373 it is the things that have piled up so far that start
to manifest themselves now
374 Put in easier terms, now you feel listless and dizzy
375 Symptoms like these, are reflections of your so far, for example
376 say, the stress you have piled up in your life
377 or the fact that you are devoted to work without even exercising now
378 such combination of factors all has led the symptoms to appear
379 it's not specifically that you are um, as I pointed out earlier um,
380 it's not like it's because your liver is bad or because your stomach is bad
381 It's not like that:
382 → Rather it is because your overall balance in the body is broken
383 P: OK
...
390 D: Such um metabolism, or say
such rhythm itself is not working well, so
391 P: Right
392 D: → Uh it's because the balance is broken.
393 P: Right
394 D: Therefore for now I think you need to get some treatment [CE]

Notice that Dr. Cho repeatedly points to Ms. Hwang's disrupted balance as a source of her complaints (lines 367, 382, and 392). He detects no particular organ group of hers in trouble, but yet the diagnosis that her overall balance is shaken helps him suggest tentative treatment options. The treatment suggestions are partly in order to start undoing the damage and partly in order to check the compatibility between her constitution that he has tentatively identified and the medications he prescribes.

Now that we have explored an interaction where the doctor's diagnosis points to a balance off the normal limit of the patient's constitution, we turn to the other type, where the doctor gives scalar, or proportionally aggravating, symptoms as the overall balance or the balance of the patient's organ group gets closer to the Axis of Illness. Such a scalar prognosis may be prevalent in all medical interactions, but what is important in a KOM prognosis is that it is not a prognosis of one particular illness but that of a spectrum of various unhealthy signs in each constitution. Thus, this section attempts to tie an excerpt in which such a scalar symptomatic prognosis is made to the KOM pathology introduced above. In no part of Excerpt 3 do the words 'balance' or 'imbalance' explicitly appear, yet the proportionality in the doctor's prognosis presupposes a more and more acutely unbalanced state from the patient's congenital (im)balance.[22]

Leading up to Excerpt 3, Dr. Song explicated the KOM organ group theory to Mr. Kim, whose main complaint is a backache. The doctor repeats the patient's condition in line 137 (after taking the patient's pulse prior to the excerpt). After a few more questions, he diagnoses the source of the patient's backache as the functionally weak kidney group (lines 148 and 149). Now, before we get to the detailed symptoms Dr. Song enumerates, notice the scalar prognoses he gives in lines 152, 160, and 164 (marked with ⇒). Line 152 indicates that if the problem resulting from the weak kidney group goes untreated, it leads to the next-level symptoms. Moreover, line 160 lists even further deteriorating symptoms now that it is 'serious' at this level. The symptoms that he enumerates are increasingly aggravating signs of proportionally deteriorating health conditions. In other words, the symptoms he lists indicate that Mr. Kim is approaching the Illness Axis. Finally, the pathologic view of the scalar departure from the Axis of Health towards the Axis of Illness is deictically encapsulated in Dr. Song's line 164, where he describes such an aggravating process as that of *–lo kakey* 'going towards' the worst conditions away from the constitutional equilibrium:

Excerpt 3

137 D: → You said you had a backache?
138 _Then um_ Do you sweat in the **armpits**?
139 P: Of course.
140 D: You do:.=
141 P: =Yes.
142 D: Does it hurt (up: and down)?\
143 P: Yes (??)
144–147 [Unintelligible]
148 D: → That's because your **kidneys** are weak?
→ Your pulse shows that the kidneys are weak.
149 → You are short of the *yang* energy {=sexual stamina}
→ and /, | sweat in the armpits/, say-
150 P: |(???)
151 D: (Next) um,
152 ⇒ If thi:s condition continues
→ you are likely to get quickly tired and quickly languid~,
153 P: So chronic fatigue:|,
154 D: |exactly, exactly
155 → Then- you may hear things in the ears or ~,
156 P: _Right_
157 D: → (You may yawn more frequently) um~, uh um then-,
158 → You may feel weak on the legs or,
159 → You may not- feel relieved {=refreshed} when you urinate: or,
160 ⇒ if it is serious, um when you are young um: uh,,
161 → it's called *yuceng~*,
162 P: _Right_
163 D: → now your semen may come out when you urinate or
164 ⇒ (You _end up going_) toward such conditions
ilen sangthaylo (ka_key toypnita_).
Be this-ATT condition-towards go-become-E
...
171 D: → Um you may develop prostate problems:~,
172 → You frequently urinate [2 secs] [N]

Now, let's examine the worsening symptoms from the pathologic view of KOM. Since the kidney group includes the reproductive organs and the urinary system, a weak performance in the kidney group entails low sexual energy (line 149) and sweaty armpits (lines 138 and 149) at the lowest threat level. If these mild conditions continue to persist with no treatment, the unbalanced axis gets closer to the Axis of Illness and worse symptoms such as general fatigue (line 152), hallucinatory noise in the ears (line 155), frequent yawning (line 157), weak lower body (line 158), and little sense of relief even after urination (line 159) are prone to develop. If the axis gets even closer to the Axis of Illness and much farther away from the congenitally stable imbalance, then even more 'serious' symptoms such as *yuceng* or involuntary seminal release into urine (lines 160 through 164) and prostate problems (line 171) are likely to trouble the patient along with frequent urination (line 172).

To summarize, unlike Excerpt 2 where Dr. Cho straightforwardly states that the patient is out of her constitutional balance, Dr. Song in Excerpt 3 provides scalar prognoses based on the patient's constitutionally weak organ group. Nonetheless, the scalar prognosis itself, along with the distal deictic verb (i.e., 'going towards such conditions') that means tilting away from the congenitally stable imbalance, illustrates that both excerpts discursively project the pathologic view of KOM presented in Figure 32.1.

Now that we have examined the interactions where the KOM pathologic view is negotiated, let's explore how undoing such damage is portrayed and how such a principle empowers the patient in KOM discourse.

Returning to healthy equilibrium toward the Axis of Health: the principle of moderation and the patient's agency for recuperation

Since the pathologic view of KOM postulates that one's health deteriorates as one drifts away from the Axis of Health through one's congenital imbalance towards the Axis of Illness, the basic goal of all KOM treatments aims to undo the damage and help the patient return to his or her healthy constitutional equilibrium. This endeavor, reinforced by the patient's personal constant monitoring of him or herself as well as the doctor's prescriptions, is called the principle of *CwungYong* 'moderation'.[23] Song explicates:

> The ultimate goal of SCM [*Sasang* Constitutional Medicine] is to view the constitution using the philosophy of the 'Golden mean' or 'Middle Path' and to guide the inherently tilted prenatal body to 'center' by postnatal efforts. This is the fundamental treatment principle of SCM as well as its method of health cultivation, which varies according to each constitution. It can be accomplished through the proper regulation of the physical body and with environmental adaptations. Moreover, SCM tries to teach people to maintain harmony with all things while maintaining a balance of body and mind.
>
> *(Song 2005: vi)*

In its narrow sense, the principle aims to counterbalance the tilted axis in order to revert to the Axis of Health. In its broad sense, however, the principle not only lays the foundation for treatment by facilitating the patient's return to the Axis of Health and undoing damage, but also emphasizes more general self-improvement and self-control not to go to extremes in almost all aspects of his or her life, including but not limited to biophysical and psychosocial factors as well as environmental and reactional factors such as chemical (e.g., medications, food, etc.) and physical ones (e.g., temperature, exercise, etc.).

Such a restorative goal under the principle is overtly negotiated in an interaction between Dr. Cho and Ms. Se, from which Excerpt 4 is taken. Among the female patient's three main complaints, fatigue (line 1101) and no menstruation (lines 1150 through 1166, particularly 1153 and 1154) have started to improve with the help of the medications Dr. Cho prescribed for her in the preceding sessions, whereas swelling has not (line 1102). Dr. Cho expressly states that the improvements are the signs of her body restoring its balance (lines 1103 and 1165). Furthermore, he argues (lines 1148 and 1149) that rectifying the disruption in balance, which turns out to have been effective, has been his treatment goal ever since she walked into his office for the first time (line 1146) and he diagnosed her problem not as an isolated condition in an organ but as an overall disruption in the equilibrium (lines 1141 to 1147). Finally, in response to her apprehension about the loss of the efficacy of the treatment when she goes off the prescription medication (lines 1151 to 1162), Dr. Cho assures her of a continuing restorative effect upon her menstrual cycle once the equilibrium in her body is restored (lines 1163 to 1166).

Excerpt 4
1101 D: Your fatigue has improved somewhat but,
1102 if your swelling and things like that improve
1103 → it means that the balance in your body itself starts to restore
...
1141 P: There doesn't seem to be any other part that is particularly bad,
1142 D: Mm
1143 P: I don't think so @@
1144 D: There isn't any. Now, |when you came in in your first visit
1145 P: |Just
1146 D: As I said when you came in in your first visit
1147 it's not that you've got one **specific** part that is bad but
1148 → the overall balance in your body is considerably disrupted
1149 → so I told you last time that we needed to correct it
1150 and your menstruation
1151 P: |That's what worries me
1152 D: |Mm
1153 You had the period, didn't you?
{lit: Your menstruation came out, didn't it}
1154 P: But
1155 D: Mm
1156 P: I was told that
1157 Um, it comes out when you take a medication
1158 D: Mm
1159 P: but in the next period it won't come out again | say
1160 D: | Mm
1161 There is a story {=rumor} like that, isn't there?
1162 P: @@ Yes, people
1163 D: Mm
1164 That's the problem {we are going to address}
1165 → Therefore, once we put your body in balance
1166 it'll come out in the next month and continue to do so [CE]

Consequently, this interaction illustrates that Dr. Cho's original treatment regimen was specifically chosen to address the disturbed balance in the patient, which he identified as the etiology to the patient's three complaints in the prior consultations. Although he makes no explicit reference to the principle itself, this interaction demonstrates that it is called into negotiation when the doctor and the patient have trouble identifying a recognizable deviance in an isolated organ, as both the participants expressly state in lines 1141 through 1148.

The interaction above illustrates that the principle operates on the biophysical factors in tandem with the reactional factors (e.g., medications), but does it also work on the psychosocial level as Song (2005) points out in the quote above? The psychosocial aspect of the principle is more fully delineated by the Association of Korean Oriental Medicine (AKOM 2000) as follows:

> The last principle is **moderation**(中庸). This means that human beings should be in the state of equilibrium [and] equanimity without fluctuation of anger, sorrow, joy and pleasure in nature and emotion without inclinations in the mind, and should be in the state of health that controls the ascents and the descents of up–down, unfasten and fasten of the interior–exterior, based on different congenital formation of the organs. In SCM [*Sasang* Constitutional Medicine], the human being can be healthy in the state of emotional moderation, physical moderation, and social life moderation. So each constitution presents its own emotional condition, physical condition and social condition in order to preserve good health. SCM has a characteristic of self-control medicine through self-control mechanism of physiology and pathology of the human body, and self-control can be obtained through efforts to polish your knowledge and deeds in real life.[24]
>
> *(http://www.koma.or.kr/eng/theory/t1_2.htm; original bold)*

Notice that the treatment goal in KOM incorporates a wide range of areas in order to restore not only one's physical equilibrium but also psychosocial equanimity. Hence, treatment is not limited to prescriptions given by the doctor, just as the identification of the patient's constitution does not solely rely on his or her biophysical and reactional factors. Equally important, if not more, are the psychosocial factors that are interdependent on them, and in so doing, the patient's own effort at restoring the equilibrium and equanimity. In other words, the principle of moderation places heavy emphasis on the patient's enhanced self-awareness and effort at self-control through abstinence, behavior modification, and mental discipline to counterbalance the tilted axis. In this sense, therefore, the principle is an empowering and existential concept that places the patient him or herself at the center of his or her own restoration.

The emphasis of the principle on the patient's own contribution to equilibrium and equanimity often blurs the boundary between what is internal medicine and what is psychological counseling or therapy. Excerpt 5 is taken from an interaction in which Dr. Song relies on the principle in order to help Ms. Kwen, whose main complaints lie in the pain in the chest, restore her equanimity as well as physical equilibrium. He eventually traces the source of her problem back to the social pressure upon her to bear a son (not presented here) and the accompanying physical damage on the liver (line 380). He explains that her anger has damaged the liver (lines 376 to 380), which is the source of her pain in the chest (lines 382 and 383). The treatment options he offers include stretching (lines 387 to 388), talking it out (line 390), and reading a sad novel for catharsis (line 392) because the descending energy of catharsis from reading a sad novel evens out the ascending energy of anger (lines 397 through 400).[25]

Excerpt 5

376 D: → |Therefore, your **anger** explodes/ you become **combative**.
377 Um the- the- then/,
378 If you **win** in the fight/,
379 Then you become a winner. If you **lose**/,
380 → you liver gets struck/
381 P: |@
382 D: |Therefore in other words,
383 That's because you've got the illness
384 P: @@
385 D: _Therefore_,
386 P: @@
387 D: → **This** um the- medi- to let go/ in order to let the stress go~/
388 → Do some stretching,
389 Or say um,
390 → Talk it out~
391 Now you can let it go like that:~
392 → Um- for catharsis m- read a sad novel or.
393 P: ,,_aha:::::~!_| [faintly]
394 D: → If you read a sad- sad novel, _it calms down.
395 → Strangely|-
396 P: |Really?
397 D: → Yes. Since {anger} is **ascending**|energy,
398 P: |Aha:::! @@@|@
399 D: → | **Descending** energy
400 → is sad|ness. If there is a sad event, it quickly dies out.[26]
401 P: |_Aha::::~!_| [faintly]
402 D: → There are such things in that respect/, mental things/?
403 P: @@
404 D: Anyway for now that's that. Let's try these prescriptions in this manner. [N]

After putting his psychosocial treatment suggestions on the table, Dr. Song sums up the discussion with a note on the mental aspects (in Ms. Kwen's illness or in KOM in general) in line 402, and goes back to the medicine-proper area of prescriptions in lines 404. Note that these suggestions are psychosocial areas that the patient herself has to work on in order to restore the equilibrium in her body and emotion, highlighting the role of the patient herself in the treatment process. The doctor gives her a prescription, but it is the patient herself who must work on the psychosocial source of her condition by actively intervening in her own life and taking a restorative and recuperative action such as reading a sad novel.

This section has explored the negotiation of the principle of moderation as a key concept in treatment considerations in KOM. To do so, the section first introduced basic pathology in KOM as a loss of one's constitutional equilibrium and subsequently demonstrated that Oriental doctors argued that the patients must restore the broken stability through the principle of moderation, which emphasizes the patient's active role in regaining the equilibrium by controlling all the elements that KOM pays attention to (particularly the psychosocial factors).

Summary and future directions

This chapter has thus far examined the negotiation of KOM pathology and recuperation under the principle of moderation in addition to the other three theoretical principles that highlighted KOM's anthropocultural anatomy and physiology. To repeat, the principle of moderation introduced the basic pathology and treatment in constitutional Oriental medicine as 'going off one's constitutional equilibrium' and the treatment process as 'restoring the equilibrium' through one's control of the balance (i.e., moderation) of biophysical, psychosocial, and reactional elements. In so doing, it also demonstrated that notions grown out of neo-Confucian humanism beyond the Taoist naturalism of Traditional Chinese Medicine laid the foundation of KOM and had a strong influence on the treatment suggestions by emphasizing the role of the patient, in rebalancing her or his broken constitutional equilibrium and equanimity.

As we have seen, the negotiation of health, illness, and treatment in KOM as the professionalized heterodox medicine in Korea illustrates certain features that are distinct from these negotiations in biomedicine as the orthodox medicine. Thus, more fine-grained research needs to be launched on what beliefs and practices are negotiated and in what manner in medicines other than biomedicine.

The findings also demonstrate that beliefs and assumptions in plural national medical systems that participants bring with them into medical interactions cannot be presumed to be always the same as those in biomedicine and thus suggest that more cross-medical understanding across various health systems be facilitated among healthcare professionals and patients. This is because differences in medical beliefs certainly raise the possibility of confusion, misunderstanding, non-compliance, or even distrust when such fundamental notions as health, illness, and treatment as well as those of the body and mind are incongruent among healthcare professionals and their patients. The Oriental doctors who participated in the current study frequently juxtaposed an introduction to KOM with a briefer version to biomedicine, possibly because of biomedical dominance even in the context where both are legal equivalents. However, they did not do that all the time, and one can only speculate how many biomedical doctors would be willing to negotiate Oriental medical beliefs and assumptions with their patients in order to improve patient compliance, let alone those in other non-professionalized medical systems. As contemporary 'state societies manifest the coexistence of an array of medical systems, or a pattern of *medical pluralism*' unlike 'simple preindustrial societies' (Baer et al. 2003: 9; original emphasis) and the resultant medically different voices or 'heteroglossia' (Bahktin 1984), such negotiation in medical encounters may be much more crucial for patient compliance than biomedical communities (or any medical communities for that matter) currently estimate.

Finally, attention to what beliefs and practices are negotiated in what manner in medicines other than biomedicine and how they intersect with orthodox biomedical interactions is imperative for effective cross-cultural medical services in multicultural societies. First, patients are more and more medically informed from multicultural sources as the world has become more and more borderless thanks to advances in communication technology and transportation. Second, a formerly homogeneous society such as Korea has become rapidly multicultural, and medical interactions in such societies are becoming increasingly more cross-medical (albeit not so overtly) as well as cross-cultural. In spite of the cross-cultural interface of various medical systems, investigations of cross-medical interactions do not appear to get the attention they deserve. The perceived universality of biomedicine and biomedical dominance seems to lead to a mistaken belief in the singular medical voice that has effectively muted out all the other medical voices. As this chapter demonstrated, we cannot assume that all participants bring with them into medical consultations only biomedical approaches to health and illness, and such an overly wishful assumption in a cross-medical interaction is likely to result in mismatches in their communication. Thus, more studies are certainly in order on how orthodox medical professionals and patients with heterodox or ethnomedical beliefs interact in multicultural societies and how participants in integrative medicine in such societies negotiate such incongruent beliefs and incompatible practices.

Related topics

Korean Oriental medical discourse; post-structuralist discourse analysis; critical medical anthropology; interactional sociolinguistics; complementary and alternative medicine (CAM).

Notes

1 This chapter is a substantially updated yet vastly reduced version based on one of the researcher's previous studies (2006). Refer to the full study for further background information and analyses of naturally occurring interactions.
2 In the case of the US medical system, Baer et al. (2003: 335) classify 'chiropractic, naturopathy, and acupuncture' as 'professionalized heterodox medical systems' and 'homeopathy, rolfing, and reflexology' as 'partially professionalized or lay heterodox medical systems'.
3 See next section for the historical background of KOM.
4 Such a dichotomous approach is certainly modernistic, as the post-modernistic take emphasizes 'emotions interacting with body' and 'return to humor theories in some medical subsystems', and 'integrate[s] orthodox and heterodox modalities' (Singer and Baer 2007: 108). This chapter, nevertheless, purposefully attempts to be modernistic for the sake of clarity and brevity.
5 Ceyma I is more commonly spelled as Je-Ma Lee (KOMS 2005; Baker 2003) or Che-ma I (KNKOMA 2009), but this study spells Korean according to the Yale Romanization Scheme (e.g., Nam 2005).
6 Kim and Huh (2005) state, '*Sasang* Constitutional Medicine (SCM) is one of only five minority medicines officially recognized by the Chinese government. The others are Mongolian, Tibetan, Uygur, and Vietnamese medicines.' Also, the Korean Oriental doctors who participated in this study are trained in, and as such, adopt SCM.
7 Furthermore, if they complete a one-year internship and a three-year residency, they can be licensed as specialist doctors in one of the eight specializations (Medical Law of Korea Ch. 6, Article 55; Presidential Edict 16616), just as biomedical specialists can as otorhinolaryngologists, ophthalmologists and so forth.
8 In this sense, the dual medical authority in Korea is a good example of 'plural national medical systems' (Singer and Baer 2007: 144) that critical medical anthropologists argue for.
9 All the participants spoke Korean, but the sample interactions below are translated into English. No morpheme-by-morpheme gloss for Korean accompanies the semi-free English translations except for one occasion in Excerpt 3, partly due to its irrelevance to this chapter and partly due to spatial constraints.
10 All the names of the participants in this study are pseudonyms. Also, the participants were told that it was simply to investigate how they 'talk' and that it would be best if they would carry on their usual business since the research agenda was hoped to emerge out of the interactions themselves.
11 The Oriental doctors wore white gowns just like biomedical doctors. The researcher in normal clothes made a visual observation of the interactions as a participant, seated in a triangular position facing the doctor and the patient, and taking notes of the participants' body movement and eye gaze as well as their dialogues. The tape-recorder with a built-in microphone was pouched in a black protective cover and placed on the doctor's desk.
12 This study centers on the talk of the participating Oriental doctors, especially on their 'clinical reasoning' (Durning et al. 2011) or 'medical diagnostic reasoning' (Cicourel 1987). The reason is

that the sample interactions are situated at the deep end of the technical frame (Goffman 1974, 1981; Kim, K.-t. 2006) that they create with the notion of *cheycil* 'constitution' in KOM, and thus the patient's contribution in this realm is limited although not impossible.

13 A full introduction to the theoretical principles as Ceyma I, the original proponent of *Sasang* Constitutional Medicine that characterizes much of contemporary KOM, initially suggested, is too daunting a task to accomplish in this short chapter. Interested readers may refer to Song (2005).

14 It is helpful to go over working propositions developed for laypeople's understanding of KOM. Among the several, yet comparable versions of the proposed working axioms, Song's (2002: 39–70; 2005: 3–17; my translations) five axioms below, which center on the principle of constitutionally different congenital formation of organs, are the most widely known:

Axiom 1: One's physique and appearance varies depending on one's constitution.
Axiom 2: A different constitution results in a different psychology.
Axiom 3: A different constitution results in differently appropriate and inappropriate foods to eat.
Axiom 4: A medication that does not match one's constitution is a poison.
Axiom 5: The diseases one is susceptible to vary according to one's constitution, as do the treatment options.

15 Thus, for example, the human body consists of four four-part interlinked systems – the Ears–Eyes–Nose–Mouth group, the Lungs–Pancreas–Liver–Kidneys group, the Chin–Chest–Naval–Abdomen group, the Head–Shoulders–Waist–Hips group – and each group has its associated traits projected in the universe, in the society, and the constitution. Ceyma I applied this overarching system to many categories such as emotions, personalities, weaknesses, and so forth, and even the four constitutions themselves are based on this principle.

16 Chong (2001) and Lee, U. (1997) argue that the four-state classificatory system itself is a significant departure from that of Traditional Chinese Medicine that consists of *yin–yang* and the five constructs (commonly known as 'phases') of wood, fire, earth, metal, and water. Lee, C. (2003) also sees the four-part system strongly influenced by Confucian philosophy rather than Taoist philosophy.

17 Kim, S.B. (1998) argues that Heaven and Human govern one's external world, whereas Nature and Order one's internal world and that Ceyma I places more emphasis on the latter two, for their control is the driving force in controlling one's psychosocial and in turn, biophysical equilibrium.

18 The *four* representative organs (excluding the heart, which is included in the anatomy in Traditional Chinese Medicine) fall under the aforementioned affairs–mind–body–objects principle.

19 In this sense, each group is more of a functional unit than an anatomical entity.

20 In its full version of the interaction from which Excerpt 1 was taken, the participants negotiate constitutionally compatible exercises for Ms. Lee. See Kim, K.-t. 2006: section 4.3.3.

21 Once again, organ *groups* to be precise.

22 Before we put a magnifying glass on Excerpt 3, it must be pointed out that the scalar prognoses in the data for the current study subsume two different patterns. In the first, the doctor discusses the patient's constitutionally aggravated symptoms and ties them to the functionally weak organ of the given constitution. In the second, the doctor focuses on the proportional aggravation of the functionally weak organ group itself without overtly associating it with the overall constitution, ending up in a more local prognosis. Nevertheless, the functionally weak organ group itself is based on the patient's identified constitution, so even without the doctor's explicit reference to the patient's constitution (i.e., as in the second type), the association is always assumed. Excerpt 3 exemplifies the second type.

23 中庸 in Chinese is also spelled as *ZhongYong* or *ChungYung* in the Chinese Romanization. *CwungYong,* literally 'the middle path', originally refers to the eponymous book commonly translated as *The Doctrine of the Mean*, one of the four Confucian scriptures, but also denotes the golden mean to remain impartial and balanced in Confucian philosophy. Being a neo-Confucian scholar, Ceyma I integrated the concept into his constitutional medicine as the main principle of treatment. However, doctors such as Kim, C.-A. (1996) who are trained only in Traditional Chinese Medicine points out that the principle is vague and underspecified.

24 The principle postulates many other important philosophical foundations than merely the treatment principle, which unfortunately are beyond the scope of this chapter. For example, as Song's description as well as that of the AKOM (2000) demonstrates, it defeats not only the mind–body dualism but also the apparent determinism in each prenatal, congenital, or genetically determined constitution by emphasizing limited, but significant self-control over one's given traits. Such a stress

on the humanistic self-improvement over naturalistic biological determinism in KOM originates from its neo-Confucian background, as pointed out previously.

25 This excerpt highlights the difference between the pathology of KOM and that of Traditional Chinese Medicine. The concept of maintaining balance has been in the latter (as well as in ancient Greco-Roman medicine) for thousands of years, but the principle of moderation in KOM is different from the idea of maintaining balance in Traditional Chinese Medicine, which sees the excess or deficiency of the *ki* (*qi* or 'vital energy') as a source of a disease (Song 2005: 107) without paying close attention to the interdependence of the organs and the emotions. KOM, in contrast, describes the organs and emotions in terms of interconnected upward or downward movement of energy rather than excess or deficiency of it. Song (2005: 107) states:

> The emotions of anger and sorrow cause physical excitement and make one's energy rise upward. Joy and pleasure will initially create emotional excitement but will later bring a person to a relaxed state. Both joy and anger cause excitement but the type of excitement is different. Excitement from joy cools quickly and drops downward, while excitement from anger does not.
>
> Joy and pleasure cause *qi* to drop downward while anger and sorrow cause *qi* to rise. The Lungs and Spleen hold the *qi* of anger and sorrow while the Kidneys and the Liver hold the *qi* of joy and pleasure. These emotions are connected to the ascending and descending energies of the internal organs.

Consequently, the vertical movements of the energy in the doctor's description reflect the principle of moderation in KOM, not that in Traditional Chinese Medicine.

26 The doctor's literal claim in lines 393 and 400 about the descending energy of sadness (or sorrow) does not work out entirely against Song's (2005: 107) explanations in the previous note, for Song states that sorrow is an ascending energy. Although it is entirely possible for the doctor to make a slip of the tongue or be mistaken or even misinformed, a more cautious reading, taking into account his argument in lines 392 and 394, shows that his 'descending energy of sadness' may refer to the descending energy of the cathartic cooling aftermath after reading a sad novel. In other words, even though sorrow itself as a static feeling is an ascending energy, the rebounding repercussion after feeling sad may be a descending energy.

Further reading

Baker, D. (2003) 'Oriental medicine in Korea.' In H. Selin (ed.) *Medicine across Cultures: History and Practice of Medicine in Non-Western Cultures* (pp. 133–153), New York: Kluwer.

Chae, H. (2003) 'Sasang typology', <http://www.chaelab.org/SasangTypology.htm> (last accessed 1 March 2011).

Kim, K.-t. (2006) 'Discourse of Oriental medicine', unpublished doctoral dissertation, Georgetown University, Washington, DC.

Na, S. (2012) 'East Asian medicine in South Korea', *Harvard Asia Quarterly*, 14(4): 44–56.

Song, I.-b. (2005) *An Introduction to* Sasang *Constitutional Medicine*, trans. J.K. Kim and M.-h. Huh, Edison, NJ: Jimoondang International.

References

AKOM. (2000) The English homepage of the Association of Korean Oriental Medicine <http://www.koma.or.kr> (accessed 3 February 2002; the English homepage is down as of 1 March 2011).

Baer, H.A., Singer, M., and Susser, I. (2003) *Medical Anthropology and the World System*, 2nd edn, Westport, CT: Praeger.

Baker, D. (2003) 'Oriental medicine in Korea.' In H. Selin (ed.) *Medicine across Cultures: History and Practice of Medicine in Non-Western Cultures* (pp. 133–153), New York: Kluwer.

Bakhtin, M.M. (1984) *Problems of Dostoevsky's Poetics*, trans. M. Holquist (ed.), Minneapolis, MN: University of Minnesota Press.

Chae, H. (2003) 'Sasang typology', <http://www.chaelab.org/SasangTypology.htm> (last accessed 1 March 2011).

Chae, H., Lyoo, I.K., Lee, S.J., Cho, S., Bae, H., Hong, M., and Shin, M. (2003) 'An alternative way to individualized medicine: psychological and physical traits of *Sasang* typology', *Journal of Alternative and Complementary Medicine*, 9(4): 519–528.

Chae, H., Park, S.H., Lee, S.J., and Koh, K.C. (2004) '*Sasang* typology from a personality perspective', *Journal of Korean Oriental Medicine*, 25(2): 151–164.

Chong, W. (2001) 'Constitutional medicine', <http://www.koreanmedicine.org/english> (last accessed 1 March 2011).

Cicourel, A.V. (1987) 'Cognitive and organizational aspects of medical diagnostic reasoning', *Discourse Processes*, 10(4): 347–367.

Durning, S., Artino, A.R. Jr, Pangaro, L, van der Vleuten, C.P., and Schuwirth, L. (2011) 'Context and clinical reasoning: understanding the perspective of the expert's voice', *Medical Education*, 45: 927–938.

Fairclough, N. (1989) *Language and Power*, New York: Longman.

Gee, J.P. (1992) *The Social Mind: Language, Ideology, and Social Practice*, New York: Bergin & Garvey.

Goffman, E.G. (1974) *Frame Analysis: An Essay on the Organization of Experience*, New York: Harper & Row.

Goffman, E.G. (1981) *Forms of Talk*, Philadelphia, PA: University of Pennsylvania Press.

Kim, C.-A. (1996) *Hanuyhak Ettehkye Hal Kesinka*? [How to Do Oriental Medicine?], Seoul, Korea: Thaywung Chwulphansa.

Kim, C. (2001) 'Sasang cheycilul almyen kenkangi pointa [You see health if you learn *Sasang* constitiutions]'. In *Yangpangi Cwuketo Mos Ttalaonun Hanpang pikyel* [*Oriental Medical Secrets that Western Medicine Cannot Compete with]*, a special issue to *New Dong-A* [*Sintonga*], 2001(1): 152–189.

Kim, J.K. and Huh, M.-h. (2005) Translators' Notes to I.-b. Song, *An Introduction to* Sasang *Constitutional Medicine*, Edison, NJ: Jimoondang International.

Kim, K.-t. (2006) 'Discourse of Oriental medicine', unpublished doctoral dissertation, Georgetown University, Washington, DC.

Kim, S.B. (1998) '*Sasanguyhakuy chelhakcek paykyeng* [Philosophical background of *Sasang* Medicine', < http://www.wooree.com/sasang_index.htm> (last accessed 1 March 2011).

KNKOMA. (2009) The English homepage of the KangNam-gu Oriental Medicine Association. <http://knkoma.or.kr/eng/> (accessed 12 June 2009; the English homepage is down as of 1 March 2013).

KOMS. (2005) 'Sasang-constitutional-medicine', Available at the English home page of Korean Oriental Medical Society <http://intl.koms.or.kr/04/03.php> (last accessed 1 March 2011).

Lee, C. (2003) *Sasang Chelhak: Momuy Chelhak Maumuy Kenkang* [*Sasang* Philosophy: Philosophy for the Body, Health of the Mind], Seoul, Korea: Chaykseysang.

Lee, U. (1997) 'Sasang Uyhakuy chelhakcek paykyeng [Philosophical background of Sasang Medicine]', *Ceysamuyhak [Hyungok Journal of Korean Medicine]*, 2(2): 435–443.

Na, S. (2012) 'East Asian medicine in South Korea', *Harvard Asia Quarterly*, 14(4): 44–56.

Nam, K.-S. (2005) *Modern Korean Syntax*, trans. S.-H. Lee and A. Boldgett, Seoul, Korea: Thaehaksa.

Singer, M. and Baer, H. (2007) *Introducing Medical Anthropology: A Discipline in Action*, Lanham, MD: AltaMira.

Song, I.-b. (2002) *Manhwalo Ponun Sasang Uyhak* [Learning Thayyangin Ceyma I's Sasang Medicine through Cartoons]. Cartoons by K. Kim, Seoul, Korea: Doosan Dong-a.

——(2005) *An Introduction to Sasang Constitutional Medicine*, trans. J.K. Kim and M.-h. Huh, Edison, NJ: Jimoondang International.

Korean laws cited

Medical Law
Medical Law Appendix 3825
Presidential Edict 16616

Appendix 32.1: Keys to transcription

<table>
<tr><td>\</td><td>Falling intonation</td></tr>
<tr><td>/</td><td>Rising intonation</td></tr>
<tr><td>~</td><td>Fluctuating intonation</td></tr>
<tr><td>_</td><td>Low tone</td></tr>
<tr><td>-</td><td>Hesitation or self- or other-initiated interruption with glottal stops</td></tr>
<tr><td>:</td><td>Lengthened syllable</td></tr>
<tr><td>?</td><td>Questions (with rising intonation contour)</td></tr>
<tr><td>(??)</td><td>Unintelligible utterances</td></tr>
<tr><td>(X)</td><td>Utterance sounds like X but mostly unintelligible</td></tr>
<tr><td>,</td><td>Pause (about 0.5 seconds)</td></tr>
<tr><td>,,,,</td><td>The number of commas indicates the duration of pause
(e.g. ,,,, indicates a pause lasting two seconds).</td></tr>
<tr><td>@</td><td>Laughter (including giggle and chuckle)</td></tr>
<tr><td>Bold</td><td>Emphatic stress or loud and high-pitched expressions</td></tr>
<tr><td>Italics</td><td>1. Romanized Korean
2. Untranslatable Korean expressions in English translations.</td></tr>
<tr><td>{X}</td><td>X is a reconstructed expression in translation from Korean to English
(e.g., elliptical subject in Korean).</td></tr>
<tr><td>X{= Y}</td><td>Y is an alternative to translation X.</td></tr>
<tr><td>[ ]</td><td>Researcher's comments and notes (e.g., non-verbal behaviours, tape counters, etc.)</td></tr>
<tr><td>A: |X|
B: |Y|</td><td>X and Y overlap.</td></tr>
<tr><td>A: I ate it =
B: =ate it?</td><td>Utterances in quick succession which are continued without a pause by two different speakers</td></tr>
<tr><td>D</td><td>Doctor</td></tr>
<tr><td>P</td><td>Patient</td></tr>
</table>

33

Midwives' communicative expertise in obstetric ultrasound encounters

Srikant Sarangi and Heidi Gilstad

Introduction

This chapter offers, from an activity analysis perspective, an account of professional expertise in the context of obstetric ultrasound encounters. Obstetric ultrasound encounters are a complex activity which involves talk between midwives (or, sonographers) and pregnant women and their companions. Such talk is routinely mediated by the visual cues in the form of the image of the foetus projected on the monitor screen towards which the participants orient during talk. In a sense, the monitor takes on a participant role and contributes to the process and outcome of the encounter. This multi-party, multi-modal activity system is typical of computer-mediated healthcare delivery. In an earlier study, Greatbatch et al. (1993) draw attention to how the computer is embedded in and coordinated with interaction between doctors and patients in primary care. They show how patients produce unsolicited turns to raise topics and concerns and how doctors provide minimal or delayed responses or abruptly shift topic, always mediated through gaze and continuation of keystrokes. More recently, Swinglehurst (2011) identifies a 'dilemma of attention' on the doctors' part when they use electronic patient records (EPR) in the primary care setting.

The use of technology in the clinical space transforms the mechanics of interaction. In our study setting concerning pregnancy care, the presence of the ultrasound technology mediates the clinical activity of the midwives. In what follows, we first begin with a brief description of routine pregnancy care, a discussion of different layers of professional expertise in the healthcare setting, followed by a review of relevant literature. We then introduce the data setting and the activity analytical framework before undertaking a micro-level analysis of the interactional data in terms of overlaying discourse types (online commentary, offline commentary, and metacommentary) vis-à-vis the key themes of normality and reassurance. The following research questions will guide our analysis:

1 How is midwifery communicative expertise manifest interactionally when examining the foetus with the help of ultrasound technology?
2 How are normality and reassurance articulated and negotiated during the physical examination phase of the ultrasound encounter?

Medicalization of pregnancy care and the ultrasound examination

Most healthcare systems in the Western world offer routine ultrasound check-up. The purpose of the ultrasound examination in the first trimester in pregnancy (11–16 weeks) is to: establish the date of pregnancy; determine the number of foetuses and identify placental structures; diagnose an ectopic pregnancy or miscarriage; examine the uterus and other pelvic anatomy; and, in some cases, at this early stage, detect foetal abnormalities. The ultrasound examination in the second trimester in pregnancy (18–28 weeks) is targeted at: confirming pregnancy date and monitor foetal growth; examining the placental structures; assisting in prenatal tests such as an amniocentesis; and examining the foetal anatomy for presence of abnormalities. Most babies are born healthy, but pregnant women's need for reassurance arises because prenatal testing underpins doubts in the first place (Rothman 1988; Rapp 2000).

There are two broad framings attempted in the ultrasound setting – medical and social – although the social frame remains subservient to the medical gaze which may be regarded, from a Foucauldian perspective, as increasing medicalization of human life (Foucault 1973). In medical terms, ultrasound technology makes visible the foetus and its uterine environment, allowing for assessment of foetal normality/abnormality. In social terms, ultrasound technology constitutes a meaningful 'social ritual' for parents to see and meet their babies (Draper 2002; Mitchell 2004). As Kuba (1995) observes, the use of ultrasound technology to obtain reassurance that the foetus is healthy is 'incredibly seductive'. Parents tend to exercise their rights via screening choices in order to seek information relevant to foetal health (Pilnick 2004; Pilnick et al. 2004). Several interview-based studies have explored the experiences of pregnant women concerning prenatal screening (Abramsky and Chapple 1994; Clement 1998) and suggest that pregnant women engage in family building, gender talk, while remaining anxious about foetal health (Harpel 2003, 2008). Our point of departure in this chapter, unlike the previous studies focusing on the experience of pregnant women, is the communicative expertise of the midwife to normalize and reassure the mother as manifest in the contingent interpretation of the foetal images generated via the ultrasound technology. We first provide a general overview of what constitutes professional expertise and within it locate the midwife's communicative expertise.

The constituents of professional expertise

With regard to the medical profession, Freidson (1970) suggests that professional expertise is constituted in a combination of scientific/technical knowledge and clinical/experiential knowledge. Sarangi (2010a), from a discourse-analytic perspective, sees these knowledge systems as interactive and cumulative, thus giving rise to an array of expert interaction systems in functionally specific ways. The additional components of this 'expertise mix', Sarangi argues, are technological knowledge (i.e., interface with expert systems) and the institutional/organizational ethos in which professional activities are embedded. Much of this expert knowledge (scientific, experiential, technological, and organizational) is discernible in the interactional/communicative level in terms of systematic history taking, diagnostic reasoning, use of evidence, offer of causal explanations, etc.

According to De Cossart and Fish (2005), medical expertise consists of propositional knowledge and procedural knowledge – both these types of knowledge fall within scientific/technical knowledge in Freidson's (1970) sense. Midwives' propositional knowledge, for instance, is manifest in the interpretation of the registered values in the medical health records and the interpretation of the visual images on the ultrasound screen. The procedural/technical knowledge of midwives is manifest in the hands-on activity of palpation, and in the use of the transducer in order to get the correct layers with the ultrasound technology.

The notion of communicative expertise offers a meta-level frame to include these four types of knowledge/expertise. From our perspective, scientific knowledge includes procedural knowledge (e.g., application of gel and handling of the transducer during an ultrasound examination) and in this sense constitutes part of technological knowledge, which is perfected via experiential knowledge. In other words, as far as professional expertise is concerned, novice and experienced midwives may show differences in how the transducer is managed, to bring up clear images on the monitor and to interpret the anatomical features of the foetus while identifying any abnormalities. We may add that midwifery expertise is mediated by not only the ultrasound expert system but also by the prevailing socio-cultural and organizational ethos of an ultrasound encounter.

Obstetric ultrasound encounter as a complex expert interaction system

Healthcare communication (e.g., between midwives and pregnant women) can be seen as an expert interaction system (Sarangi 2010a) that embeds complex configurations of participant frameworks and different levels of professional expertise. Obstetric ultrasound encounters are particularly complex because of the inclusion of technology, as an expert system, which mediates the encounter in significant ways. As Shortliffe (1986) points out, the expert system is designed to capture and make available the cumulative knowledge of experts in the field. The midwife, as an expert interpreter of the visual images generated through ultrasound technology, can derive significant information about foetal well-being, far beyond the information that is available about the foetus without the visualizing technology. The scientific or propositional knowledge of the midwife is thus enhanced through the use of ultrasound technology, which assumes relevance for the prospective parents. It is quite conceivable that at the levels of interpretation and communication surrounding ultrasound technology, healthcare professionals such as physicians, midwives, sonographers, and radiographers may vary considerably. Pregnant women, as clients, may be ambivalent about the procedure in itself – experiencing it as both normal routine while remaining anxious about potential risks to the foetus as well as childbirth.

Relevant literature

Our review of literature is in two parts. Given our focus on the physical examination phase of the ultrasound encounter, we draw on relevant studies which address the physical examination phase in primary and tertiary healthcare settings. Empirical studies concerning ultrasound encounters are sparse; we therefore, in the second part, summarize discourse-analytic studies relating to pregnancy care, whether or not the encounter involves physical examination using the ultrasound technology.

In the context of primary care, Heath (1986) characterizes the physical examination phase of the medical consultation as a nonvocal activity, which may partly explain why this phase of the consultation has had little appeal for discourse/communication researchers. Heath's main interest is how the physical examination is accomplished through visual orientation. According to him, physical examination is also marked by contradictory demands:

> For the patient the concern is to attend and cooperate whilst remaining insensitive to much of the actual examination – the proddings, touching, and the like it may entail –

> whereas the doctor has specifically to examine parts of the body as an object yet maintain a concern for the patient as a person.
>
> *(Heath 1986: 100–101)*

Heath refers to what he calls 'middle-distance look' as a way of managing the contradiction present in the activity. As we will see, the ultrasound examination in the midwifery setting is far from nonvocal: it is constitutive of talk (especially, online commentaries, offline commentaries, and metacommentaries). Instead of the 'middle-distance look' parents are invited to join the midwife in seeing the image of the foetus on the monitor.

Heritage and Stivers (1999) distinguish between two kinds of online communication during physical examination in primary care settings: online explanations of medical procedures and online commentary – the latter referring to the communication behaviour of healthcare practitioners with regard to what they see or feel during the physical examination. Examples of online explanation are: 'let's check your sinuses and see how they look today'; 'hold your breath again'; 'can you open your mouth wide for me'. Examples of online commentary are: 'that's a little bit red back there'; 'there may be a little bit of lymph node swelling on this side compared to the other side'; 'I don't see any fluid'. According to Heritage and Stivers, online commentary can be characterized by four interactional features: (i) it is subordinate to the main activity of the examination and occurs while the physician is doing the physical examination or between the successive elements in the examination; (ii) it is usually a reporting of mild or absent signs of risk, and works as a reassurance to the patient (the absence of signs of risk is often modified with evidential formulations, through the use of verbs such as *see, feel, appear, seem*, or *hear*, which downgrade the claims (Chafe 1986)); (iii) it is presented either as reports of observations or as assessments of what is observed; and (iv) it is usually not addressed directly to the patient, and it is usually not responded to directly by the patient (the lack of response may be due to physical limitations, or due to the use of medical tools and expert systems that require a particular expertise to enable interpretation).

The above characterization conflates almost every dimension of talk that is characteristic of physical examination (see also Mangione-Smith et al. 2003). As we will see, in the ultrasound encounters, far from being a subordinate activity, the reporting of what is to be seen and what is seen are constantly upgraded with evaluative comments, metacomments, and invitations for joint seeing.

In his work in the primary care physical examination setting, Sarangi (2010b) draws a useful distinction between online commentary and offline commentary. Through the use of offline commentaries, 'the doctor steps outside the physical examination phase and offers explanations of various kinds' (Sarangi 2010b: 89; see Ragan 1995 for a parallel account in the context of obstetrical-gynaecological examination). The following are examples of offline commentary: 'children usually have this'; 'sometimes, with this kind of bronchitis in babies, because the airways are already tightening because babies are small and it swells up, we run into little problems with breathing'. The offline commentary generally serves an educational purpose for the patient and, in this sense, unlike online commentaries, is specifically targeted at the addressee. As Sarangi (2010b) suggests, the onset of offline commentaries can be mapped on to the two complementary roles that the doctor occupies in the medical consultation: the therapeutic role as the dispenser of treatment; and the pedagogic role as the educator of patients. In paediatric encounters, while educating the parents, the doctor also has to maintain his/her activity-specific discourse role of talking to the children, affectively and instructionally, as direct addressees rather than as overhearing audience (Tannen and Wallat

1993). In paediatric consultations, according to Sarangi (2010b: 90), 'both online commentaries and offline commentaries function rhetorically: the parent remains both the overhearing audience and the primary addressee in anticipation of future action plans'. On occasions, offline commentaries influence the decisional outcomes such as non-prescription of antibiotics for children.

What Heritage and Stivers (1999) refer to as online explanation of medical procedure can be better captured under the broad notion of metacommentary. Bateson (1972) suggests that we continuously interpret the situations we take part in with regard to verbal and nonverbal linguistic signals to see how these frame the activity (see also Goffman 1974 on frame and footing and Gumperz 1982 on contextualization cues). In their examination of paediatric consultations, Tannen and Wallat (1993) report how metacommunicative signals function as indicators of frame shifts. In the primary care setting, Heath (1986) shows how nonverbal cues serve a metacommunicative function in directing the patients what to do or about the status of their health. As Watzlawick et al. (1967: 53) observe: 'The ability to metacommunicate appropriately is not only the *condition sine qua non* of successful communication, but is intimately linked with the enormous problem of awareness of self and others.' As we will see in our analysis of ultrasound encounters, metacommentaries can either be prospectively or retrospectively framed in the organization of the physical examination phase of the consultation activity.

Among others, Måseide (2007, 2011) explores the distinctive medical examination phase involving bronchoscopy (pre- and post-examination phases) in thoracic wards. While the examination is instrumental and routine, involving collaborative teamwork (surgeons, nurses, radiographer, anaesthetist), he (2011) highlights the analytic themes of frame and footing shifts as moral tensions arise when the patient has to be attended to as both a physical object and as a social (lived) body – similar to what we have seen with Heath's (1986) observations earlier. Such tensions require the enactment of deference and demeanour strategies. Within the examination, the doctor refers to what is seen, and not to how it might be interpreted from the patient's perspective, thus reducing the patient's participation status and discursive rights – similar to what we may find in ultrasound encounters.

To summarize, three discourse types are relevant when analyzing communicative expertise in obstetric ultrasound: online commentary, offline commentary, and metacommentary. The occurrence of online commentary with or without assessment of 'normality' may be indicative of the routine reassurance procedure, which may be accompanied by minimal response tokens from the pregnant women.

In the context of preventive maternal care, Bredmar and Linell (1999) focus on how normality, as the organizing principle for understanding pregnancy, is managed in talk between midwives and expectant mothers. In specifically looking at symptom-exploring sequences and reporting of measurements and test results, they suggest that normality is manifest at two levels: (i) pregnancy in general is normal; and (ii) the individual woman's pregnancy is normal. With regard to reporting of measurements and test results, which is of relevance for our present purposes, such talk balances the conversational task of reassuring with the act of medical surveillance. On the one hand, the midwife transforms identifiable symptoms into normal physical responses and neutralizes unexpected deviations from the normal. On the other hand, she has to highlight any deviations and intervene as appropriate. In responding to expectant mothers' concerns about deviant values, midwives tend to extend the boundary of what constitutes the normal range. In an earlier study, Linell and Bredmar (1996) connect such topical sensitivity on the part of the midwives to facework. Two types of topic dominate the first scan encounter. The first topic relates to lifestyle (e.g., smoking, drinking, and sexually transmitted diseases) and the second concerns serious diseases and disabilities with strongly intimidating aspects (malformation of the foetus/baby). The interactional features range from pauses to reduction of topic prominence to deferral of topics to mitigating vocabulary, etc. In our data analysis, we will draw upon notions of normality as well as facework selectively.

Methodology and analytical framework

The present study derives from the doctoral project (Gilstad 2012) that constituted part of a large-scale Norwegian educational training programme in South Africa with the goal of developing propositional and procedural expertise of midwives. The data mainly comprise communication between three advanced midwives (who had undergone training through the educational programme at the Nelson Mandela School of Medicine in Durban) and 12 pregnant women. The obstetric ultrasound encounters (a total of 13) involving the three midwives – Nivedita (4 encounters), Nobuntu (3 encounters) and Nonkululeko (6 encounters which included a repeat consultation) – took place in three different hospitals in the rural areas of KwaZulu-Natal in South Africa. The duration of the encounters ranged between 12 to 55 minutes. One of the hospitals had a separate ultrasound room. The ultrasound encounters in the two other hospitals took place in a designated area of the maternity ward and the general ward respectively, only separated by curtains.

Prior to the observation of the ultrasound encounters, as part of our secondary data corpus, interviews with the cohort of advanced midwives who participated in the educational training programme led to the selection of the three midwives. These three midwives also regularly used the obstetric ultrasound technology as part of the scan encounters in the two years following their educational training. The three midwives agreed to be observed in their clinic settings and gave consent for video-recording.

The pregnant women attending the ultrasound clinic were approached prior to the clinical encounter with a request to participate in the present study. Of the 13 approached, 12 agreed to participate and signed the informed consent form (two of the pregnant women signed with a fingerprint). In one of the hospitals, the pregnant women were literate in English and Zulu. In the two other hospitals, the pregnant women were Zulu-speaking, but largely illiterate and came from rural areas with little or no English proficiency. Generally, the pregnant women spoke their mother tongue, Zulu, and although several of them understood English, the advanced midwives switched between English and Zulu. The talk in English in the video recordings was transcribed by the researcher, while the talk in Zulu was transcribed and translated by a professional Zulu translator.

It is worth adding that in addition to the advanced midwife and the pregnant woman, the Norwegian researcher, as part of the training evaluation protocol, was co-present in the clinic setting which led to the overuse of English for the benefit of the researcher and perhaps at the expense of the pregnant woman. There were occasions where the researcher explicitly prompted for English translations. This scenario made specific communicative demands on the midwives in terms of participation structure.[1]

The study was approved by the respective hospital administrations as well as by the Ethics Committee at the University in KwaZulu-Natal. The names of the pregnant women and the advanced midwives are anonymized in order to protect their confidentiality.

Our analytic approach derives from the theoretical notion of 'activity types', premised upon Wittgenstein's (1958) notion of language game. As Linell (2001: 236) points out:

> One crucial point [for Wittgenstein] was that linguistic actions are, by their very nature, embedded in more comprehensive wholes. Accordingly, an important argument for the concept of Activity Type, or language game, is that elementary utterances, communicative acts, cannot be fully understood without reference to this overarching concept.

Following Levinson (1979), the ultrasound encounter can be recognized as a distinctive activity type with constraints on structure and participation. The concept of 'hybrid activity type' (Sarangi 2000) applies to the ultrasound encounter under investigation because of its dual pedagogical and clinical framing, made particularly salient due to the co-presence of the researcher. The advanced midwives were trying to display their 'acquired' professional expertise through the educational training programme prior to the recording of their clinical activity. This became apparent in the ways in which they oriented to the researcher through their talk, especially marked in the switches from Zulu into English and vice versa throughout the encounter.

Based on the notion of activity type, Sarangi (2010a: 178) develops the framework of activity analysis which 'pays attention to the flexible nature of the relationship between form and content of a given encounter' (see also Sarangi 2010c). Of particular relevance in this chapter is the notion of 'discourse type'. According to Sarangi (2000), while activity type is a means of characterizing settings (e.g., a medical consultation, a service encounter, a university seminar), discourse type is a way of characterizing the forms of talk (e.g., medical history taking, promotional talk, interrogation, troubles telling, explanation, etc). In the analysis we pay specific attention to three discourse types already discussed: 'online commentary' (Heritage and Stivers 1999), 'offline commentary' (Sarangi 2010b), and 'metacommentary' (Bateson 1972). (See Appendix 33.1 at the end of this chapter for illustrative examples.)

Data analysis

Given that the ultrasound encounter has not been previously studied from a discourse-analytic perspective, it is useful to begin with the structural mapping (Sarangi 2010c) of this activity type in order to locate the physical examination phase. Our data corpus suggests that the obstetric ultrasound encounter is typically structured as follows: pre-examination phase,[2] physical examination phase, and post-examination phase, each with distinctive sub-phases (see Table 33.1). While the three key phases are consistently sequential, there is some level of variation at the level of sub-phases.

In terms of interactional mapping (Sarangi 2010c) of representative encounters across the three midwives, the physical examination phase routinely included the three discourse types – online commentaries, offline commentaries, and metacommentaries – with online commentaries and metacommentaries occupying more prominence than offline commentaries. It is to be acknowledged that the co-presence of the researcher and the pedagogic framing of the encounter will have contributed to the higher occurrence of metacommentaries.

The physical examination phase is a crucial component of the ultrasound encounter and is the focus of our analysis. In what follows we offer detailed analysis of two illustrative examples, both taken from the physical examination phase (Phase II), and organized along a cline of communicative complexity (see Appendix 33.2 for transcription conventions).

Table 33.1 The phase structure of the ultrasound encounter

Phase I		PRE-EXAMINATION
	Sub-phases:	
		Initial greeting Introduction of participants Informed consent
Phase II		PHYSICAL EXAMINATION
	Sub-phases:	
		Preparatory routine Examination of the maternal anatomy and the uterus Examination of the anatomy of the foetus Measurements
Phase III:		POST-EXAMINATION PHASE
	Sub-phases:	
		Talk about delivery Summary of findings Farewell

Example 1 (Nivedita – Salome)
As contextual background, Nivedita has an ultrasound machine that is not calibrated for measurements, and she is not able to provide the pregnant woman with the information she would like to. Nivedita therefore attempts to compensate for this technical deficit communicatively. The extract begins when she prepares the pregnant woman for the application of the gel to her abdomen.

Nivedita:
Ok. This is going to be a bit cold, but …
What I am gonna do is … I am gonna look at what's happening, and don't get
worried. As soon as I am ready, I will allow you to see as well. ((Puts gel on
the abdomen)) ((Somebody is talking in the background. CTG making noise))
((Concentrating in silence))
OK? ((Looking at Salome)) looking down on … the uterus. The top of the
uterus. That is what we are looking for, isn't it? Where the head is. ((Looking
back to the screen))
Yes. I am looking at the bottom now. ((Pointing at the screen)) And I can see
the head. And the bladder. That is what we were looking at. But I will show
you. ((Pointing at the screen)) ((Concentrating in silence)) ((Working with the
transducer on the abdomen))
((Looking at Salome)) Ok. What I was trying to do was to get an overview of
the whole foetus.
And what we saw was that the head was at the bottom. And the there was
water around the baby's head. And we saw the placenta was there.
Anterior … on the frontal wall. Anterior means frontal on the top of the
uterus. And normal placenta … placenta is afterbirth … it is normal for it to be
at the top ( ). Now we found that the placenta was there and there was
enough fluid and there was a live baby. And just general … how the baby is
situated in the presentation … presentation means where the head is.
In any pregnancy you ( ) exactly where the head is, but as the pregnancy

progresses, you want to see that the head is at the lower part of the uterus.
So that when you deliver if the baby comes out … if you have a normal
delivery, the head comes out first.

Salome:

Yeah.

Nivedita:

Cause any other position…can be difficult to deliver. We might have to ask
you to have a caesarean section. But we saw now that the head is ok.

The opening long turn, which appears as a monologue, is highly interactive because of Nivedita's task-orientation that includes the mediating role of the ultrasound technology. It is in two distinct parts – the first part (lines 1–12) focusing on the physical examination task itself and the second part (lines 13–25) offering an account of what has been seen and what needs explaining. Nivedita seems to move between online commentaries, offline commentaries, and metacommentaries with ease.

The preparatory sub-phase of physical examination is marked by 'this is going to be a bit cold' (line 1) – anticipating the application of gel to the abdomen which is delayed until after the metacommentary (lines 2–3). This metacommentary, which is framed prospectively, serves three functions: it explicates the physical examination activity; it offers some reassurance to Salome; and it anticipates Salome's active participation in the form of joint seeing.

As expected, the online commentaries co-occur with the physical activity of ultrasound examination, typically bounded by pointers to the screen, but not always including Salome in this seeing. The onset of the online commentaries marked by 'looking down on … the uterus' (line 6) is meant to follow the foetal anatomy – sequentially from top of the uterus to head to bottom to bladder, etc. Nivedita then uses a metacomment in a rhetorical question format – 'That is what we are looking for, isn't it? Where the head is' (line 7) – which is presumably targeted at the co-present researcher in orienting to the pedagogical frame of the activity, while signalling her relatively novice status in using ultrasound technology. This metacomment is followed by a further metacomment framed both retrospectively and prospectively, with Salome as the designated addressee: 'That is what we were looking at. But I will show you' (lines 10–11).

Unlike the first part, the second part of Nivedita's monologue is rich in talk, which is triggered by the boundary marker 'ok' (line 13). She turns to Salome with a retrospective metacommentary, documenting what has been seen so far: 'Ok. What I was trying to do was to get an overview of the whole foetus' (lines 13–14). Subsequently, she evaluates, in a summarizing manner, what she has observed: 'And what we saw was that the head was at the bottom. And the there was water around the baby's head. And we saw the placenta was there' (lines 15–16).

The rest of the second part is framed as offline commentaries, i.e., explanations marked by expressions such as 'X means'; 'if X then Y', etc. The first offline commentary concerns the anterior and the placenta (lines 17–19) which attempts normalization, combined with reassurance in the form of a retrospective metacommentary as evidence: 'we found that the placenta was there and there was enough fluid and there was a live baby' (lines 19–20). It is likely that this offline commentary is directed at both the pregnant woman and the researcher. The next offline commentary (lines 20–21) is offered in more general terms and concerns how the baby is situated in the presentation; what this means as the pregnancy progresses; and what the preferred positioning of the head is. The final offline commentary (lines 22–25) is also framed in general terms using the hypothetical construction: 'if you have a normal delivery, the head comes out first'. These offline commentaries, taken together, may be seen as having both educational and reassurance functions as far as the pregnant woman is concerned. But such offline commentaries are also likely to be targeted at the co-present researcher as part of displaying advance midwifery expertise within a pedagogical frame. This ambiguity in interpretation stems from the fact that what counts as an online-/offline-/meta-commentary is not simply a linguistic categorization but is heavily dependent on how the midwife orients – verbally and gesturally – to the hybrid activity type (with its pedagogical and clinical frames) and who the addressee is (whether it is the pregnant woman or the researcher). In other words, what may count as an offline commentary aimed at the pregnant woman may have been intended as a metacommentary for the attention of the researcher, depending on the use of linguistic jargons, pronominal address forms, and shifts in gaze. However, it is safe to argue that the offline commentaries such as the ones identified above can fulfil the dual purpose of demonstrating propositional/procedural expertise as well as communicative expertise.

In the above example we have considered a 'normal' scenario and how different discourse types (online commentaries, offline commentaries, and metacommentaries) are configured as part of midwifery communicative expertise. Our next example involves Nobuntu as the midwife and another pregnant woman, Jabulile, where there is a surprising noticing of a twin pregnancy and the encounter is marked by constant code-switching (Zulu represented in italics, followed by English translation).

Example 2 (Nobuntu – Jabulile)

Nobuntu:
01 ((Looking at the screen)) --- There's something that I'm...I'm catching here.
02 ((Pointing at the screen)) ---Do like this ---
03 ((Transducer following the left side of the abdomen)) --- OK ---
04 ((Moves transducer from below the abdomen and up to the right side of the
05 abdomen))
06 *Nansi inhliziyo yengane, nansi intamo yakhe bese kuba ikhanda.*
(Here's the baby's heart and here is the neck and then the head)
07 *Kunelinye ikhanda la, uyalibo?*
(There's another head in there, can you see it?)
Jabulile:
08 *Uyaguquka ....*
(Is the baby turning?)
Nobuntu:
09 *Nangu la ....* (Here it is ...) ------ ((Pointing at the screen)) --------
Jabulile:
10 *Owesibili? ... Hhayi, angifune ma-twins ...*
(Is it the second one? No I don't want any twins ...)
Nobuntu:
11 *Ehhe ..* (Yes.)
Jabulile:
12 *Hhayi bo, ngeke kuphume ama-twins la, ngiyawesaba, ngiwesaba kabi.*
(No way! I cannot give birth to twins, I'm scared of them, and I'm really scared ...)
Nobuntu:
13 ((Looking at Jabulile)) ___ ((Laughing)) --- ((Looking at the researcher))
14 I am just saying to her--- ((Adding gel on the abdomen)) --- I am not

sure…there is something I have seen…I thought it was a single baby…But
when I see it properly, I see two fetal hearts. --- ((Indicating two with two
fingers)) ---

Researcher:
Two foetuses?

Nobuntu:
((Looking at the screen)) --- This is the first. --- ((Indicating on the screen.
Moves the transducer from the left side to the right side to get the image of
the other foetus. The head appears)) --- Maybe look at the head. ---((Pointing
at the screen)) ------- That's the head. And we move here, and there is
another __((Short glimpse at the researcher before turning back to look at
the screen)) __ There is another one.

Researcher:
((Laughing)) another

Nobuntu:
((Looking at Jabulile)) _______ They are both facing down.
Awuthi ngibone ukuthi zingaki lezingane zakho ezisesiswini
(Let me see how many babies you have in your belly ...)

Jabulile:
Hhayi, hhayi....Musa ukungishayisa ngovalo ...
(No! ... No! ... Please don't scare me ... I'm really terrified now...)
((Smiles, turns her head towards the camera, turns her head back to the
screen.)) __

Nobuntu:
((Looking at the screen)) _ _ _Angikushayisi ngovalo, ngikutshela into
engiyibonayo. Angithi siyabona sobabili, nawe uyangibonisa. Ngikutshengisa
ikhanda. Nami angiso phela ukuthi.....ngithi ngibona sengathi. ---((Pointing at
the screen)) --- Khona kuyenzeka ukuthi ngingaboni kahle njengomuntu
osafunda ...
(I'm not trying to terrify you, I'm just telling you what I see. We are both looking at it and you are confirming what I see and I have shown you the babies' heads. Well, I'm not saying that I'm completely certain which is why I said, 'it seems'... At times I don't see properly because I'm still learning ...) .

Jabulile:
((Looking at the screen)) _ _ *Hhayi, ngibona ukuthi uyabona.*
(No, I'm sure you can see properly)

In lines 6–7, Nobuntu orients explicitly to Jabulile with online commentaries using Zulu. The noticing of something 'unusual' ('there's another head in there') is treated almost the same way as noticing 'usual' anatomical features of the foetus, resulting in an invitation to seeing. In lines 10 and 12, Jabulile voices her anxiety about giving birth to twins but this is responded to by Nobuntu in a light-hearted manner, signalling attendance to facework (line 13). Here laughter becomes a boundary marker for issuing a metacommentary with an element of uncertainty – the use of English signalling a switch to the researcher as the primary addressee. In her response, the researcher expresses surprise (two foetuses?', line 18) which occasions an online commentary (lines 19–24) addressed to her in the pedagogical frame. Nobuntu then returns to Jabulile by switching to Zulu and adopts the same light-hearted tone in the ensuing discussion of multiple pregnancies.

In lines 26–27, Nobuntu orients specifically to Jabulile and underscores that there is still some uncertainty about her finding: '(trans: Let me see how many babies you have in your belly ...)'. When Jabulile responds with anxiety, Nobuntu explicitly includes Jabulile in her online commentary when interpreting what can be seen on the screen in lines 31–35: '(trans: We are both looking at it and you are confirming what I see and I have shown you the babies' heads)'. This is followed by a qualification that her expertise is limited, that she is not certain, and that she is still in the process of learning how to use the ultrasound technology competently.

Conclusion

Our analysis demonstrates that an obstetric ultrasound encounter calls for communicative expertise. A key finding derived from the present study is that professional expertise of the advanced midwives is not limited to the propositional and procedural knowledge of conducting the obstetric ultrasound examination instrumentally. An equally important part of their professional expertise is the communicative expertise. The communicative expertise not only includes their context sensitivity, but also their strategic deployment of certain discourse types in order to manage their professional conduct informatively and ethically, for example by including the pregnant women in the medical examination and by informing them iteratively throughout the encounter. The communicative expertise is constituted in three discourse types: online commentaries, offline commentaries, and metacommentaries, each with distinctive linguistic characteristics and serving specific communicative functions such as reassuring the pregnant woman and normalizing the foetus and childbirth.

The online commentaries mainly refer to the condition of the foetus and the pregnancy, with the explicit function of reporting what appears on the screen, often accompanied with assessments of the condition and/or accompanied by invitations for joint seeing. The offline commentaries are propositional elaborations, explaining what evidence is observable on the screen, backed by scientific knowledge gained through educational training. Both online and offline commentaries, by default, perform a normalization function, unless warranted by a detection of potential abnormalities. The metacommentaries, primarily concerned with the framing of the activity of the ultrasound examination itself, fall into two categories: prospective and retrospective. Such metacommentaries operate both at the level of the activity type (i.e., participant structure) and at the level of specific task/action, facilitating the inclusion and involvement of the pregnant women as designated addressees and consequently making them feel that they have ownership of what is happening with the pregnancy.

As we have seen, the three different discourse types – online commentaries, offline commentaries, and metacommentaries – operate in interweaving ways. Communicating what is seen, in the context of midwifery practice, fulfils the institutional and professional requirements, while maintaining relational and ethical propriety during the encounter. A closer examination of the examples suggests that there are variations across individual performances – both in terms of occurrence and distribution of the three different discourse types – and this can be explained with reference to differential levels of expertise and experience, while acknowledging the hybrid nature of the encounter with its dual pedagogical and clinical framing. Communicative expertise, in our data setting, extends to the midwife's ability and willingness to include the pregnant women in the physical examination process via 'joint seeing'.

Recommendations for practice

The present study, with its focus on the examination phase of the obstetric ultrasound examination, has provided insights about how advanced midwives communicate to pregnant women the findings originating from the scan procedure. Their professional, technological expertise in conducting scans and in interpreting the scan images on the monitor has to be translated into language – what we have indentified as three discourse types: online commentaries, offline commentaries, and metacommentaries. These discourse types can be seen as a form of metalanguage underpinning midwifery communicative expertise that all midwives can be made aware of in their educational training and routine practice. Once midwives, and by extension sonographers, understand the distinctive forms these discourse types take in actual ultrasound scan encounters, they will be able to reflect on the functions such discourse types can serve in a given encounter. The analysis of ultrasound encounters by paying attention to the constituent discourse types has the potential for revealing differential professional practice (e.g., between experienced and inexperienced midwives vis-à-vis literate and illiterate pregnant women) and for improving communicative expertise of midwives more generally. In stressing that communicative expertise is integral to midwifery propositional and procedural expertise, this study offers important insights into the interplay of corollary discourse types.

Future directions

The design of the present study turned out to be complex – being part of an evaluation of an educational training programme for advanced midwives – with co-present researcher assuming a ratified participant status and thus influencing the interactional trajectory as manifest, among other things, in code-switching. The data therefore does not accurately represent how midwives in this South African rural setting communicate their expertise to the pregnant women. Future studies should aim for more 'pure' data to ascertain the structure and substance of the ultrasound encounter. The co-presence of the researcher, representing the educational training arm of the research project, is a clear limitation of the present study.

Our analysis focuses on the use and function of three discourse types – online commentary, offline commentary, and metacommentary. Future studies should go beyond this analytical framework and take into account the multimodal communication pathways that are characteristic of the ultrasound scan encounter. There are not many studies about communicative expertise in relation to medical technologies. However, modern health care is increasingly being technologized with regard to preventive, diagnostic, and curative medicine. The extent to which visualization technologies, accompanied by communication trajectories, enable the healthcare professionals to synchronously inform and reassure patients should be part of a future research agenda.

Of equal importance are the dynamic aspects of the interactional trajectories, highlighting the (non)participation of the pregnant women, as well as the management of situations where foetal complications arise and are in need of being expertly communicated by the midwives to anxious would-be parents.

Related topics

Ultrasound scan encounter; activity type; discourse type; online commentary; offline commentary; metacommentary.

Notes

1 Our focus here is the communicative expertise of the midwives, i.e., how they notice, formulate, and explain what is seen during the ultrasound scan. As part of the evaluation of the educational training programme, the Norwegian researcher's presence in the scan encounter became a necessity. In the data analysis section we will see how the midwives chose to orient to the researcher when communicating their expertise.

2 In this pre-examination phase, the introduction of participants, especially the researcher vis-à-vis the pregnant woman, was foregrounded. As part of the research agenda, the informed consent procedure had to be managed within the encounter. In this respect, the pre-examination phase may not resemble routine ultrasound encounters.

Further reading

Bredmar, M. and Linell, P. (1999) Reconfirming normality: the constitution of reassurance in talks between midwives and expectant mothers, in S. Sarangi and C. Roberts (eds) *Talk, Work and Institutional Order: Discourse in Medical, Medication and Management Settings*, 237–270, Berlin: Mouton de Gruyter. (This paper deals with encounters between pregnant women and midwives, with a focus on how different formulations of normality, including unexpected deviations, by both midwives and pregnant women can function as reassurance.)

Heritage, J. and Stivers, T. (1999) Online commentary in acute medical visits: a method of shaping patients' expectations. *Social Science & Medicine*, 49(11): 1501–1517. (This paper consolidates the notion of online commentary as a key feature of the physical examination phase which can serve to pre-empt patient resistance if there were to be a 'no problem' diagnosis. Following Sarangi (2000), online commentaries can be regarded as a discourse type which co-occurs with other discourse types such as offline commentaries and metacommentaries in the physical examination phase (see Sarangi 2010b).)

Sarangi, S. (2000) Activity types, discourse types and interactional hybridity: the case of genetic counselling, in S. Sarangi and M. Coulthard (eds) *Discourse and Social Life*, 1–27, London: Pearson. (This paper revisits the important notion of activity types and suggests that activity types are composed of discourse types, i.e., distinct forms of talk/text, which contribute towards interactional hybridity as well as role hybridity (see Sarangi 2010b).)

——(2010a) Healthcare interaction as an expert communicative system: an activity analysis perspective, in J. Streeck (ed.) *New Adventures in Language and Interaction*, 167–197, Amsterdam: Benjamins. (This paper demonstrates how expertise is manifest at the interactional level (i.e., communicative expertise) in healthcare encounters, drawing on other dimensions of professional knowledge such as scientific/technical knowledge and clinical/experiential knowledge.)

——(2010c) Practising discourse analysis in healthcare settings, in I. Bourgeault, R. DeVries, and R. Dingwall (eds) *The SAGE Handbook of Qualitative Methods in Health Research*, 397–416, London: Sage. (This paper offers an integrated discourse analytic approach – inclusive of activity analysis and accounts analysis – for the study of healthcare encounters.)

References

Abramsky, L. and Chapple, J. (eds) (1994) *Prenatal Diagnosis: The Human Side*, London: Chapman and Hall.

Bateson, G. (1972) *Steps to an Ecology of Mind: Collected Essays in Anthropology, Psychiatry, Evolution, and Epistemology*, Chicago, IL: University of Chicago Press.

Bredmar, M. and Linell, P. (1999) Reconfirming normality: the constitution of reassurance in talks between midwives and expectant mothers, in S. Sarangi and C. Roberts (eds) *Talk, Work and Institutional Order: Discourse in Medical, Medication and Management Settings*, 237–270, Berlin: Mouton de Gruyter.

Chafe, W. (1986) Evidentiality in English conversation and academic writing, in W. Chafe and J. Nichols (eds) *Evidentiality: The Linguistic Coding of Epistemology*, Norwood, NJ: Ablex.

Clement, S. (ed.) (1998) *Psychological Perspectives on Pregnancy and Childbirth*, Edinburgh: Churchill Livingstone.

de Cossart, L. and Fish, D. (2005) *Cultivating a Thinking Surgeon. New Perspectives on Clinical Teaching, Learning and Assessment*, Shrewsbury, UK: TFM Publishing.

Draper, J. (2002) 'It was a real good show': the ultrasound scan, fathers and the power of visual knowledge, *Sociology of Health and Illness*, 24(6): 771–795.

Foucault, M. (1973) *The Birth of the Clinic*, trans. A. Sheridan, London: Tavistock Publications.

Freidson, E. (1970) *Profession of Medicine: A Study of the Sociology of Applied Knowledge*, New York: Dodd, Mead.

Gilstad, H. (2012) Obstetric Ultrasound Expertise as Manifest in Encounters between Midwives and Pregnant Women: A Case Study from KwaZulu-Natal in South Africa. Unpublished Doctoral Thesis, NTNU, Trondheim, Norway.

Goffman, E. (1974) *Frame Analysis: An Essay on the Organisation of Experience*, New York: Harper & Row.

Greatbatch, D., Luff, P., Heath, C., and Campion, P. (1993) Interpersonal communication and human–computer interaction: an examination of the use of computers in medical consultations, *Interacting with Computers*, 5(2): 193–216.

Gumperz, J.J. (1982) *Discourse Strategies*, Cambridge: Cambridge University Press.

Harpel, T.S. (2003) *'You can see your future': Ultrasound and the Pregnancy Experience*, Purdue, IN: Purdue University Press.

——(2008) Fear of the unknown: ultrasound and anxiety about foetal health, *Health*, 12(3): 295–312.

Heath, C. (1986) *Body Movement and Speech in Medical Interaction*, Cambridge: Cambridge University Press.

Heritage, J. and Stivers, T. (1999) Online commentary in acute medical visits: a method of shaping patients' expectations, *Social Science & Medicine*, 49(11): 1501–1517.

Kuba, L. (1995) The prenatal testing roller coaster: one mother's story, *Journal of Perinatal Education*, 4: 19–22.

Levinson, S.C. (1979) Activity types and Language, *Linguistics*, 17: 365–399.

Linell, P. (2001) *Approaching Dialogue*, Amsterdam: John Benjamins.

Linell, P. and Bredmar, M. (1996) Reconstructing topical sensitivity: aspects of face-work in talks between midwives and expectant mothers, *Research on Language and Social Interaction*, 29(4): 347–379.

Mangione-Smith, R., Stivers, T., Elliott, M., McDonald, L., and Heritage, J. (2003) Online commentary during the physical examination: a communication tool for avoiding inappropriate antibiotic prescribing?, *Social Science & Medicine*, 56(2): 313–20.

Måseide, P. (2007) The role of signs and representations in the organisation of medical work: X-rays in medical problem solving, in R. Iedema (ed.) *The Discourse of Hospital Communication: Tracing Complexities in Contemporary Healthcare Organisations*, New York: Macmillan.

——(2011) Institutional bodies and social selves: the discourse of medical examinations in hospital settings, in C.N. Candlin and S. Sarangi (eds) *Handbook of Communication in Organisations and Professions*, Berlin: Mouton De Gruyter.

Mitchell, L.M. (2004) Women's experiences of unexpected ultrasound findings, *Journal of Midwifery and Women's Health*, 49: 228–234.

Pilnick, A. (2004) 'It's just one of the best tests that we've got at the moment': the presentation of nuchal translucency screening for foetal abnormality in pregnancy, *Discourse & Society*, 15(4): 451–465.

Pilnick, A.M., Fraser, D.M., and James, D.K. (2004) Presenting and discussing nuchal translucency screening for foetal abnormality in the UK, *Midwifery*, 29(1): 89–93.

Ragan, S.L. (1995) Educating the patient: interactive learning in an OB-GYN context, in G.H. Morris and R.J. Chenail (eds) *The Talk of the Clinic: Explorations in the Analysis of Medical and Therapeutic Discourse*, 185–207, Hillsdale, NJ: Erlbaum.

Rapp, R. (2000) *Testing Women, Testing the Fetus: The Social Impact of Amniocentesis in America*, New York: Routledge.

Rothman, B.K. (1988) *The Tentative Pregnancy: Prenatal Diagnosis and the Future of Motherhood*, London: Pandora.

Sarangi, S. (2000) Activity types, discourse types and interactional hybridity: the case of genetic counselling, in S. Sarangi and M. Coulthard (eds) *Discourse and Social Life*, 1–27, London: Pearson.

——(2010a) Healthcare interaction as an expert communicative system: an activity analysis perspective, in J. Streeck (ed.) *New Adventures in Language and Interaction*, 167–197, Amsterdam: Benjamins.

——(2010b) Reconfiguring self/identity/status/role: the case of professional role performance in healthcare encounters, *Journal of Applied Linguistics and Professional Practice*, 7(1): 75–95.

——(2010c) Practising discourse analysis in healthcare settings, in I. Bourgeault, R. DeVries, and R. Dingwall (eds) *The SAGE Handbook of Qualitative Methods in Health Research*, 397–416, London: Sage.

Shortliffe, E. (1986) Medical expert systems, knowledge tools for physicians, *Western Journal of Medicine*, December: 830–839.

Swinglehurst, D. (2011) Opening up the 'black box' of the electronic patient record: a linguistic ethnographic study in general practice, *Communication & Medicine*, 8(1): 3–15.

Tannen, D. and Wallat, C. (1993) Interactive frames and knowledge schemas in interaction: examples from a medical examination/interview, in D. Tannen (ed.) *Framing in Discourse*, New York: Oxford University Press.

Tegnander, E. and Eik-Nes, S.H. (2006) The examiner's ultrasound experience has a significant impact on the detection rate of congenital heart defects at the second-trimester foetal examination, *Ultrasound Obstetrics and Gynaecology*, 28(1): 8–14.

Watzlawick, P., Beavin, J.H., and Jackson, D.D. (eds) (1967) *Pragmatics of Human Communication*, London: Faber & Faber.

Wittgenstein, L. (1958) *Philosophical Investigations*, Oxford: Blackwell.

Appendix 33.1: Illustrative examples of online commentary, offline commentary, and metacommentary

Communication behaviour	*Description*	*Examples*
Occurrence of online commentary (ONC)		
Reporting	Online commentaries during the physical examination that reports without assessing	'I can see the heart.'
(Levels of sophistication of reporting)	Online commentaries with more detailed level of reporting without assessing	'I can see the position of the heart, I can see the rhythm of the heart, I can see the four chambers, I can see the sizes of the two atria, I can see the sizes of the two ventricles, I can see that the left ventricle forms an apex.' (Tegnander and Eik-Nes 2006: 31)
	Online commentaries with highly detailed level of reporting without assessing	'I can see the moderator band in the right ventricle, I can see the two atrioventricular valves, I can see the two septa and the atrioventricular valves form an "offset cross" in the middle of the heart and I can see that the two pulmonary veins connect to the left atrium.' (Tegnander and Eik-Nes 2006: 31)
Assessing	Online commentary accompanied by assessment	'I see the heart, and I see that it is ok.'
(Level of sophistication of assessing)	Detailed online commentary accompanied by assessment	'I can see that the position of the heart is in the middle of the thorax with the apex pointing left, which is the normal position. I can see the rhythm of the heart is regular with 150 beats a minute, which is normal.'
Invitations for seeing (IS)	Online commentary accompanied by invitation for seeing	'Can you see?'

Communication behaviour	Description	Examples
	Online commentary accompanied by invitation for seeing with more detailed level of reporting	'Can you see that I am pointing at the heart and respectively the four chambers?'
	Online commentary accompanied by invitation for seeing with highly detailed level of reporting	'Now I am pointing at the two pulmonary veins that connect to the left atrium of the heart. Can you see?'
Occurrence of offline commentary (OFC)		
Explications	Offline commentaries referring facts	'The heart has four chambers.'
Educational (more sophisticated explanations)	Offline commentaries referring facts in a more elaborate manner	'The heart occupies a third of the thoracic area.'
	Offline commentary referring facts in a highly detailed manner	'The rhythm of the heart is regular between 120 and 160 beats/minute. Short periods of bradycardia are normal in the second trimester of the pregnancy; bradycardia means that the heart beats at a slow rate.'
Occurrence of metacommentary (MC)		
MC (level of sophistication of metacommentary)	Metacommentary referring the present action	'I am just showing her the heart.'
Prospective metacommentary (PMC)	Metacommentary referring the coming action	'Now I will look at the heart.'
(Level of sophistication of prospective metacommentary)	Metacommentary referring the detailed level of the coming action	'I shall identify the position of the heart, the four chamber view, and measure the rhythm.'
	Metacommentary referring the highly detailed level of the coming action	'I will compare the sizes of the two atria and the two ventricles, and look at the position of the tricuspid valve and the mitral valve in relation to the apex.'
Retrospective metacommentary (RMC)	Metacommentary referring the previous action	'Now I have seen the heart.'
(Level of sophistication of retrospective metacommentary)	Metacommentary referring the detailed level of the previous action	'I have identified the position of the heart, the four chamber view, and measured the rhythm.'
	Metacommentary referring the highly detailed level of the previous action	I have compared the sizes of the two atria and the two ventricles, and looked at the position of the tricuspid valve and the mitral valve in relation to the apex.

Sources: Gilstad (2012), with additional examples taken from Tegnander and Eik-Nes (2006); the coding scheme suggested by Mangione-Smith et al. (2003) has been expanded.

Appendix 33.2: Transcription conventions

Symbol	*Explanation*
(name)	The name of a person or persons, clinic or a hospital, anonymized.
(.)	A dot in parentheses indicates a tiny gap, probably no more than one-tenth of a second. Several dots indicate a longer gap.
WORD	Capitals, except at the beginnings of lines, indicate especially loud sounds relative to the surrounding talk.
( )	Empty parentheses indicate the transcriber's inability to hear what was said. The length of the parenthesized space indicates the length of the untranscribed talk. When the inaudible talk is Zulu, this is marked: (inaudible Zulu). Parenthesized speaker designation indicates inability to identify a speaker.
(word)	Parenthesized words are possible hearings or speaker identifications. The translations between Zulu and English, and English and Zulu, are parenthesized, and the spoken utterances appear immediately before the parenthesis.
(( ))	Double parentheses contain the transcriber's descriptions and researcher's observations rather than, or in addition to, transcriptions.
____________	The continuous line immediately above or below the transcribed talk and/or silence indicates that the participant is gazing at the face of the co-participant. (...) If the fragment involves more than two persons, the person being gazed at is indicated on the line.
_ _ _ _ _ _ _	The longer dashes are used to indicate that the participant is looking at a particular object. Frequently, a series of lengthy dashes is accompanied by a description, such as 'records', 'fingers', 'camera', to indicate what object is being looked at. In this project the following descriptions: _ _ _ ((Looking at the screen))_ _ _ and _ _ _ ((Pointing at the screen))_ _ _ are recurring in the transcripts.
,,,,,,,,,,,,,,,,,,,,	A series of commas indicates that the party is turning away from a participant.
....	A series of dots indicates that the participant is turning towards a co-participant. In multiparty interactions, when one participant moves his/her gaze from one person to another, the notation of dots and commas becomes ambiguous because the person is simultaneously moving away from one co-participant and towards another. On occasions, dots and commas are also used to capture gaze moving towards and away from particular objects.
--------------	Close dashes are used to represent movement. They are accompanied by a description to indicate what type of movement it is. (...) If necessary, additional dashed lines above and below the transcribed talk are used to represent other movements in relation to where they begin and end in the talk and/or gaps.

34

Genetic counseling in multicultural and multilingual contexts

Olga Zayts and Alison Pilnick

Introduction

In recent years there has been a proliferation of research in medical sociology, medical anthropology, and medical education examining the role of culture in genetic counseling (e.g., Awwad et al. 2008; Lehtinen 2005; Lewis 2002; Nukaga and Cambrosio 1997). This trend may be attributed to an increasing understanding of and demand for genetic counseling across healthcare specialties, as well as to 'changing communicative ecology' (Roberts 2009a: 243) of health care in general and genetic counseling, in particular. Genetic counseling encounters involving participants from diverse cultural and linguistic backgrounds are increasingly becoming everyday realities due to globalization of health care and an increasing migration of professional workforce and clients around the world. A common theme emerging from these studies is that culture has a significant impact on the decision-making and the outcomes of genetic counseling. While the existing studies undoubtedly provide useful insights into the role of culture, they do not address how culture is brought about in communication in the *actual* counseling process.

Communication-based studies have highlighted the predominantly communicative nature of genetic counseling. It has been described as a 'hybrid' (Sarangi 2000) activity that resembles both other forms of psychosocial counseling and traditional medical encounters. While specific practices of counseling may vary across and within countries (Arribas-Ayllon et al. 2011), certain characteristics of the activity, however, appear typical across contexts. For example, 'traditional' medical encounters are typically organized around the presence of an acute health problem (e.g., Heritage and Maynard 2006) that is presented by the patient, whereas in genetic counseling there is usually no acute or existing medical condition to be addressed and professionals instead engage in a considerable amount of talk about possible future scenarios (Arribas-Ayllon et al. 2011). Descriptions of principal activities from the genetic counseling literature (e.g., Clarke 1997; Harper 2010) outline a wide range of topics that may be covered in a counseling session, such as discussing diagnostic and clinical aspects of a genetic condition, taking family and pedigree information, explaining inheritance patterns and the clients' risks, providing psychosocial support to those affected by the condition and the family, providing information on available options, including genetic testing, and facilitating decision-making. It follows that genetic counseling addresses complex medical, psychosocial, moral, and educational issues. The differences in the cultural and linguistic backgrounds of the participants may have an impact on communication processes; but while communication in genetic counseling has been the subject of a significant number of detailed studies, those studies have mainly been conducted in mono-cultural and monolingual settings and have not specifically addressed issues of the cultural and linguistic diversity. There, therefore, exists a significant gap in the literature: studies of the communicative processes of genetic counseling have not addressed these issues; and those wider studies that have addressed them have not done so at a sufficient level of communicative detail to shed light on how and why difficulties might arise. In this chapter we focus on how these two groups of studies may be brought together to examine genetic counseling in multicultural and multilingual contexts.

Historical perspectives

Studies of multicultural and multilingual genetic counseling

This section offers an overview of studies in several broad fields, between which certain parallels can be drawn. While a detailed discussion of the concept of culture goes beyond the scope of this chapter, we note that there exist many typologies of culture that offer different degrees of elaboration of what it is (see, for example, Carter and Qureshi's (1995) typology in respect to multicultural counseling and training). In the vast majority of existing studies on multicultural genetic counseling in the medical sociology, medical anthropology, medical education, and genetic counseling literature, culture refers to geo-political or ethnic boundaries. There appear to be two distinct groups of studies. The first includes studies that draw heavily on a wider anthropological and sociological literature on culture in healthcare deliveries. These studies focus on cultural beliefs and attitudes of clients coming from non-Western backgrounds and how these beliefs and attitudes impact the counseling process. Awwad et al. (2008), for example, examine prenatal decision-making among native Palestinians and first-generation Palestinian Americans using interview data in which participants were asked to imagine themselves in hypothetical premarital and prenatal situations. The similarities (e.g., sharing information about an affected pregnancy with their nuclear families only) are explained in terms of common cultural roots; and the differences (e.g., being more comfortable with sharing information with close friends and clients in similar circumstances in the case of Palestinian Americans, but not native Palestinians) are attributed to acculturation. The main shortcoming of these studies is that they offer 'homogenized group stereotypes without [giving] attention to intragroup variation and individual differences' (Ota Wang 2001: 208). Culture is seen as a static, easily identifiable entity and the originating source of differences and challenges in genetic counseling.

The second group is notably smaller and includes studies that take a step back from the position of cultural homogeneity and cultural stereotyping, essentially highlighting the multifaceted nature of culture (e.g., Clarke and Parsons 1997; Lewis 2002; see also Ota Wang 2001 who offers a comprehensive review and criticism of the first approach). They note that multicultural genetic counseling implies '[a shift] from learning about cognitive (e.g., between-group differences) information about visible racial-cultural groups to an integrated cognitive-affective racial-cultural identity (within-group/individual variation) perspective integrating social, historical, and political, etc. frameworks' (Ota Wang 2001: 212). This position of the complex multifaceted nature of culture has translated into recent educational research. In medical education, multicultural competence (that is also referred to as culturally appropriate/culturally sensitive genetic counseling – e.g., Weil and Mittman 1993; Steinberg

Warren 2011) is generally understood as the skills necessary to work effectively and sensitively with clients from diverse cultural backgrounds (Holcomb-McCoy and Myers 1999; Ota Wang 1994). What comes across strongly in these studies is that general counseling skills are not sufficient for conducting multicultural counseling. The common components of multicultural awareness proposed by medical educators include knowledge of ethnocultural groups and ethnocultural self-awareness. By talking about the counselor's self-awareness, these studies expand the focus from the 'cultural' client (McCrae and Johnson 1991, cited in Ota Wang 1998: 9; Middleton et al. 2007) to include the professional with his or her own cultural beliefs and attitudes into the counseling process (Ota Wang 1998). Weil (2001) adds that it is also important to consider the institutional and the social barriers to service. Sodowsky et al. (1994) note the importance of the multicultural counseling relationship that forms part of the counselor's competence.

While acknowledging that medical educators have been incredibly prolific in producing frameworks and guidelines for multicultural genetic counseling training, we note several limitations of these studies (many of which are also acknowledged by the medical educators and genetic counselors themselves). Clarke (1997) suggests that in addition to educating about different cultures, there is a need to explore the ways in which these different cultures are *experienced*. Lewis (2002) notes that the lack of empirical data on multicultural genetic counseling 'makes it difficult to document the extent of challenges to multicultural genetic counseling and their effects on the counseling experiences' (Lewis 2002: 194). Indeed, the studies that we have reviewed have routinely ignored the role of language and communication in multicultural counseling. In order to gain a better understanding of the role of culture in genetic counseling, it is important to capture the actual processes, or the 'interior of practice' (Biesecker and Peters 2001: 192) through which culture is enacted, negotiated, and/or contested in real time through talk. To achieve this, appropriate methodological tools are required that are offered by communication-based approaches.

Communicative approaches to culture

In the discussion of communicative approaches to culture, a distinction between multicultural/cross-cultural and intercultural genetic counseling is important (Sarangi 2012). Sarangi (ibid.) notes that either of the first terms is preferred in the medical literature to refer to 'patterns of behavior or accounts of experiences across distinct cultural borders', and the term 'intercultural' is used in communication-based literature in the analysis of 'situated encounters between two or more participants who represent different linguistic and cultural backgrounds'. As our focus in this chapter is on situated analysis of genetic counseling between participants from different cultural backgrounds, hereafter we use the term intercultural genetic counseling. The particular focus on language use in the analysis of intercultural encounters should be noted since many communication-based studies start with a premise that when participants do not share culture, they also do not share linguistic backgrounds. This is probably why there appears to be a strong tendency to view intercultural encounters as problematic and bound to miscommunications. Sarangi (1994 [2011]) offers a systematic overview of two main communication-based approaches to intercultural communication: interactional sociolinguists (e.g., Gumperz 1982; Gumperz and Tannen 1979) and cross-cultural pragmatics (e.g., Blum-Kulka et al. 1989). Sarangi (1994 [2011]) notes that in contrast to anthropological studies (and one can expand it to sociological, educational, and genetic counseling studies that we have reviewed above) that draw heavily on examples from hypothetical cultural encounters, and, therefore, offer analyses that are disconnected from real life encounters, the two communicative approaches rely on data from real life interactions. These approaches, therefore, offer insights into the actual communicative processes of intercultural encounters. This is achieved through close engagement with interactional data that, following the data collection (typically, audio- or video-recording), are coded and transcribed with different level of detail using some conventional transcription systems (for a review of different approaches to transcribing discourse data see Edwards 2001). The analyses of interactional data may also be supported and informed by ethnographic data (e.g., participant observation; interview data). Despite this close attention to the subtleties of communicative processes, both interactional sociolinguistics and cross-cultural pragmatics have been criticized for overemphasizing the cultural differences as the cause of communicative problems and downplaying or ignoring other important contextual variables (for a review of these approaches see also Roberts and Sarangi 1993; Sarangi 2012).

More recent studies in sociolinguistics, pragmatics, and discourse analysis, although not specifically dealing with healthcare encounters, offer a more dynamic, multifaceted outlook on culture (for an overview, see Sarangi 1994 [2011]; Sarangi 1995 [2009]; Senft et al. 2009). Studies that specifically focus on intercultural healthcare encounters are fewer but their number is growing (e.g., Roberts 2004, 2009b; Roberts et al. 2005). These studies stress the interplay of contextual variables in intercultural encounters, such as institutional context or individual differences that may account for communicative difficulties. Intercultural encounters are thus approached from the viewpoint of making sense of 'complex institutional processes in which the shifting nature of "culture" is embedded' (Sarangi 1994 [2011]). Culture is, thus, not assumed a significant variable in these encounters *a priori*, unless participants are orienting themselves to it in an interaction in more or less explicit ways.

The language proficiency of the participants is also approached from a more dynamic perspective: it is acknowledged that it is not an 'either–or matter' (Roberts 2009b); participants from non-native backgrounds may display different levels of proficiency and may not necessarily be 'linguistically deprived' in their patient/client roles. On the other hand, these studies offer evidence that if misunderstandings do occur in intercultural encounters, they are more likely to be attributed to participants' linguistic rather than cultural backgrounds (e.g., Roberts et al. 2005). The language issues in intercultural encounters 'challenge much of the received wisdom about good communication skills in the healthcare literature' (Roberts 2009a: 250). For example, increased talk (e.g., explanation-giving; elicitation of patient concerns) and patient-directed listening have traditionally been seen as patient-centered techniques; in intercultural encounters, they are, however, more likely to generate further misunderstandings (ibid.). We should also acknowledge a growing number of studies in various healthcare sites that specifically focus on encounters with patients with limited language proficiency that include an interpreter as one of the participants (e.g., Bolden 2000; Davidson 2000). These studies note a complex role of interpreters as 'cultural brokers, mediators and advocates' (Meyer et al. 2003: 78) and that provision of interpreters, whether formal (trained interpreters) or informal (family members, friends, or hospital staff) may exacerbate rather than facilitate the delivery of healthcare services to multicultural patient populations.

The studies that we reviewed in this section have been mainly conducted in primary care settings. In what follows we first review a critical issue in genetic counseling communication, before examining how this dynamic, communication-based approach to culture and language may be applied to the analysis of intercultural genetic counseling.

Critical issues and topics of genetic counseling communication: focus on nondirectiveness

In intercultural genetic counseling encounters the issues of intercultural communication may intersect in complex ways with general psychosocial issues of genetic counseling (Weil and Mittman 1993). To illustrate this point, we focus on the nondirective approach to genetic counseling that has been the crux of much debate in both medical and communication-based studies.

Traditionally understood as the withholding of counselor's advice to clients (Kessler 1997) and providing genetic information in a neutral and value-free manner, nondirectiveness was widely endorsed by genetic counseling communities around the world by the late 1980s (Wertz and Fletcher 1988). More skeptical positions, however, were soon put forward questioning nondirectiveness in both its ideology and practice (e.g., Anderson 1999; Gervais 1993; Shiloh 1996). The approach has been questioned as potentially requiring a complete suspension of expert professional judgment (Pilnick and Zayts 2012). The dilemma many counselors have reported is finding a balance between upholding nondirectiveness while simultaneously ensuring the best possible support for their clients (Burke and Kolker 1994; Brunger and Lippman 1995; Bower et al. 2002). Nondirectiveness followed rigidly has been criticized for the lack of responsiveness and empathy to clients' needs (Sarangi 2010). As a result of these criticisms, several models of genetic counseling were formulated (Kessler 1997; Elwyn et al. 2000; Weil 2003; McCarthy Veach et al. 2007), each in part describing to what extent nondirectiveness should count as a guiding principle of genetic counseling. Central to all these accounts is the idea that the principle of unqualified client autonomy may not *always* be in the best interests of the client and, therefore, may conflict with the principle of beneficence.

Communication-based studies of genetic counseling have noted specific challenges that professionals may face in adhering to nondirectiveness in the actual counseling process. Benkendorf et al. (2001), for example, observe that many genetic counselors conflate nondirectiveness with the use of indirect speech (see also Zayts and Kang 2009). Such an attempt at 'best practice', however, may actually lead to undesirable outcomes by hindering the clients' understanding of provided information. For example, when counselors use generic nouns, such as 'some people' or 'most people', clients may face difficulties in inferring which utterances apply to them or, indeed, they may assume that 'what most people do' is what they should also do (Benkendorf et al. 2001; Pilnick 2002). On the other hand, the overt use of indirect speech does not preclude professionals from steering their clients in the direction of a particular decision. Pilnick (2008), elaborating on Anspach (1993, cited in Pilnick 2008), identifies several means by which the interactional context may impact decision-making despite the professionals' nondirectiveness. For example, the sequential location of talk about optional genetic tests immediately following the discussion of other, more routine tests may lead to conflation of two different groups of tests by clients. There is also an ongoing discussion about information-giving vis-à-vis advice-giving in genetic counseling (e.g., Sarangi 2002; Sarangi and Clarke 2002; Sarangi et al. 2004) that suggests that in this professional context *any* information given by professionals may be perceived as (directive) advice by clients.

The interactional subtleties of directive versus nondirective counseling may potentially present additional challenges in intercultural genetic counseling encounters, as suggested by the data from our study of prenatal screening in Hong Kong that we discuss in the next section.

Current contributions and research

Main research methods and data

Our data come from a large-scale communication-based study of prenatal screening for Down Syndrome in Hong Kong that has been ongoing since 2006. In our study we have applied both conversation and discourse analytic techniques. The analyses presented in this chapter use conversation analysis (ten Have 2007) that is concerned with '*the interactional accomplishment of particular social activities*' (Drew and Heritage 1992: 17, original emphasis). These activities are analyzed with regards to their context, social organization, and alternative means of accomplishment (Drew and Heritage 1992). In our study, we have employed ethnographic methods, drawing on extensive participant observation, interviews with participants prior to and following prenatal screening encounters, and institutional documents regulating screening services that the research team was given access to.

The prenatal screening encounters we examine are part of routine prenatal services. The screening is organized as a multi-stage activity: women are first introduced to it through information leaflets and a 15-minute video about Down Syndrome, followed by face-to-face consultations with hospital staff to discuss screening (nuchal translucency and maternal blood tests), diagnostic testing (CVS or amniocentesis), the implications of different tests, and a woman's personal risks. While screening presents a safer option in comparison to diagnostic testing, which carries a small risk of miscarriage (0.5 to 1 percent), the detection rate is higher with diagnostic testing. In addition, screening can only give a probabilistic rather than a definitive or diagnostic result. Therefore, further consultations are arranged to discuss diagnostic testing for those women who receive 'positive' screening results after the initial screening.

The dataset that we draw on comprises more than 120 consultations, with 90 percent being intercultural encounters. Hong Kong provides a particularly rich site to investigate issues of intercultural communication, due to the diversity of the city's population both culturally and linguistically. While the Chinese population in Hong Kong accounts for 95 percent of the population (Census and Statistics Department of Hong Kong SAR 2007), there is ethnic diversity within this group. In addition, the remaining 5 percent of the expatriate community come from very diverse backgrounds. The professionals in our study (one nurse and four doctors) are all Hong Kong Chinese. The clients originate from more than 20 countries around the world, including the UK, the US, France, Spain, Italy, Denmark, Japan, Nepal, Thailand, and Mainland China among others. Therefore, in these consultations either English or Chinese are used as native or non-native languages of the participants. In three cases, the clients' partners perform the role of informal interpreters; no professional interpreters are involved in the consultations.

All consultations were transcribed using transcription conventions traditionally used in conversation analytic research (Atkinson and Heritage 1984). The Chinese data transcripts were translated into English independently by two research assistants and verified by a bilingual research team member.

As our previous research has begun to show, the cultural diversity of participants can be highly consequential to the provision of prenatal screening services, as both clients and health professionals negotiate different culturally influenced ideas, assumptions, and expectations about the screening process and outcomes (Pilnick and Zayts 2012). Our interest in the Hong Kong context is particularly strong, because the genetic counseling profession and, therefore, the tenets guiding the profession are still being established and negotiated by the professionals in this region (Zayts et al. 2012).

Intercultural genetic counseling in Hong Kong: cases from prenatal screening for Down Syndrome

In our previous research (Pilnick and Zayts 2012; Zayts et al. 2012) we have noted that Chinese doctors and nurses appear in some instances to be quite directive in these consultations, both explicitly by assuming that testing will take place and more implicitly through what information they offer or decide to withhold in particular circumstances. Based on previous research on intercultural communication that includes Chinese speakers, one may explain this directiveness solely on the basis of a hierarchical relationship between the interlocutors: in particular, that interlocutors in higher positions tend to use directive expressions (Lee-Wong 1999), while interlocutors in lower positions take on a listener's role (Gao and Ting-Toomey 1998) and use indirect language (Young 1994; Gao et al. 1995). The presumed applicability of these findings could easily be extended to interactions including Chinese medical professionals and clients from other Asian backgrounds. Example 1, which presents a consultation between a Hong Kong Chinese doctor and a Filipina patient who has received a positive screening report, illustrates our point about professionals being directive in these interactions.

Example 1[1]
The consultation is conducted in English.

D: So emm you understand that we tell you before the .h we told you before
that the blood test comes back er: to be positive.
W: Yeh.
D: That means the Down Syndrome screening test is positive. Em it's about em
one em: The- the risk is about umm one in two hundred thirty five. Hh
That means in two hundred and four- thirty four babies will be normal.
And e: ah one of the- out of the two hundred twenty five could be
having the Down Syndrome. .hh
((W nods))
D: Ok? To- to con<u>firm</u> whether there is- your baby is eh Down Syndrome or not,
so we need to put a needle into your tummy and then got some water
around the baby and test for the eh chromosome .hh to test whether
the baby is having the Down Syndrome, okay?
W: Mm:
D: You just have the e: needle, .hh (.) okay?
W: °Okay.° ((while nodding))

This example comes from the beginning of the consultation. Having delivered the screening test results, the doctor explicitly suggests that the woman should take amniocentesis 'to confirm' the diagnosis (lines 10–13; and 15). This suggestion is extremely directive as it assumes that further testing will take place, which is exacerbated by the use of the modal 'need to'. Used in the final turn position, the particles 'okay' (turns 13 and 15) mark the turn boundaries and assume the woman's agreement with the suggestion rather than elicit her opinion about further testing. Unsurprisingly, the woman in this consultation opts for taking amniocentesis.

Despite the seemingly obvious explanation of hierarchical relationships, our previous research (Zayts et al. 2012) has suggested that other contextual factors should be taken into account in explaining the directiveness of the doctor's discourse: in particular, the specifics of prenatal screening in Hong Kong that is delivered by obstetric nurses and doctors who also provide regular prenatal services may account for why 'medical' issues (that is, testing) rather than 'counseling' agenda prevail in these encounters. A 15-minutes' time-slot assigned to prenatal screening encounters may also prevent the professionals from exploring women's concerns and preferences. It is equally important to examine the professionals' directiveness as a conjointly constructed phenomenon. Noticeable in Example 1 is the woman's minimal verbal participation in the interaction and that she makes no attempt to get more actively involved in the decision-making. In our corpus we have observed a curious paradox: if women do not themselves elicit information about the 'meaning' of the test results and what they should do on the basis of it, then professionals appear to be able to provide this meaning and a suggested course of action. If women explicitly elicit advice regarding which tests to pursue, however, the professionals refrain from doing so, as Example 2, which presents an interaction between a Hong Kong Chinese nurse and a Filipina patient, demonstrates:

Example 2[2]
(abridged from Zayts and Schnurr 2011, 2012)
Context: the extract comes from the beginning of the decision-making stage after the nurse has delivered the information about available screening and testing options. The consultation is conducted in English.

N: Or, can you decide today? Or you want- you prefer to talk to your
husband first?
W: It's ok, which is the best for me? [I(h)] (h)don't k(h)now.
N: [Naa,] see, (.) Naa, see now whether
you want to have the, the first thing, is (.) you decide you want to have
test, or no test, ok? And the second thing is whether you want to have
direct test, or indirect test. Whether you want to have an accurate test,
or whether you want to have a safe test. If you want to have a safe test,
then you need to undergo the screening test. But if you think that I
want to have an accurate test, then you need to undergo the, the::, the::,
the other test.
(10) ((W is looking at the papers in front of the N))
W: °huh huh huh .hhh° ((chuckle))

The framing of the woman's question (line 3) suggests that her difficulty with making a decision relates to 'not knowing' what would be the best decision in her circumstances (rather than 'not understanding' provided information that may be the case with non-native speaking clients). In contrast to Example 1 where the doctor is extremely directive in suggesting further testing to the woman, in this example the nurse responds to the request for guidance indirectly by summarizing the information about available choices that she had previously delivered (not included in the example) rather than giving direct advice (lines 4–11). The nurse also explicitly states that the decision lies with the woman. We note a number of discursive strategies that may be aimed at facilitating the comprehension of information: the choices are presented in a dichotomous manner (e.g., to have a test or not to have a test); screening and diagnostic tests are characterized with easily understandable descriptors 'safe' and 'accurate'; and the information is personalized to the woman's specific situation (e.g., *you* decide, *you* want). The information about the various options, however, is also 'packaged' within one turn which makes it a very complex information unit to process. It is perhaps not surprising then that the nurse's avoidance to address the woman's question by simply repeating the information does not lead to the woman's decision. Instead there is a long pause (10 seconds in line 12) followed by the woman's laughter that may signal that she is still encountering difficulties in reaching a decision. This consultation brings to mind Bosk's vivid metaphor that 'the dark side of patient autonomy [is] patient abandonment' (1992: 158). In this example by giving the woman autonomy to make her own decision, the nurse does not appear to provide sufficient support to enable the decision-making.

One possible explanation for why professionals are directive in some cases and not others may be that explicit requests for advice highlight the phenomenon of directiveness and make the professionals aware of it in their responses. We would also like to put forward the idea that professionals may also be making assumptions about the 'burden' of decision-making and a woman's ability to carry this 'burden' better or worse than others. One may be tempted to link these assumptions solely to the clients' cultural backgrounds, in line with previous anthropological studies that have noted that '[for] people whose backgrounds may be quite rich in cultural resources, but not forged with the tools of scientific literacy, ... the model of isolated, individual decision-making may present more *burdens* than benefits' (Rapp 1993: 193, author's emphasis). For example, the clients' compliance with the professionals' directiveness and their requests for advice in the examples that we have analyzed may then be explained simply by the fact that the clients are of Asian backgrounds and that Filipino clients in our corpus are predominantly employed as domestic workers in Hong Kong, have a limited family support network and may, therefore, have more reasons than others to seek help (see Zayts and Schnurr 2012). While the cultural background may serve as one of the explanations, we would like to take our analysis one step further: in interactional terms, our evidence suggests that professionals make judgments about these women's ability to deal with the 'burden' of decision-making, at least partly, on the basis of the lack of or minimal responses or uptake of information from the clients in these encounters. In other words, elicitations of advice signal that women are engaged in the decision-making and responsive to the information provided by the professional, so that they are able to 'carry the burden' of decision-making autonomously. The imperfect 'mapping' of the professionals' directiveness to the clients' cultural background becomes evident in those interactions where clients become more engaged in the decision-making as an interaction progresses, as an interaction between a Hong Kong Chinese nurse and a Mainland Chinese woman who has received a positive screening report in Example 3 demonstrates.

Example 3[3]

The consultation is conducted in Cantonese, a non-native language of the client.

D: <h right h> (.) hh I think you mainly consider this one (.) Sometimes the chance
Is (.) just a ↑bit higher=
W: =°just a bit higher°
D: Then second, the ultrasound is normal .hh third, (.) you have to balance (.)
the risk of miscarriage caused by amniocentesis. .h Fourth, you have to consider (.)
hh em: (.) the baby, I mean if=
W: °Umm°
D: if the baby has Down Syndrome (.) are you really unable to take care of him. (.)
Something like that. .hh
W: I think (.) I can't accept it. (.) I can't take care of him. hehehe ((looking at D and
smiling embarassingly))
D: Eh:: hmm (.) you have to consider how much you understand the syndrome. (.)

13 Fifth (.) we can't guarantee that the baby is hundred percent normal even if you have
14 the amniocentesis or ultrasound. (.) We just test the things we have to know.
15 W: I see. ((nodding))
16 D: If the baby is born, (.) we discover he has another problem (.) we can't say
17 if we can accept it or not, right? So, (.) if you think you can accept an abnormal baby
18 (.) then take it.
19 (0.2)
20 W: I'm afraid that I really can't take care of the baby if he has any problems.
21 huh huh huh
22 D: °Do you? Are you looking after one child? °
23 W: Yes. I am living with my son. (.) I'm single.
24 D: °I see°. How old is he?
25 W: He's in primary three.
26 D: °That means you have to look after two children alone? °
27 W: Yes, (.) I have to work (.) so my mum helps me with this.
28 (0.3)
29 D: Okay. (0.2) Perhaps you may discuss it with your mother.
30 W: Mmm
31 (0.2)
32 D: It's not that urgent to decide now. (.)
33 Do you have the number of ((nurse's name))?

At the beginning of this example the doctor appears quite equivocal about testing. By highlighting three factors, that the woman's risk is only slightly higher than what would be considered normal for her age group, that the result of the ultrasound examination is normal, and that further testing presents a risk of miscarriage, she creates a context in which testing is presented as not a favored option. This is continued with the doctor's statement that the woman has to consider 'if the baby has Down Syndrome are you really unable to take care of him' (line 8), where the emphasis on 'really' suggests a contrast between what might be ideal and what is practically possible. The doctor in this example is being directive in that she appears to be quite strongly steering the woman away from testing. In line with our previous argument, then, it could be that this doctor is acting on the assumption that the woman needs this 'steering' in the decision-making. The woman's response that she could neither accept nor take care of a child with a disability (line 10) is not immediately accepted by the doctor as a rationale for undergoing testing. Instead, the doctor suggests by her utterance in line 12 ('you have to consider how much you understand the syndrome') that the woman's response is not necessarily based on full information. The doctor then adds further to her list of factors to consider, by stating that no test can guarantee a 'normal' child (lines 13–14). This utterance serves to build an argument that not being able to accept a child with Down Syndrome is not a sufficient justification to pursue further testing. Despite the doctor' directiveness, however, the woman continues to pursue her point of being unable to care for a child with Down Syndrome. She evokes the specifics of her own situation: that she is single and already has one child, whom her mother helps her to care for. At this point, the doctor, who until then appears to have strongly favored the option of not pursuing amniocentesis and has twice rejected the woman's expressed inability to care for a disabled child as a rationale for pursuing it, suggests that the issue should be discussed with the woman's mother (line 29) and that a future appointment is possible. In this interaction, we see a shift from a more to a less directive stance by the doctor. While the woman's active engagement with the decision-making and responsiveness to the doctor's suggestions have failed to bring about an offer of testing, they appear to have served as the stimulus for preserving this possibility.

These three examples demonstrate the complexity of genetic counseling communication in intercultural contexts and how the professional tenet of nondirectiveness is evoked and negotiated by the participants of these encounters. Our findings are in contrast to previous studies of prenatal screening involving speakers from the same linguistic and cultural backgrounds in the UK (e.g., Pilnick 2008) that have noted that professionals actively avoid being directive. In our setting the professionals shift between being very directive and more nondirective. And while it is tempting to explain the directiveness of the professionals' discourse in terms of the social hierarchy and cultural backgrounds of the participants, our data suggest that this explanation does not hold for all clients in the study and point to something more subtle at the interactional level. In particular, based on the situated analysis of these encounters, we have highlighted that it is participants' moment-by-moment interactional behavior that may be accountable for the directiveness of the genetic professionals. Furthermore, the directiveness is co-constructed by the participants of these encounters in that professionals take on a more directive stance on the basis of lack of responses and/or uptake of information by women. We have also highlighted other contextual variables in these encounters, such as the specifics of the prenatal screening activity in Hong Kong that may account for the directiveness of the professionals. As a concluding remark, in intercultural encounters, the differences in participants' cultural backgrounds may not necessarily account for all observable interactional challenges, as in our analysis the fact that participants come from various Asian backgrounds does not solely explain why some encounters are more or less directive.

Recommendations for practice

In this chapter we have examined intercultural genetic counseling in the context of Hong Kong, focusing on how the professional tenet of nondirectiveness is negotiated by the participants of these encounters. Our analysis has demonstrated that in analyzing intercultural genetic counseling one has to go beyond focusing on participants' cultural backgrounds and consider the multifaceted nature of communicative encounters and other contextual variables. In other words, cultural diversity does not offer an unequivocal explanation of the observable differences in communication. In particular, the directiveness of our example encounters may be attributed to the specifics of prenatal screening activity in Hong Kong where it is run by the obstetric doctors and nurses, the short time allocated to these consultations, and the participants' interactional behavior in these encounters.

The position of going 'a step ahead' of focusing solely on culture has strong implications for practice and training of medical professionals that we believe may be extended to various healthcare specialties. Revisiting the concept of multicultural competence, in addition to the knowledge of ethnocultural groups and self-awareness, professionals and medical students also need to acquire the analytic ability to reflect on the complex nature of communicative encounters. They need to recognize the 'diversity within the diversity': that patients/clients of similar cultural backgrounds may display a wide range of language proficiency, cultural beliefs and assumptions about health and illness issues, as well as different degrees of assimilation into a 'host' culture. Likewise medical professionals may also display a range of cultural attitudes and beliefs as to their professional roles and the degree of engagement with patients/clients' health-related issues. Also important is the understanding that culture as a contextual variable becomes important only when and if participants are orienting themselves to it in an interaction. These ideas are summed up in Sarangi's (2012) call for the move from 'passive awareness [about cultural issues] towards developing critical analytic sensibility'.

In terms of developing this 'critical analytic sensibility', we believe that our analysis has shown the potential contribution that communication-based approaches may make to the medical curricula and professional training. Roberts (2004) notes that in the current curricula, issues of cultural and linguistic diversity are dealt with sporadically and rather generally. While medical curricula are overcrowded with many 'non-medical' disciplines looking to contribute to them, we see the value of introducing the students and professionals to the basics of communication-based analyses of real-life intercultural healthcare encounters. This will imply a gradual move from a more traditional prescriptive 'communication skills approach' to a more dynamic and reflective approach.

Future directions

In the Introduction to this chapter we have noted that genetic counseling varies within and across countries. This observation holds for multicultural genetic counseling that will display differences across different cultural contexts. Our research began to outline the specifics of multicultural genetic counseling in the socio-cultural context of Hong Kong. Clearly, more empirical research is needed in various cultural contexts to shed further light on genetic counseling in culturally and linguistically diverse societies.

Acknowledgments

The research reported here was fully supported by a grant from the Hong Kong Research Grants Council of the Hong Kong Special Administrative Region, China (project no. HKU 754609 H). Our thanks are due to all participants of the project who allowed us to video- and audio-record their interactions and to the medical research team who continue to engage in an ongoing dialogue with us about their practices, in particular to Ms. Vivian Chan, Dr. H.Y.M. Tang, and Dr. C.P. Lee.

Related topics

Genetic counseling communication; multicultural and multilingual genetic counseling; intercultural communication; conversation analysis; prenatal screening; Hong Kong.

Notes

1 The study that is quoted in this chapter has obtained a standard Ethics approval. The participants were anonymized and all identifying information was removed from the data.
2 An extended version of this example is also analyzed in Zayts and Schnurr 2011, 2012.
3 This example is also analyzed in Pilnick and Zayts 2012.

Further reading

Pilnick, A. and Zayts, O. (2012) '"Let's have it tested first": choice and circumstances in decision-making following positive antenatal screening in Hong Kong', *Sociology of Health and Illness*,

34(2): 266–282. Republished in N. Armstrong and H. Eborall (eds) (2012) *The Sociology of Medical Screening: Critical Perspectives, New Direction,* Chichester: Wiley-Blackwell.

Roberts, C. (2009) 'Intercultural communication in healthcare settings', in H. Kotthoff and H. Spencer-Oatey (eds) *Handbook of Intercultural Communication*, New York: Mouton de Gruyter.

Sarangi, S. (1994) 'Intercultural or not? Beyond celebration of cultural differences in miscommunication analysis', *Pragmatics*, 4(3): 409–427. Republished in Zhu Hua (ed.) (2011) *The Language and Intercultural Communication Reader*, London: Routledge.

——(2000) 'Activity types, discourse types and interactional hybridity: the case of genetic counselling', in S. Sarangi and M. Coulthard (eds) *Discourse and Social Life*, London: Pearson.

Zayts, O. and Schnurr, S. (2012) '"You may know better than I do": negotiating advice-giving on Down Syndrome screening in a Hong Kong prenatal hospital', in M.A. Locher and H. Limberg (eds) *Advice in Discourse*, Amsterdam: John Benjamins.

References

Anderson, G. (1999) 'Nondirectiveness in prenatal genetics: patients read between the lines', *Nursing Ethics*, 6(2): 126–136.

Anspach, R. (1993) *Deciding Who Lives: Fateful Choices in the Intensive Care Nursery*, Berkeley, CA: University of California Press.

Arribas-Ayllon, M., Sarangi, S., and Clarke, A. (2011) *Genetic Testing: Accounts of Autonomy, Responsibility and Blame,* London: Routledge.

Atkinson, J.M. and Heritage, J. (eds) (1984) *Structures of Social Action: Studies in Conversation Analysis,* Cambridge: Cambridge University Press.

Awwad, R., Veach, P.M., Bartels, D.M., and LeRoy, B.S. (2008) 'Culture and acculturation influences on Palestinian perceptions of prenatal genetic counseling', *Journal of Genetic Counseling*, 17: 101–116.

Benkendorf, J.D., Prince, M.B., Rose, M.A., De Fina, A., and Hamilton, H.E. (2001) 'Does indirect speech promote non-directive genetic counseling? Results of a sociolinguistic investigation', *American Journal of Medical Genetics,* 106: 199–207.

Biesecker, B.B. and Peters, K.F. (2001) 'Process studies in genetic counseling: peering into the black box', *American Journal of Medical Genetics,* 106: 191–198.

Blum-Kulka, S., House, J., and Kasper, G. (eds) (1989) *Cross-cultural Pragmatics: Requests and Apologies*, Norwood, NJ: Ablex.

Bolden, G.B. (2000) 'Toward understanding practices of medical interpreting: interpreters' involvement in history taking', *Discourse Studies*, 2(4): 387–419.

Bosk, C.L. (1992) *All God's Mistakes: Genetic Counseling in a Pediatric Hospital*, Chicago, IL: Chicago University Press.

Bower, M.A., Veach, P.M., Bartels, D.M., and LeRoy, B.S. (2002) 'A survey of genetic counselors' strategies for addressing ethical and professional challenges in practice', *Journal of Genetic Counseling,* 11(3): 163–186.

Brunger, F. and Lippman, A. (1995) 'Resistance and adherence to the norms of genetic counseling', *Journal of Genetic Counseling,* 4(3): 151–167.

Burke, B.M. and Kolker, A. (1994) 'Directiveness in prenatal genetic counseling', *Women and Health,* 22(2): 31–53.

Carter, R.T. and Qureshi, A. (1995) 'A typology of philosophical assumptions in multicultural counseling and training', in J.G. Ponterotto, J.M. Casas, L.A. Suzuki, and C.M. Alexander (eds) *Handbook of Multicultural Counseling*, Thousands Oak, CA: Sage.

Census and Statistics Department of Hong Kong SAR (2007) 'Census information: population by ethnicity 2001 and 2006', Online. Available HTTP: <http://www.censtatd.gov.hk/hong_kong_statistics/statistical_tables/index.jsp?tableID=139&ID=&subjectID=1> (accessed 12 October 2011).

Clarke, A. (1997) 'Introduction', in A. Clarke and E. Parsons (eds) *Culture, Kinship and Genes: Towards Cross-Cultural Genetics,* Basingstoke: Macmillan.

Clarke, A. and Parsons, E. (eds) (1997) *Culture, Kinship and Genes: Towards Cross-Cultural Genetics,* Basingstoke: Macmillan.

Davidson, B. (2000) 'The interpreter as institutional gatekeeper: the sociolinguistic role of interpreters in Spanish–English medical discourse', *Journal of Sociolinguistics,* 4(3): 379–405.

Drew, P. and Heritage, J. (eds) (1992) *Talk at Work: Interaction in Institutional Settings,* Cambridge: Cambridge University Press.

Edwards, J.A. (2001) 'The transcription of discourse', in D. Schiffrin, D. Tannen, and H.E. Hamilton (eds) *The Handbook of Discourse Analysis*, Malden, MA: Blackwell.

Elwyn, G., Gray, J., and Clarke, A. (2000) 'Shared decision making and non-directiveness in genetic counselling', *Journal of Medical Genetics,* 37: 135–138.

Gao, G. and Ting-Toomey, S. (1998) *Communicating Effectively with the Chinese*, Thousand Oaks, CA: Sage.

Gao, G., Ting-Toomey, S., and Gudykunst, W. (1995) 'Chinese communication process', in M.H. Bond (ed.) *The Handbook of Chinese Psychology*, Hong Kong: Oxford University Press.

Gervais, K.G. (1993) 'Objectivity, value neutrality, and nondirectiveness in genetic counseling', in D.M. Bartels, B. LeRoy, and A.L. Caplan (eds) *Prescribing our Future: Ethical Challenges in Genetic Counseling,* New York: Aldine de Gruyter.

Gumperz, J. (1982) *Discourse Strategies*, Cambridge: Cambridge University Press.

Gumperz, J. and Tannen, D. (1979) 'Individual and social differences in language use', in C. Fillmore, D. Kempler, and W. Wang (eds) *Individual Differences in Language Ability and Language Behavior*, London: Academic Press.

Harper, P.S. (2010) *Practical Genetic Counseling*, 7th edn, London: Hodder Arnold.

ten Have, P. (2007) *Doing Conversation Analysis: A Practical Guide,* London: Sage.

Heritage, J. and Maynard, D.W. (eds) (2006) *Communication in Medical Care: Interactions between Primary Care Physicians and Patients,* Cambridge: Cambridge University Press.

Holcomb-McCoy, C.C. and Myers, J.E. (1999) 'Multicultural competence and counselor training: a national survey', *Journal of Counseling and Development*, 77: 294–302.

Kessler, S. (1997) 'Psychological aspects of genetic counselling. XI. Nondirectiveness Revisited', *American Journal of Medical Genetics,* 72: 164–171.

Lee-Wong, S.M. (1999) *Cross-Cultural Communication: Politeness and Face in Chinese Culture,* Frankfurt am Main: Peter Lang.

Lehtinen, E. (2005) 'Information, understanding and the benign order of everyday life in genetic counselling', *Sociology of Health and Illness*, 27(5): 575–601.

Lewis, L.J. (2002) 'Models of genetic counseling and their effects on multicultural genetic counseling', *Journal of Genetic Counseling,* 11(3): 193–212.

McCarthy Veach, P., Bartels, D.M., and LeRoy, B. (2007) 'Coming full circle: a reciprocal-engagement model of genetic counseling practice', *Journal of Genetic Counseling,* 16: 713–728.

McCrae, M.B. and Johnson, S.D. (1991) 'Toward training for competence in multicultural counselor education', *Journal of Counseling and Development,* 70: 131–135.

Meyer, B., Apfelbaum, B., Pöchhacker, F., and Bischoff, A. (2003) 'Analyzing interpreted doctor–patient communication from the perspectives of linguistics, interpreting studies and health sciences', in L. Brunette, G.L. Bastin, I. Hemplin, and H. Clarke (eds) *The Critical Link 3: Interpreters in the Community,* Amsterdam: John Benjamins.

Middleton, A., Robson, F., Burnell, L., and Mushtaq, A. (2007) 'Providing a transcultural genetic counseling service in the UK', *Journal of Genetic Counseling*, 16(5): 567–582.

Nukaga, Y. and Cambrosio, A. (1997) 'Medical pedigrees and the visual production of family disease in Canadian and Japanese genetic counselling practice', *Sociology of Health and Illness,* 19(19B): 29–55.

Ota Wang, V. (1994) 'Cultural competency in genetic counseling', *Journal of Genetic Counseling*, 3: 267–277.

——(1998) 'Introduction', *Journal of Genetic Counseling*, 7(1): 3–13.

——(2001) 'Multicultural genetic counseling: then, now, and in the 21st century', *American Journal of Medical Genetics*, 106: 208–215.

Pilnick, A. (2002) '"There are no rights and wrongs in these situations": identifying interactional difficulties in genetic counselling', *Sociology of Health and Illness*, 24(1): 66–88.

——(2008) '"It's something for you both to think about": choice and decision making in nuchal translucency screening for Down's sydrome', *Sociology of Health and Illness*, 30(4): 511–530.

Pilnick, A. and Zayts, O. (2012) '"Let's have it tested first": choice and circumstances in decision-making following positive antenatal screening in Hong Kong', *Sociology of Health and Illness*, 34(2): 266–282. Republished in N. Armstrong, and H. Eborall (eds) (2012) *The Sociology of Medical Screening: Critical Perspectives, New Direction,* Chichester: Wiley-Blackwell.

Rapp, R. (1993) 'Amniocentesis in sociocultural perspective', *Journal of Genetic Counseling*, 2(3): 183–196.

Roberts, C. (2004) 'Presentation of self and symptoms in primary care consultations involving patients from non-English speaking backgrounds', *Communication and Medicine*, 1(2): 159–170.

——(2009a) 'Intercultural communication in healthcare settings', in H. Kotthoff, and H. Spencer-Oatey (eds) *Handbook of Intercultural Communication*, New York: Mouton de Gruyter.

——(2009b) 'Mince or mice? Misunderstanding and patient safety in a linguistically diverse community', in B. Hurwitz and A. Sheikh (eds) *Health Care Errors and Patient Safety*, Oxford: Blackwell.

Roberts, C. and Sarangi, S. (1993) 'Culture revisited in intercultural communication', in T. Boswood, R. Hoffman, and P. Tung (eds) *Perspectives on English for Professional Communication*, Hong Kong: City University of Hong Kong.

Roberts, C., Moss, R., Wass, V., Sarangi, S., and Jones, R. (2005) 'Misunderstandings: a qualitative study of primary care consultations in multilingual settings and educational implications', *Medical Education*, 39(5): 465–475.

Sarangi, S. (1994) 'Intercultural or not? Beyond celebration of cultural differences in miscommunication analysis', *Pragmatics*, 4(3): 409–427. Republished in Zhu Hua (ed.) (2011) *The Language and Intercultural Communication Reader*, London: Routledge.

——(1995) 'Culture', in J. Verschueren, J.-O. Ostman, and J. Blommaert (eds) *Handbook of Pragmatics*, Amsterdam: John Benjamins. Republished in G. Senft, J.-O. Ostman, and J. Verschueren (eds) (2009) *Culture and Language Use. Handbook of Pragmatics Highlights*, vol. 2, Amsterdam: John Benjamins.

——(2000) 'Activity types, discourse types and interactional hybridity: the case of genetic counselling', in S. Sarangi and M. Coulthard (eds) *Discourse and Social Life*, London: Pearson.

——(2002) 'The language of likelihood in genetic counseling discourse', *Journal of Language and Social Psychology*, 21(1): 7–31.

——(2010) 'Professional values in interaction: non-directiveness, client-centredness and other-orientation in genetic counselling', in S. Pattison, B. Hannigan, R. Pill, and H. Thomas (eds) *Emerging Values in Healthcare: The Challenge for Professionals*, London: Jessica Kingsley.

——(2012) 'The intercultural complex in healthcare encounters: a discourse analytical perspective', in N.G. Patil and C. Lam (eds) *Making Sense in Communication*, Hong Kong: Institute of Medical and Health Sciences Education.

Sarangi, S. and Clarke, A. (2002) 'Zones of expertise and the management of uncertainty in genetics risk communication', *Research on Language and Social Interaction*, 35(2): 139–171.

Sarangi, S., Bennert, K., Howell, L., Clarke, A., Harper, P., and Gray, G. (2004) 'Initiation of reflective frames in counselling for Huttington disease predictive testing', *Journal of Genetic Counselling*, 13(2): 135–155.

Senft, G., Ostman, J.-O., and Verschueren, J. (eds) (2009) *Culture and Language Use. Handbook of Pragmatics Highlights*, vol. 2, Amsterdam: John Benjamins.

Shiloh, S. (1996) 'Decision-making in the context of genetic risk', in T. Marteau and M. Richards (eds) *The Troubled Helix: Social and Psychological Implications of the New Human Genetics*, Cambridge: Cambridge University Press.

Sodowsky, G.R., Taffe, R.C., Gutkin, T.B., and Wise, S.L. (1994) 'Development of multicultural counseling inventory: a self-report measure of multicultural competencies', *Journal of Counseling Psychology*, 41: 125–136.

Steinberg Warren, N. (2011) 'Introduction to the special issue: towards diversity and cultural competence in genetic counseling', *Journal of Genetic Counseling*, 20: 543–546.

Weil, J. (2001) 'Multicultural education and genetic counseling', *Clinical Genetics*, 59: 143–149.

——(2003) 'Psychosocial genetic counselling in the post-nondirective era: a point of view', *Journal of Genetic Counseling*, 12(3): 199–211.

Weil, J. and Mittman, I. (1993) 'A teaching framework for cross-cultural genetic counseling', *Journal of Genetic Counseling*, 2(3): 159–169.

Wertz, D.C. and Fletcher, J.C. (1988) 'Attitudes of genetic counselors: a multinational survey', *American Journal of Human Genetics*, 42: 592–600.

Young, L.W.L. (1994) *Crosstalk and Culture in Sino-American Communication*, New York: Cambridge University Press.

Zayts, O. and Kang, M.A. (2009) '"So, what test do you prefer?" Negotiating politic behavior in an L2 prenatal genetic counselling setting in Hong Kong', *Journal of Politeness Research: Language, Behaviour, Culture,* 5(1): 33–52.

Zayts, O. and Schnurr, S. (2011) 'Laughter as a medical provider's resource: negotiating informed choice in prenatal genetic counseling', *Research, on Language and Social Interaction,* 44(1): 1–20.

——(2012) '"You may know better than I do": negotiating advice-giving on Down Syndrome screening in a Hong Kong prenatal hospital', in M.A. Locher and H. Limberg (eds) *Advice in Discourse,* Amsterdam: John Benjamins.

Zayts, O., Wake, V.Y., and Schnurr, S. (2012) 'Chinese prenatal genetic counseling discourse in Hong Kong: health care providers' (non)directive stance, or who is making the decision?' in Y. Pan and D. Gazdar (eds) *Chinese Discourse and Interaction: Theory and Practice,* London: Equinox.

35

Interpreting in the healthcare setting

Access in cross-linguistic communication

Claudia V. Angelelli

Introduction

In multilingual societies cross-linguistic communication is increasingly frequent, especially when it relates to accessing health care. Speakers of the societal language and members of linguistic minorities need to communicate. Both in urban and rural areas, effective communication between speakers who do not share a language is enabled by interpreters. In addition, in certain countries the existence of many indigenous languages, coupled with the development of effective public services, has contributed to the need for healthcare interpreting as a means to access health services.

In a healthcare encounter, when patient and provider do not share a language, a healthcare interpreter coordinates the talk and enables communication. These three co-participants, that is patients seeking care, providers supplying it, and healthcare interpreters coordinating the talk, belong to different speech communities (Angelelli 2000; Hymes 1974). Members of these diverse cultural groups and speech communities often understand health, disease, pain, and healthcare practices differently. In addition, in some medical settings (e.g., mental health) or countries (e.g., the United States), it is often the case that linguistic minorities are vulnerable groups and, therefore, power differentials between providers and patients become salient. An exception to this is medical treatment that has evolved into a field called medical tourism. In countries like Mexico or Korea, for example, health care and surgeries are provided to foreign visitors at affordable costs. In 'medical tourism' interaction the power differentials between providers and patients are not so salient, even when issues arising from cultural and linguistic diversity are still present. In all cases, however, healthcare interpreting assures every person access to communication, since it is through interpreting that patients obtain language access.

Definitions

Healthcare interpreting: can be defined as a special type of interpreting that facilitates communication between users of health services and providers of health services who do not share the same language (either spoken or signed). It occurs mainly in settings such as hospitals, clinics, and doctor offices and involves the communication of signed, verbal and non-verbal messages in real time. The language of one user group (the provider) is mainly the societal language(s) of the country. The language of the patient is the non-societal language, i.e., the language of the specific ethnic group. Healthcare interpreting serves the latter user group to ensure their access to public services.

Interpreted communicative event: occurs among three participants: a speaker of a non-societal language (for example a patient seeking health care), a speaker of the societal language (generally the service provider – for example a physician, a nurse, or a hospital administrator), and an interpreter who facilitates the communication in either consecutive or simultaneous mode. These three parties should interact for the encounter to be considered an interpreted communicative event. Interaction can occur face to face or remotely.

Healthcare interpreter: a professional who holds a degree in interpreting or a related field, or has specific qualifications or credentials, and exhibits interpreting skills, demonstrates experience, observes the code of ethics of the profession, and is able to carry out an assignment successfully. The job of an interpreter is to communicate a message constructed in a source language, be it spoken or signed, into a target language, spoken or signed, in real time and conveying every semantic element (content, intention, form, gist, gesture, pauses, silences, and tone) of the message. Healthcare interpreters engage in interactive types of communication that usually follow a bi-directional and dialogic pattern. These individuals are proficient in two or more languages (spoken or signed) and are able to facilitate communication. In these events, interpreters work mostly consecutively but they may also interpret simultaneously, with or without equipment (using *chuchotage*), when working with large groups (e.g., a family consultation with several specialists). Sometimes they work face to face and sometimes remotely using technology such as video or teleconferencing. These individuals may be members of the community for which they interpret, which can make it difficult for the interpreters to adhere to professional ethics and standards of practice.

Ad-hoc interpreter: does not hold a degree in interpreting, nor have any other qualifications or credentials, and may or may not have any experience in performing the task at hand, and may or may not observe any code of ethics, although this person may exhibit the ability to speak both the source and target languages and volunteer to perform the role of an interpreter, or be directed to do it by the pertaining authority (e.g., the case of bilingual employees in hospitals). Speakers of the non-societal language cannot always access services through interpreters, mostly due to lack of availability. Therefore, in the absence of quality interpreting, users of non-societal languages often resort to ad-hoc interpreters to communicate with speakers of societal languages. These include bilingual service providers (e.g., teaching assistants, laboratory technicians, receptionists) as well as family members (including minors) or friends who are asked to step in and to help broker communication with various degrees of success. This may lead to serious consequences that undermine equal access to services.

End users of community interpreting services: belong to two distinct groups and they may not necessarily coincide with the party requesting the interpreting service. One group is formed by speakers of the societal language who are offering healthcare services (e.g., providers, administrators, educators, patient advocates). In addition to the knowledge of the societal language, these individuals have knowledge of the subject matter (e.g., health care, insurance, law). The other group generally is formed by linguistic and ethnic minorities, individuals who do not speak the societal language and who need to communicate with speakers of the societal language in order to access services. End users should be encouraged to request professional/qualified interpreters to provide them with interpreting services. In the case of a hospital, for example, the two end users are the provider and the patient interacting, and the party requesting the service may have been a member of the administrative staff.

'Chuchotage': is simultaneous interpreting done in the form of 'whispering' and used in circumstances when technical equipment is not available or the audience is too small to justify using booths.

Consecutive interpreting: in this kind of interpreting, the rendering of a speech into the target language occurs at different intervals and the speaker pauses during the interpreted rendition. The intervals can be arranged beforehand between speakers and interpreter. Consecutive interpreting generally requires ability in note-taking.

Note-taking: a way of conceptualizing information by using symbols, arrows, and sometimes words and used to aid the interpreter's memory and attention by noting important concepts, links, and data such as dates and figures. Note-taking is neither shorthand, nor regular writing. Note-taking requires education and experience. It is generally not mastered by ad-hoc interpreters.

Simultaneous interpreting: where the rendering of speech into another language occurs at the same time as the speaker is delivering the speech. It may require the use of special equipment and booths.

Interpreting should not be confused with translation. While translation involves the communication of a written/video/electronic message into another language in written/video/electronic form and a certain period of time is allocated for the task, interpreting involves the communication of oral or signed messages in real time. In addition to the difference between written and oral form and the time constraints, interpreting conceptualizes communication as the result of human interaction. As such, community interpreting means brokering both the content and meaning of messages. Meaning is formed not only by words but also by body language, facial expressions and gestures, intonation contours, and other paralinguistic features used during an interpreted communicative event. Interpreting may occur across a wide range of social factors (gender, ethnicity, socio-economic class, education, age, and nationality).

Critical issues and topics

Initially, most discussions on interpreting have centered on issues of cognitive and linguistic abilities; most of them concerning students' performance and selection, and their abilities to perform as conference interpreters. During the 1990s the discussions turned more to naturalistic settings and topics included more types of interpreting such as legal, medical, educational, and community. They also reflected the growing pains of those fields as they struggled to become recognized professions. Perhaps one of the issues that has attracted more attention from both researchers and practitioners has been the role that interpreters play in the interpreted communicative event. Since the 1990s we have witnessed a shift in the perception of the interpreter's role, from a language conduit (Reddy 1979) to an essential partner in a cross-cultural conversation or co-constructor in the interaction (Roy 2000; Wadensjö 1998) to a co-participant with agency (Angelelli 2001, 2004a, 2004b).

In its inception, interpreting was conceptualized as an exchange between two speakers who did not share a language with an invisible interpreter facilitating it. This may be due, in part, to the great impact of the Theory of Meaning (see below) at the time. The conceptualization of an interpreter as a ghost (Kopscinscki 1994), or invisible participant (Angelelli 2001), considers accuracy over all other aspects that can be attributed to the message (intention of the parties, goal of the communicative event, and context of the interaction). This model portrays an invisible interpreter who is a mere conduit or channel between two speakers who do not share a common language. It assumes no interaction between interpreter and speakers, and no direct interaction between speakers except through the interpreter. Additionally, by overlooking the social and cultural factors brought by the interpreter and the parties to the interaction (Angelelli 2001, 2003) it also assumes that interpreting can indeed happen in a social vacuum (Wadensjö 1998: 8). According to this invisible model, the interpreter is seen as a language modem. In addition, this model assumes that in any given utterance there is only one meaning, which is not subject to co-construction by all participants to the interaction (including the interpreter) but rather that meaning exists independent of the parties. This conceptualization of the interpreter as a conduit (Reddy 1979) or a ghost (Collado Aís 1998) is still prevalent, especially among practitioners and trainers, both in sign and spoken languages. In sign language, for example, practitioners recurrently use the terms *channel, machine, telephone, window*, or *bridge* to explain what they do (Roy 1993 in Pöchhacker and Shlesinger 2002: 351). Roy also explains the evolution of the various descriptions used among the professionals working with American Sign Language (ASL), from the interpreter as a helper (which encompasses the professional role as well as the social and personal) to the interpreter as a conduit to the interpreter as a communication facilitator (as ASL professionals turned to the field of communications for possible answers on their role). Although this description at first glance appears to be more inclusive than the previous one, it still conveys 'the conduit notion in the disguise of communication-facilitator' (ibid.). The last description used is that of interpreters as bilingual, bicultural specialists. According to this description, the interpreter's role includes an awareness of dialectal and regional language varieties and socio-cultural pragmatics.

Various professional associations of healthcare interpreting have produced codes of ethics (e.g., the California Healthcare Interpreting Association in 2002; the *Code of Ethics for Medical Interpreters and Translators* by Stanford Hospital and Clinics in 1985; *Medical Interpreting Standards of Practice* by the Massachusetts Medical Interpreters Association (renamed the International Medical Interpreters Association) in 1995; and the National Council of Interpreters in Healthcare in 2004) in which they describe (or prescribe) the role of the interpreter in a medical setting. The California Healthcare Interpreting Association (CHIA) was the first one to base their code on empirical research (Angelelli 2006; Angelelli et al. 2007). It recognizes that the interpreter has multiple roles as a party in the patient/clinician interaction in addition to the message converter role portrayed in earlier writings. 'Message converter' is the first role discussed in the California Healthcare Interpreting Association (CHIA) Standards (2002: 36). The second role of 'message clarifier' (36–37) includes gaining more information from a speaker to explain a message or concept in an alternate or more easily understood manner to facilitate communication. The third role, 'cultural clarifier' (37–38), involves confirming and providing cultural information, particularly about cultural health beliefs. 'Transparency' is defined in the CHIA glossary as,

> The idea that the interpreter keeps both parties in the interpreting session fully informed of what is happening, who is speaking, and what the interpreter is doing … Whenever interpreters intervene by voicing their own thoughts and not the interpreted words of one of their clients, it is critical that they ensure that a) the message is conveyed to all parties and b) everyone is aware that the message originates from the interpreter.
>
> *(CHIA 2002: 51)*

The fourth role, 'patient advocate' (38–42), prohibited for the court interpreter, may be required in the healthcare setting to support the health and well-being of the patient. For example, an interpreter may witness instances of discrimination or disparities to access health care on the part of limited-English-speaking patients. The latter may not be familiar with the healthcare systems and services available to them and their healthcare rights (e.g., eligibility and enrollment, making appointments, understanding procedures). These factors make it difficult for patients themselves to advocate for their own rights. In these cases, 'interpreters are often the only individuals to recognize the problem and advocate for the patient' (41).

Unlike statements in codes of ethics that tend to be prescriptive in nature, descriptive research shows that interpreters impact the nature of the interaction. They are present, they acknowledge they have agency, and they exercise it (Angelelli 2004a, 2004b, 2006, 2011). Around the 1990s, studies utilizing a sociolinguistics lens illustrated crucial differences in the participatory role of interpreters, and these differences depend upon the nature of the interpreted communicative event (Angelelli 2000, 2004a, 2004b, 2011; Metzger 1999; Roy 1989, 2000; Wadensjö 1995, 1998). The fact that the interpreter constructs, co-constructs, repairs, and facilitates the talk during an interpreted encounter proves her role as a co-participant. Speakers and interpreters co-construct conversations in what is referred to by Wadensjö as a *pas de trois* (1998: 10).

Current contributions and research

Observations of interpreters at work show that in the social environments in which they work, they interact with the parties for whom they interpret (Angelelli 2004a, 2004b, 2007; Bolden 2000; Davidson 1998, 2000, 2001; Metzger 1999; Roy 1989; Valero 2005; Wadensjö 1995, 1998). Well-documented studies of interpreters in the courtroom (Berk-Seligson 1990), in the hospital (Angelelli 2004a; Davidson 2000; Metzger 1999), in schools (Roy 2000), the immigration office, and the police station (Wadensjö 1995 and 1998) as well as of young interpreters in the community (Valdés, Chavez and Angelelli 2000; Valdés et al. 2003) are evidence of the *visibility* or agency (Angelelli 2001, 2003, 2004a, 2004b) of interpreters. These studies have challenged the notion of neutrality by studying the participation of interpreters during interactions (Davidson 2000, 2001; Metzger 1999) and by considering interpreting as a special case of interaction (Wadensjö 1998) or discourse process (Roy 2000) in which interpreters are co-participants who share responsibility in the talk and exercise their agency (Angelelli 2001).

Researchers (Angelelli 2004a, 2004b; Bolden 2000; Davidson 2000, 2001; Metzger 1999; Wadensjö 1998) have studied a variety of strategies and behaviors performed by interpreters as they provide their renditions of original utterances produced by parties requiring interpreting services. Wadensjö's taxonomy of interpreters' renditions (1998: 106–108) is based on a comparison of the propositional context present in the original utterance and the rendition rather than on the different types of equivalences (lexical, grammatical, and pragmatic) (1998: 42). She also looks at the interpreter's role in coordinating talk and how that coordination can be implicit (interpreter's talk) or explicit (request for clarification or requests to observe turn-taking order) (1998: 107–108). This taxonomy and classification of coordination are essential for us to see interpreters' participation in the communicative event. Based on Hymes's taxonomy of speech (1974) and comparing conference interpreters to community/medical interpreters, Angelelli (2000) argues that in a conference setting speakers and listeners (e.g., country member representatives in a meeting at NATO or the United Nations) share the psychological setting or scene, the same speech community and do not share the same language. Conference interpreters are only temporary guests in that speech community. Alternatively in a medical setting, providers and patients do not share the psychological setting or scene (Hymes 1974), as they do not belong to the same *speech community.* Interpreters belong to the speech community of one of the two interlocutors. Some of the interpreters further studied by Angelelli (2001, 2004a) are physicians in their countries of origin while others have more in common with the speech communities of patients. Therefore the medical scene is more accessible or evident for the interpreter as she explores it not so much as an outsider does but as a 'discovering' party. The interactions among parties allows for clarification. In doing this, interpreters exercise their agency (Angelelli 2004a) as they participate in cross-linguistic communication. Angelelli identifies the following behaviors on the part of the interpreters: exploring answers, expanding and summarizing statements, brokering comprehension and explaining technical terms, bridging cultural gaps, expressing affect, perpetuating or brokering power differentials between patients and providers, and replacing interlocutors (2004a: 78). She argues that as the interpreter becomes the owner of text, visibility increases. When this happens, the interpreter's role is highly consequential. Triggered by social factors such as gender, race, ethnicity, age, and socio-economic status, interpreters increasingly claim text ownership and, in so doing, they impact the medical or personal information exchanged during an interpreted communicative event. They also impact the provider–patient relationship (Angelelli 2004a). In the following excerpt we see examples of text ownership that impact the provider–patient relationship. The patient is suffering from pain. The doctor needs to find out more information about the reported pain. To do that, the doctor also needs to have the patient rate the pain on a pain scale. In this way the doctor can make an informed decision for treatment and medicine. The interpreter, Joaquín, is brokering the 1–10 pain scale for the doctor (Angelelli 2004a: 94–95):

1	Dr.	In a scale from one to ten, how would she rate her pain?
2 ►	Ii Int.	*A ver Señora Rita, en una escala de uno a diez, ¿que número le pondría a su dolor? Por ejemplo, si el uno es que está para irse a bailar y no tiene nada y el diez es que se está muriendo, dónde estaría el dolor?* (Let's see Mrs. Rita, in a scale from one to ten, what number would you assign to your pain? For example, if one is a pain that would allow you to go dancing, you almost don't feel anything and ten is so painful that you are dying from that pain…)
3	Pat.	*¿Cómo dice?* (What did you say?)
4	Int.	*Qué... ¿qué número le daría a su dolor?* (What… what number would you give to your pain?)
5	Pat.	*Pos... a mi me duele mucho.* (Well… it hurts a lot)
6 ►	Int.	*¿cuánto es mucho señora? ¿mucho que se está muriendo del dolor?* (How much is a lot Ma'am? Does a lot mean you are dying from the pain?)

7 Pat. Pos…no… muriendo no, pero…
(Well…no… not dying… but…)
8 Int. ¿Qué cosas puede hacer con el dolor?
▶ (Which things can you do when you are in pain?)
9 Pat. Pos no sé… cuando me duele mucho me siento.
(Well, I don't know… when it is very hard I sit down)
10 Int. Pero ¿puede cocinar con el dolor?
▶ (But, can you cook when you are in pain?)
11 Pat. A veces me pega fuerte y no
(Sometimes it is very hard and I can't)
12 Int. Y, esas veces, ¿siente como que se va a morir o no tanto?
▶ (And at times, does it feel like you are going to die or it is not so hard?)
13 Pat. No, morir no, nomás pega fuerte
(No, not like I'm going to die, it's just hitting me hard)
14 Int. ¿Le ponemos un ocho o un nueve?
▶ (Do we give it an eight or a nine?)
15 Pat. Pos yo no sé, pos sí…
(I don't know… yes)
16 Int. When it is most painful it would be close to an eight, doctor
▶
17 Dr. Okay

As we can see from the transcript, the doctor's question (line 1) is not responded to immediately after it is asked. It takes 14 turns between interpreter and patient before the interpreter gets back to the doctor on line 16. In addition, there is much of the patient–interpreter conversation that did not surface in the interpreter's rendition to the doctor.

Studies on the cognitive or linguistic aspect of interpreting have allowed us to gain some understanding of this complex communicative event (de Bot 2000; Paradis 2000; Russo 2011; Swayer 2004; Szabo 2006). A deeper knowledge of the complexities involved in healthcare interpreting resulted from studying the interpreted communicative event as a social act, and examining the interpreter's multifaceted role within that event. Social and sociological perspectives have allowed us to explore the agency or power that interpreters hold (Angelelli 2003, 2004a; Davidson 2000; Metzger 1999; Wadensjö 1998), previously overlooked under the guise of the interpreter's neutrality (Metzger 1999). Additional insights were gained by studying this communicative event embedded within an institution which is itself embedded in society (Angelelli 2006; Davidson 2001). Furthermore, the notion of neutrality was challenged by emphasizing the need for codes of ethics that would incorporate situations where interpreters act as advocates for patients (CHIA 2002: 38–43).

This notion of advocacy can be exemplified by the study on the role of interpreters for aboriginal languages, when Kaufert and Putsch (1997) discuss the challenges of monolingualism in medical practice, which is increasingly multicultural, placing heavy emphasis on the aspects of clinical communication that involve power and dominance. They state that 'health care interpretation often occurs across major gulfs of culture, class, and language; and therefore it is unlike interpretation in the courts or in business or international negotiation. Attempts to encourage mutually shared understanding require the health care interpreter to engage in explanation, cultural brokerage, and mediation, when these actions are necessary' (1997: 75). The importance of taking into consideration the historical and institutional context in which interpreters perform their job, in order to better analyze their actions and their role was also underscored by Davidson (1998). In later work, he refers to interpreters as gatekeepers for the minority-language speakers for whom they interpret, stating that these interpreters align with healthcare providers, making them active participants in the diagnostic process (Davidson 2001).

In sum, research on communication in the healthcare setting facilitated by interpreters indicates that the difficulties in interpreted conversations lie in the construction of reciprocal understanding, the accurate transformation of semantic and pragmatic content, and the role of the interpreter as linguistic facilitator (Angelelli 2004a, 2006, 2010, 2011; Bolden 2000; Davidson 1998, 2000, 2001; Metzger 1999; Wadensjö 1998). For healthcare providers, the interpreter is the instrument that keeps the patient on track; for the patient the interpreter is a co-conversationalist (Davidson 1998).

Main research methods

For many years, theory and research on interpreting have studied mostly the conference venue, focusing on information processing skills, and these studies were mostly experimental and/or quasi-experimental (Gile 2001). This research could not account for the complexities that interpreters face when they work in healthcare interpreting, brokering and facilitating communication between members of different levels of society, or in the courts where party interactions or interpreters' interventions are closely regulated. Because findings from conference interpreting have influenced heavily the field of healthcare interpreting in its inception, it is helpful to look at the different periods, the various methods used, and the profiles of researchers studying conference interpreting.

Specifically in the healthcare setting, various empirical studies have been conducted on interpreted medical discourse (Angelelli 2004a, 2011; Bolden 2000; Davidson 1998, 2000, 2001; Kaufert and Putsch 1997; Metzger 1999; Wadensjö 1995, 1998). Most of these have been qualitative in nature with a few exceptions that have used mixed paradigms or a few quantitative studies (Angelelli 2001, 2003, and 2004b respectively). They have studied different ethnic groups and vary both in the types of questions asked and the number of encounters analyzed. Focusing on aboriginal interpreters and using interviews, Kaufert and Putsch (1997) look at the interpreter's dilemmas and consider day-to-day workplace pressures and ethical decisions, focusing on informed consent and end-of-life decisions mediated by interpreters. Also using interviews as part of a larger ethnographic study Angelelli (2004a) interviewed 10 participants to discuss their role. Many of these interpreters turn to the use of metaphors to describe their jobs. The only traditional view is that of interpreters as multifaceted bridges; the other metaphors clearly point to a more visible and proactive role. These medical interpreters compare their work to that of a detective who searches for the necessary answer, a miner who excavates until the answer is found, and a *diamond connoisseur* who must possess the ability to distinguish relevant information (diamonds) from the less relevant information (dirt). During this study, the tension between the role prescribed by professional associations, as stated in professional codes of ethics and/or standards of practice, and the role described by interpreters in their own words (which illustrates their own perception) becomes evident.

Several studies have used discourse analysis as a lens to study interactions. While examining English–ASL medical interviews, Metzger (1999) applies frame theory and Goffman's (1981) concept of footing to analyze the interpreter's influence on interpreted interactions in two interpreting cases. She concludes that interpreters can misrepresent the source message footings by using their own renditions and utterances, thus giving them powerful influence over the discourse that is interpreted. Also studying ASL interlocutors and using Goffman's framework of roles, Roy (1993, 2000) analyzes an interpreted (ASL–English) encounter between a deaf student and a professor. She demonstrates that the interpreter is an active participant in the interaction, because of 'the shifts interpreters make from relaying messages to managing and coordinating talk' (2000: 111). In the two instances analyzed by Roy, the interlocutor directly addresses the interpreter, and the interpreter responds directly back to the interlocutor. The author focuses on turn-taking as she analyzes the role of the interpreter, whom she says takes 'responsibility for the flow and maintenance of communication (2000: 121). In another school setting, this time with young immigrant bilingual Spanish/English high-school students, Valdés et al. (2000) examine the performance of 25 participants from two high schools who act as interpreters between a mother and the school principal. The study reveals that young interpreters, considered ad-hoc interpreters, exhibit many of the same characteristics displayed by experienced and professional interpreters in terms of strategies. It also demonstrates the agency displayed by these youngsters as they deal with offensive remarks and face-threatening acts.

Studying spoken languages, Davidson (1998) looks at the construction of reciprocity and meaning in interpreted conversations between Spanish-speaking patients and English-speaking healthcare providers. He states that the various parties to the interpreted communicative encounter see the role of the interpreter differently. For example, the physician sees the interpreter as a human instrument (who helps keep the patient and thus, the conversation) on track. However, the patient sees the interpreter as a co-conversationalist. Davidson attributes the difficulties that occur during interpreted encounters to both the construction of reciprocal understanding and the inaccurate transformation of semantic and/or pragmatic content. Targeting a different ethnic group and also using medical interviews as the object of study, Bolden (2000) analyzes interactions between English-speaking doctors and Russian-speaking patients. She challenges the non-participatory nature of interpreters by demonstrating that interpreters orient toward obtaining medically relevant information from patients and conveying that information to providers. Also using discourse analysis Wadensjö (1995) looks at how responsibility 'for the progression and the substance of interaction is distributed in and through talk' (1995: 112). Her analysis shows that the interpreter's role during the interaction goes beyond a traditional channel that simply conveys information. She argues that interpreters co-construct meaning together with the interlocutors, and that responsibility during interpreting is shared by all parties to the conversation.

Recommendations for practice

As evident from the discussion above, complex layers of meaning are embedded in conversations about pain, illness, and medicine. The complexity multiplies in the healthcare setting when interpreters are needed to bridge the discourse communities of the provider (and medicine) and the patient, not only by interpreting the languages spoken, but also by bridging cultures coordinating talk, and seeking answers to questions that providers and patients raise as they communicate with one another.

Currently there are no universally agreed rules for healthcare interpreters working in different types of encounters (e.g., diabetic education, mental health). Nor is there a universally accepted definition of interpreting competence, or subset of competencies that constitute ability in healthcare interpreting (Angelelli 2008b). Healthcare interpreters range from certified professionals in other areas related to language professions (e.g., court interpreting, translation, language teaching) to bilingual professionals in other areas who are assigned dual roles (e.g., a bilingual nurse or lab technician) to non-professionals or ad-hoc interpreters (patients' friends, family members – including children). As discussed above, there are various codes of ethics and standards of practice. There is, however, little empirical evidence of how these codes reflect the realities of the practices at hand (c.f. Angelelli 2006; Angelelli et al. 2007). This is an area that requires attention and it would benefit from researchers and practitioners working together (Angelelli 2008a; Roy 2000).

Additionally, to bridge the gap between theory and practice we need to pay special attention to the education (and training) of healthcare interpreters (Angelelli 2008b). Some schools that offer interpreting courses and many professional associations offering training teach from experiential knowledge. Oftentimes courses do not provide students with the context and framework in which the practice is grounded. In the United States there are limited educational opportunities for healthcare interpreters to pursue. By bringing theory and research to bear in the education of healthcare interpreters, students will become aware of the role they may or may not choose to play and of the responsibility emerging from the power they have as interpreters. They will learn how to use their interpersonal skills effectively, and the responsibilities and duties that arise from their tasks. Students need to learn that healthcare interpreters, like interpreters in general, are co-participants who share responsibility for effective communication (Roy 2000). This responsibility needs to be made explicit to students (Angelelli 2006: 28). Additionally, an integral education in interpreting would affect how student interpreters are assessed and certified (Angelelli 2007, 2008a), and the measurement of skills would also be comprehensive. Student interpreters need to gain awareness (Angelelli 2006:40–41; 2008a, 2008b) on the nature of situated practices, and the specifics of the healthcare setting. They must be able to contextualize the type of interactions in which they will participate.

In addition to the recommendations for teaching and professional associations, a word must be said about the importance of meaningful testing and assessment in this area, both for professional and educational purposes. The need for qualified healthcare interpreters is increasing exponentially. However, less than 25 percent of US hospitals are either staffed with skilled interpreters (Flores et al. 2003) – be they on-site or working remotely via teleconference or video-conference – or have the adequate screening mechanisms in place to determine who can perform the job. Current tests need to target not only the information processing and lexical abilities of interpreters, but also the sociolinguistic competence and the role of the interpreter. The language interpreter in general, and the healthcare interpreter in particular, needs to exhibit at least an advanced/superior proficiency level in both languages as well as an ability to use those languages under pressure to convey messages in a socio-culturally appropriate way (Angelelli 2007, 2008a). Yet, our understanding of the language competencies used by these individuals is only incipient, as these superior L1/L2 users have seldom been studied (Angelelli 2008b), and little is known on the development of language competencies beyond the advanced level in general. A basic assumption is that healthcare interpreters must be able at a minimum: (a) to understand what both interlocutors say (using both formal and informal registers); (b) to relay information in both registers, and (c) to understand material written in the two languages of the interaction. In addition, the role that interpreters are expected to play in interactions needs to be tested with meaningful instruments (Angelelli 2003) rather than assumed.

Future directions

Healthcare interpreting is a complex communicative event, a site of linguistic and cultural contact. Over the last 25 years, it has been establishing itself as a professional type of interpreting. Several codes of ethics and standards of practice have been developed and researchers have turned their attention to the little connection that exists between research and practice (Angelelli 2008a, 2010; Valero Garcés and Martin 2008).

Further research could shed some light on the tensions arising between the code of ethics that prescribes what interpreters should do in their practice and what the interpreters actually do. In addition, further research is needed to develop a comprehensive aptitude scale and test on healthcare interpreting, to actually assure that individuals who broker communication for linguistic minorities are up to the task. This scale and this test should also reflect the use of new technologies (e.g., video conferencing) currently in place in some healthcare settings.

In sum, nearly every hospital in our country receives patients with limited-English proficiency. As a result, we see an increasing need for professional interpreters in the medical setting. In the absence of qualified interpreters, healthcare organizations in the US have been forced to resort to creative solutions in order to bridge the linguistic barrier between providers seeking to assist patients and patients seeking help. Further studies are necessary to see if current solutions are enabling meaningful access to equal quality of health care for linguistic minorities.

Related topics

Access to services; agency; code of ethics; community interpreters; conference interpreters; healthcare interpreter; invisibility; linguistic diversity; linguistic minorities; agency; role; visibility.

Further reading

Chun, A., Nguyen, E., Agger-Gupta, N., Angelelli, C., Green, C.E., Haffner, L., et al. (2002) *California Standards for Healthcare Interpreters: Ethical Principles, Protocols and Guidance on Roles and Intervention*. Santa Barbara, CA: California Healthcare Interpreters Association (CHIA) and The California Endowment. (Available online at: http://www.calendow.org).

Metzger, M. (1999) *Sign Language Interpreting: Deconstructing the Myth of Neutrality*. Washington, DC: Gallaudet University Press.

Valdés, G. and Angelelli, C. (2003) Interpreters, interpreting, and the study of bilingualism. *Annual Review of Applied Linguistics*, 23: 58–78.

Valero Garcés, Carmen and Martin, Anne (eds) (2008) *Building Bridges: The Controversial Role of the Community Interpreter*. Amsterdam: John Benjamins.

References

Angelelli, C.V. (2000) Interpreting as a communicative event: a look through Hymes' lenses. *Meta. Journal des Traducteurs*, 45(4): 580–592.

——(2001) Deconstructing the invisible interpreter: a critical study of the interpersonal role of the interpreter in a cross-cultural/linguistic communicative event. *Dissertation Abstracts International*, 62(09), 2953. (UMI No. AAT 3026766).

——(2003) The interpersonal role of the interpreter in cross-cultural communication: survey of conference, court, community and medical interpreters in the US, Canada and Mexico. In Louise Brunette, George Bastin, Isabelle Hemlin, and Heather Clarke (eds) *Critical Link 3: Interpreters in the Community* (pp. 289–302). Amsterdam: John Benjamins.

——(2004a) *Medical Interpreting and Cross-cultural Communication*. Cambridge: Cambridge University Press.

——(2004b) *Revisiting the Interpreter's Role*. Amsterdam: John Benjamins.

——(2006) Validating professional standards and codes: challenges and opportunities. *INTERPRETING: International Journal of Research and Practice in Interpreting*, 8(2): 175–193.

——(2007) Accommodating the need for medical interpreters: the California Endowment Interpreter Testing Project [This work was made possible by The California Endowment Grant G00005318]. *The Translator*, 13(1): 63–82.

——(2008a) The role of the interpreter in the healthcare setting: a plea for a dialogue between research and practice. In Carmen Valero Garcés and Anne Martin (eds) *Building Bridges: The Controversial Role of the Community Interpreter* (pp. 139–152). Amsterdam: John Benjamins.

——(2008b) Longitudinal studies and the development of assessment for advanced competencies. In Lourdes Ortega and Heidi Byrnes (eds) *The Longitudinal Study of L2 Advanced Capacities.* Second Language Acquisition Research Series. (pp. 264–278). New York: Routledge.

——(2010) A glimpse into the socialization of bilingual youngsters as interpreters: the case of Latino bilinguals brokering communication for their families and immediate communities. In *MonTI Monografías de Traducción e Interpretación* Volume 2 (pp. 81–96).

——(2011) Can you ask her about chronic illnesses, diabetes and all that? In C. Alvstad, A. Hild, and E. Tiselius (eds) *Methods and Strategies of Process Research Integrative Approaches in Translation Studies* (pp. 231–246). [John Benjamins Translation Library 94]. Amsterdam: John Benjamins.

Angelelli, C., Agger-Gupta, N., Green, C., and Okahara, L. (2007) The California Standards for Healthcare Interpreters: Ethical Principles, Protocols and Guidance on Roles and Intervention. In Cecilia Wadensjö, Birgitta Dimitrova, and Anna-Lena Nilsson (eds) *The Critical Link 4: The Professionalization of Interpreting in the Community* (pp. 167–180). Amsterdam: John Benjamins.

Berk-Seligson, S. (1990) *The Bilingual Courtroom: Court Interpreters in the Judicial Process.* Chicago, IL: University of Chicago Press.

Bolden, G. (2000) Toward understanding practices of medical interpreting: interpreters' involvement in history taking. *Discourse Studies*, 2(4): 387–419.

California HealthCare Interpreting Association. CHIA (2002) *California Standards for Healthcare Interpreters: Proposed Ethical Principles, Protocols and Guidance on Interpreter Interventions and Roles*. Sacramento, CA: The California Endowment.

Collado Aís. A.(1998) Quality assessment in simultaneous interpreting: the importance of non-verbal communication. In F. Pöchhacker and M. Shlesinger (eds) (2002) *The Interpreting Studies Reader* (pp. 326–336). New York: Routledge.

Davidson, B. (1998) Interpreting medical discourse: a study of cross-linguistic communication in the hospital clinic. Doctoral Dissertation, Stanford University, Stanford, CA.

——(2000) The interpreter as institutional gatekeeper: the social-linguistic role of interpreters in Spanish–English medical discourse. *Journal of Sociolinguistics*, 4(3): 379–405.

——(2001) Questions in cross-linguistic medical encounters: the role of the hospital interpreter. *Anthropological Quarterly*, 74(4): 170–178.

de Bot, K. (2000) Simultaneous interpreting as language production. In B. Dimitrova and K. Hyltenstam (eds) *Language Processing and Simultaneous Interpreting* (pp. 65–89). Amsterdam: John Benjamins.

Flores, G., Laws, M.B., Mayo, S.J., Zuckerman, B., Abreu, M., Medina, L., et al. (2003) Errors in medical interpretation and their potential clinical consequences in pediatric encounters. *Pediatrics*, 111(1): 6–14.

Gile, D. (2001) Conference and simultaneous interpreting. In M. Baker (ed.) *Routledge Encyclopedia of Translation Studies* (pp. 40–45). London: Routledge.

Goffman, I. (1981) *Forms of Talk*. Philadelphia, PA: University of Pennsylvania Press.

Hymes, D. (1974) *Foundations in Sociolinguistics*. Philadelphia, PA: University of Pennsylvania Press.

Kaufert, J. and Putsch, R. (1997) Communication through interpreters in healthcare: ethical dilemmas arising from differences in class, culture, language and power. *Journal of Clinical Ethics*, 8(1): 71–87.

Kopscinscki, A. (1994) Quality in conference interpreting: some pragmatic problems. In M. Snell-Hornby, F. Pöchhacker, and K. Kaindl (eds) *Translation Studies – An Interdiscipline* (pp. 189–198). Amsterdam: John Benjamins.

Massachusetts Medical Interpreters Association. (1995) *Medical Interpreting Standards of Practice.* Boston, MA: Massachusetts Medical Interpreters Association.

Metzger, M. (1999) Sign *Language Interpreting: Deconstructing the Myth of Neutrality* (pp. 1–9). Washington, DC: Gallaudet University Press.

National Council on Interpreting in Health Care. (2012) Available HTTP. <http://www.ncihc.org/> (accessed February 2, 2012).

Paradis, M. (2000) Prerequisites to a study of neurolinguistic processes involved in simultaneous interpreting. A synopsis. In B. Dimitrova and K. Hyltenstam (eds) *Language Processing and Simultaneous Interpreting* (pp. 17–24). Amsterdam: John Benjamins.

Reddy, M. (ed.) (1979) *The Conduit Metaphor: A Case of Frame Conflict in our Language about Language*. Cambridge: Cambridge University Press.

Roy, C. (1989) A sociolinguistic analysis of the interpreter's role in the turn exchanges of an interpreted event. Unpublished Dissertation, Georgetown University, Washington, DC.

——(1993) The problem with definitions, descriptions and the role of metaphors of interpreters. In F. Pöchhacker and M. Shlesinger (eds) (2002) *The Interpreting Studies Reader* (pp. 344–353). New York: Routledge.

Roy, C.B. (2000*) Interpreting as a Discourse Process*. New York: Oxford University Press.

Russo, Mariachiara. (2011) Aptitude testing over the years. *Interpreting,* 13(1): 5–30.

Stanford Hospital and Clinics Interpreter Services Department. (1985) *Code of Ethics for Medical Interpreters and Translators*. Stanford, CA: Stanford Hospital and Clinics.

Swayer, D. (2004) *Fundamental Aspects of Interpreter Education: Curriculum and Assessment*. Amsterdam: John Benjamins.

Szabo, C. (2006) Language choice in note-taking for consecutive interpreting: a topic revisited. *INTERPRETING: International Journal of Research and Practice in Interpreting,* 8(2): 129–148.

Valdés, G., Chavez, C., and Angelelli, C. (2000) Bilingualism from another perspective: the case of young interpreters from immigrant communities. In A. Roca (ed.) *Research on Spanish in the United States: Linguistic Issues and Challenges* (pp. 42–81). Somerville, MA: Cascadilla Press.

Valdés, G., Chavez, C., Angelelli, C., Enright, K., Garcia, D., and Gonzalez, M. (2003) The performance of the young interpreters on the scripted task. In Guadalupe Valdés *Expanding Definitions of Giftedness. The Case of Young Interpreters from Immigrant Communities* (pp. 119–164). Mahwah, NJ: Lawrence Erlbaum.

Valero Garcés, C. (2005) Doctor–patient consultations in dyatic and triatic exchanges. *Interpreting,* 7(2): 193–210.

Valero Garcés, C. and Martin, A. (eds) (2008) *Building Bridges: The Controversial Role of the Community Interpreter* (pp. 139–152). Amsterdam: John Benjamins.

Wadensjö, C. (1995) Dialogue interpreting and the distribution of responsibility. *Hermes, Journal of Linguistics,* 14: 111–129.

——(1998) *Interpreting as Interaction*. London: Longman.

36

The contribution of provider–patient communication to health disparities

Carma L. Bylund and Emily B. Peterson

Introduction

Widespread disparities exist among individuals living in the United States in terms of overall health status, disease incidence and mortality rates, time of diagnosis, and co-morbidities. Generally speaking, individuals of minority race, less education, and lower income experience worse health and health outcomes than do white, educated, middle-upper income individuals.

A well-known example of racial cancer disparities is in breast cancer: white American women have higher incidence rates of breast cancer than African American women, but African American women have a higher mortality rate than white women from breast cancer even when controlling for socio-economic status (SES) (CDC 2010a). Further, African Americans have higher incidence rates and mortality rates than whites for colorectal cancer (CDC 2010b), and African American men have higher incidence and mortality rates than white men for lung and prostate cancer (CDC 2010c, 2010d). African Americans are nine times more likely than whites to be diagnosed with AIDS (CDC 2009). Recent nationwide studies have found striking racial and ethnic disparities related to type 2 diabetes, including age of diagnosis, overall incidence rates (both diagnosed and undiagnosed), and morbidity and mortality rates after diagnosis. Type 2 diabetes is most prevalent among American Indians and Alaskan Natives, with diabetes prevalence in some groups representing over half of the population (Nsiah-Kumi et al. 2009). Additionally, non-Hispanic blacks are 1.6 times as likely and Hispanic/Latino Americans are 1.5 times as likely to have diabetes than non-Hispanic whites of similar age (Mensah et al. 2005).

A variety of explanations have been offered as the cause for such disparities. After a brief overview of these factors, we focus specifically on what has been called communication disparities, or the notion that healthcare providers communicate with patients differently depending on the same factors that predict health disparities.

The chapter begins with a review of the evidence about health disparities, including a focus on three diseases. We then provide a detailed review of the literature on disparities in healthcare communication and consider potential causes for such disparities. Finally, we overview potential solutions to these communication disparities. We use the term *provider* when referring to patients' communication with their healthcare providers more generally, and use the term *doctor* when referring to specific research that used doctors as subjects.

Historical perspectives

Health disparities

The Minority Health and Health Disparities Research and Education Act in the US (2000) defined a population to have health disparities 'if there is a significant disparity in the overall rate of disease incidence, prevalence, morbidity, mortality or survival rates in the population as compared to the health status of the general population'.

Health disparities are prevalent in multiple disease contexts and using multiple indicators. Due to the extent of health disparities in the US, the National Institutes of Health established the Office of Research on Minority Health in 1990, and in 2000 established the National Institute on Minority Health and Health Disparities, with the goal 'to promote minority health and to lead, coordinate, support, and assess the NIH effort to reduce and ultimately eliminate health disparities' (NIMHD 2011). In the following sections, we provide a brief overview of some key findings in the literature grouped into three major causes for health disparities: biological differences, individual-level differences, and systems-level differences. Examples for these factors will come from three major disease contexts: cancer, HIV/AIDS, and type 2 diabetes.

Biological differences

The research literature suggests that biological differences may be at least a partial cause of racial disparities. For example, one study examined nearly 20,000 adult cancer patients who were enrolled in randomized, Phase III cancer treatment clinical trials (Albain et al. 2009). The patients were receiving standardized care through the trials and the researchers statistically controlled for SES, thus being able to isolate the effects of race. When researchers compared the African American patients in the group to all other patients, an interesting pattern emerged: Higher mortality rates were present for African American patients with sex-specific cancers (e.g., breast, prostate), but not for other types of cancers.

Individual-level barriers

While biological factors have been shown to explain some of the causes of differences in prevalence and incident rates in certain disease contexts, another major factor is the interpersonal and individual-level differences that affect quality of care and prevention participation. Two of these factors will be examined below: medical non-adherence and provider visits.

For HIV patients, a main factor related to the behavioral dimension is rates of anti-retroviral treatment non-adherence. Compared with their white counterparts, African Americans with HIV are less likely to adhere to antiretroviral treatment utilization and adherence (Johnson et al. 2009). Medical mistrust may influence this phenomenon, as a recent study found that 64 percent of African American men with HIV held at least one genocidal or treatment-related conspiracy belief (e.g., HIV is a manmade virus, there is a cure for AIDS that is being withheld), and that such beliefs were significantly associated with non-adherence (Bogart et al. 2010).

Once with a provider, African American patients with HIV/AIDS are less verbally dominant than white patients, although they show similar levels of provider trust and satisfaction (Beach et al. 2010; Sohler et al. 2007). Studies in primary care settings often show differences in levels of racially discordant providers' patient-centeredness and emotional tone with African American patients, but this disparity seems to fade somewhat after the AIDS diagnosis (Johnson et al. 2004; Beach et al. 2010).

The same phenomenon is present for patients with type 2 diabetes. In a study of diabetic retinopathy, a microvascular complication causing blindness in patients, researchers found that racial and ethnic populations are at high risk for this complication, yet are not being adequately screened or treated for the condition (Nsiah-Kumi et al. 2009). Provider–patient communication factors again seemed to play a dominant role in screening and treatment rates for diabetic retinopathy. For example, one study explored barriers to compliance with diabetic retinopathy screening guidelines (Mukamel et al. 1999). The most prominent factor for screening was the average number of primary care physician (PCP) visits each patient had. This suggests that an increase in contact may lead to more time for interaction and education of the patient. In fact, an increase of one monthly visit to the PCP increased the odds of screening by 28 percent in diabetes patients.

While an individual's preferences or medical mistrust may influence his or her average number of primary care physician visits, socio-economic barriers or other system-level factors also play a primary role to a patient's access to physicians. These differences are discussed in the following section.

System-level barriers

A final barrier or difference that causes racial health disparities are societal or system-level issues that are related to a patient's culture and socio-economic status. SES is often measured using income, education, occupation, and health insurance status.

The relationship between SES and indicators of health is not a 'threshold model' where everyone above a certain level of SES achieves the same health benefits that are higher than those below that level. Instead it is a continuous model, where as income and education increase, generally so do major health indicators (Barr 2008). This pattern is also apparent when looking at health disparities in other countries. Two major issues related to SES, health insurance status and access to health care, are discussed below followed by a brief discussion on cultural-level differences.

An individual's health insurance status (private, Medicaid, or uninsured) is a primary factor in health disparities. Health insurance status can play a major role in explaining disparities as it is associated with prevention, screening, and consequently early detection, stage of diagnosis, and survival (Ward et al. 2008). One disease context where this is very evident is cancer. The insured are significantly more likely than the uninsured to receive screening for breast and colorectal cancer (ACS 2001). Lack of screening consequently leads to later stage diagnosis. One study of 3.7 million individuals with cancer found that those patients who were uninsured or Medicaid-insured were significantly more likely to present with advanced- stage cancer than those who were privately insured with cancers that can be detected early by screening or system assessment showing the largest differences (Halpern et al. 2008).

Health insurance status has been shown to be a predictor for another major system-level barrier related to health disparities: access to care. Generally speaking, African Americans and Latinos with HIV/AIDS tend to receive care from sites with limited resources, longer travel and wait times, and less provider continuity than whites, and the trend continues with patients living with HIV/AIDS (Korthuis et al. 2008). Additionally, individuals from ethnic/minority backgrounds have not been proportionately represented in AIDS clinical trials, which may be due to lack of knowledge about the trials, fear of being 'a guinea pig', or because they were not offered enrollment by their provider (Sullivan et al. 2007). Lack of access to preventative care services has also been hypothesized as a cause of high cancer prevalence rates. Among Medicare patients with early-stage non-small cell lung cancer, African Americans had significantly lower rates of surgical treatment than did whites, and African American patients also had a lower survival rate (Bach et al. 1999). However, among patients who had surgery, there were no differences in mortality between African American and white patients.

Although these issues play a dominant role in health disparities, racial disparities in risk factors do not fully explain disparities in the disease. In fact, racial disparities in type 2 diabetes are often most prominent when common risk factors are not a significant contributing factor. One study found that racial/ethnic disparities in type 2 diabetes were most pronounced in normal and overweight groups, and least pronounced in obese and severely obese groups of similar SES status (Zhang et al. 2009). This suggests that other causes may additionally be contributing to the unequal racial distribution of type 2 diabetes incidence rates. For example, acculturation and psychosocial stress have been shown to increase insulin resistance, regardless of weight (Bjorntorp 2001). Because of this, Zhang et al. (2009) called for culturally tailored programs, specifically for Mexican Americans and Native Americans who are at greatest risk of developing type 2 diabetes.

A similar disparity exists for individuals with HIV/AIDS. While an individual's risky behavior is often linked to HIV/AIDS incidence rates, one study found that young African American adults are at high risk of HIV infections even when they engaged in normative behaviors (Hallfors et al. 2007). In response to these findings, Kraut-Becher and colleagues (2008) called for a closer look at cultural or macro-level factors instead of solely individual-level factors such as non-normative behaviors (Muula 2007).

Current contributions and research

Communication disparities and possible causes

Racial communication disparities

The presence of racial communication disparities in health care has also been acknowledged as a potential contributor to health disparities, given the link between provider–patient communication and health outcomes (Epstein and Street 2007; Ashton et al. 2003; Gordon et al. 2006a, 2006b). Most research on communication disparities has used patient race as the predictive variable, although many have also controlled for SES and other patient demographics.

Doctors communicate differently with different patients (Epstein and Street 2007; Bao et al. 2007; Street 2001). Several explanations could potentially exist for this variance. First, doctors may be appropriately responding to patients' needs, such as a doctor involving one patient more in decision-making than another because of the patient's expressed preferences for involvement. Second, doctors could have biases based on prejudicial attitudes, such as a doctor involving a highly educated patient more in decision-making than a less educated patient, without discovering patient preferences. An important third explanation is that patients' own communication and attitudes influence the communication process as well.

Studies show a continual pattern of poorer patient-centered communication when doctors communicate with non-white patients than with white patients. In a study of patients visiting thoracic surgery or oncology clinics, African American patients perceived their doctors' communication to be less informative, less supportive, and less partnering than did white patients (Gordon et al. 2006a). In another study of cancer patients, African American patients reported poorer communication with their doctors than did white patients. However, patient income seemed to explain much of this difference (Manfredi et al. 2010). In a primary care setting, African American patients rated their doctors' visits as significantly less participatory than white patients, even when controlling for patient demographics and length of the doctor–patient relationship (Cooper-Patrick et al. 1999).

African Americans and Latinos tend to utilize healthcare services that need a doctor's order less than whites (Ashton et al. 2003), even when access to healthcare services are held constant. In a study on cancer screening, non-white patients and less educated patients were less likely to have received counseling from their doctors about colorectal cancer screening than were white and more educated patients (Wee et al. 2005). Further, when a recommendation for screening was given, there was no difference in race between the white and non-white patients in terms of adherence. Because Hispanic patients and less educated patients were also less likely to have been screened, this is a prime example of how a communication disparity can directly impact a health outcome.

Other research has gone beyond patient self-report measures to assess actual doctor–patient interactions, through recording and coding these interactions. In a study of primary care interactions and using the Roter Interaction Analysis System (RIAS), researchers found white patients and African American patients had different communication processes with their doctors (Johnson et al. 2004). Overall, doctors dominated the conversation more, were less patient-centered, and showed less affect with African American patients than white patients. Another study showed doctors to be more contentious with African American rather than white and Hispanic patients (Street et al. 2007). In addition, the doctors in the study perceived African American patients to be less effective communicators and less satisfied with their care. The researchers explored whether this difference existed because the African American patients were also more contentious and displayed less positive affect than white and Hispanic patients, but did not find this to be so. There was, however, some effect of the physician's race on perceptions of patients such that African American physicians did not perceive African American patients as poorly as did other physicians.

Other research has found similar results in contexts other than primary care. Gordon and colleagues audio recorded and coded interactions between a group of patients and their companions with pulmonary nodules or lung cancer at a VA hospital (Gordon et al. 2006b). They found that in consultations with African American patients doctors used fewer information-giving utterances and there were also fewer utterances indicating patient or companion participation. The researchers then controlled for the frequency with which patients and companions sought information from the doctor, and found that the differences in information-giving disappeared. Further coding of information-giving utterances demonstrated that doctors self-initiated information-giving equally between African American and white patients, but information-giving prompted by patients happened less frequently with African American than white patients. This highlights the fact that interpersonal communication is influenced by both parties, and that while communication racial disparities may still be influenced by doctors, they are also influenced by patients (Gordon et al. 2006b).

Beach and colleagues examined the different experiences of white patients and Hispanic patients during HIV care using audio recording and RIAS. Overall, Hispanic patients received less patient-centered care and less psychosocial talk from their providers than did non-Hispanic white patients (Beach et al. 2010). Interestingly, the Hispanic patients did not perceive their care more negatively than did the white patients.

Another study examined patients who had high levels of depressive symptoms, finding that African American patients had less overall depression talk in their interactions with doctors than did white patients. The African American patients also had less rapport-building conversations than did white patients. These differences remained, even after adjusting for education (Ghods et al. 2008).

In summary, self-reports and coded interactions from multiple studies in various contexts show a similar overall pattern that doctors' communication with non-white patients is poorer than with white patients. Each of these methods has its strengths and limitations. Self-reported patient surveys can capture patients' perspectives on their communication with their doctors and provide important information about the importance of a variety of healthcare communication functions. However, such surveys do not give the researchers a clear and objective description of the interaction. Audio or video recordings of the interaction would allow researchers to identify specific communication behaviors. For example, if patients consistently report a particular doctor to be empathic in her interactions with patients, without audio or video recordings there is no way to identify what the doctor is doing that is perceived as empathic.

There are also some limitations to the studies reviewed above as a group. Not all of the studies reported controlling for the clustering effect of a doctor seeing multiple patients. In the studies where self-report data from patient surveys were analyzed (Manfredi et al. 2010; Wee et al. 2005), this is understandable; however, one study that recruited patients from a specific group of doctors in clinics did not report whether the effect of the doctor was controlled for (Levinson et al. 2008). Despite these limitations and the need for further research, it seems clear that non-white patients have poorer overall communication with their doctors. We will now consider two possible causes of this phenomenon: Doctors' assumptions and biases, and patients' assumptions and mistrust.

Doctor assumptions and biases

There is considerable evidence that doctors' attitudes and diagnoses vary based solely on patient's sociodemographic characteristics, even when researchers control for income, insurance coverage, and disease severity (Bertakis et al. 1993; Martin et al. 1998). For example, Van Ryn and Burke (2000) found that doctors rated their coronary artery disease (CAD) African American patients as more at risk for a number of factors, including noncompliance with cardiac rehabilitation and substance abuse. Additionally, they reported less affiliative feelings toward African American patients than toward white patients. Finally, the doctors in the study rated their African American coronary artery disease patients as less intelligent than white patients even when controlling for patient sex, age, income, and education. Perhaps most disturbing, doctors in the study rated African American patients as significantly less educated than white patients, even when controlling for the patient's actual level of education. These unfounded assumptions and biases toward African American patients from white doctors are directly observable on medical care, including amount of follow-up and medical care (Tischler 1966) and mammogram screening recommendations (Bao et al. 2007). Research on doctor bias and communication is in its infancy, but it is easy to see how biases may affect communication, consequently affecting medical outcomes.

However, doctors are not always aware of their biases. Research has shown that unconscious or implicit bias can affect doctors' clinical judgments and decision-making, possibly even more than overt prejudice. Green and colleagues (2007) were the first to directly test implicit race bias among doctors. Using the Implicit Association Test (IAT), the authors measured the amount of time it took for doctors to match hypothetical African American and white patients to specific attributes or characteristics. They found that while there were no differences in doctors' self-reported preferences for African American or white patients, there were significant implicit biases found in the IAT test with negative characteristics (e.g., uncooperative or 'bad') more strongly associated with African Americans than whites. Importantly, as the degree of doctor implicit bias against African American patients increased, the likelihood to recommend the patient for thrombolysis treatment decreased.

Implicit biases are often related to issues of perceived adherence and cooperation levels of ethnic groups and are often manifested through a decreased likelihood to recommend the patient for transplants, therapies, or clinical trials. For example, doctors perceived African Americans as being less adherent to the treatment guidelines for highly active antiretroviral therapy, an HIV treatment, and reported less willingness to prescribe the therapy to African American patients (Bogart et al. 2001). Similar results have been found in other medical specialties, with doctors significantly less likely to recommend African American patients for renal transplants (Ayanian et al. 1999), cardiac catheterization (Schulman et al. 1999), and coronary heart disease treatment (Fincher et al. 2004).

Patient assumptions and mistrust

Although doctors' stereotypes of minorities and resulting communication changes have a clear link to quality of care given, another important possible factor in explaining communication and health disparities is the mistrust that many African American patients have toward doctors and the healthcare system. A defining moment between these two groups was the Tuskegee syphilis study. In 1932, researchers enrolled poor African American men with syphilis in the study, which was conducted to determine the effects of syphilis on the human body. The participants were never told they had syphilis, and even after penicillin became the standard cure in the 1940s, the men were not told about or offered the medication (Freimuth et al. 2001). Matthews et al. note, 'the legacy of the Tuskegee experiments is still monumental for many African Americans, particularly in the absence of information about the current regulation of research studies, including clinical trials' (2002: 215).

Given this history, it is unsurprising that some African Americans today exhibit low levels of trust toward their white doctors. Additionally, trust is of great importance to African American patients because of 'a cultural belief that a doctor must know a patient to provide good medical care. ... Viewing the doctor–patient relationship as a business may create feelings among African American patients of their bodies as a commodity of an easily quantifiable value versus that of a human being' (Collins et al. 2002: 132), which may result in fears of exploitation. For example, Freedman found that some African American women believe that white doctors overlook diseases prevalent in the African American community (Freedman 1998), while Matthews and colleagues describe a sentiment of mistrust of doctors and that the medical community will continue to use African Americans as medical experiments, like Tuskegee (Matthews et al. 2002). As one African American patient put it, 'No, I'm not going up there 'cause all they do is lie. They just want to use us as guinea pigs' (Matthews et al. 2002: 214).

This mistrust has strong implications for health outcomes, and contributes to disparity of care in this population. One study found that participants strongly preferred treatments that they knew about independently from their doctors (e.g., mastectomy), as opposed to treatments they perceived as experimental (e.g., lumpectomy) but in reality were the highest standard of care offered to all patients (Matthews et al. 2002). Additionally, this mistrust is often manifested in doctor–patient communication through patient reticence and lack of questions, which doctors may in turn interpret as passivity or low intelligence, thus exacerbating the problem (Gordon et al. 2005). When these barriers to effective communication interact, 'a scenario may unfold where physicians may be less engaged with African American patients, and the patient does little to prompt more from the doctor' (Gordon et al. 2005: 1022).

Recommendations for practice: improving communication disparities

The research literature, as summarized above, points to the conclusion that communication disparities exist and that both doctors and patients contribute to these. In the final section of this chapter, we address three possible ways to address such: having racial concordance in healthcare interactions, mitigating the effect of provider implicit bias, and improving healthcare communication through skills training interventions.

Racial concordance

Unsurprisingly, many of the health disparities between African American and white patients seem to disappear when the doctor and the patient are racially concordant (i.e., of the same race). Gordon and colleagues (2006b) found that patients in racially concordant consultations received more information from their doctors, primarily because they engaged more in communicative behaviors, like asking questions or expressing concerns. The authors concluded that, 'while not directly negating the possibility that racial disparities in medical care are due to doctor biases or patient preferences, [the findings] suggest that disparities in medical care are related in part to the communicative dynamics of the encounter, particularly the degree to which patients are actively involved' (Gordon et al. 2006b: 1318).

This hypothesis is consistent with previous research examining racial concordance that suggests that technical issues of care (e.g., amount of information giving, screening recommendations) may be less important to the outcomes of patient care than interpersonal rapport. Cooper and colleagues (2003) found significant differences in length visit, rate of speech, and patient satisfaction between racially concordant and discordant doctor–patient dyads. However, they did not find any difference between the actual participatory decision-making between the two groups, suggesting 'that race concordance has an independent effect on patients' judgment of the visit regardless of the verbal nature of the medical dialogue' (Cooper et al. 2003: 911). In other words, patients interpreted the same medical dialogue differently, depending on if they were experiencing interaction through a racially concordant or racially discordant context.

Increasing the number of minorities practicing medicine is important to increase the diversity of providers and give minority patients more ability to choose racially concordant providers (Smedley 2003); however, it is not realistic or even desirable for this to be the only solution to racial communication disparities.

Mitigation of the effect of implicit bias

A second method by which racial communication disparities might be improved is to lessen the effect of providers' implicit bias on health care. The goal is not to eliminate the biases, as these are very resistant to change, but to help providers realize that they have biases so that they can manage them effectively (Burgess et al. 2007). Several researchers and medical educators have proposed strategies for doing this (Teal et al. 2012).

For instance, based upon social cognitive psychology, Burgess and colleagues recommended several strategies that might be useful in working to overcome the negative effects of implicit bias in health care (Burgess et al. 2007). These include focusing on a person's individual attributes rather than the attributes of the groups to which they belong; helping providers recognize their biases and to understand the normal process of psychological bias; increasing providers' abilities and confidence to interact successfully and build partnerships with patients who are dissimilar from them; and increasing empathy. They conclude that these strategies need to be empirically tested in healthcare settings.

Teal and colleagues tested a discussion-based intervention to help third-year medical students become aware of their implicit biases and to develop strategies to manage these biases, finding that it was a feasible intervention and that it changed students' intentions on strategy use to mitigate bias (Teal et al. 2010). Stone and Moskowitz also outline important components of a workshop with medical students on this topic (Stone and Moskowitz 2011).

Increasing patient-centered healthcare communication

Improving healthcare communication may also be an effective method by which to reduce racial communication disparities in health care. Emerging literature shows that patient-centered healthcare communication may be able to counteract the effects of racial communication disparities. Beach and colleagues tested the hypothesis that patient-centered communication can overcome racial biases/differences through a study with third-year medical students who were randomly assigned to interact with either an African American or a white standardized patient (Beach et al. 2007). Before the interaction, students received a survey assessing their attitudes toward patient-centered medicine. Patient-centered students used better communication in the standardized patient assessment with African American patients than did non-patient centered students. There was no difference between the two groups of students in their communication with white patients. However, patient-centered students still performed more poorly with African American than white patients, suggesting that racial communication disparities may not be able to be completely eliminated by the use of patient-centered communication (Beach et al. 2007).

Further adding to this body of evidence is a recent study that examined a group of African American patients with hypertension who interacted with either an African American doctor or a white physician (Schoenthaler et al. 2012). In the race-discordant interactions, patients' self-report of collaborative communication with the doctor resulted in better adherence than did patients' self-report of non-collaborative communication.

Street and colleagues (2008) also found that doctors can overcome the barriers inherent in racially discordant doctor–patient interactions through the use of patient-centered communication, noting 'a physician who is skilled in informing, showing respect, and supporting patient involvement can transcend issues of race and sex to establish a connection with the patient that in turn contributes to greater patient satisfaction, trust and commitment to treatment' (Street et al. 2008: 203).

As these studies seem to indicate the importance of patient-centered communication in overcoming racial communication disparities in health care, both doctor-focused and patient-focused interventions designed to help improve patient-centered communication may help to decrease racial communication disparities.

A primary doctor-focused intervention is communication skills training. Communication skills training has been shown to be effective in improving doctors' communication with patients, and thus their patient-centeredness (Brown et al. 2010; Bylund et al. 2010; Back et al. 2007; Cegala and Broz 2002). Best practices in communication skills training include experiential learning through role plays (Kurtz et al. 1998) that simulate a real consultation using an actor taking the role of a patient. The process of role play provides an opportunity for trainees to practice new skills and receive feedback about their performance from their facilitator and peers.

Patient-focused communication interventions focus on improving patients' communication skills globally, using patient communication skills training or focus specifically on improving patients' question asking, through the implementation of question prompt lists. Cegala and colleagues have studied patient communication training interventions, training patients in information-giving skills, asking questions, checking information, and expressing concerns (Cegala et al. 2000a, 2000b; Post et al. 2001). Results from these studies show that training patients to more effectively communicate with their doctors improves their participation in the encounter and health-related behaviors as well as affecting healthcare outcomes. Question prompt lists for patients have demonstrated effectiveness in improving patients' question-asking abilities and some patient outcomes (Brown et al. 1999; Shields et al. 2010).

More research needs to be done on patient-focused communicated interventions with minority patients. One study found that receipt of a communication skills workbook had a strong and significant effect on white patients, but minimal to no effect on African American patients (Post et al. 2001). The authors suggest that such findings may be explained by the fact that a workbook intervention involves minimal interpersonal contact, thus failing to address cultural factors. Cultural and language barriers may also make recruiting minority patients to patient communication skills training studies difficult (Bylund et al. 2011).

Conclusion

Health disparities are prevalent and pervasive in the US across various disease contexts. The multifaceted causes of health disparities need further study; however, the research is clear that racial communication disparities are a substantial contributor to health disparities. The causes of such disparities need further study, with a focus on both provider and patient factors.

As researchers and educators continue to develop and disseminate communication training interventions for providers and patients, a continual focus on how these interventions are addressing biases and encouraging patient-centered communication will be an important priority. Through careful and thoughtful work in this area, communication researchers can help to make a real difference in reducing health disparities.

Related topics

Communication disparities; race; social-economic status; cancer health disparities; bias; patient-centered care.

Further reading

Barr, D. A. 2008. *Health disparities in the United States,* Baltimore, MD, Johns Hopkins University Press.

Bylund, C. L., Brown, R. F., Bialer, P. A., Levin, T. T., Lubrano Di Ciccone, B., and Kissane, D. W. 2011. Developing and implementing an advanced communication training program in oncology at a comprehensive cancer center. *Journal of Cancer Education,* 26, 604–611.

Gordon, H. S., Street, R. L., Kelly, P., Souchek, J., and Wray, N. P. 2005. Physician–patient communication following invasive procedures: an analysis of post-angiogram consultations. *Social Science & Medicine,* 61, 1015–1025.

Post, D. M., Cegala, D. J., and Marinelli, T. M. 2001. Teaching patients to communicate with physicians: the impact of race. *Journal of the National Medical Association,* 93, 6–12.

Teal, C. R., Gill, A. C., Green, A. R., and Crandall, S. 2012. Helping medical learners recognise and manage unconscious bias toward certain patient groups. *Medical Education,* 46, 80–88.

References

2000. Minority Health and Health Disparities Research and Education Act. United States Public Law 106–525.

ACS. 2001. *www.cancer.org* [Online]. American Cancer Society.

Albain, K. S., Unger, J. M., Crowley, J. J., Coltman Jr., C. A., and Hershman, D. L. 2009. Racial disparities in cancer survival among randomized clinical trials patients of the Southwest Oncology Group. *Journal of the National Cancer Institute,* 101, 984–992.

Ashton, C. M., Haidet, P., Paterniti, D. A., Collins, T. C., Gordon, H. S., O'Malley, K. J., et al. 2003. Racial and ethnic disparities in the use of health services. *Journal of General Internal Medicine,* 18, 146–152.

Ayanian, J. Z., Cleary, P. D., Weissman, J. S., and Epstein, A. M. 1999. The effect of patients' preferences on racial differences in access to renal transplantation. *New England Journal of Medicine,* 341, 1661–1669.

Bach, P. B., Cramer, L. D., Warren, J. L., and Begg, C. B. 1999. Racial differences in the treatment of early-stage lung cancer. *New England Journal of Medicine,* 341, 1198–1205.

Back, A. L., Arnold, R. M., Baile, W. F., Fryer-Edwards, K. A., Alexander, S. C., Barley, G. E., et al. 2007. Efficacy of communication skills training for giving bad news and discussing transitions to palliative care. *Archives of Internal Medicine,* 167, 453–460.

Bao, Y., Fox, S. A., and Escarce, J. J. 2007. Socioeconomic and racial/ethnic differences in the discussion of cancer screening: 'between-' versus 'within-' physician differences. *Health Services Research,* 42, 950–970.

Barr, D. A. 2008. *Health disparities in the United States,* Baltimore, MD, Johns Hopkins University Press.

Beach, M. C., Rosner, M., Cooper, L. A., Duggan, P. S., and Shatzer, J. 2007. Can patient-centered attitudes reduce racial and ethnic disparities in care? *Academic Medicine,* 82, 193–198.

Beach, M. C., Saha, S., Korthuis, P. T., Sharp, V., Cohn, J., Wilson, I. B., et al. 2010. Differences in patient–provider communication for Hispanic compared to Non-Hispanic White patients in HIV care. *Journal of General Internal Medicine,* 25, 682–687.

Bertakis, K. D., Callahan, E. J., Helms, L. J., Azari, R., and Robbins, J. A. 1993. The effect of patient health status on physician practice style. *Family Medicine,* 25, 530–535.

Bjorntorp, P. 2001. Do stress reactions cause abdominal obesity and comorbidities? *Obesity Reviews,* 2, 73–86.

Bogart, L. M., Catz, S. L., Kelly, J. A., and Benotsch, E. G. 2001. Factors influencing physicians' judgments of adherence and treatment decisions for patients with HIV disease. *Medical Decision Making,* 21, 28–36.

Bogart, L. M., Wagner, G., Galvan, F. H., and Banks, D. 2010. Conspiracy beliefs about HIV are related to antiretroviral treatment nonadherence among African American men with HIV. *JAIDS – Journal of Acquired Immune Deficiency Syndromes,* 53, 648–655.

Brown, R. F., Butow, P. N., Boyer, M. J., and Tattersall, M. H. N. 1999. Promoting patient participation in the cancer consultation; evaluation of a prompt sheet and coaching in question asking. *British Journal of Cancer,* 80, 242–248.

Brown, R. F., Bylund, C. L., Lubrano Di Ciccone, B., Diamond, C., Eddington, J., and Kissane, D. 2010. Patient-centered communication skills training for oncologists: describing the content and efficacy of training. *Communication Education,* 59, 236–249.

Burgess, D., Van Ryn, M., Dovidio, J., and Saha, S. 2007. Reducing racial bias among health care providers: lessons from social-cognitive psychology. *Journal of General Internal Medicine,* 22, 882–887.

Bylund, C. L., Brown, R. F., Gugeun, J. A., Diamond, C., Bianculli, J., and Kissane, D. W. 2010. The implementation and assessment of a comprehensive communication skills training curriculum for oncologists. *Psycho-Oncology,* 19, 583–593.

Bylund, C. L., Goytia, E. J., D'Agostino, T. A., Bulone, L., Horner, J. A., Li, Y., et al. 2011. Evaluation of a pilot communication skills training intervention for minority cancer patients. *Journal of Psychosocial Oncology,* 29, 347–358.

CDC. 2009. HIV/AIDS Surveillance Report, 2009. Atlanta, GA: US Department of Health and Human Services.

CDC. 2010a. *Breast cancer rates by race and ethnicity* [Online]. Centers for Disease Control and Prevention. Available: http://www.cdc.gov/cancer/breast/statistics/race.htm [Accessed December 13, 2011].

——2010b. *Colorectal cancer rates by race and ethnicity* [Online]. Centers for Disease Control and Prevention. Available: http://www.cdc.gov/cancer/colorectal/statistics/race.htm [Accessed December 13, 2011].

——2010c. *Lung cancer rates by race and ethnicity* [Online]. Centers for Disease Control and Prevention. Available: http://www.cdc.gov/cancer/lung/statistics/race.htm [Accessed December 13, 2011].

——2010d. *Prostate cancer rates by race and ethnicity* [Online]. Centers for Disease Control and Prevention. Available: http://www.cdc.gov/cancer/prostate/statistics/race.htm [Accessed December 13, 2011].

Cegala, D. J. and Broz, S. L. 2002. Physician communication skills training; a review of the theoretical backgrounds, objectives and skills. *Medical Education,* 36, 1004–1016.

Cegala, D. J., Marinelli, T., and Post, D. 2000a. The effects of patient communication skills training on compliance. *Archives of Family Medicine,* 9, 57–64.

Cegala, D. J., Marinelli, T. M., Mcclure, L., and Post, D. M. 2000b. An examination of factors affecting patients' participation in primary care medical interviews. Acapulco: Health Communication Top Three Program.

Collins, T. C., Clark, J. A., Petersen, L. A., and Kressin, N. R. 2002. Racial differences in how patients perceive physician communication regarding cardiac testing. *Medical Care,* 40, I27–I34.

Cooper, L. A., Roter, D. L., Johson, R. L., Ford, D. E., Steinwachs, D. M., and Powe, N. R. 2003. Patient-centered communication, ratings of care, and concordance of patient and physician race. *Annals of Internal Medicine,* 139, 907–915.

Cooper-Patrick, L., Gallo, J. J., Gonzales, J. J., Vu, H. T., Powe, N. R., Nelson, C., and Ford, D.E. 1999. Race, gender and partnership in the patient–physician relationship. *Journal of the American Medical Association,* 282, 583–589.

Epstein, R. and Street, R. L., Jr. 2007. *Patient-centered communication in cancer care: promoting healing and reducing suffering*, Bethesda, MD, National Cancer Institute.

Fincher, C., Williams, J. E., Maclean, V., Allison, J. J., Kiefe, C. I., and Canto, J. G. 2004. Racial disparities in coronary heart disease: a sociological view of the medical literature on physician bias. *Ethnicity and Disease,* 14, 360–371.

Freedman, T. G. 1998. 'Why don't they come to Pike Street and ask us?': Black American women's health concerns. *Social Science & Medicine,* 47, 941–947.

Freimuth, V. S., Quinn, S. C., Thomas, S. B., Cole, G., Zook, E., and Duncan, T. 2001. African Americans' views on research and the Tuskegee Syphilis Study. *Social Science & Medicine,* 52, 797–808.

Ghods, B. K., Roter, D., Ford, D. E., Larson, S., Arbelaez, J. J., and Cooper, L. A. 2008. Patient–physician communication in the primary care visits of African Americans and whites with depression. *Journal of General Internal Medicine,* 23, 600–606.

Gordon, H. S., Street, R. L., Kelly, P., Souchek, J., and Wray, N. P. 2005. Physician–patient communication following invasive procedures: an analysis of post-angiogram consultations. *Social Science & Medicine,* 61, 1015–1025.

Gordon, H. S., Street Jr., R. L., Sharf, B. F., Kelly, A., and Souchek, J. 2006a. Racial differences in trust and lung cancer patients' perceptions of physician communication. *Journal of Clinical Oncology,* 24, 904–909.

Gordon, H. S., Street, R. L., Jr., Sharf, B. F., and Souchek, J. 2006b. Racial differences in doctors' information-giving and patients' participation. *Cancer,* 107, 1313–1320.

Green, A. R., Carney, D. R., Pallin, D. J., Ngo, L. H., Raymond, K. L., Iezzoni, L. I., and Banaji, M. R. 2007. Implicit bias among physicians and its prediction of thrombolysis decision for black and white patients. *Journal of General Internal Medicine,* 22, 1231–1238.

Hallfors, D. D., Iritani, B. J., Miller, W. C., and Bauer, D. J. 2007. Sexual and drug behavior patterns and HIV and STD racial disparities: the need for new directions. *American Journal of Public Health,* 97, 125–132.

Halpern, M. T., Ward, E. M., Pavluk, A. L., Schrag, N. M., Blan, J., and Chen, A. Y. 2008. Association of insurance status and ethnicity with cancer stage at diagnosis for 12 cancer sites: a retrospective analysis. *Lancet Oncology* 9, 222–231.

Johnson, M. O., Chesney, M. A., Neilands, T. B., Dilworth, S. E., Remien, R. H., Weinhardt, L. S., et al. 2009. Disparities in reported reasons for not initiating or stopping antiretroviral treatment among a diverse sample of persons living with HIV. *Journal of General Internal Medicine,* 24, 247–251.

Johnson, R. L., Roter, D., Powe, N. R., and Cooper, L. A. 2004. Patient race/ethnicity and quality of patient–physician communication during medical visits. *American Journal of Public Health,* 94, 2084–2090.

Korthuis, P. T., Saha, S., Fleishman, J. A., McGrath, M. M., Josephs, J. S., Moore, R. D., et al. 2008. Impact of patient race on patient experiences of access and communication in HIV care. *Journal of General Internal Medicine,* 23, 2046–2052.

Kraut-Becher, J., Eisenberg, M., Voytek, C., Brown, T., Metzger, D. S., and Aral, S. 2008. Examining racial disparities in HIV: lessons from sexually transmitted infections research. *Journal of Acquired Immune Deficiency Syndromes,* 47, S20–S27.

Kurtz, S., Silverman, J., and Draper, J. 1998. *Teaching and Learning Communication Skills in Medicine,* Abingdon, Radcliffe Medical Press.

Levinson, W., Hudak, P. L., Feldman, J. J., Frankel, R. M., Kuby, A., Bereknyei, S., and Braddock, C. H. 2008. 'It's not what you say ... ': Racial disparities in communication between orthopedic surgeons and patients. *Medical Care,* 46, 410–416.

Manfredi, C., Kaiser, K., Matthews, A. K., and Johnson, T. P. 2010. Are racial differences in patient–physician cancer communication and information explained by background, predisposing, and enabling factors? *Journal of Health Communication,* 15, 272–292.

Martin, R., Gordon, E. E., and Lounsbury, P. 1998. Gender disparities in the attribution of cardiac-related symptoms: contribution of common sense models of illness. *Health Psychology,* 17, 346–357.

Matthews, A. K., Sellergren, S. A., Manfredi, C., and Williams, M. 2002. Factors influencing medical information seeking among African American cancer patients. *Journal of Health Communication,* 7, 205–219.

Mensah, G. A., Mokdad, A. H., Ford, E. S., Greenlund, K. J., and Croft, J. B. 2005. State of disparities in cardiovascular health in the United States. *Circulation,* 111, 1233–1241.

Mukamel, B. D., Bresnick, H. G., Wang, Q., and Dickey, F. C. 1999. Barriers to compliance with screening guidelines for diabetic retinopathy. *Opthalmic Epidemiology,* 6, 61–72.

Muula, A. S. 2007. Male circumcision to prevent HIV transmission and acquisition: what else do we need to know? *AIDS and Behavior,* 11, 357–363.

NIMHD. 2011. *Vision and Mission* [Online]. National Institute on Minority Health and Health Disparities. Available: http://www.nimhd.nih.gov/about_ncmhd/mission.asp [Accessed December 13, 2011].

Nsiah-Kumi, P., Ortmeier, S. R., and Brown, A. E. 2009. Disparities in diabetic retinopathy screening and disease for racial and ethnic minority populations: a literature review. *Journal of National Medical Association,* 101, 430–437.

Post, D. M., Cegala, D. J., and Marinelli, T. M. 2001. Teaching patients to communicate with physicians: the impact of race. *Journal of the National Medical Association,* 93, 6–12.

Schoenthaler, A., Allegrante, J. P., Chaplin, W., and Ogedegbe, G. 2012. The effect of patient–provider communication on medication adherence in hypertensive black patients: Does race concordance matter? *Annals of Behavioral Medicine,* 43(3), 372–382.

Schulman, K. A., Berlin, J. A., Harless, W., Kerner, J. F., Sistrunk, S., Gersh, B. J., et al. 1999. The effect of race and sex on physicians' recommendations for cardiac catheterization. *New England Journal of Medicine,* 340, 618–626.

Shields, C. G., Ziner, K. W., Bourff, S. A., Schilling, K., Zhao, Q., Monahan, P., et al. 2010. An intervention to improve communication between breast cancer survivors and their physicians. *Journal of Psychosocial Oncology,* 28, 610–629.

Smedley, B. D., Stith, A.Y., and Nelson, A.R. 2003. *Unequal treatment: Confronting racial and ethnic disparities in healthcare,* Washington, DC, National Academy Press.

Sohler, N. L., Fitzpatrick, L. K., Lindsay, R. G., Anastos, K., and Cunningham, C. O. 2007. Does patient–provider racial/ethnic concordance influence ratings of trust in people with HIV infection? *AIDS and Behavior,* 11, 884–896.

Stone, J. and Moskowitz, G. B. 2011. Non-conscious bias in medical decision making: what can be done to reduce it? *Medical Education,* 45, 768–776.

Street, R. 2001. Active patients as powerful communicators: the linguistic foundation of participation in heatlh care. In Robinson, W. and Giles, E. (eds) *Handbook of language and social psychology.* Chichester: John Wiley.

Street, R. L., Gordon, H., and Haidet, P. 2007. Physicians' communication and perceptions of patients: Is it how they look, how they talk, or is it just the doctor? *Social Science & Medicine,* 65(3), 586–598.

Street, R. L., Jr., O'Malley, K. J., Cooper, L. A., and Haidet, P. 2008. Understanding concordance in patient–physician relationships: personal and ethnic dimensions of shared identity. *Annals of Family Medicine,* 6, 198–205.

Sullivan, P. S., McNaghten, A. D., Begley, E., Hutchinson, A., and Cargill, V. A. 2007. Enrollment of racial/ethnic minorities and women with HIV in clinical research studies of HIV medicines. *Journal of the National Medical Association,* 99, 242–250.

Teal, C. R., Shada, R. E., Gill, A. C., Thompson, B. M., Fruge, E., Villareal, G. B., and Haidet, P. 2010. When best intentions aren't enough: helping medical students develop strategies for managing bias about patients. *Journal of General Internal Medicine,* 25, 115–118.

Teal, C. R., Gill, A. C., Green, A. R., and Crandall, S. 2012. Helping medical learners recognise and manage unconscious bias toward certain patient groups. *Medical Education,* 46, 80–88.

Tischler, G. 1966. Decision-making processes in the emergency room. *Archives of General Psychiatry,* 14, 69–78.

Van Ryn, M. and Burke, J. 2000. The effect of patient race and socio-economic status on physicians' perceptions of patients. *Social Science & Medicine,* 50, 813–828.

Ward, E., Halpern, M., Schrag, N., Cokkinides, V., Desantis, C., Bandi, P., et al. 2008. Association of insurance with cancer care utilization and outcomes. *CA: A Cancer Journal for Clinicians,* 58, 9–31.

Wee, C. C., McCarthy, E. P., and Phillips, R. S. 2005. Factors associated with colon cancer screening: the role of patient factors and physician counseling. *Preventive Medicine,* 41, 23–29.

Zhang, Q., Wang, Y., and Huang, E. S. 2009. Changes in racial/ethnic disparities in the prevalence of Type 2 diabetes by obesity level among US adults. *Ethnicity & Health,* 14, 439–457.

37

Analyzing ethics-in-interaction in medical decision-making

Ellen Barton and Andrew Winckles

Introduction

Ever since Hippocrates enjoined physicians to guard the confidentiality of medical and social information, ethics has been interpolated in health communication. The history of medicine is thus also the history of medical ethics, and as medicine professionalized, so did its understanding and standards of ethics (Baker and McCullough 2009). In American medicine today, bioethics is considered the top-down set of principles – autonomy, beneficence/non-maleficence, justice – that should normatively underlie decision-making (Beauchamp and Childress 2001).[1] Medical decision-making with ethical dimensions, however, most often takes place in interaction among real people, in real time, in (semi-)ordinary language that is often more indirect than direct, and in complex contexts that are institutional and asymmetrical. Yet the actual language of medical decision-making with ethical dimensions has rarely been studied in the literature, and a bottom-up perspective on ethics as interactional and rhetorical is only beginning to emerge in discourse studies (Barton 2011).

In discourse studies, our research program on ethics-in-interaction investigates one central question: what are the linguistic means by which ethical issues are raised, explored, negotiated, justified, and settled (or not) in medical decision-making? Based on observational and interactional data (field notes, informal discussions with key informants, and transcripts), projects in this research program describe ethically charged communicative events in medicine such as end-of-life discussions and offers to participate in medical research, the two discourses of decision-making with ethical dimensions we analyze in this chapter.

Theoretical and methodological frameworks

Our theoretical framework for research on ethics-in-interaction utilizes Sarangi and Roberts' (1999) distinction between the institutional order and the interactional order (see also Candlin and Sarangi 2011). Briefly, institutional orders seek to regulate professional practices, including communication and decision-making, in order to achieve accountability to the policies of the institution. Examples of institutional orders in medicine include the incorporation of bioethics in professional codes, systems of federal and state regulations, and a wide variety of hospital policies and protocols for ethics consults. Interactional orders are the conventionalized discourses of particular communicative events where decision-making actually takes place, such as end-of-life discussions in surgical intensive care units or offers to participate in clinical trials in oncology encounters. Considerable tension often exists between the bioethically oriented policies of institutional orders and the clinically oriented practices of interactional orders: physicians work actively and systematically to patrol and control certain interactional orders, including the two discourses we examine here, so this framework allows the exploration of complex theoretical concepts revolving around authority, accountability, professionalism, agency, boundaries, control, persuasion, and resistance.

Our methodological framework in this research program is what Roberts and Sarangi (2005) call theme-oriented discourse analysis, with theme defined as the connection between the analysis of linguistic conventions in medical discourse(s) and 'professional concerns in medicine' (639). Applied to research on ethics-in-interaction, our methodological reasoning for using discourse analysis goes as follows. Schön (1983) describes practitioners across professions as enacting 'thought-in-action' – expertise and experience incorporated into everyday actions, extended, for our purposes, to interaction. In an intriguing paper, McGrath et al. (2006) suggest that physicians enact medical ethics relatively unself-consciously in everyday clinical practices, again extended for our purposes to the interaction of shared decision-making with patients and families.[2] Shared decision-making with ethical dimensions often takes place within conventionalized discourse events – repeated and rhetorical institutional/interactional genres such as end-of-life discussions and offers to participate in clinical trials.

To analyze decision-making sequences, we look at the ways that physicians as well as patients/families conventionally index the medical and ethical bases for their decisions. Index is a term we coined from Peräkylä's (1998) analysis of the linguistic conventions physicians use to indicate the basis for a diagnosis, either directly or inferentially (*it's X, it seems like/may be X, the tests showed X*). What we have found is that indexing is often an expression of medical as well as ethical accountability: physicians index traditional medical ethics as well as bioethics, and patients/families index principles of their own lay ethics, with interaction blending these perspectives into a hybrid discourse of ethical decision-making often summed up by all parties as *the right decision*.

Emerging themes from research on ethics-in-interaction

The importance of these theoretical and methodological frameworks is that they use theme-based discourse analysis as a bottom-up discovery process to describe the ethical assumptions, questions, issues, dilemmas, and reasoning physicians and patients/families actually bring to medical decision-making. In this chapter we present two discourse analyses of decision-making in end-of-life discussions and offers to participate in clinical trials, drawing from each analysis to illustrate the emerging themes of our research program on ethics-in-interaction, as follows:

1 Interactional attention to ethical issues is distributed across communicative events rather than concentrated in specific decision-making sequences.
2 Physicians and patients/families index the medical and ethical bases for their decisions, sometimes differently and sometimes similarly.
3 Decision-making is less often an explicit sequence and more often an implicit trajectory of interactional alignment or non-alignment.

4 The use of persuasion is a key ethical issue for physicians, sometimes reflecting the tension between bioethics and traditional medical ethics.
5 Research on ethics-in-interaction disseminates information that points to unethical as well as ethical ways of managing the interaction of ethically charged decision-making discourses.

In Sample Analysis I, we describe indexing in end-of-life discussions with respect to themes 1–3. In Sample Analysis II, we describe indexing in offers to participate in clinical trials with respect to themes 3 and 4. We conclude with a discussion of theme 5 and a set of suggestions for future research on ethics-in-interaction in health communication.

Sample analysis i: end-of-life decision-making

The data for our project on end-of-life (EOL) discussions consisted of a corpus of 20 EOL discussions from a Surgical Intensive Care Unit (SICU). In practice, EOL discussions are a goal-based institutional and interactional genre in medicine: physicians do not initiate an EOL discussion unless the goal is to move from therapeutic to palliative care, thereby allowing the patient to die (see Cassell 2005 for an ethnography of the SICU where these discussions took place). In the study corpus, 14 discussions reached a decision to withdraw life support from the patient, and 6 discussions did not reach such a decision.

Barton et al. (2005) found that EOL discussions have four phases with distinct structures and functions:

- *Phase 1 Opening* – physicians and families co-construct the traditional role structure of a medical encounter, with the physician in the interactional lead.
- *Phase 2 Description of current status* – physicians present medical information about the patient in the form of a problem list, culminating in an inferential summary statement of terminal status.
- *Phase 3 Shared decision-making* – physicians and families co-construct short and inferential decision-making sequences regarding the withdrawal of life support.
- *Phase 4 Logistics of dying* – physician and families co-construct a hybrid medical–lay discourse of palliative/comfort care.

Phase 3 is the shortest section of the EOL discussion, with inferential decision-making more a function of an implicit trajectory of interactional alignment or non-alignment than explicit decision-making sequences (Barton 2006). Goodwin and Goodwin (1992) define alignment as interlocutors taking an evaluative stance in interaction, analyzing agreement as a feature displaying positive alignment. In Phase 3 of EOL discussions, we found multiple features of alignment and non-alignment, including agreement or disagreement, positive or neutral continuers, latching, repetition, silence, and, most importantly, the use of these features in uptake (or lack of uptake) to bids for decision-making. Uptake is a concept from early speech act theory, defined interactionally by Edmondson (1981: 81) as an utterance that links back to a previous speaker's utterance, validating it (or not) as a contribution to the discourse (e.g., the use of *right* in conversation as alignment, or the use of silence to indicate non-alignment).

Example A is from an EOL discussion with multiple features of alignment and uptake in inferential decision-making.

Example A – Phases 2–3 with trajectory of alignment

(1) P: And this has gone on for a few days now and she's shown no improvement at all, zero. [...] [W]e can very confidently say that we don't think she's ever going to get better. We can keep her body alive on the machine for a very long period of time, but==

(2) F: ==but she is going now.

(3) P: And it sounds like that's not what she would want.

(4) F: No.

(5) P: Everybody is in agreement with that [...] Based upon what everybody said, her to her doctors and all of you to me, it sounds like it's not what she would want.

(6) F: No.

In (1), the physician ends Phase 2 with an inferential summary statement of terminal status indexed to medical futility, followed by a Phase 3 bid for inferential decision-making ending with the single word but==. In (2), the family member provides latched agreement using the same word, then reformulating and indexing terminal status in lay language. This latched agreement serves as the inferential decision, further indexed by the physician's bid for alignment upon the patient's wishes in (3): note here that the use of the definite pronoun *that* provides evidence that the end-of-life decision has been made. In (4), the family member provides agreement, indicating alignment to the indexing of the patient's wishes, and the physician and family member repeat and align to consensus upon an elaborated version of the patient's wishes in (5)–(6), with the physician again using a definite pronoun – *it* – to refer to the end-of-life decision that has been made within the trajectory of alignment in this Phase 3.

In contrast, Example B is from an EOL discussion with multiple features of non-alignment and a failed bid for inferential decision-making.

Example B – Phases 2–3 with trajectory of non-alignment

(1) P: So when someone in the--experiences all of these, um, complications of the sepsis in the face of the strong medications that we are using, um, we feel like it is important to try to touch base with the family and clarify the goals of treatment and what you imagined the goals of treating her to be.

(2) F: OK.

(3) P: Does that make sense? What questions can I answer to help that make sense?

(4) F: [silence]

As in Example A, the physician ends Phase 2 with an inferential summary statement in (1), followed by a Phase 3 bid for inferential decision-making. Unlike the previous example, the physician here uses medically oriented language rather than hybrid medical–lay language. To someone familiar with medical discourse, *all of these complications of the sepsis in the face of strong medications* inferentially indexes medical futility; similarly, *clarify the goals of treatment* inferentially refers to changing the goals of treatment from therapeutic to palliative care. In (2), however, the family member responds with *OK*, a neutral continuer providing overt agreement to a discussion about the goals of treatment only, with no uptake of the physician's bid for inferential decision making. In (3), the physician retreats from her bid, with a marked and awkward pre-closing sequence which is met in (4) with silence – again, no uptake. Whether the non-alignment in this example is based on a lack of understanding of the implications of the medical language in (1) or an unwillingness to participate in decision-making at this point in the discussion, this trajectory of non-alignment in Phase 3 does not end in a decision to withdraw life support from the patient.

From an analysis of the decision-making sequences in the 14 discussions in the corpus that reached a decision to withdraw life support, Table 37.1 shows how physicians and families indexed their medical and ethical bases for the EOL decision. In the analysis, we found that physicians take the interactional lead in EOL decision-making, as shown in Example A, indexing first in bids for decision-making; families often mirror that indexing in a trajectory of alignment in discussions that reach a decision to withdraw life support. In decision-making, both physicians and families can index multiple factors, so the numbers in Table 37.1 indicate the number of times each factor was indexed (and thus add up to more than the number of discussions).

In these decision-making sequences, physicians most frequently index medical futility (9), the patient's wishes (8), and consensus upon the decision (7). Families mirrored the indexing in terms of the patient's wishes most often (7), and indexed consensus (3) and medical futility (2) to a lesser extent.

One interesting difference between physician and family indexing is that families also index any end-of-life papers that the patient may have (*I can tell you want he wants. He has signed papers.*). Physicians did not index end-of-life papers, which may initially seem surprising and problematic, as physicians are ethically enjoined to follow the patient's wishes in these advance directives. However, studies have found that in the emergent care situations typical in intensive care units, physicians are more oriented to a patient's clinical situation in particular than advance directives in general (Danis 1994): for example, a patient may have an advance directive against full life support, but a physician will not follow that directive if s/he believes that a short or even prolonged course on full life support would be the best clinical decision for the patient, at that particular moment of clinical care.

There are similarities and differences in Phase 3 indexing in the six discussions in the corpus that did not reach a decision to withdraw life support, as shown in Table 37.2. Like the discussions that did reach a decision to withdraw life support, physicians were in the interactional lead in the decision-making sequences, indexing first in bids for decision-making, with some mirroring by families. However, in Phase 3 of the discussions that did not reach an end-of-life decision, as shown in Example B, there was less alignment, even when families mirrored the physician's indexing. Again, through multiple indexing the numbers in Table 37.2 add up to more than the number of discussions.

In these decision-making sequences, physicians again index medical futility (5) and the patient's wishes (4) most frequently. In response, families also index the patient's wishes (2) and futility (2) to a lesser extent, but not necessarily in alignment with the physician. For example, in one decision-making sequence a family member indexed futility in response to a bid for inferential decision-making (P: *Has he been sort of going downhill slowly and this is*

Table 37.1 Indexing in discussions with a decision to withdraw life support

	Physician indexing	*Family indexing*	*Total*
Medical futility	9	2	11
Patient's wishes	8	7	15
Consensus	7	3	10
EOL papers	0	3	3
Recommendation	1	0	1

Table 37.2 Indexing in discussions with no decision to withdraw life support

	Physician indexing	*Family indexing*	*Total*
Medical futility	5	2	7
Patient's wishes	4	2	6
Consensus	1	0	1
Quality of life	1	0	1
EOL papers	0	1	1
Recommendation	0	0	0

sort of the end? F: *It definitely is.*), but he then turned the discussion back to a Phase 2 description of a particular medical problem, and the decision-making sequence did not continue.

In sum, the analysis of indexing in Phase 3 decision-making sequences in the whole corpus indicates that physicians index futility as the primary medical dimension of the decision, but they also index ethical dimensions of shared decision-making in terms of the patient's wishes and the medical–lay consensus upon the decision, thereby incorporating principles of traditional medical ethics as well as bioethics in a hybrid medical–lay discourse of shared EOL decision-making. As Examples A and B show, however, family contributions are minimal in Phase 3, especially when the discussion is non-aligned. Phase 3 decision-making could thus be seen as primarily physician-directed, with little interactional attention to the family's understanding and participation in an ethically grounded end-of-life decision. However, it is in Phase 4 that families often review the end-of-life decision and also index the ethical bases for their alignment (or non-alignment) with the decisions made (or not) earlier in Phase 3.

In their review of the end-of-life decision, families index two ethical principles: the loss of consciousness and/or the loss of personhood. In a sub-study of nine discussions from the EOL corpus where the families indicated high satisfaction with the end-of-life decision, Barton (2007) found that families raised the topics of consciousness and/or personhood six times. Example C indexes the loss of consciousness.

Example C – Phase 4 with a trajectory of alignment

(1) F: If she's not in any pain, if she's not struggl[ing] with--if I'm standing there I don't want to see her going through this because that would make me feel that I made the wrong choice if she's trying to catch on--

(2) P: Right. We will keep her pain free. If it turns out that she's off the ventilator and she's having what looks like difficulty breathing, we can make that more comfortable. We can make her totally comfortable.

(3) F: Write orders on the chart, make her comfortable, write that if she's having a problem make her comfortable.

In (1), the family member indexes a lay definition of consciousness – *trying to catch on* – as the basis for *the wrong choice*, thereby implying that an ethical condition for an end-of-life decision requires the complete and permanent loss of consciousness. The physician reformulates the family member's concern in terms of the goals of comfort care in (2); in (3), the family member's repetition and direction to *write orders on the chart* indicate his alignment with using the treatments of palliative care to allow the patient to die.

In another example, a family member indexes loss of personhood as the condition for ethical end-of-life decision-making.

Example D – Phase 4 in a trajectory of alignment

(1) F: If you had known her, you would know that we're doing the right thing.

(2) P: And that's important. And again I want everybody to know that from the doctors' standpoint we're doing the right thing.

In (1) the family member indexes personhood (*if you had known her*) as the ethical basis for *doing the right thing* in decision-making. In (2) the physician indexes the consensus of the family and the medical team in his aligned repetition.

In discussions that do not reach a decision to withdraw life support, however, a truncated and hypothetical Phase 4 can continue a trajectory of non-alignment from Phase 3.

Example E – Phase 4 in a trajectory of non-alignment

(1) F: [to daughter on phone] She's dying, I know what's going on. Well, I have to make a decision to pull the plug. I hate to--

(2) P: You don't have to do that yet.

Here in (1) the family member indexes a lay formulation of medical futility (*she's dying*) but then predicts a solo and reluctant end-of-life decision, not indexed to the patient's wishes or to any alignment or consensus between the family and the medical team. In (2) the physician does not take up her inferential end-of-life decision *to pull the plug*, immediately retreating in response to the lack of alignment in what would be non-shared decision-making.

Emerging themes

In terms of the themes of the research program on ethics-in-interaction, the discourse analysis of EOL discussions illustrates themes 1–3 particularly well. Theme 1 suggests that interactional attention to ethical issues is distributed across communicative events rather than concentrated in specific decision-making sequences. As we have seen, in EOL discussions Phase 3 is where decision-making takes place; however, interactional attention to ethical issues is distributed across Phases 2, 3, and 4. Theme 2 suggests that physicians and patients/families index the medical and ethical bases for their decisions, sometimes differently and sometimes similarly. In EOL discussions, physicians index medical futility and the patient's wishes as the medical and ethical bases for the decision to withdraw life support in Phases 2 and 3. To use Mishler's (1984) term, in Phase 4 families articulate a lay ethics of EOL decision-making from their own lifeworld, indexing the loss of personhood and consciousness. If the physician and the family are aligned, it is in Phase 4 that they co-construct a hybrid medical/lay discourse of *the right decision* with multiple and repeated indexing. Finally, theme 3 suggests that medical and ethical decision-making is less often an explicit sequence and more often an implicit trajectory of interactional alignment or non-alignment. What we have seen in Phase 3 is that the language in decision-making sequences is typically short, indirect, and inferential, with a trajectory of alignment in support of shared decision-making to withdraw life support, as in Example A, and a trajectory of non-alignment in resistance to bids for end-of-life decision-making, as in Example B.

Sample analysis ii: offers to participate in clinical trials

The data for our project on offers to participate in cancer clinical trials consisted of a corpus of 22 encounters in medical oncology selected from a larger set (Albrecht et al.

2008). In the corpus, 13 offers resulted in a preliminary decision to participate in the trial, and 9 offers did not.

Clinical trials are the gold standard for medical research evaluating new treatments in cancer care; however, too few patients enroll in trials, creating a significant barrier to progress in research and clinical care (Nass, Moses, and Mendelsohn 2010). Offering participation in a trial is fraught with ethical issues for physicians since it fundamentally changes the dynamics of a medical encounter from what is known to what is unknown – open questions in research and clinical care. The chief ethical issues at stake in recruitment to clinical trials include what is called in bioethics the therapeutic misconception: the blurring of the lines between (standard) treatment and (experimental) research if a physician unduly influences patients to think that the research treatment is known to be clinically beneficial (Beauchamp and Childress 2001).

From the perspective of bioethics, offers to participate in clinical trials should not use persuasion, as this would constitute undue influence: 'physicians should be completely objective in discussing [the trial] and should not use persuasion to obtain consent' (American Medical Association 1998). From the perspective of traditional medical ethics, however, the venerable *Harrison's Principles of Internal Medicine* notes, 'As part of broader social responsibilities, the physician should encourage patients to participate in ethical and properly approved clinical investigations' (Kasper et al. 2005: 5). The National Comprehensive Cancer Network (2013) has recently blended these two traditional principles into one statement: '[P]atients enrolled in clinical trials receive the best management of care.' The bioethics perspective thus licenses a discourse of autonomous decision-making, while the traditional medical ethics perspective licenses a discourse of persuasive decision-making. In order to manage this tension between two institutional orders within the interactional order of offers to participate in clinical trials, physicians often construct offers as a hybrid discourse drawing upon both perspectives.

Barton (2007) found that offers to participate in clinical trials within oncology encounters are a distinct, flexibly structured topic that usually includes the following elements, not always in the same order and often repeated throughout the development of the topic: purpose of the trial; procedures (e.g., scanning, drug regimens, etc.); benefits; risks; consent; questions; and logistics (e.g., setting up tests, appointments, etc.). As in end-of-life discussions, preliminary decision-making sequences for or against trial participation are often short and sometimes inferential, with agreement and other features such as repetition solidifying an interactional trajectory of alignment, and deferral or other features such as silence constructing a trajectory of non-alignment. As in the EOL discussions, physicians and patients/families sometimes index the medical and ethical bases for their bids and decisions.

Example F includes both a deferral in response to perceived non-alignment as well as subsequent decision-making within a trajectory of alignment.

Example F – Preliminary decision-making

(1) P: What do you think?
(2) Pt: [silence]
(3) P: I'm not asking you now to whether you want to commit to being on the study.
(4) Pt: I would like to [participate in] the study.
(5) P: OK, then what I'm gonna do is I'm gonna ask the research nurses to come down, go over your chart with me, talk with you, and if you're eligible get you enrolled. OK?
(6) Pt: OK.

(7) P: Do you have any questions about it?
(8) Pt: None that I can think of it.

Here, the physician's bid for decision-making in (1) is met in (2) with silence. In (3), taking silence for non-alignment, the physician defers the decision. In (4), however, the patient makes an overt decision statement to participate in the trial, indexing his understanding that this is participation in medical research. Continuing within this trajectory of alignment, the physician begins arranging the logistics of the trial in (5)–(8), indexing eligibility, and then begins to close the topic by soliciting patient questions.

From an analysis of the decision-making sequences in the 13 encounters in which the patient made a preliminary decision to participate in the clinical trial, Table 37.3 shows how patients and families indexed their medical and ethical bases for the decision. Through multiple indexing, the numbers in Table 37.3 add up to more than the number of discussions.

Although the numbers are small, there is a notable pattern here: patients/families index treatment-related factors (recurrence/survival, treatment/starting treatment, physician recommendation for trial treatment) much more often (11/16, 69 percent) than they index their understanding of participation in research (5/16, 31 percent).

The four examples in G illustrate each of these types of treatment-related indexing.

Example G – Treatment-related indexing
(i) Recurrence/survival/quality time
(1) Pt: OK. I'm trying--I'm willing to do whatever's necessary to have me on this planet for a while.

(ii) Starting treatment
(1) Pt: All right, well, we'll start the procedure.

(iii) Physician recommendation
(1) Pt: Well the only thing I would say is whatever you recommend I'm going along with it.

(iv) Combined indexing -- treatment, research, and survival
(1) Pt: OK. Well I want the radiation, the treatment. And I'm willing to go along if it's--
(2) P: To be part of the study?
(3) Pt: To be part of the study, and go on and get it over with. At least I'll be--at least in another few months I'll be seventy and my dad lived to be seventy-eight.

Table 37.3 Patient/family indexing in encounters with a preliminary decision to participate in a clinical trial

	Patient/family indexing
Recurrence/survival/quality time	5 (31%)
Treatment/starting treatment	5 (31%)
Physician recommendation	1 (6%)
Research (participation)	5 (31%)
Total	16 (99%)

In sum, patients appear to make treatment decisions in these sequences, selecting the trial as their best treatment option, with much less consideration of the decision as one to participate in research.

In end-of-life decision-making, families often mirror the physician's indexing, particularly with respect to the patient's wishes, creating and maintaining a trajectory of alignment. In trial offers, it is often the physician who mirrors the patient's indexing for reasons to participate in the trial. However, in this mirroring physicians face a substantive ethical task: as shown above, patients index their decision primarily in terms of selecting what seems to be the best treatment option, which raises the issue of the therapeutic misconception, so physicians have to construct a hybrid discourse of treatment and research within the ongoing trajectory of alignment in decision-making, in order to bring attention to the ethical issue at hand – making sure the patient understands the distinction between standard treatment and experimental treatment.

Table 37.4 shows how physicians mirrored and indexed reasons for participation in a clinical trial after the patient made a preliminary decision to do so. Again, through multiple indexing, the numbers in Table 37.4 add up to more than the number of discussions.

The first five factors in Table 37.4 – treatment, trial logistics, recurrence/survival, physician recommendation, and questions – are treatment-related, which physicians indexed 12 times (67 percent of the total). The last two factors in Table 37.4 – research and consent – are research-related, and physicians indexed these factors 6 times (33 percent of the total). Compared to Table 37.3, Table 37.4 shows that physicians mirrored the patients' proportion of treatment vs. research categories: both patients and physicians indexed treatment about twice as often (69 percent for patients and 67 percent for physicians) as research (31 percent for patients and 33 percent for physicians). However, in 7 encounters, half of the total of encounters in which a decision to participate in the trial was made, physicians did not let the patients' decisions indexed only to treatment stand alone by constructing a hybrid discourse of treatment and research that indexes the ethical perspectives of bioethics as well as traditional medical ethics.

One linguistic means in constructing such a hybrid discourse is the use of reformulation, as in Example H.

Table 37.4 Physician indexing in encounters with a preliminary decision to participate in a clinical trial

	Physician indexing
Treatment/starting treatment	4 (22%)
Logistics of trial	5 (27%)
Recurrence/survival/quality time	1 (6%)
Physician recommendation	1 (6%)
Questions	1 (6%)
Research (good trial/good candidate)	4 (22%)
Consent	2 (11%)
Total	18 (100%)

Example H – Reformulated decision-making

(1) Pt: No, definitely, there's no doubt--. And, I definitely want to participate because I don't know [throws up hands] whether the cancer's still in my body or what.
(2) P: That's--
(3) Pt: So, I gotta participate.
(4) P: Yeah, well I think it's a good idea [...] for you to have further treatment.
(5) Pt: True.
(6) P: And, I think this trial is worthwhile participating in.

In (1)–(3), the patient indexes his decision to enroll in the trial in terms of research participation as well as recurrence of the cancer. In response, the physician first creates a trajectory of alignment with the agreement token *yeah*, but then reformulates the patient's decision into two parts: the treatment decision to *have further treatment* in (4) and only then an affirmation of the decision to participate in the trial indexed to its scientific merits as *worthwhile* research in (6). Note that the physician provides no explicit uptake of the patient's indexing to recurrence, as that might create or strengthen the therapeutic misconception. In this hybrid discourse, the physician separates the treatment decision from the decision to participate in the trial, thereby satisfying the traditional medical ethics standard of providing the best treatment for the patient as well as the bioethics standard of separating research from treatment in order to avoid the therapeutic misconception.

In constructing this hybrid discourse of medical and ethical decision-making, physicians also index consent, often in combination with logistics, as in Example I.

Example I – Physician indexing consent

(1) Pt: All right, well, we'll start the procedure.
(2) P: OK, well, let me go get you the consent form. I'll let you look that over. And I'll have [one] of my coordinators come and talk to you, work on getting things scheduled and organized for you.

After the patient indexes her decision to participate in the trial in terms of a treatment decision, the physician creates a trajectory of alignment in (2) with the agreement token *OK*, but then indexes consent as the necessary next step, thereby satisfying the medical and bioethical principles that treatment within a research protocol requires informed consent.

Note that in both Examples H and I, physicians follow the agreement tokens (*Yeah*, *OK*) with *well* as a discourse marker of non-alignment, an indication that the patient's treatment decision cannot stand alone.[3] Examples H and I also illustrate an interesting difference between Tables 37.3 and 37.4: although patients and physicians index participation in research and treatment at roughly the same proportion in decision-making sequences, physicians do not mirror patient indexing in terms of recurrence/survival. Patients indexed recurrence/survival 6 times, but physicians mirrored this only 2 times, perhaps as an important way to avoid the therapeutic misconception.

Emerging themes

In terms of the themes of the research program on ethics-in-interaction, the discourse analysis of clinical trial offers illustrates themes 3 and 4. Theme 3 suggests that medical and ethical decision-making is less often an explicit sequence and more often an implicit trajectory of interactional alignment or non-alignment. As we saw in end-of-life decision-making, the language of decisions to participate (or not) in clinical trials is typically short and sometimes inferential within a co-constructed trajectory of alignment, as shown in Example F. Theme 4 suggests that the use of persuasion is (and, according to both bioethics and traditional medical ethics, should be) a key ethical issue for physicians, particularly in the avoidance of the therapeutic misconception. For patients, the decision to participate in a clinical trial understandably foregrounds treatment over research, as shown in Table 37.3; physicians, however, may construct a hybrid discourse in order to contextualize that decision in terms of the ethical dimensions of offering participation in clinical trials to patients, as shown in examples H and I.

Summary and future directions

To return to the central question of this research program on ethics-in-interaction, we hope to have shown that discourse analysis can usefully describe how ethical issues are explored and negotiated throughout medical encounters in a complex co-construction of alignment or non-alignment, with both physicians and patients/families indexing the medical and ethical bases for their decisions. More specifically, in the end-of-life project, the discourse analysis above provides a better understanding of the ethical basis for end-of-life decision-making and the means for the physician and the family to co-construct consensus upon *the right decision* in Phase 4. This research thus suggests that Phase 4 has a significant ethical function: it is not only a discussion of the logistics of dying, but also an important review of the end-of-life decision from the perspective of the ethics of the family lifeworld, a review in which the physician provides considerable ethical reassurance. In the clinical trials project, the discourse analyses provide a better understanding of the reasons patients decide to participate in trials: patients index this decision primarily as a medical one, a decision to choose the best treatment option for themselves. This research also suggests, however, that physicians can contextualize that treatment decision more broadly by reformulating those decisions in terms of research, thereby addressing the ethical issues of this special kind of decision-making.

Thinking more critically, however, our final emerging theme (5) notes that discourse analyses can disseminate information that points to unethical as well as ethical ways of managing the interaction of medical decision-making. In the EOL project, for example, a better understanding of Phase 4 as providing ethical reassurance to families could suggest that physicians appropriate the topics of consciousness and personhood, thereby shortening a lengthy discussion and manipulating families to satisfaction with a decision that they have not reasoned out on their own, by articulating and developing their own ethical perspectives on the decision at hand. In the clinical trials project, detailed descriptions of successful persuasive strategies could allow physicians to deploy persuasion without meaningful ethical contextualization, again short-circuiting the patient's consideration of what is involved in participation in research. In sum, while we hope the information that discourse analysis provides would lead to more ethical health communication, we cannot guarantee that our research will always have that effect.

Nevertheless, we are more optimistic than pessimistic, hoping that research on ethics-in-interaction contributes both to better understanding and delivery of health communication, particularly in terms of the multiple ethical perspectives that bear upon difficult and complex decisions in health care. Obviously, there remains a tremendous amount of descriptive research to be done. End-of-life discussions and offers to participate in clinical trials are just two communicative events that are complex linguistically and ethically, and there are hundreds more, from relatively straightforward treatment recommendations to ethics consults where there is conflict within or among hospital administrators, clinical staff, patients, or families. Of great importance in the development of research in this area, too, is the need to look at ethics-in-interaction in other clinical interactions besides the well-studied duo of physician–patient: nurses, for instance, face complex ethical issues in their discourse with patients and families, as do social workers, chaplains, emergency personnel, and others. The multiple sites of healthcare delivery also deserve investigation of ethics-in-interaction: the studies above collected data from academic hospital settings, but there are many other settings in which ethically charged decision-making takes place, such as community hospitals, free clinics, and private practice. There are also many other configurations of participants, such as intercultural encounters and encounters across lines of ethnicity and socio-cultural groups. The studies above looked at American medical encounters in English, but it would be important to extend this research program to settings in other countries and other languages, describing the many social and cultural traditions of the interpolation of ethics in health communication.

Acknowledgments

We would like to thank the principal investigators on these two projects for providing data and support: SICU (Surgical Intensive Care Unit) Care at End of Life (R01 NR05124, Timothy Buchman, PI, Washington University); Effects of Physician Communication on Patient Accrual to Clinical Trials (R01 CA075003, Terence Albrecht, PI, Wayne State University).

We would like to thank the Wayne State University Office of the Vice President for Research for supporting Andrew Winckles' work on this project.

We also would like to thank Susan Eggly, Wayne State University School of Medicine (Communication and Behavioral Oncology) for many helpful discussions of offers to participate in clinical trials.

Related topics

Ethics; end of life; clinical trials; ethics-in-interaction; decision-making.

Notes

1 Critiques, defenses, and rapprochements of principlism in bioethics abound in the literature (Baker and McCullough 2009). Space precludes a full review of this literature, so we remain neutral in this chapter on the possible contributions of discourse analysis to the debates of this contested territory; however, see Barton (2008).

2 Shared decision-making is defined by Charles et al. (1997): 'at least two participants, the clinician and patient be involved; both parties share information; both parties take steps to build a consensus about the preferred treatment; and an agreement is reached on the treatment to implement' (681).

3 See Schiffrin (1987) on *well* as a discourse marker that indicates non-alignment.

Further reading

Barton, E., 2011. Speaking for another: ethics-in-interaction in medical encounters. In C. Candlin and S. Sarangi (eds) *Handbook of Communication in Organizations and Professions*. Berlin: Mouton de Gruyter, pp. 215–234.

Barton, E., and Eggly, S., 2009. Ethical or unethical persuasion? The rhetoric of offers to participate in clinical trials. *Written Communication*, 26: 295–319.

Roberts, C. and Sarangi, S., 2005. Theme-oriented discourse analysis of medical encounters. *Medical Education*, 39: 632–460.
Sarangi, S. and Candlin, C.N., 2011. Professional and organizational practice: a discourse/communication perspective. In C. Candlin and S. Sarangi (eds) *Handbook of Communication in Organizations and Professions*. Berlin: Mouton de Gruyter, pp. 3–58.
Sarangi, S. and Roberts, C., 1999. The dynamics of interactional and institutional orders in work-related settings. In S. Sarangi and C. Roberts (eds) *Talk, Work and Institutional Order: Discourse in Medical, Mediation and Management Settings*. Berlin: Mouton de Gruyter, pp. 1–60.

References

Albrecht, T., Eggly, S., Gleason, M., et al., 2008. Influence of clinical communication on patients' decision-making on clinical trials. *Journal of Clinical Oncology*, 10: 3324–3332.
American Medical Association, 1998. Clinical investigation (E-2.07). Retrieved July 17, 2012, from AMA Code of Medical Ethics Current Opinions website: http://www.ama-assn.org/ama/pub/physician-resources/medical-ethics/code-medical-ethics/opinion207.page
Baker, R. and McCullough, L. (eds), 2009. *The Cambridge World History of Medical Ethics*. New York: Cambridge University Press.
Barton, E., 2006. Trajectories of alignment and the situated ethics of end-of-life discussions in American medicine. In M. Gotti and F. Salager-Meyer (eds) *Advances in Medical Discourse Analysis: Oral and Written Contexts*. New York: Peter Lang, pp. 23–42.
——2007. Situating end-of-life decision making in a hybrid ethical frame. *Communication & Medicine*, 4: 131–140.
——2008. Further contributions from the ethical turn in composition/rhetoric: analyzing ethics in interaction. *College Composition and Communication*, 59: 596–632.
——2011. Speaking for another: ethics-in-interaction in medical encounters. In C. Candlin and S. Sarangi (eds) *Handbook of Communication in Organizations and Professions*. Berlin: Mouton de Gruyter, pp. 215–234.
Barton, E., Aldridge, M., Trimble, T., and Vidovic, J., 2005. Structure and variation in end-of-life discussions in the surgical intensive care unit. *Communication & Medicine*, 2: 3–20.
Beauchamp, T. and Childress, J., 2001. *Principles of Biomedical Ethics*, 5th edn. New York: Oxford University Press.
Candlin, C.N. and Sarangi, S. (eds), 2011. *Handbook of Communication in Organizations and Professions*. Berlin: Mouton de Gruyter.
Cassell, J., 2005. *Life and Death in Intensive Care*. Philadelphia, PA: Temple University Press.
Charles, C., Gafni, A. and Whelan, T., 1997. Shared decision-making in the medical encounter: what does it mean? (or it takes at least two to tango). *Social Science & Medicine*, 44(5): 681–692.
Danis, M., 1994. Following advance directives. *Hasting Center Report*, 24: 521–523.
Edmondson, W., 1981. *Spoken Discourse: A Model for Analysis*. London: Longman.
Goodwin, C. and Goodwin, M., 1992. Assessments and the construction of context. In A. Duranti and C. Goodwin (eds) *Rethinking Context: Language as an Interactive Phenomenon*. Cambridge: Cambridge University Press, pp. 147–190.
Kasper, D., Braunwald, E., Hauser, S., Longo, D., Jameson, J.L., and Fauci, A.S. (eds), 2005. *Harrison's Principles of Internal Medicine*, 16th edn. New York: McGraw-Hill Medical.
McGrath, P., Henderson, D., and Holewa, H., 2006. Ethics and communication in the real world of acute medicine: Australian findings. Paper presented at the COMET (Communication, Medicine, and Ethics) Conference, Cardiff University, Wales.
Mishler, E.G., 1984. *The Discourse of Medicine: Dialectics of Medical Interviews*. Norwood, NJ: Ablex Publishing.
Nass, S., Moses, H., and Mendelsohn, J., 2010. A national cancer clinical trials system for the 21st century: reinvigorating the NCI cooperative group program. Washington DC: Institute of Medicine. Retrieved December 10, 2013 from http://iom.edu/Reports/2010/A-National-Cancer-Clinical-Trials-System-for-the-21st-Century-Reinvigorating-the-NCI-Cooperative.aspx
National Comprehensive Cancer Network, 2013. NCCN Guidelines for Patients: Clinical Trials Frequently Asked Questions. Retrieved December 10, 2013 from http://www.nccn.org/patients/resources/clinical_trials/faq.aspx

Peräkylä, A., 1998. Authority and accountability: the delivery of diagnosis in primary health care. *Social Psychology Quarterly*, 61(4): 301–320.
Roberts, C. and Sarangi, S., 2005. Theme-oriented discourse analysis of medical encounters. *Medical Education*, 39: 632–640.
Sarangi, S. and Roberts, C., 1999. The dynamics of interactional and institutional orders in work-related settings. In S. Sarangi and C. Roberts (eds) *Talk, Work and Institutional Order: Discourse in Medical, Mediation and Management Settings*. Berlin: Mouton de Gruyter, pp. 1–60.
Schiffrin, D., 1987. *Discourse Markers*. Cambridge: Cambridge University Press.
Schön, D., 1983. *The Reflective Practitioner: How Professionals Think in Action*. New York: Basic Books.

38

Physician–patient communication about cancer clinical trials

Richard F. Brown

Introduction

Historical background

Today, many cancer patients are survivors as a result of improvements in the efficacy of new treatments made over the past 30 years. Cancer clinical trials are crucial to the advancement of treatment. The success of such research relies on recruiting voluntary cancer patients to clinical trials. The US National Cancer Institute (NCI) has identified low rates of patient accrual to cancer clinical trials as one of the greatest barriers to the development of effective cancer treatments. Recruitment to cancer trials is particularly difficult due to their experimental nature, design, and, in some cases, the poor prognoses of the patient population targeted for recruitment to these trials and the low probability of personal benefit for patients compared to the treatment risks.

Types of cancer clinical trials

According to the US National Cancer Institute, cancer clinical trials are generally categorized into one of the following phases of research: *Phase I trials* are initial studies with humans that usually enroll limited numbers of people. Their main purpose is to evaluate dosage safety and the frequency and method by which new drugs should be administered (e.g., either orally or by injection into the bloodstream or muscle). *Phase II trials* are designed to further evaluate drug and dosage safety and to begin assessing the impact of drugs in treating specific types of cancer. *Phase III trials* test new drugs, new drug combinations, or new surgical procedures by comparing them against current standards of care. A participant will usually be randomly assigned to the standard (control) group or the new treatment group. Phase III trials often require, by design, large numbers of enrollees and data may be collected at multiple clinical sites (http://www.cancer.gov/clinicaltrials/learningabout).

Informed consent

Strict codes of ethical human subject research now guide experimentation. This 'strong protectionism' is typified by concurrent third-party monitoring of consent and study procedures, disclosure of financial arrangements and conflicts of interest, training of researchers in research ethics, and independent review of the decision-making capacities of potential subjects (Moreno 2001). It is apparent in such legislation that there is an erosion of the researcher's self-regulation in the conduct of experiments involving human subjects.

Strong patient protection has been operationalized through the concept of informed consent underpinned by ethical principles of justice, autonomy, beneficence, and non-maleficence (for a full description of these ethical concepts and their application in the clinical trial communication setting please see Brown et al. 2010; Brown and Albrecht 2010). Informed consent is an *autonomous* action taken by a patient giving permission for a physician to undertake a medical plan (Finklestein et al. 1993). In order to join a clinical trial, patients must provide informed consent. Informed consent is intended to protect patient autonomy and ensure that patients have an active role in making treatment decisions (Cahn 1980; Finklestein et al. 1993; Kirby 1983; Lebacqz and Levine 1977).The informed consent process involves the physician presenting *a set of information* to the patient and making an appraisal about the patient's response to the information, including the degree to which the patient understands the set of information (Beauchamp and Childress 1989). The World Health Organization (WHO) (Cox et al. 2006) and US Federal Regulations (US Department of Health and Human Services 1991 (Revised 2009)) specify that human subjects must be informed about the clinical trial's aims, methods, anticipated benefits, and potential side effects, as well as their rights to refuse or withdraw from the clinical trial. Informed consent requires that patients understand this set of information and be competent to weigh possible courses of action.

However, the information delivered to patients often appears to be unclear. The complex language and excessive detail of some information statements and consent forms may confuse rather than enhance patient understanding (Grossman et al. 1994). Furthermore, while these are vetted by institutional ethics committees, the type and amount of information provided by physicians in the process of seeking informed consent is not monitored, and the impact of that information provision on patient accrual to clinical trials and other outcomes is not clear. Research focusing on patient understanding of clinical trial information across trial types shows that the WHO recommendations are not always followed (Cox et al. 2006).

Physician–patient communication challenges to informed consent

High quality communication has been identified as key to achieving informed consent (Hall 2001); however, there is mounting evidence about the communication challenges present in physician–patient consultations about clinical trials (Agrawal et al. 2006; Albrecht et al. 2009; Albrecht et al. 2003b; Brown et al. 2004b; Brown et al. 2010; Fallowfield et al. 2002; Fallowfield 1995). The research literature suggests that physicians omit critical information or the information is poorly presented (Meropol et al. 2003; Cox 2002; Daugherty et al. 2009; Brown et al. 2007; Brown et al. 2004a). Consequently, patients often misunderstand the rationale for trials, fail to recall that they are receiving their treatment within a clinical trial (Cox et al. 2006; Penman et al. 1984; Joffe et al. 2001), and may overestimate their likely chance of receiving benefit from trial medications (Cox et al. 2006; Cohen et al. 2001).

Few studies have described the specific content of clinical trial discussions. In one study comparing informed consent to Phase III adult and pediatric oncology trials, Simon et al. (2004) note that in most adult cases (69.4 percent) the physician described the concept of randomization. The risks of the study were described in 67.9 percent of cases but numerical information was provided in only 39.7 percent of the cases. Conversely, numerical information about possible benefits of the study was provided in 79.5 percent of cases. The physician described that participation was voluntary in less than half of cases (44.3 percent) and patients were informed that they could withdraw at any time in 30 percent of cases (Simon et al. 2004). Jenkins et al. 2005 also describe the content of consultation discussions when patients are approached by their physicians to participate in randomized clinical trials. Of note, in 48 percent of these consent discussions the term 'randomization' was not used whereas 'side effects' (87.8 percent) and 'treatment choices' (83 percent) were commonly described. Information leaflets were not given to 28 percent of the patients and patient understanding of information about the trial was checked in only 17 percent of the consultations. The duration of consent consultations was less than 15 minutes, and most patients signed the consent document at the first consultation where the clinical trial was discussed (Jenkins et al. 2005).

The imperative for physicians to involve patients in treatment decision-making has intensified over the past decade, particularly in response to changes in ethical mandates about informed consent (Breitsameter 2010; Charles and Gafni 2010) and evidence that offering patients more participation in decision-making results in better patient outcomes than offering less (Brown et al. 2012a; Gattellari et al. 2001). Yet many physicians do not routinely involve patients in clinical decision-making (Albrecht et al. 2003a; Brown et al. 2004b; Brown et al. 2010), are not negotiable when making final treatment decisions (Tomamichel et al. 1995), and rarely elicit or meet their patients' decision-making preferences (Ford et al. 2003; Gattellari et al. 2001; Sutherland et al. 1989; Brown et al. 2007; Brown and Albrecht 2010). Physicians; however, are concerned that involving patients in information seeking and decision-making may be overly burdensome, leading to confusion and raising anxiety, particularly for patients who prefer passivity (Kaplan et al. 1996).

Current issues

Minority recruitment to clinical trials

Low rates of patient accrual to cancer clinical trials remain one of the greatest barriers to the development of effective new treatments. Approximately 20 percent of adult cancer patients are eligible to participate in cancer clinical trials but only 2.5–9 percent actually do so (Comis et al. 2003; Korn et al. 2010). The mortality rates for African Americans from all cancers is 33 percent higher than for white Americans and African Americans have the lowest five-year survival rates when compared with all other ethnic groups (Adams-Campbell et al. 2004). Yet even lower rates of enrollment have been reported in minority populations compromising the generalizability of trial results (Bartlett et al. 1984) and threatening external validity as a result of selection bias (Britton et al. 1999). Further, differential representation in enrolled populations may lead to a failure to identify important positive or negative treatment effects among minorities.

The National Cancer Institute and the American Cancer Society, and private associations such as the American Society for Clinical Oncology (ASCO), have recognized the unequal burden of cancer in African American populations and the low representation in clinical trials and many studies and systematic reviews have detailed barriers to minority recruitment (Ford et al. 2007). In their June 2009 policy statement regarding minority recruitment to clinical trials ASCO identified barriers at all levels of the healthcare system including institutional, physician, and patient barriers. It has been suggested that effort now be expended in developing strategies and interventions to address these barriers (Ford et al. 2007; Fouad 2009).

Therapeutic misconceptions in early phase clinical trials

Although the hope for a personal therapeutic response is the stated main reason cancer patients join a Phase I study, less than 5 percent experience any personal benefit and there are substantial risks of side effects. This patient misunderstanding is at the heart of ethical questions about the validity of patient informed consent to Phase I studies and the possibility of raising false hope in an already vulnerable patient population. Cancer patients are asked to consider participation in Phase I clinical trials at one of the worst times imaginable; patients may be learning of a recurrence or that a treatment has failed, both causing great anxiety for the patient and their family members. Phase I clinical trial decision-making poses a unique challenge for physicians as the likelihood of benefit to individual patients is very low, yet there is a significant possibility that they will experience serious side effects and patients asked to participate in dose escalation studies may hope for enrollment in the high dose stage of the study and risk the possibility of toxicity (Daugherty et al. 1995).

The communication skills of physicians need to be of a high order in order to convey information sensitively and help patients navigate difficult treatment decisions. Although there are now studies exploring cancer patient treatment decision-making generally, and a few studies that have detailed decisions about participation in Phase II and III clinical trials, there are no data that comprehensively detail patient decision-making about Phase I clinical trial participation.

Patient–family communication and discordance about treatment options

Discussions about clinical trials are rarely conducted with the patient alone as approximately 80 percent of cancer patients attend appointments accompanied by at least one family member (Street and Gordon 2008). Those patients who are unaccompanied frequently consult with a family member or other important individual who are influential in the treatment decision-making process. Little is known about the role of family members in clinical trial communication and the impact on outcomes such as decision-making and ongoing trust in the clinician. One study by Albrecht et al. showed that patient–family member congruence influenced patient decision-making about joining a trial (Albrecht et al. 2008).

Family members can aid communication in consultations. Studies have shown that physicians give more information (Labrecque et al. 1991) and physician–patient understanding is increased (Schilling et al. 2002) when a family member is present versus when the patient is alone. Family members can aid patient recall, promote more patient participation in the consultation, and verify patient information (Street and Gordon 2008). On the other hand there is evidence that patients can be more passive in consultations where a family member is present (Greene et al. 1994) and the physicians may direct the conversation towards the family member (especially in cases where the patient is elderly or cognitively impaired) (Beisecker 1996). Concern has been expressed that family members may exert undue influence on patient decision-making and have divergent values and priorities from the patient (Clayman et al. 2005) both of which may serve to undermine patient autonomy and threaten valid informed consent (Ho 2008). Although physicians generally welcome the inclusion of family members in the consultation, they are concerned about their intervention in decision-making processes and worry about challenges to their professional authority (Ho 2008). Thus it is likely physicians have difficulty determining the degree to which they should draw the family member into the treatment discussion.

Sample analysis

Developing a communication typology to guide physicians' discussions about clinical trials

Prior communication research has usefully described the nature of the information contained within informed consent discussions and patient/physician perceptions of this difficult process. However, little research has been conducted that (a) explores interventions designed to assist in the communication process or (b) systematically defines optimal communication content and process to ensure ethical informed consent. In the research study described for this sample analysis we aimed first to develop a typology to describe physician–patient interactions that occur when participation in Phase II and III clinical trials are discussed. Second, we aimed to develop ethical strategies for discussing participation of eligible patients in Phase II and III clinical trials (Brown and Albrecht 2010; Brown et al. 2004a).

To gather information about the range of communication styles oncologists used to discuss clinical trials with their patients, a qualitative analysis of audiotaped consultations containing discussions of Phase II and III clinical trials between nine medical and radiation oncologists (five male and four female) working at two university teaching hospitals and their patients was conducted. This research was conducted in two stages.

Stage 1

Sixteen audiotape transcripts that were part of an existing library of transcripts of over 300 initial consecutive oncology consultations collected as part of a previous research project were analyzed (Brown et al. 2001). The transcripts were analyzed by a panel including experts in ethics, cancer medicine, and psycho-oncology. The analysis was initially limited to an exploration of the language used to seek informed consent to clinical trials.

The transcripts were analyzed using the constant comparative method proposed by Glaser (Glaser and Strauss 1967) and supported by the qualitative research software Non Numerical Unstructured Data by Indexing, Searching and Theorizing (NUD*IST) (NUD*IST 1997). Meetings of the research team were conducted at weekly intervals during which themes were identified and discussed. Initially, as the methodology requires, only a few transcripts were analyzed. Once an exhaustive analysis of this original dataset was complete, further small samples of transcripts were analyzed. The themes that emerged from these data were compared with those from the original dataset and if necessary new thematic categories were defined. This process continued until no new themes emerged.

Stage 2

In order to ensure that an exhaustive analysis had been conducted and that *theoretical saturation* or *redundancy* (Miles and Huberman 1984) had been reached, a further 10 consultations in which clinical trials were discussed with one of four medical oncologists were audiotaped with patient consent. It was apparent from the Stage 1 analysis that there were difficulties in exploring the clinical trial discussion in isolation from other aspects of the consultation discourse. Therefore, the aim of Stage 2 was to conduct an expanded analysis allowing an exploration of the structure of the whole consultation. In particular, (a) the framework within which doctor–patient communication had been established at the beginning of the consultation, (b) the types of strategies employed by the oncologist to introduce and encourage a positive approach to clinical trials and ensure understanding prior to the specific trial discussion, and (c) the implications of gaining prior informed consent to standard treatment on the subsequent clinical trial discussion. An identical procedure to that utilized in Stage 1 was used to analyze the transcripts of the audiotapes of this patient sample.

Expert linguists, who formed part of the research team, analyzed a subset of seven (or approximately 25 percent) of the 26 transcripts to explore the type of language used in offering clinical trials as treatment options, in particular coercive and non-coercive elements. The sample was selected at random using random number lists generated by the Statistical Program for Social Sciences (SPSS). A Systemic Functional Linguistics approach was taken (Eggins 1994; Halliday 1994). This model theorizes the relation between a text and its context as one of mutual realization between different strata (levels of organization) of language, building on the work of Malinowski (1923) among others.

These four strata are: context of culture, context of situation, semantic level, and lexico-grammar. To demonstrate this approach, the four strata are listed below and illustrated in terms of their application to the context of offering clinical trials.

Context of culture

Patterning at this level distinguishes societies and groups at the broadest level, and it is within the *context of culture* that each context of situation has its particular significance. For instance in Western culture, the medical context is seen as a predominantly scientific context rather than a religious one, but tensions between the value, purpose, and structure of scientific knowledge, vis-à-vis lay knowledge, or religious and ethical knowledge, are crucial to understanding how offering participation in an experiment may – or may not – count as care.

Context of situation

By being systematic about the relevant dimensions of this specific context of situation – how it is both like and unlike other forms of social process and interaction (including the technological environment such processes assume) – we can establish in a non-ad hoc way why it is that wording that in one place might seem quite suitable can be anathema (or even illegal) at another point in the same interaction, or in a similar consultation (Butt and Moore 2002). The context of situation studied here is that of consultations between oncologists and their patients, and more particularly those in which trials are offered as treatment options. Any context of situation can be described synoptically as a configuration of specific types of activity, relation, and contact (Butt 1983; Halliday and Hasan 1985). It can also be modeled dynamically in terms of the moves or phases by which it typically unfolds (its Generic Structure Potential – see Halliday and Hasan 1985). Considerable variation in the configuration and phasing of these consultations is possible, however some variations are likely to introduce coercion.

Semantic level (system of meanings)

In the context of oncology consultations, critical areas of meaning include *risk, choice, agency, actual/potential, inclination/obligation,* along with concepts particular to medicine such as *equipoise* which are usually highly technical and often contentious (Lilford 2001).

Each of these concepts can be seen as a dimension of the 'meaning potential' which may or may not be actualized in any given instance of the context, and, where actualized, may take various forms in terms of words and grammar. Sometimes these wording differences put a crucial spin on semantics. For example, physicians often take options in the semantics of spatial proximity, which tend to indicate that the oncologist is the owner of, or possesses control of, the clinical trial in which the patient has been invited to participate, and this tends to foreground the physician's agency. Clusters of semantic choices like these can construe the *context of situation* as one with quite a hierarchical *relation* between physician and patient, which may influence the treatment decision. The example below indicates how language can be used that promotes patient agency in the consultation.

> *Avoid:*
> *Physician*: '**We** will develop a treatment plan **for you** by the end of this session. **I'll** let your surgeon know what **I have decided**, and **I can organize** you to start treatment by next week. For the chemotherapy, **we** will be putting a cannula **into your arm** for about an hour, and **then you can go home**.'
>
> *Rather:*
> *Physician*: 'OK, so you're happy with that decision? You would like to go ahead with chemotherapy? If you like, I'll introduce you to our chemo nurse, who can talk to you a bit more about the chemotherapy, and explain how it will all work. Basically, you will have to come in once every three weeks. You will have a drip in your arm, and the anti-cancer drugs will go through the drip and then spread around your system, and that will take about an hour, each time.'

Lexico-grammar (systems of wording)

To continue the example above, *wording* such as 'You can *join us* on the trial', or 'If you *come* onto the trial' realizes the *semantics* of positioning the trial in close spatial proximity to the physician, which indicates to patients that the physician is the owner of the trial, or is some kind of agent of the trial. Of note, where such wording patterns are used by physicians with high frequency, or where different aspects of the wording used (e.g., proximity and transitivity) invoke the same semantic motif (e.g., physician as agent), patients will be more likely to pick up on this 'semantic drift' (Butt 1983).

Results

The broad analyses of the data described above, including the specific linguistic analysis, resulted in the identification of four key themes which formed the basis of a set of ethical strategies to guide physicians' communication about gaining informed consent to cancer clinical trials. These were: (a) shared decision-making strategies, (b) the sequence of moves in the consultation, (c) the type and clarity of the information provided, and (d) disclosure of controversial information and coercion.

These data have been published in full elsewhere: however, we present limited data here about coercion, as this was a particular focus of the linguistic analysis (Brown et al. 2004a). The analysis revealed language used by oncologists, who may be quite unaware of their ramifications that may encourage or perhaps coerce patients into participating in clinical trials.

Physician preferences

If the physicians do not explicitly state their views on clinical trial participation, while acknowledging patient choice, patients may feel unspoken pressure to participate. Preferences may be covertly suggested in many ways, for example by spending more time talking about the trial treatment versus standard treatment, by minimizing versus maximizing side effects and/or benefits of one or other treatment, or by differential use of agency (patient active in one treatment, passive in the other) and proximity (patient will be part of the team if they join the trial, or offered standard treatment). Another subtle example of this is where probabilities are presented as group statistics in one treatment and as personalized in another. For example, 'most patients will lose their hair on this treatment' (group) versus 'it is most likely that you will lose your hair on this treatment' (personalized). Subtle differences such as these may influence patient decisions.

Terms

Physicians commonly use the term 'you are eligible for this trial'. This phrase, however, can imply that the patient is 'lucky' to have been selected, or should be hopeful that their disease status allows them to participate in the trial. We suggest using the phrase 'the trial is suitable for you'. This is a subtle yet powerful delineation. Making it clear that a trial is 'suitable' for the patient objectifies the trial and does not imply the patient should aim to meet a set of criteria.

Appealing to altruism

A common motivation for patients to enter clinical trials is a sense of making a contribution to medical knowledge which will benefit others, or altruism. Finding the balance between recognizing and appreciating patient altruism and using it in a coercive fashion can be difficult. Once again, the terms used can make a difference. Thus the use of terms such as '*You* can benefit future generations' is perhaps more coercive than 'This will help us find the answer to this question'.

Framing

Coercion may also occur when the potential value of a clinical trial treatment is presented with a positive frame versus negative framing for the standard treatment (or vice versa). Patient preferences for framing of prognostic information should be negotiated. Research suggests that some patients prefer positively framed information ('you have a 70 percent chance of cure') as this encourages a positive outlook, while others prefer negatively framed information ('you have a 30 percent chance of the cancer coming back') as this emphasizes the importance of additional treatment (Brown et al. 2004a).

To this point the focus of this chapter has been on Phase II and III clinical trials. More recently, we conducted an exploratory study to extend our knowledge of communication strategies oncologists employ in discussions about clinical trials to the Phase I setting. This study aimed to gain a better understanding of oncologist–patient interactions through analysis of conversational data from audio recordings of Phase I clinical trial discussions (Brown et al. 2010). Although there was some common ground between communication in Phase I and the Phase II and III settings, there were distinct differences. For example, oncologists used persuasive communication and limited patients' decisions in Phase I consultations as compared to Phase II and III consultations. For example, in one instance the oncologist raised the question of the patient's eligibility for the Phase I study at the end of the consultation once the study had been fully described and the patient was hopeful that the trial would be suitable by saying,

> *Physician*: 'And then if you're … no pressure you know. No matter what happens I'll do the best for you, but just so you understand, from this clinical trial standpoint, this is a multi-centered study, meaning other centers are also available. So we have this spot for a few days and then we have to give it up if we don't find somebody. So right now this spot is yours, if you are eligible.'

Future directions

Patient-focused interventions

Improving physician communication is necessary, but not sufficient to achieve the best possible communication in a clinical trial discussion. The physician–patient interaction is a dynamic, socially constructed, and reciprocal process that relies on at least two participants. Thus, while this chapter has focused on training clinicians as a means of improving communication, we now turn attention to patient-focused interventions as future directions for communication research in this area.

Decision aids

Decision aids (DAs) have been developed to help patients make sense of complex information and arrive at a shared decision by clarification of patients' values and treatment preferences. Patients need to understand all treatment options, including respective benefits and limitations. Typical information includes information on the disease/condition; probabilities of outcomes tailored to personal health risk factors; an explicit values clarification exercise; information on others' opinions; a personalized recommendation on the basis of clinical characteristics and expressed preferences; and guidance or coaching in the steps of decision-making and in communicating with others.

Other researchers (Juraskova et al. 2008) have successfully piloted a DA to assist breast cancer patients in clinical trial decision-making. Future research could usefully develop, test, and evaluate DAs that target (a) post-consultation clinical trial decision-making, and (b) involve patients and family members together balancing the advantages and disadvantages of the clinical trial. Further, the content of the DA could be developed as a collaborative effort between researchers, minority community groups, and other stakeholders involved in increasing the participation of minorities in therapeutic cancer clinical trials.

Question prompt lists

One patient-focused intervention with potential to improve communication is a Question Prompt List (QPL). QPLs are simple and inexpensive interventions to aid patients to be active participants in consultations by asking questions. QPLs are easily disseminated. The goal of a QPL is to increase knowledge of novel topics, and to stimulate patients to raise these with their physician or to use the QPL as a reminder. Our early work in the general oncology setting (Brown et al. 2001), and that of others in primary care (Kinnersley et al. 2007), demonstrated that using the QPL, coupled with physician endorsement of question asking, (a) encouraged patients to ask questions about sensitive and difficult topics such as prognosis, diagnosis, and issues surrounding end-of-life care, and (b) improved patient outcomes (Brown et al. 2001; Butow et al. 1994; Roter 1977; Clayton et al. 2007). Recent implementation studies have found that a high proportion, 50–65 percent, of patients made use of a QPL when it was offered as part of routine clinical practice (Dimoska et al. 2012; Geest et al. 2006). Although QPLs have been shown to be an effective means of promoting active patient participation in other settings (Brown et al. 2001; Brown et al. 1999; Clayton et al. 2007), there are no studies demonstrating their efficacy in the context of achieving high quality informed consent to cancer clinical trials.

To fill this gap we have conducted initial pilot testing of a clinical trial focused QPL. The results of preliminary focus groups revealed that the QPL was comprehensive and could prompt patients to consider novel issues, gain salient information, and be better informed for future trial discussions and to help make a trial decision (Brown et al. 2011a; Brown et al. 2011b). The results of feasibility and utility testing revealed that the QPL increased patient questions about realistic benefits from treatment, thus potentially helping with issues of therapeutic misconceptions (Brown et al. 2012b).

Each individual trial protocol presents different communication challenges as patients are tasked with learning trial specific terminology, facts and statistics, for example side effects profiles, the names of experimental agents, and trial regimens. In Phase III randomized trials, patients are faced with understanding complex trial processes such as chance allocation to treatment arms. Patients who have some understanding of specific clinical terminology and processes are better able to discuss individual health topics and thereby to participate more fully in trial decision-making, resulting in improved patient outcomes (Street et al. 2005). The potential for additional benefit of customized QPLs, which provide questions focused on a specific clinical trial and thereby personalize trial information, has not been explored. These results suggest that future research is warranted to demonstrate the efficacy of the clinical-trial focused QPL and customized QPLs that target individual clinical trials.

Summary

The literature clearly demonstrates that low rates of accrual to cancer clinical trials impede progress towards effective new treatments. Optimizing physician–patient communication is key to improving the quality of informed consent, thereby potentially improving trial accrual, adherence to, and completion of, therapeutic treatment regimens. Linguistic analysis of physician–patient conversations about clinical trials has been a critical tool to further our understanding of this complex communication challenge. The provision of effective, inexpensive, communication aids that are easy to disseminate and help meet ethical mandates for informed consent could be a great service to cancer patients, clinicians, and those involved in the design and conduct of therapeutic clinical trials.

Related topics

Physician–patient communication; informed consent; clinical trials; question prompt lists.

Further reading

Albrecht, T.L., Eggly, S.S., Gleeson, M.E.J., et al. (2008) 'Influence of clinical communication on patients' decision-making on participation in clinical trials', *Journal of Clinical Oncology*, 26: 2666–2673.

Brown, R.F., Butow, P.N., Butt, D.G., et al. (2004) 'Developing ethical strategies to assist oncologist in seeking informed consent to cancer clinical trials', *Social Science & Medicine*, 58: 379–390.

Brown, R.F., Bylund, C.L., Li, Y., et al. (2012) 'Testing the utility of a cancer clinical trial specific Question Prompt List (QPL-CT) during oncology consultations', *Patient Education and Counseling*, 88(2): 311–317.

Kirby, M.D. (1983) 'Informed consent: what does it mean?', *Journal of Medical Ethics*, 9: 69–75.

References

Adams-Campbell, L.L., Ahaghotu, C., Gaskins, M., Dawkins, F.W., Smoot, D., Polk, O.D., Gooding, R. and Dewitty, R. (2004) 'Enrolment of African Americans onto clinical treatment trials: study design barriers', *Journal of Clinical Oncology*, 22: 730–734.

Agrawal, M., Grady, C., Fairclough, D.L., Meropol, N.J., Maynard, K. and Emanuel, E.J. (2006) 'Patient decision-making process regarding participation in Phase I oncology research', *Journal of Clinical Oncology*, 24: 4479–4483.

Albrecht, T.L., Penner, L.A. and Ruckdeschel, J.C. (2003a) 'Understanding patient decisions about clinical trials and the associated communication processes; a preliminary report', *Journal of Cancer Education*, 18: 210–14.

Albrecht, T.L., Ruckdeschel, J.C., Riddle, J.C., Blanchard, C.G., Penner, L.A., Coovert, M.D. and Quinn, G. (2003b) 'Communication and decision-making about cancer clinical trials', *Patient Education and Counseling*, 50: 39–42.

Albrecht, T.L., Eggly, S.S., Gleeson, M.E.J., Harper, F.W.K., Foster, T.S., Peterson, A.M., Orom, H., Penner, L.A. and Ruckdeshel, J.C. (2008) 'Influence of clinical communication on patients' decision-making on participation in clinical trials', *Journal of Clinical Oncology*, 26: 2666–2673.

Albrecht, T.L., Penner, L.A., Cline, R.J.W., Eggly, S. and Ruckdeschel, J.C. (2009) 'Studying the process of clinical communication: issues of context, concepts and research directions', *Journal of Health Comunication*, 14: 47–56.

Bartlett, E.E., Grayson, M., Barker, R., Levine, D.M., Golden, A. and Libber, S. (1984) 'The effects of physician communications skills on patient satisfaction; recall, and adherence', *Journal of Chronic Diseases*, 37: 755–764.

Beauchamp, T.L. and Childress, J.F. (1989) *Principles of Biomedical Ethics*, Oxford: Oxford University Press.

Beisecker, A.E. (1996) 'The influence of a companion on the doctor–elderly patient interaction', *Health Expectations*, 1: 55–70.

Breitsameter, C. (2010) 'Medical decision-making and communication of risks: an ethical perspective', *Journal of Medical Ethics*, 36: 349–352.

Britton, A., McKee, M. Black, N., Macpherson, K., Sanderson, C. and Bain, C. (1999) 'Threats to the applicability of randomised trials, exclusions and selective participation', *Journal of Health Services Research Policy*, 4: 112–121.

Brown, R.F. and Albrecht, T.L. (2010) 'Enrolment in clinical trials', in Kissane, D., Bultz, B., Butow, P.N. and Finlay, I.G. (eds) *Handbook of Communication in Oncology and Palliative Care*, New York: Oxford University Press.

Brown, R.F., Butow, P.N., Boyer, M.J. and Tattersall, M.H.N. (1999) 'Promoting patient participation in the cancer consultation; evaluation of a prompt sheet and coaching in question asking', *British Journal of Cancer*, 80: 242–248.

Brown, R.F., Butow, P.N., Dunn, S. and Tattersall, M.H.N. (2001) 'Promoting patient participation and shortening cancer consultations: a randomized trial', *British Journal of Cancer*, 85: 1273–1279.

Brown, R.F., Butow, P.N., Butt, D.G., Moore, A. and Tattersall, M.H.N. (2004a) 'Developing ethical strategies to assist oncologist in seeking informed consent to cancer clinical trials', *Social Science & Medicine*, 58: 379–390.

Brown, R.F., Butow, P.N., Ellis, P., Boyle, F. and Tattersall, M.H.N. (2004b) 'Seeking informed consent to cancer clinical trials: describing current practice', *Social Science & Medicine*, 58: 2445–2457.

Brown, R.F., Butow, P.N., Boyle, F. and Tattershall, M.H.N. (2007) 'Seeking informed consent to cancer clinical trials: evaluating the efficacy of communication skills training', *Psycho-Oncology*, 16: 507–516.

Brown, R.F., Bylund, C.L., Siminoff, L.A. and Slovin, S.F. (2010) 'Seeking informed consent to Phase I cancer clinical trial: identifying oncologists' communication strategies', *Psycho-Oncology*, 20: 361–368.

Brown, R.F., Shuk, E., Butow, P.N., Edgerson, S., Tattersall, M.H.N. and Ostroff, M.H.N. (2011a) 'Identifying patient information needs about cancer clinical trials using a question prompt list', *Patient Education and Counselling*, 84: 69–77.

Brown, R.F., Shuk, E., Butow, P.N., Leighl, N., Edgerson, S., Ostroff, J. and Tattersall, M.H.N. (2011b) 'Enhancing decision-making about participation in cancer clinical trials: development of a question prompt list', *Supportive Care in Cancer*, 19: 1227–1238.

Brown, R.F., Butow, P.N., Wilson-Genderson, M., Bernhard, J., Ribi, K. and Juraskova, I. (2012a) 'Meeting the decision-making preferences of patients with breast cancer in oncology consultations: impact on decision-related outcomes', *Journal of Clinical Oncology*, 30(8): 857–862.

Brown, R.F., Bylund, C.L., Li, Y., Edgerson, S. and Butow, P.N. (2012b) 'Testing the utility of a cancer clinical trial specific Question Prompt List (QPL-CT) during oncology consultations', *Patient Education and Counseling*, 88(2): 311–317.

Butow, P.N., Dunn, S.M., Tattersall, M.H.N. and Jones, Q.J. (1994) 'Patient involvement in the cancer consultation; evaluation of a question prompt sheet', *Annals of Oncology*, 5: 199–204.

Butt, D.G. (1983) 'Semantic drift in verbal art', *Australian Review of Applied Linguistics*, 6: 38–48.

Butt, D.G. and Moore, A.R. (2002) 'Risk and meaning potential; why a network?' Sociolinguistics Symposium 12, Ghent.

Cahn, C.H. (1980) 'Consent in psychiatry. The position of the Canadian Psychiatric Association', *Canadian Journal of Psychiatry*, 25: 78–84.

Charles, C. and Gafni, A. (2010) 'Shared treatment decision-making and the use of decision aids', in Kissane, D., Bultz, B., Butow, P.N. and Finlay, I.G. (eds) *Handbook of Communication in Oncology and Palliative Care*, New York: Oxford University Press.

Clayman, M.L., Roter, D., Wissow, L.S. and Bandeen-Roche, K. (2005) 'Autonomy related behaviors of patient companions and their effect on decision-making activity in geriatric primary care', *Social Science & Medicine*, 60: 1583–1591.

Clayton, J.M., Butow, P.N., Tattersall, M.H.N., Devine, R.J., Simpson, J.M., Aggarwall, G., Clark, K.J., Currow, D.C., Elliott, L.M., Lacey, J., Lee, P.G. and Noel, M.A. (2007) 'Randomized controlled trial of a prompt list to help advanced cancer patients and their caregivers to ask questions about prognosis and end-of-life care', *Journal of Clinical Oncology*, 25: 715–723.

Cohen, L., De Moor, C. and Amato, R.J. (2001) 'The association between treatment specific optimism and depressive symptomatology in patients enrolled in a Phase I cancer clinical trial', *Cancer*, 91: 1949–1955.

Comis, R.L., Miller, J.D., Aldige, C.R., Kreps, L. and Stoval, E. (2003) 'Public attitudes towards participation in cancer clinical trials', *Journal of Clinical Oncology*, 21: 830–835.

Cox, A.C., Fallowfield, L.J. and Jenkins, V.A. (2006) 'Communication and the informed consent process in Phase I trials: a review of the literature', *Supportive Care in Cancer: Official Journal of the Multinational Association of Supportive Care in Cancer*, 14: 303–309.

Cox, K. (2002) 'Informed consent and decision-making: patients' experiences of the process of recruitment to phases 1 and 2 anti-cancer drug trials', *Patient Education and Counselling*, 46: 31–38.

Daugherty, C., Kass, N.E., Roter, D., Larson, S., Sugarman, J., Kasza, M., Ratain, M.J. and Hlubocky, F.J. (2009) 'A study of physician investigator (PI) disclosure of alternatives of care and prognostic information to advanced cancer patients (ACP) enrolling in Phase I trials', *Journal of Clinical Oncology*, 27: suppl;abstr 6508.

Daugherty, C.K., Ratain, M.J. and Siegler, M. (1995) 'Pushing the envelope: informed consent to phase I trials', *Annals of Oncology*, 6: 321–323.

Dimoska, A., Butow, P.N., Lynch, J., Hovey, E., Agar, M., Beale, P. and Tattersall, M.H.N. (2012) 'Implementing patient question-prompt lists into routine cancer care', *Patient Education and Counseling*, 86(2): 252–258.

Eggins, S. (1994) *An Introduction to Systemic Functional Linguistics*, London: Pinter.

Fallowfield, L. (1995) 'Can we improve the professional personal fulfilment of doctors in cancer medicine', *British Journal of Cancer*, 71: 1132–1133.

Fallowfield, L., Jenkins, V., Farewell, V., Saul, J., Duffy, A. and Eves, R. (2002) 'Efficacy of a Cancer Research UK communication skills training model for oncologists: a randomised controlled trial', *Lancet*, 359: 650–656.

Finklestein, D., Karsh-Smith, M. and Faden, R. (1993) 'Informed consent in medical ethics', *Archives of Opthamology*, 111: 324–326.

Ford, G.F., Howerton, M.W., Lai, G.Y., Gary, T.L. Bolen, S., Gibbons, M.C., Tilburt, J., Baffi, C., Tanputukpongse, T.P., Wilson, R.F., Powe, N.R. and Bass, E.B. (2007) 'Barriers to recruiting underrepresented populations in cancer clinical trials: a systematic review', *Cancer*, 112: 228–242.

Ford, S., Schofield, T. and Hope, T. (2003) 'Are patients' decision-making preferences being met?', *Health Expectations*, 6: 72–80.

Fouad, M. (2009) 'Enrolment of minorities in clinical trials: did we overcome the barriers?', *Contemporary Clinical Trials*, 30: 103–104.

Gattellari, M., Butow, P.N. and Tattersall, M.H.N. (2001) 'Sharing decisions in cancer care', *Social Science & Medicine*, 52: 1865–1878.

Geest, T.A., Wetzels, R., Wensing, M., Castel, O.C. and Olsen, F. (2006) 'Evaluation of an intervention designed to enhance involvement of older patients in their own care', *European Journal of General Practice*, 12: 3–9.

Glaser, B.J. and Strauss, A.L. (1967) *The Discovery of Grounded Theory: Strategies for Qualitative Research,* New York: Adline.

Greene, M.G., Majerovitz, S.D., Adelman, R.D. and Rizzo, C. (1994) 'The effects of the presence of a third person on the physician–older person medical interview', *American Geriatrics Society*, 42: 413–419.

Grossman, S.A., Piantodosi, S. and Cohavey, C. (1994) 'Are informed consent forms that describe clinical oncology research protocols readable by most patients and their families?', *Journal of Clinical Oncology*, 12: 2211–2215.

Hall, A. (2001) 'The role of effective communication in obtaining informed consent in medical research', In Loyal, L. and Tobias, J.S. (eds) London: BMJ Books.

Halliday, M.A.K. (1994) *An Introduction to Functional Grammar*, 2nd edn, London: Edward Arnold.

Halliday, M.A.K. and Hasan, R. (1985) *Language, Context and Text: Aspects of Language in a Social–Semiotic Perspective,* Waurn Ponds, Vic.: Deakin University Press.

Ho, A. (2008) 'Relational autonomy or undue pressure? Family's role in medical decision-making', *Scandinavian Journal of Caring Science*, 22: 128–135.

Jenkins, V., Fallowfield, L., Solis-Trapala, I., Landridge, C. and Farewell, V. (2005) 'Discussing randomised clinical trials of cancer therapy:evaluation of a Cancer Research UK training programme', *British Medical Journal*, 330: 400–406.

Joffe, S., Cook, E., Francis, V., Cleary, P.D., Clark, J.W. and Weeks, J.C. (2001) 'Quality of informed consent: a new measure of understanding among research subjects', *Journal of the National Cancer Institute*, 93: 139–147.

Juraskova, I., Butow, P., Lopez, A., Seccombe, M., Coates, A., Boyle, F., McCarthy, N., Reaby, L. and Forbes, J.F. (2008) 'Improving informed consent: pilot of a decsion aid for women invited to participate in a breast cancer prevention trial (IBIS-II DCIS)', *Health Expectations*, 11: 252–262.

Kaplan, S.H., Greenfield, S., Gandek, B., Rogers, W.H. and Ware, J. (1996) 'Characteristics of physicians with participatory decision-making styles', *Annals of Internal Medicine*, 124: 497–504.

Kinnersley, P., Edwards, A., Hood, K., Cadbury, N., Ryan, R., Prout, H., Owen, D., Macbeth, F., Butow, P. and Butler, C. (2007) 'Interventions before consultations for helping patients address their information needs', *Cochrane Database of Systematic Reviews*: CD004565.

Kirby, M.D. (1983) 'Informed consent: what does it mean?', *Journal of Medical Ethics*, 9: 69–75.

Korn, E.L., Freidlin, B., Mooney, M. and Abrams, J.S. (2010) 'Accrual experience of National Cancer Institute Cooperative Group phase III trials activated from 2000 to 2007', *Journal of Clinical Oncology: Official Journal of the American Society of Clinical Oncology*, 28: 5197–5201.

Labrecque, M.S., Blanchard, C.G., Rucjdeschel, J.C. and Blanchard, E.B. (1991) 'The impact of family presence on the physician–cancer patient interaction', *Social Science & Medicine*, 33: 1253–1261.

Lebacqz, K. and Levine, R.J. (1977) 'Respect for persons and informed consent to participate in cancer research', *Journal of Clinical Research*, 25: 101–107.

Lilford, R.J. (2001) 'Equipoise is not synonymous with uncertainty', *British Medical Journal*, 323: 574.

Malinowski, B. (1923) 'The problem of meaning in primative language', in Ogden, C.K. and Richards, I.A. (eds) *The Meaning of Meaning*, New York: Harcourt Brace.

Meropol, N.J., Weinfurt, C.B., Balshem, A., Benson, A.B., Castel, L., Corbett, S., Diefenbach,M., Gaskin, D.J., Li, Y., Manne, S., Marshall, J., Rowland, J.H., Slater, E., Sulmasy, D.P. Echo, D.V., Washington, S. and Schulman, K.A. (2003) 'Perceptions of patients and physicians regarding Phase I cancer clinical trials: implications for physician–patient communication', *Journal of Clinical Oncology*, 21: 2589–2596.

Miles, M.V. and Huberman, M.A. (1984) *Qualitative Data Analysis: A Sourcebook of New Methods*, London: Sage.

Moreno, J.D. (2001) 'Goodbye to all that: the end of moderate protectionism in human subjects research', *Hastings Centre Report*, 31: 9–17.

NUD*IST 1997. Software for qualitative data analysis. 4 ed. Melbourne: Qualitative Solutions and Research.

Penman, D., Holland, J. and Bahna, G. (1984) 'Informed consent for investigational chemotherapy: patients' and physicians' perceptions', *Journal of Clinical Oncology*, 2: 849–855.

Roter, D. (1977) 'Patient participation in the patient–provider interaction: the effects of patient question asking on the quality of interaction, satisfaction and compliance', *Health Education Monographs*, 5: 281–315.

Schilling, L.M., Scatena, L., Steiner, J.F., Albertson, G.A., Lin, C.T., Cyran, L. Ware, L. and Anderson, R.J. (2002) 'The third person in the room: frequency, role, and influence of companions during primary care medical encounters', *Journal of Family Practice*, 51: 685–690.

Simon, C.M., Siminoff, L.A., Kodish, E.D. and Burant, C. (2004) 'Comparison of informed consent process for randomized clinical trials in pediatric and adult oncology', *Journal of Clinical Oncology*, 22: 2709–2717.

Street, R.L. and Gordon, H.S. (2008) 'Companion participation in cancer consultations', *Psycho-Oncology*, 17: 244–251.

Street, R.L., Jr., Gordon, H.S., Ward, M.M., Krupat, E. and Kravitz, R.L. (2005) 'Patient participation in medical consultations: why some patients are more involved than others', *Medical Care*, 43: 960–969.

Sutherland, H.J., Llewellyn-Thomas, H.A., Lockwood, G.A. and Tritchler, D.L. (1989) 'Cancer patients: their desire for information and participation in treatment decisions', *Journal of the Royal Society of Medicine*, 82: 260–263.

Tomamichel, M., Sessa, C., Herzig, S., De Jong, J. Pagani, O., Willems, Y. and Cavalli, F. (1995) 'Informed consent for phase I studies: evaluation of quantity and quality of information provided to patients', *Annals of Oncology*, 6: 363–369.

US Department of Health and Human Services. 1991 (Revised 2009) *45 Code of Federal Regulations: Federal Policy for the Protection of Human Subjects ('Common Rule')* [Online]. Available: http://www.hhs.gov/ohrp/humansubjects/commonrule/. Last accessed December 9, 2013.

39

Medical interaction analysis systems

Coding challenges when applied to communication in palliative care

Lee Ellington, McKenzie Carlisle, and Maija Reblin

Introduction

In our lifetimes, we have witnessed tremendous advances in detection, prevention, and even curing of disease. However, less attention and resources have been directed towards advancing health care for those approaching end of life. Although palliative and hospice care services are becoming increasingly integrated into healthcare systems, there is still room for improvement. In 2010, only 41.9 percent of US deaths were served by hospice (NHPCO 2011), and with an aging US population, the need for these services will only continue to grow. Within the general field of health care, there is significant emphasis on a patient-centered, biopsychosocial approach to care, and it could be argued that there is no other healthcare specialty where a holistic approach is more urgently needed than when providers, patients, and families are in need of palliative or end-of-life care.

Palliative care is a specialized healthcare service for individuals with serious illnesses and their families. The focus of care is on the provision of comfort and enhancing quality of life, and can be invoked at any point across the disease continuum. Falling under the rubric of palliative care, hospice care is targeted for those patients and families who are no longer seeking curative therapy. At the core of successful palliative care is effective communication, requiring advanced skills in attending to the whole family's medical, psychosocial, and spiritual concerns. However, our knowledge about communication needs and approaches to support patients, families, individual providers, and healthcare teams remains in the early stages of development. One strategy to increase this knowledge base and to understand the impact of communication on care outcomes is to conduct research on healthcare interactions in palliative and hospice care.

Chapter focus and overview

This chapter examines the application of interaction analysis systems to palliative care encounters. These systems operationalize both the content and the process of interactions between providers, patients, and families and rely largely on quantitative statistical interpretations of patterns of communication behaviors. Often, the content-focused coding is directed at the clinical mission of the encounters (e.g., *caregiver provision of information on symptom management*), whereas the process is captured by coding relationship dynamics (e.g., *provider response to patient emotional concerns*). These approaches are designed to be applied to large datasets and often coders are trained to code directly from the voice or visual recordings without the aid (or cost) of transcription. The purpose of this chapter is not to compare quantitative coding systems to health communication approaches within linguistics or in the qualitative spectrum. Rather, we will present different interactional analysis systems that have been applied in the palliative care context, describe the specific operationalizations of communication behaviors, note strengths and weaknesses of each approach, and, finally, discuss future research directions.

In this chapter, we first discuss the widely used medical communication coding scheme, Roter Interaction Analysis, applied to full palliative care encounters. Next we discuss coding approaches to capturing hospice team communication. This is followed by a discussion of coding approaches that target specific behaviors salient to palliative care: emotional dialogue and the provision of bad news. All sections include a discussion of strengths and limitations. We end with a general discussion of the challenges in studying communication in palliative care and directions for future research.

The Roter Interaction Analysis System (RIAS)

RIAS was designed to represent patient–provider exchanges, where each individual is equal and has expertise to share (Detmar et al. 2001; Roter and Larson 2002). The system was derived from social exchange theories related to interpersonal influence, problem solving, reciprocity, and empowerment (Roter 2010b; Roter and Larson 2002).

RIAS is applied to utterances, the smallest unit of expression to which a meaningful code can be assigned. This unit is a single thought which may be expressed as a simple sentence, clause, or even a single word. Each utterance is assigned one of 40 mutually exclusive and exhaustive categories that reflect the form (e.g., information giving, closed-/open-ended questions, partnership building) and content (e.g., medical condition, lifestyle behaviors, psychosocial topics) of the dialogue. The communication categories can be broadly viewed as reflecting socio-emotional components of a medical exchange, such as paraphrasing and showing concern, as well as task-focused components, like giving directions and asking for clarification (Roter and Larson 2002). Although the majority of codes are equally applicable to both health professionals and patients, six categories are health professional-specific (e.g., asking for patient opinion or self-disclosure), and one category is patient-specific (requesting service or medication). In addition to verbal code categories, speakers may be rated on separate scales reflecting emotional tone, including anger, anxiety, dominance, interest, friendliness, engagement, sympathy, and hurry (Roter 2010b; Roter and Larson 2002).

RIAS codes can be used individually or summarized in a number of ways. There are useful frameworks for organizing the individual codes, such as the Four-Function Communication Model (Roter 2000) which allows for the integration of patient communication behaviors into visit functions and the identification of a distinct activation and engagement function. Ratios can also be calculated, such as the ratio of open- to closed-ended questions to analyze the tenor of a conversation. Composite scores, such as patient-centeredness scores, can also be computed to reflect health professional versus patient communication control (Roter and Hall 2004).

RIAS in palliative care

Initially applied to the primary care environment, RIAS is now utilized in other areas, such as palliative care settings. Roter and Larson (2002) posit that the adaptive nature of RIAS allows users to tailor the system for capturing unique contextual dimensions of the situation of interest. Below we describe how researchers have applied RIAS to palliative care interactions, including adaptations and additions to the original system.

Researchers often supplement RIAS codes by including additional content-based items or interaction categories. This approach has been used to describe physicians' best and usual practices in communication about advance directives (Roter et al. 2000), to assess health-related quality of life in outpatient palliative chemotherapy (Detmar et al. 2001), and to explore treatment decision-making processes in palliative radiotherapy (Verhaak et al. 2000). Verhaak et al.'s study (2000) demonstrates the use of the full RIAS with supplemental categories. They added three additional physician codes to the existing RIAS categories: *treatment information, information about abstaining from treatment,* and *asking patient opinion about treatment.* Although these additional codes would have been captured in broad RIAS coding categories (biomedical information and ask opinion), the authors' primary objective was to understand specific processes related to treatment decision-making. Findings demonstrated little support for shared decision-making, as evidenced by oncologists' talk being predominantly focused on biomedical information, with radiotherapy being presented as the only option. In the majority of interviews (75 percent), oncologists did not ask for patient/proxy opinions regarding treatment. By coding the entire encounter with RIAS supplemented by additional communication behavior codes, researchers can use a relatively large set of interactions to explore elements of the patient-centered process, as well as specific provider competencies.

RIAS codes can also be combined to represent communication behaviors not specific to the original system. In a series of studies, Timmermans and colleagues (2005; 2006; 2007) applied RIAS to videotaped consultations with radiation oncologists and their cancer patients. They combined individual codes into categories to examine decision-making processes, a process not originally outlined in RIAS. For example, they examined patient question asking and information provision related to decision-making (e.g., patient question asking: *Doc, would you recommend this treatment to your family member?*). Their findings suggest that although patients exhibit differences in verbal engagement in decision-making about palliative versus curative radiation treatment, the consultations are largely physician driven and decision-making is typically not an explicit process.

RIAS applied to the hospice setting

Caregiving for palliative care patients is increasingly shifting to family members, and this is especially true in the hospice setting, where patients typically spend their final days at home (NHPCO 2011). Family caregivers have multiple informational, physical, and emotional concerns and often communicate patient needs. Effective communication between providers and caregivers has the potential to enhance symptom management for the patient, reduce caregiver burden and distress (Lunney et al. 2003), and improve bereavement adjustment (Stroebe et al. 2007). Surprisingly, there have been few systematic studies conducted on provider–family caregiver communication. An exception includes recent preliminary work using RIAS coding of audio recordings to describe communication between hospice nurses and patient/caregivers in the home.

Ellington et al.'s pilot study was conducted to study the nature and content of communication during in-home hospice nurse visits, and assess the fit of RIAS to this context. Hospice nurses and family caregivers (and patients when able) were invited to participate. Hospice visits were audiotaped by nurses wearing small, unobtrusive digital recorders around their necks and recorded from just before entering the home until leaving. The researchers combined individual RIAS codes to create composite categories to reflect visit tasks and processes (e.g., nurse–caregiver partnering, lifestyle, humor, providing psychosocial information). Results showed that nurses devote more talk to providing information on physical care than any other topic (22 percent), while also engaging in talk directed towards building partnerships with caregivers and patients (17 percent) ('How do you think you could tell your kids about this?'), rather than telling them what to do (4 percent) ('You need to make sure your family is informed.'). While nearly a third to half of caregiver/patient talk was related to physical care and lifestyle (physical assessment, discussion of hobbies, biographical information, etc.), there were also expressions of humor (e.g., letting a grandchild paint the toes of the patient) and distress (e.g., 'I don't want to go on without my husband.'), indicating that the dying process can be a time of both joy and sadness (Ellington et al. 2012).

In applying RIAS to family caregiver dialogue in the home hospice setting, the authors confronted some challenges. For example, they noted that although RIAS has the capacity to distinguish between multiple speakers (Ellington et al. 2006; Pieterse et al. 2005; Roter 2010b), often multiple family members served as caregivers, talking to each other, and to the nurse. At a practical level, at times it was difficult for coders to discern who was talking and this increased coder burden. Additionally, the home context generated dialogue that 'exploded' the lifestyle category. This category depicts talk about an individual's way or habits of living and pertains to family and home situations, health habits (e.g., exercise, smoking, and diet habits), and self-care issues (Roter 2010a). The home setting prompted broad discussion of these and other related topics ranging from activities of daily living to reminiscing. It may be important in home-based encounters to disentangle topics within the lifestyle category to elucidate the interpersonal role they serve.

Advantages and limitations of RIAS

A major advantage of RIAS is that it is designed to be applied directly to audio/video recorded interactions; thus, time and money that may have been spent on transcription are bypassed. This resource saving makes RIAS logistically plausible for coding the large number of interactions needed to adequately power clinical trials (Roter 2010b). RIAS allows for coding both content and process of the interactions, which is critical for assessing the range of topics and emotions inherent in conversations at end of life. From recordings, coders can take the interaction context into consideration. The system is also designed to capture the complete dialogue of an encounter and thus provides a comprehensive, albeit general, indication of the exchange. While RIAS gives an overview of communication patterns, an integrated approach combining RIAS with qualitative methods may provide researchers with a more dimensional and in-depth representation of the interaction (Chou et al. 2011).

While perhaps burdensome for coders, RIAS codes can be applied to multiple parties, but with an important caveat: the system is strictly designed to only capture talk between providers and other individuals (e.g., provider–patient or provider–caregiver talk) and does not allow for inter-family or inter-provider communication (e.g., caregiver–patient or physician–nurse interaction). Therefore, potentially important dialogue about care may not be reflected in the analysis. This system also only allows the application of one code per unit of speech, making it impossible to examine multidimensional aspects of a communication. Most individuals who utilize RIAS rely on it to demonstrate frequency or relative dominance of communication behaviors. Its ability to aid in interpreting relative weight or importance beyond the amount of dialogue devoted to a specific domain or communication behavior is limited. In addition, there is evidence to suggest that RIAS accurately captures non-verbal affect (e.g., voice tone) (Hall et al. 1981; Roter and Larson 2002). With the increasing movement in health communication research away from audio recording to video, interactional analysis systems in general are likely to improve in their sensitivity to capturing all non-verbal behaviors.

Coding the team context: palliative care and teams

Health care can be improved when healthcare team members communicate effectively with each other and with patients (Haynes et al. 2009; Williams et al. 2007). Overwhelmingly, the majority of studies examining healthcare team communication use qualitative methodology (Real and Pool 2011). Interaction analysis systems have been designed for, and are typically used in, the study of dyadic communication, but palliative and hospice care is optimally a team approach. To address team communication, a group of researchers are engaged in a series of projects using communication coding schemes to explore and improve communication in hospice interdisciplinary team (IDT) meetings and involve family caregivers in the process.

In one study, researchers examined relational communication control in hospice IDT meetings (Wittenberg-Lyles et al. 2009). Communication control consists of interactions that establish the right to define, direct, and delimit actions; in this case, these actions are specific to the IDT members in their attempts to share information and contribute to decision-making. The researchers recorded hospice IDT conferences and applied the Family Relational Communication Control Coding System (Heatherington and Friedlander 2011) to identify three control types. The first code type was a *one-up*, which is an interaction in which a team member is attempting to gain control of the exchange. The second code was a *one-down*, or an interaction in which an individual allows another to have control of the exchange. A final code was a *one-across*, or when a team member neutralizes control of the exchange. Results from coding suggested that a majority of the team communication was aimed at gaining control of the information exchange.

This same group of researchers have presented a theoretical framework and rationale for an intervention to promote family caregivers' active participation in hospice IDT meetings via videophone and coded it using different approaches (Wittenberg-Lyles et al. 2010b). For example, using intervention pilot data, the researchers applied Street and colleagues' active participation verbal behavior coding scheme (Street et al. 2003; Street and Millay 2001) to recorded IDT meetings. Active caregiver participation was examined on three forms of speech: asking questions (e.g., *Should I make an appointment?*), expressing concerns (e.g., *I'm worried that she* [patient] *might be getting too much* [pain medication]), and assertive utterances (e.g., *I'd like to get your opinion on that*). A participation score was then calculated for the caregiver, based on the sum of utterances in these three categories. Additionally, the researchers coded for the hospice team participation (coded statements collapsed across team members), which included partnership building utterances (e.g., asking the caregiver a question), supportive utterances (e.g., telling the caregivers they are doing a good job), team-prompted caregiver participation, and caregiver-initiated active participation. Findings demonstrated that family caregivers were only minimally active in IDT meetings. As expected, *team-prompted* caregiver participation showed a positive relationship with caregiver participation. The least common behavior expressed by the team was support or praise of the caregiver's role.

In summary, these researchers have used different quantitative approaches to describe interpersonal dynamics among hospice team members during their regular IDT conferences. These tools have aided in the examination of the roles the team and family caregivers play in caregiver participation and in the development of a care plan. Advancing the science on healthcare team communication is critical to fully support the increasing numbers of family caregivers providing day-to-day care in their home for dying patients.

Targeted behavioral coding systems

Many researchers examine conversations for specific dialogue. Instead of coding the entire interaction, these systems zero-in on operationalized target behaviors. Coders search the dialogue to indicate whether the behavior occurs or not, and sometimes rate the behavior (e.g., rate severity of emotion (Kennifer et al. 2009)) or further categorize the behavior (e.g., treatment-related, disease-related, or testing- related prognostic talk (Rodriguez et al. 2010)). Discussed in detail below are two of the most widely studied communication behaviors in palliative care encounters: dialogue surrounding patient emotional expression and the giving of bad news.

Systems for coding emotion in palliative care encounters

There has been a surge of interest in the last decade by health communication scholars in identifying empathic opportunities expressed by the patients. Provider empathy has been linked to increased satisfaction with care, information recall, adherence, and reduced litigation (Beckman et al. 1994; Bellet and Maloney 1991; Eide et al. 2004; Jansen et al. 2009). As expected, when patients are supported in their emotional expression, they have reduced levels of distress (Mauksch et al. 2008; Schofield et al. 2003; Uitterhoeve et al. 2007). Patient expression of an emotion or personal concern is considered an *empathic opportunity* for healthcare provider response (Suchman et al. 1997). Multiple approaches and coding schemes have been developed to capture patients' expression of emotions or personal concern and the nature of the provider's response (e.g., Bylund and Makoul 2005). An application to palliative care has been conducted by researchers based largely at Duke University, North Carolina, US. In the Study of Communication Oncologist–Patient Encounters Trial (SCOPE), this team conducted an intervention to improve oncologists' empathic responses to patients with advanced cancer. From audio-recorded conversations between oncologists and patients, researchers identified empathic opportunities and oncologist responses (Tulsky et al. 2011).

Coding patient expression of emotion

SCOPE researchers first identified expressions of patients' emotional concerns using Suchman's definition of empathic opportunities: 'direct and explicit description of an emotion by a patient' (Suchman et al. 1997). Direct or explicit emotional expression was defined as the patient labeling their emotion: *'I have been very sad since I got the bad news.'* Implicit or indirect expression of emotion was defined as when a patient referred to an affective state either in words, or in tone or pace of talking, but not specifically by labeling it: *'I guess this is it for me ... the end.'* The authors found that nearly two-thirds of the empathic opportunities were direct and one-third was indirect. Even though these were patients with advanced disease, only 47 percent of patients expressed emotional concerns during their appointments with their oncologist.

Building upon these initial findings, Anderson et al. (2008) identified patients' direct expressions of negative emotions in the past, present, or future tense and categorized them according to common psychological definitions for primary emotions (e.g., fear, sadness). They found anxiety (46 percent of the instances) followed by fear (25 percent) to be the most commonly expressed primary emotions. Depression (12 percent) and anger were less common (9 percent), followed by 8 percent of emotions that did not fit into the primary categories.

Coding provider response to emotion

Rather than examine communication behaviors in isolation, health communication researchers who study patient emotional expression are interested in how the provider responds. Consistent with research outside of palliative care, researchers have examined if physicians respond empathically and foster a deepening in the conversation or block further discussion (Pollak et al. 2010; Pollak et al. 2007; Shields et al. 2009; Tulsky et al. 2011). For example, SCOPE researchers (Pollak et al. 2010; Pollak et al. 2007) coded oncologist 'continuers' by applying the NURSE mnemonic (Fischer et al. 2000; Smith 2002) developed for teaching communication skills: **N**ame, **U**nderstand, **R**espect, **S**upport, and **E**xplore. The authors collapsed their continuer findings across the five behaviors. They found that when patients raised an empathic concern, the majority of the time oncologists terminated the discussion (73 percent) and only used a 'continuing' behavior 27 percent of the time. In more recent analysis, they found that physicians who received a tailored communication intervention showed slight, but significant, difference from the physicians in the control condition for using 'continuing' behaviors (34 percent vs. 22 percent (Tulsky et al. 2011).

Coding the delivery of bad news

Considerable training resources have been devoted to delivering bad news for oncologists and palliative care providers (Back et al. 2005). A widely used, step-wise clinical protocol (SPIKES: Baile et al. 2000)) for delivering bad news has also been used as a basis for coding schemes to assess palliative care interactions (Shields et al. 2009). For example, to assess the impact of an intensive communication skills training workshop, Back et al. audiotaped oncology fellows' encounters with standardized patients before and immediately after the training (Back et al. 2007). Using content-based coding, they quantified communication behaviors related to giving bad news and to transitioning patients to palliative care. They used five of the six steps in the SPIKES model: (1) setting preparation (not assessed); (2) assessment of perception; (3) invitation to disclose; (4) sharing knowledge; (5) response to emotion; and (6) summarize plan (Baile et al. 2000). Interestingly, the standardized patients were trained to remain silent for 20 seconds after hearing the bad news, and the number of seconds providers remained silent was interpreted as an indication of their attention to patients' emotion. For transitions to palliative care, the team developed a step-wise coding system: (1) assessment of understanding; (2) elicitation of goals and values; (3) query concerns; (4) response to emotions; (5) care plan; and (6) check for understanding. The coders were instructed to code provider emotional response separately using the NURSE mnemonic discussed previously. In bad news encounters, oncology fellows showed improvement on all of the SPIKES model steps except summarization (step 6). They also exhibited improvement and skill acquisition in emotion responsiveness, including maintaining increased silence, and showed improvement on all of the transitions to palliative care communication skills except for checking for understanding.

Advantages and limitations of targeted behavioral coding systems

In examining emotional expression, responsiveness, and delivery of bad news in palliative care, teams have developed coding systems based on prior literature and best communication practices typically defined by clinical teams. The advantage of this approach is that the research is focused on a specific construct or specific interchange. The identified target of interaction is often deemed as important for patient outcomes by psychological literature, as well as more recent findings in patient–provider interaction research. As compared to full-encounter coding schemes, the specific focus allows for decreased coder training time, relatively rapid coding of encounters, and increases in the likelihood of strong inter-coder reliability. A major disadvantage of targeting a specific element of conversation is that the behavior is examined out of context from the full encounter. Isolating a communication behavior decreases our confidence in its meaning and relevance to patient outcomes. Additionally, researchers are unable to determine whether targeted behaviors are enacted at the expense of other important elements of communication.

Challenges in conducting communication research in palliative care

For a multitude of reasons, the study of interpersonal communication in palliative care is fraught with challenges. Researchers and clinicians must confront the barriers of both social and medical stigma associated with death and dying. These barriers include the often complicated transition from active curative treatment to comfort care within current medical systems. Additionally, patients and families are often overwhelmed at these times, and the added perceived burden of participating in research seems untenable to them. For these reasons and others, researchers have struggled with conducting in-depth research with the palliative care population (Kutner et al. 2010; Ransom et al. 2006).

For direct observation communication research in particular, the end-of-life context presents novel dilemmas. Traditional dyadic communication coding methods may be stretched when applied to palliative care encounters. First, in palliative care, patients and their families are viewed as the unit of care, rather than simply the patient alone. Multiple family members may be involved in care and decision-making and may serve as a proxy for patient symptoms and concerns at different times. Second, palliative and hospice care are inherently interdisciplinary and at their best utilize a team approach. For example, federal law requires hospice agencies to provide interdisciplinary team care. Finally, common communication coding schemes that aptly capture primary care outpatient encounters may not fully encompass the dynamics typical to palliative care. The palliative care provider addresses a range of concerns from past, present, and future across domains of the physical, psychosocial, and spiritual. As such, many of the current medical communication coding schemes may only generally capture the wide range of topics and processes often evident in palliative care.

Directions for future research

Despite challenges, the systematic study of palliative and hospice care communication is essential to advance the research and inform end-of-life clinical care. Coding of palliative care provider and patient/family encounters is still in an early phase with much work to do and contributions to make, including future research applications of interactional analysis systems and content-based coding schemes. To date, the majority of the research has examined interactions in clinics and hospitals on cancer patients and their physicians, thus there is need to broaden the target of our observations. New interdisciplinary research teams are turning their attention to palliative care communication and expanding the paradigm of '*who, when* and *where*' in their study of end-of-life care.

Less attention has been paid to non-physician members on the palliative and hospice care teams. An exception includes Dr. Susie Wilkinson, who has devoted her career to the study and improvement of nurse communication in oncology and palliative care (Mohán et al. 2010; Wilkinson 1991; Wilkinson et al. 1999; 2002; 2008; 1998; 2003). The End-of-Life Nursing Education Consortium (ELNEC), a train-the-trainer program, which includes evidenced-based curriculum on communication, presents another opportunity to broaden the focus of communication to nurses. ELNEC has trained over 13,000 nurses nationally and has been presented in over 70 countries internationally (AACN 2012). ELNEC raises exciting opportunities for the study of nurse communication at national and international levels.

In terms of future research on the palliative care consumer, there is much work to be done to broaden our understanding beyond communicating with patients, to communicating with families and supportive others. Research teams are expanding to the study of family caregiver and home hospice nurse communication (Cloyes et al. 2012; Ellington et al. 2012) and caregivers with the hospice team communication (Wittenberg-Lyles et al. 2010a; 2010b). Inherent in this is the necessity to attend to diversity in ethnicity, culture, socio-economics, and spiritual beliefs (Northhouse et al. 2010).

Our current approaches are hampered in representing the dynamic behavioral interactions within and across visits. Researchers currently attempt to capture reciprocity in relationships by carving out a single, targeted exchange. Given the advantages of digital coding technology and the use of newer statistical tools (e.g., augmented latent growth curve analysis), researchers will be able to advance modeling of reciprocity and demonstrate the trajectory of interactional processes within a visit, as well as across the course of visits.

Interactional analysis systems and content-based coding schemes are best at describing broad patterns of behaviors and processes within interactions. The depth, context, and nuances of interactions can be difficult to capture using these systems. It is common for researchers to make a first pass of coding an encounter with an interactional analysis system while simultaneously digitally marking segments, based on a priori decisions, for secondary qualitative analysis and reporting their results separately. Using mixed method approaches for study design and interpretation of findings is likely to further both our depth and breadth of understanding of interactions in the palliative care context.

It is critical to establish the relationship between palliative care communication and patient/family caregiver outcomes and move forward using findings to create more tailored care. For instance, Temel and colleagues found that early palliative care consultations, as compared to standard care, led to improvements in metastatic lung cancer patients' quality of life and mood and resulted in longer survival (Temel et al. 2010). It is likely that only some components of a consultation serve as the primary mechanism for patient/family outcomes. If identified, these elements may be used to target patients most at risk. Additionally, certain patient and family factors may dictate a tailored communication approach. Future research would benefit from applying existing biopsychosocial and communication theories to guide tailoring of provider communication and the identification of the salient components of communication to improve patient and family outcomes.

Conclusions

This chapter outlines the use of several existing interactional analysis systems and quantitative coding schemes for examining patient–provider encounters in palliative care and provides suggestions for their application in future research. These systems generally show adequate to strong reliability and demonstrate clinical relevance. The choice to use a particular system depends on various factors (Butow and Ford 2010). First and foremost, the research questions will dictate a choice of system. For example, researchers conducting early work in an understudied area may want to capture the general descriptive nature of the exchange and use a system with well-established validity and reliability, such as RIAS. However, if researchers are interested in a specific behavior, using a previously developed targeted behavioral coding scheme may be the optimal and most efficient approach. The conceptual or theoretical model will also inform the choice of approach, as researchers will want to ensure that the key constructs can be readily operationalized. Finally, these systems are particularly applicable to large datasets. Although such an endeavor may require significant research resources for data collection and coding, the ability to establish relationships between communication behaviors and clinical outcomes has the potential to provide the necessary evidence base to improve palliative care. Each approach has merit, but their usefulness depends on the fit to specific research objectives.

Related topics

Hospice and palliative care communication; interaction analysis; patient–provider communication; communication coding.

Further reading

Chou, W.S., Abramson, K., and Ellington, L. (2013) 'End-of-life communication in cancer care'. In B. Carr and J.L. Steele (eds) *Psychological Aspects of Cancer: A Guide to Emotional and Psychological Consequences of Cancer, Their Causes and Their Management,* New York: Springer.

Fine, E., Reid, M.C., Shengelia, R., and Adelman, R.D. (2010) 'Directly observed patient–physician discussions in palliative and end-of-life care: a systematic review of the literature', *Journal of Palliative Medicine,* 13: 595–603.

Kisane, E., Bultz, B., Butow, P., and Finlay, I. (2010) *Handbook of Communication in Oncology and Palliative Care*, New York: Oxford University Press.

Wittenberg-Lyles, E., Goldsmith, J., Ferrell, B., and Ragan, S. (2013) *Communication in Palliative Nursing*, New York: Oxford.

References

AACN. (2012) American Association of Colleges of Nursing. Online. Available HTTP: <http://www.aacn.nche.edu/elnec/elnec-connections> (accessed 1 July, 2012).

Anderson, W.G., Alexander, S.C., Rodriguez, K.L., Jeffreys, A.S., Olsen, M.K., Pollak, K.I., et al. (2008) '"What concerns me is ... " Expression of emotion by advanced cancer patients during outpatient visits', *Support Care Cancer*, 16(7): 803–811.

Back, A., Arnold, R., Baile, W., Tulsky, J., and Fryer-Edwards, K. (2005) 'Approaching difficult communication tasks in oncology', *CA: A Cancer Journal for Clinicians,* 55: 164–177.

Back, A., Arnold, R., Baile, W., Fryer-Edwards, K., Alexander, S., Barley, G., et al. (2007) 'Efficacy of communication skills training for giving bad news and discussing transitions to palliative care', *Archives of Internal Medicine,* 167: 453–460.

Baile, W., Buckman, R., Lenzi, R., Glober, G., Beale, E., and Kudelka, A. (2000) 'SPIKES – A six-step protocol for delivering bad news: application to the patient with cancer', *Oncologist,* 5: 302–311.

Beckman, H., Markakis, K., Suchman, A., and Frankel, R. (1994) 'The doctor–patient relationship and malpractice: lessons from plaintiff depositions', *Archives of Internal Medicine,* 54: 1365–1370.

Bellet, P. and Maloney, M. (1991) 'The importance of empathy as an interviewing skill in medicine', *Journal of the American Medical Association,* 266: 1831–1832.

Butow, P. and Ford, S. (2010) 'Issues in coding cancer consultations: interaction analysis systems'. In D.W. Kissane, B.D. Bultz, P.N. Butow, and I.G. Finlay (eds) *Handbook of Communication in Oncology and Palliative Care* (pp. 707–715), New York: Oxford University Press.

Bylund, C.L., and Makoul, G. (2005) 'Examining empathy in medical encounters: an observational study using the empathic communication coding system', *Health Communication,* 18: 123–140.

Chou, W.S., Han, P., Pilsner, A., Coa, K., Greenberg, L., and Blatt, B. (2011) 'Interdisciplinary research on patient–provider communication: a cross-method comparison', *Communication and Medicine,* 8: 29–40.

Cloyes, K.G., Berry, P.H., Reblin, M., Clayton, M.F., and Ellington, L. (2012) 'Exploring communication patterns among hospice nurses and family caregivers: a content analysis of in-home speech interactions', *Journal of Hospice and Palliative Nursing,* 14(6): 426–437.

Detmar, S.B., Muller, M.J., Wever, L.D., Schornagel, J.H., and Aaronson, N.K. (2001) 'The patient–physician relationship. Patient–physician communication during outpatient palliative treatment visits: an observational study', *Journal of the American Medical Association,* 285: 1351–1357.

Eide, H., Quera, V., Graugaard, P., and Finset, A. (2004) 'Physician–patient dialogue surrounding patients' expression of concern: applying sequence analysis to RIAS', *Social Science & Medicine,* 59: 145–155.

Ellington, L., Baty, B.J., McDonald, J., Venne, V., Musters, A., Roter, D., et al. (2006) 'Exploring genetic counseling communication patterns: the role of teaching and counseling approaches', *Journal of Genetic Counseling,* 15: 179–189.

Ellington, L., Reblin, M., Clayton, M.F., Berry, P., and Mooney, K. (2012) 'Hospice nurse communication with cancer patients and their family caregivers', *Journal of Palliative Medicine,* 15: 262–268.

Fischer, G., Arnold, R., and Tulsky, J. (2000) 'Talking to the older adult about advance directives', *Clinics in Geriatric Medicine,* 16: 239–254.

Hall, J.A., Roter, D.L., and Rand, C.S. (1981) 'Communication of affect between patient and physician', *Journal of Health & Social Behavior,* 22: 18–30.

Haynes, A., Weiser, T.G., Berry, W.R., Lipsitz, S.R., Breizat, A.H., Dellinger, E.P., et al. (2009) 'A surgical safety checklist to reduce morbidity and mortality in a global population', *New England Journal of Medicine,* 360: 491–499.

Heatherington, L. and Friedlander, M. (2011) *Family relational communication control coding system: Coding manual.* Online. Available HTTP: <http://www.softa-soatif.com/docusofta/other%20 instruments/FRCCCS.doc> (accessed 8 December 2011).

Jansen, J., van Weert, J.C.M., de Groot, J., van Dulmen, S., Heeren, T.J., and Bensing, J.M. (2009) 'Emotional and informational patient cues: the impact of nurses' responses on recall', *Patient Education and Counseling,* 79: 218–224.

Kennifer, S., Alexander, S., Pollak, K., Jeffreys, A., Olsen, M., Rodriguez, K., et al. (2009) 'Negative emotions in cancer care: do oncologists' responses depend on severity and type of emotion?', *Patient Education and Counseling,* 76: 51–56.

Kutner, J., Smith, M., Mellis, K., Felton, S., Yamashita, T., and Corbin, L. (2010) 'Methodological challenges in conducting a multi-site randomized clinical trial of massage therapy in hospice', *Journal of Palliative Medicine,* 13: 739–744.

Lunney, J.R., Foley, K.M., Smith, T.J., and Gelband, H. (2003) *Describing Death in America: What We Need to Know*, Washington, DC: National Academies Press.

Mauksch, L., Dugdale, D., Dodson, S., and Epstein, R. (2008) 'Relationship communication and efficiency in the medical encounter: creating a clinical model from a literature review', *Archives of Internal Medicine,* 168: 1387–1395.

Mohan, D., Alexander, S.C., Garrigues, S., Arnold, R., and Barnato, A. (2010) 'Communication practices in physician decision-making for an unstable critically ill patient with end-stage cancer', *Journal of Palliative Medicine,* 13: 949–956.

NHPCO. (2011) *NHPCO Facts and Figures: Hospice Care in America.* Online. Available HTTP: <http://www.nhpco.org/i4a/pages/index.cfm?pageid=5994> (accessed 1 July 2012).

Northhouse, L., Katapodi, M., Song, L., Zhang, L., and Mood, D. (2010) 'Interventions with family caregivers of cancer patients', *CA: A Cancer Journal for Clinicians,* 60: 317–339.

Pieterse, A.H., van Dulmen, A.M., Beemer, F.A., Ausems, M.G., and Bensing, J.M. (2005) 'Tailoring communication in cancer genetic counseling through individual video-supported feedback: a controlled pretest–posttest design', *Patient Education and Counseling,* 60: 326–335.

Pollak, K.I., Arnold, R.M., Jeffreys, A.S., Alexander, S.C., Olsen, M.K., Abernethy, A.P., et al. (2007) 'Oncologist communication about emotion during visits with patients with advanced cancer', *Journal of Clinical Oncology*, 25(36): 5748–5752.

Pollak, K.I., Arnold, R., Alexander, S.C., Jeffreys, A.S., Olsen, M.K., Abernethy, A., et al. (2010) 'Do patient attributes predict oncologist empathic responses and patient perceptions of empathy?', *Support Care Cancer,* 18: 1405–1411.

Ransom, S., Azzarello, L.M., and McMillan, S.C. (2006) 'Methodological issues in the recruitment of cancer pain patients and their caregivers', *Research in Nursing & Health,* 29: 190–198.

Real, K. and Pool, M.S. (2011) 'Health care teams: communications and effectiveness'. In T.L. Thompson, R. Parrott, and J.F. Nussbaum (eds) *The Routledge Handbook of Health Communication,* 2nd edn (pp. 100–116), New York: Taylor & Francis.

Rodriguez, K., Bayliss, N., Alexander, S., Jeffreys, A., Olsen, M., Pollak, K., et al. (2010) 'How oncologists and their patients with advanced cancer communicate about health-related quality of life', *Psycho-Oncology,* 19: 490–499.

Roter, D. (2000) 'The enduring and evolving nature of the patient–physician relationship', *Patient Education and Counseling,* 39: 5–15.

——(2010a) *RIAS Manual*, Baltimore, MD: Johns Hopkins University.

——(2010b) 'The Roter Interaction Analysis System (RIAS): applicability within the context of cancer and palliative care'. In D.W. Kissane, B.D. Bultz, P.N. Butow, and I.G. Finlay (eds) *Handbook of Communication in Oncology and Palliative Care* (pp. 717–726), New York: Oxford University Press.

Roter, D. and Larson, S. (2002) 'The Roter Interaction Analysis System (RIAS): utility and flexibility for analysis of medical interactions', *Patient Education and Counseling,* 46: 243–251.

Roter, D. and Hall, J.A. (2004) 'Physician gender and patient-centered communication: a critical review of empirical research', *Annual Review of Public Health,* 25: 497–519.

Roter, D., Larson, S., Fischer, G., Arnold, R., and Tulsky, J. (2000) 'Experts practice what they preach: a descriptive study of best and normative practices in end-of-life discussions', *Archives of Internal Medicine,* 160: 3477–3485.

Schofield, P., Butow, P., Thompson, J., Tattersall, M., Beeney, L., and Dunn, S. (2003) 'Psychological responses of patients receiving a diagnosis of cancer', *Annals of Oncology,* 14: 48–56.

Shields, C., Coker, C., Poulsen, S., Doyle, J., Fiscella, K., Epstein, R., et al. (2009) 'Patient-centered communication and prognosis discussions with cancer patients', *Patient Education and Counseling,* 77: 437–442.

Smith, R. (2002) *Patient-Centered Interviewing*, Philadelphia, PA: Lippincott Williams & Wilkins.

Street, R.L., Jr. and Millay, B. (2001) 'Analyzing patient participation in medical encounters', *Health Communication,* 13: 61–73.

Street, R.L., Jr., Krupat, E., Bell, R.A., Kravitz, R.L., and Haidet, P. (2003) 'Beliefs about control in the physician–patient relationship: effect on communication in medical encounters', *Journal of General Internal Medicine,* 18: 609–616.

Stroebe, M., Schut, H., and Stroebe, W. (2007) 'Health outcomes of bereavement', *The Lancet,* 370: 1960–1973.

Suchman, A., Markakis, K., Beckman, H., and Frankel, R. (1997) 'A model of empathic communication in the medical interview', *Journal of the American Medical Association,* 277: 678–682.

Temel, J., Greer, J., Muzikansky, A., Gallagher, E., Admane, S., Jackson, V., et al. (2010) 'Early palliative care for patients with metastatic non-small-cell lung cancer', *New England Journal of Medicine,* 363: 733–742.

Timmermans, L.M., van der Maazen, R.W., Verhaak, C.M., van Roosmalen, M.S., van Daal, W.A., and Kraaimaat, F.W. (2005) 'Patient participation in discussing palliative radiotherapy', *Patient Education and Counseling,* 57: 53–61.

Timmermans, L.M., van der Maazen, R. W.M., Leer, J.W.H., and Kraaimaat, F.W. (2006) 'Palliative or curative treatment intent affects communication in radiation therapy consultations', *Psycho-Oncology,* 15: 713–725.

Timmermans, L.M., van Zuuren, F.J., Rwm, Leer, J.W.H., and Kraaimaat, F.W. (2007) 'Monitoring and blunting in palliative and curative radiotherapy consultations', *Psycho-Oncology,* 16: 1111–1120.

Tulsky, J.A., Arnold, R.M., Alexander, S.C., Olsen, M.K., Jeffreys, A.S., Rodriguez, K.L., et al. (2011) 'Enhancing communication between oncologists and patients with a computer-based training program: a randomized trial', *Annals of Internal Medicine,* 155: 593–601.

Uitterhoeve, R., de Leeuw, J., Bensing, J., Heaven, C., Borm, G., Demulder, P., et al. (2007) 'Cue-responding behaviours of oncology nurses in video-simulated interviews', *Journal of Advanced Nursing,* 61: 71–80.

Verhaak, C.M., Kraaimaat, F.W., Staps, A.C., and van Daal, W.A. (2000) 'Informed consent in palliative radiotherapy: participation of patients and proxies in treatment decisions', *Patient Education and Counseling,* 41: 63–71.

Wilkinson, S. (1991) 'Factors which influence how nurses communicate with cancer patients', *Journal of Advanced Nursing,* 16:, 677–688.

Wilkinson, S., Roberts, A., and Aldridge, J. (1998) 'Nurse–patient communication in palliative care: an evaluation of a communication skills programme', *Palliative Medicine,* 12: 13–22.

Wilkinson, S., Bailey, K., Aldridge, J., and Roberts, A. (1999) 'A longitudinal evaluation of a communication skills programme', *Palliative Medicine,* 13: 341–348.

Wilkinson, S., Gambles, M., and Roberts, A. (2002) 'The essence of cancer care: the impact of training on nurses' ability to communicate effectively', *Journal of Advanced Nursing,* 40: 731–738.

Wilkinson, S.M., Leliopoulou, C., Gambles, M., and Roberts, A. (2003) 'Can intensive three-day programmes improve nurses' communication skills in cancer care?', *Psycho-Oncology,* 12: 747–759.

Wilkinson, S., Perry, R., Blanchard, K., and Linsell, L. (2008) 'Effectiveness of a three-day communication skills course in changing nurses' communication skills with cancer/palliative care patients: a randomised controlled trial', *Palliative Medicine,* 22: 365–375.

Williams, R.G., Silverman, R., Schwind, C., Fortune, J.B., Sutyak, J., Horvath, K.D., et al. (2007) 'Surgeon information transfer and communication: factors affecting quality and efficiency of inpatient care', *Annals of Surgery,* 245: 159–169.

Wittenberg-Lyles, E.M., Oliver, D.P., Demiris, G., and Regehr, K. (2009) 'Exploring interpersonal communication in hospice interdisciplinary team meetings', *Journal of Gerontological Nursing,* 35: 38–45.

Wittenberg-Lyles, E., Parker Oliver, D., Demiris, G., Washington, K.T., Regehr, K., and Wilder, H.M. (2010a) 'Question asking by family caregivers in hospice interdisciplinary team meetings', *Research in Gerontological Nursing,* 3: 82–88.

Wittenberg-Lyles, E., Parker Oliver, D., Demiris, G., and Baldwin, P. (2010b) 'The ACTive Intervention in Hospice Interdisciplinary Team Meetings: exploring family caregiver and hospice team communication', *Journal of Computer-Mediated Communication,* 15: 465–481.

40

Donation solicitation in interaction

Telephone requests for human tissue donations

Elizabeth M. Bishop

Introduction and definitions

In this chapter, I analyse a novel healthcare communication, the telephone solicitation for a human tissue donation. The calls, initiated by an organ procurement organization's (OPO) trained donation solicitor, rather than the healthcare provider herself, are made to the decedent's proxy, the 'next-of-kin', in the early hours after the decedent's death. The organizational goal is to procure as much tissue as possible, but without seeming overly aggressive which could turn the public against future donation solicitations. The OPO solicitors, correspondingly, present themselves as 'Family Support' or 'Family Service' Coordinators[1] telephoning to facilitate an altruistic opportunity, rather than solicitors requesting a donation. In spite of this indirect approach, tissue donation rates remain low and Family Support Coordinators – allied health professionals such as pastoral counselors, medical technicians, and social workers – describe their jobs as 'very stressful' (Weathersbee, interview).

The cause of low donation rates and employee stress may seem obvious given the substantive context, calling grieving family members in the middle of the night to solicit a tissue donation from their deceased loved one. And while this context cannot be ignored, to fully understand the tissue donation solicitation interaction we must also consider the generic conversational context. This context includes the inherent difficulty of maintaining social solidarity while making a request of another person – whether intimate or stranger – over the telephone.

In the pages that follow, I describe the historical background and review relevant studies of organ and tissue donation and then use conversation analytic methods to detail how tissue donation solicitations are actually made in interaction between the tissue donation centre employee and the family of the recently deceased. Through this analysis, I suggest potential sources of trouble that could impact the solicitation outcome. I argue that by analyzing the concrete, unfolding moments of these social interactions rather than relying on traditional social scientific studies of 'altruistic inclinations' or 'donor role identities', we can more completely understand tissue donation solicitation outcomes and recommend targeted interventions to increase donation rates.

Historical perspectives

Over 113,000 American men, women, and children currently sit on the national organ waiting list. Eighteen will die each day, waiting for a transplant (Donate Life America 2012). The shortage of transplantable organs and tissues has as yet few sustainable solutions (Koh et al. 2007). Though the vast majority of Americans (95 percent) report that they support the donation of organs for transplantation, and a large majority (78 percent) report they would be at least somewhat likely to have their organs donated after their death (Gallup 2005), actual donation consent rates remain at approximately 50 percent of eligible donors for organs (Siminoff et al. 2001) and 35 percent for tissues (Rodrigue et al. 2003). These numbers remain low despite the efforts of the US Organ Procurement and Transplantation Network (OPTN) and its affiliated agencies, and a plethora of federally funded initiatives including legislative attempts to further protect donors' rights to designate their organs for donation after their death; increased spending on donor education; and adopting less stringent donor requirements (Kaserman and Barnett 2002).

Critical issues and topics

Some scholars argue that low consent rates reflect a lack of altruism in the American public that will only be changed by offering a financial incentive to donate (Barnett and Kaserman 2000; Epstein 2006; Satel 2006). Others, going back to Titmuss's (1971) classic study of blood donation, disagree and argue that financial markets may actually *decrease* donations by driving altruists out of the market and replacing them with egoists, or by 'crowding out' various civic virtues that lead the majority of people to donate (Healy 2006b: 10). In the Institute of Medicine report on organ donation, in fact, scholars and policymakers continue to strongly recommend *against* financial incentives (Childress and Liverman 2006).

In 2011, there were 8,127 deceased and 6,017 living solid organ donors resulting in 28,535 organ transplants, given that multiple organs were procured from single donors. In addition, more than 42,000 corneal grafts were prepared for distribution to eye tissue banks (Donate Life America 2012). Though living organ donors constitute nearly half (42 percent) of all donors, most of the education, research, and legislative efforts focus on the challenge of procuring donations from the recently deceased (or soon to be deceased, in the case of solid organ donors).

To understand the challenge of increasing donations from deceased donors, it is important to note that the donation solicitation is not made of the donors, but of their proxy, the surviving 'next-of-kin' (Haddow 2004; Morgan 2004; Rodrigue et al. 2003; Siminoff et al. 2001; Verble and Worth 2000; Zink and Wertlieb 2006). This practice, long established within American common law (Peters 1986), follows from the notion of the decedent's right to a decent burial, which is interpreted as a family's right to determine what happens to the body between death and burial (May et al. 2000; Muyskens 1978). In practice, this means that identifying yourself as an organ and tissue donor on your driver's license or donor card is no guarantee that donation will occur after your death. Rather, the donation decision remains the purview of the surviving family member(s).

Due to these practical realities of organ and tissue donation, there have been intensive legislative efforts to codify state laws to better protect individuals' rights to designate the disposition of their organs and tissues after their death. However, these efforts – codified in the 1968 Uniform Anatomical Gift Act (UAGA) and its 1987 and 2006 revisions (National Conference of Commissioners on Uniform State Laws 2012) – have failed and will most likely continue to fail. As legal scholars note, 'the history of American case law on the disposition of cadavers hardly gives reason for optimism concerning the ultimate triumph of decedent's wishes over family objections [to donation] under judicial review' (Peters 1986: 247). Indeed, organ procurement organization solicitors continue to defer to the family of the deceased for the final donation decision (Healy 2006a; Kurtz et al. 2007). This means that the 'altruistic inclination' to donate is at best some combination of the inclinations of the decedent, the 'next-of-kin', and the other family members involved in the decision-making process.

Current contributions and research

Under the current system of deferring to the family, a significant number of donations are lost when the family declines donation. At least in theory, enforcing the UAGA and removing the family from the decision would recapture lost donations and increase the pool of transplantable organs and tissues.

A system that purportedly does this is in place in many countries outside of the United States (Healy 2006a). In this system of '*presumed consent*', the donation organization is authorized to procure organs and tissues at an individual's death unless that individual specifically *opted out* of donation while living (e.g., by signing on to a non-participant registry).

Spain – with its high rate of organ donation and presumed consent laws – has long been considered the presumed consent case, par excellence. However, as Healy (2004, 2006b) discovered, in Spain and the 15 other Organization for Economic Co-operation and Development (OECD) countries with presumed consent laws, families are actually consulted and allowed to make the final donation decision, just as in the United States. In fact, of the 16 OECD countries with presumed consent laws, only Austria practises a strong form of presumed consent (Healy 2004, Healy 2006b).

Healy (2004) argues instead that regional, national, and international organ donation rates vary extensively not because of any variation in altruistic motives or a 'donor role identity' (Callero 1985; Callero et al. 1987; Lee et al. 1999; Piliavin and Callero 1991), but because of the logistical efforts of organ procurement organizations (OPO). These efforts include the investment in more staff that is better trained in 'the crucial process of requesting consent from families' (Healy 2006b: 1042–1043). However, the organizational perspective – just as donor role identity theory – is not designed to illuminate the tissue donation solicitation interaction between OPO staff and donor families.

After their extensive meta-analysis of organ donation studies, Institute of Medicine committee members also agreed that, '(c)ommunication and the relational aspects of the donation process are instrumental in creating a positive environment for considering and consenting to donation' (Childress and Liverman 2006: 107). Unfortunately, recent studies that claim to explore the organ and tissue donation interaction, including those from Scotland (Haddow 2004), Greece (Bellali and Papadatou 2007), and the US (Rodrigue et al. 2006), do not look directly at the interaction itself but rely instead on interviews in which family members recollect their organ donation experience. Additionally, when studies claim to analyze the actual interaction surrounding donation, and even suggest that '(p)roblems with the ways in which families are asked about donation' account for high refusal rates (Siminoff et al. 1995: 16), they neglect any investigation of actual interactions as they unfold. While these studies suggest *who* should approach the family about donation, they are not devised to study the concrete ways in which the donation solicitation actually occurs in a social interaction. While the literature concentrates mostly on organ rather than tissue donation solicitation, the issues are the same: to fully understand the donation solicitation process, it is necessary to examine actual, real-time interaction between donation centre employees as they solicit a donation from family members who may or may not give their consent (Weathersbee and Maynard 2009).

Main research methods

The data analyzed in this study were collected as part of a wider study I conducted with Douglas W. Maynard (Weathersbee and Maynard 2009) on the 'Tissue Centre', a pseudonym for one of the largest organ, eye, and tissue recovery, processing, and distribution programs in the nation. From this office, located in a large US city, personnel initiate tissue solicitation calls to families located in multiple – including local and national – geographical regions. These telephone calls are routinely recorded and archived as digital audio files for legal as well as quality control purposes.

In this chapter, I analyze extracts from the 131 (74 percent) initial solicitation calls placed during a six-month period in 2004 to the contact number for the decedent's 'next-of-kin'. I transcribed each of these calls according to conversation analytic conventions (see Appendix 40.1 at the end of this chapter) and use general analytic procedures for the conversation analysis field as outlined in Clayman and Gill (2004) and ten Have (1999). For this analysis, I also incorporate field notes from observations I conducted in the Tissue Centre over two separate, three-day periods[2] along with interviews with the Family Support Coordinators and the Tissue Centre Director. While this particular methodological approach to exploring the tissue donation solicitation interaction improves my analysis, I acknowledge a 'limited affinity' (Maynard 2003: ch. 3) between ethnography and conversation analysis. Accordingly, I use my field observations and interviews judiciously, to 'describe settings and identities [and] explicate unfamiliar terms or courses of action' (Maynard 2003: 73–76).

Data analysis

The Tissue Centre (TC) is staffed 24 hours a day, seven days a week with one to two Family Support Coordinators and two to three triage personnel who receive the initial death notification from the hospital nursing staff or the medical examiner's office (in the case of decedents who did not die in the hospital). During these triage calls, staff collect pertinent information on the decedent, including time and cause of death; next-of-kin's contact information; and emotional state of the family members. They also make a determination, based on the cause of death, as to what tissues the decedent is able to donate. The resulting donor file is given to the Family Support Coordinator to review and initiate the call to the decedent's next-of-kin.

In the section that follows, I describe a sample of audio-recorded telephone interactions between the Tissue Centre's Family Support Coordinators and the decedent's next-of-kin. In my analysis, I compare the institutional tissue call practices with ordinary telephone call practices, and focus on the call opening and the reason for the call sequences. Through this analysis, I suggest potential sources of trouble that may impact tissue donation solicitation call outcomes.

Telephone call openings

Telephone conversations – like other types of 'speech exchange systems' – are organized by a turn-taking system of talk (Sacks et al. 1974: 696) whose turns 'hang together' as 'sequences' (Schegloff 2007: 2). In his classic study of call openings, Schegloff (1986b) identified four core, opening sequences to ordinary telephone calls: summons/answer, identification, greeting, and 'Howareyou' types. These sequences are vehicles for important social actions (Schegloff 1979, 1986b) such as opening or closing the gate to further interaction ('gatekeeping'); constituting or reconstituting relationships; and establishing what gets talked about in what order (Schegloff 1986b: 113).

As outlined in Table 40.1, the opening sequences of the tissue solicitation calls demonstrate the 'context-free' or generic practices of the core call opening sequences (Schegloff 1986b) along with 'context-sensitive variations' specific to the Tissue Centre (Weathersbee and Maynard 2009) that make reference to the 'various places, times, and identities of parties to interaction' (Sacks et al. 1974: 699).

Summons/answer and identification/recognition sequence

The tissue donation solicitation calls begin with a summons/answer and identification/recognition sequence that starts, as ordinary calls do, with the ringing phone. As Schegloff notes, the ring is itself a 'socially and interactionally shaped product' in that persons who hear the ringing phone are oriented to such things as how quickly to pick up the phone or if at all, depending on whether or not the phone actually 'belongs' to them (1986b: 118–120). The orderliness of these sequences owes much to the conduct of the call recipient who will typically answer in the United States by using several forms of greeting such as, 'Yeah/Yes' or 'Hi' when they are fairly confident of who is calling, or 'Hello' if they are not. Otherwise, the recipient may do a self-identification or self-formulation in the greeting if they are answering on behalf of another person or persons or business (Schegloff 1986b: 123). For example, instead of 'Hi' the recipient might say, 'Smith residence'. This demonstrates that call recipients are oriented not only to the sound of the phone but to the caller's interests in confirming that they have reached the correct destination (Schegloff 1986b).

The call recipient's answer to the summoning phone at line 2 in Extract 1 ('Huhlo:: hh') is followed by the Family Support Coordinator's short in breath at line 3, then an affirmative acknowledgement of the summons' answer ('Yes'), and a form of what Schegloff (1979) calls a 'switchboard request' (30). This particular formulation is a bit indirect, but is analyzable (by call recipient and analyst) as a request for a specific recipient. The call recipient, accordingly, responds immediately at line 4 and confirms her identity as the targeted recipient. The sound stretching and rising intonation at the end of line 4 indicate that the recipient is not recognizing the caller.

Table 40.1 Comparison of ordinary and tissue solicitation call opening sequences

Ordinary calls	*Tissue solicitation calls*
Summons/answer	Summons/answer
Identification/recognition	Identification/recognition
Greeting	Epistemic display
How are you (HAY)	Condolence

Extract 1

1 ((ringing phone))
2 A: Huhlo:: hh
3 C: .hh Yes I'm >tryin ta reach< Sandy Severson please?
4 A: This is she:::?
5 C: Ma'a::m my name is Dana (.) and I'm a Family Support
6 Coordinator with Regional Donor Service::s.
7 A: .hhh Yes Ma'am=

The Family Support Coordinator responds at line 5 with a deferential title ('Ma'am') in place of the recipient's name – typical especially in this local region of the United States – and proceeds to identify herself by first name, title, and institutional affiliation, marking this as a business call from a stranger. The recipient hesitates at the start of line 7 with a slightly longer in breath than the Family Support Coordinator produced at the start of line 3, indicating some trouble, then completes the identification/recognition sequence with an affirmative ('Yes') and mirrors the deferential title ('Ma'am') that the Family Support Coordinator used at line 5.

Through this identification/recognition sequence, the Family Support Coordinator and the decedent's 'next-of-kin' have established their 'individual or categorical identity' (Whalen and Zimmerman 1987: 173) and moved to confirm one another's co-presence. In doing so they have reached what Goffman referred to as a 'state of ratified mutual participation' (Schegloff 1986b: 129), and opened the gate for further interaction. These opening moments are especially important in solicitation calls where call recipients can initiate a blocking move including hanging up the phone, that 'unilaterally disable[s] pursuit' (Maynard and Schaeffer 1997: 53) of the solicited item.

Greeting versus epistemic display sequence

With the gate open for further interaction, what typically follows in ordinary conversation between those who can be recognized or are suspected to be known acquaintances is a 'greeting' sequence (Schegloff 1986b). The tissue solicitation calls, however, are between unacquainted others, so an ordinary call greeting sequence will not typically be initiated (Maynard and Schaeffer 1997). Instead, the identification/recognition initiates what we call an 'epistemic display' sequence regarding the death of the potential donor (Weathersbee and Maynard 2009). This context-sensitive turn embodies a 'practical epistemology' (Whalen and Zimmerman 1990) that includes an exhibit of how a party came to know about the event under discussion.

The epistemic display sequence demonstrated in Extract 2 at lines 9–10 includes two sub-parts demonstrating both 'how-we-know' ('the ho:spital informed us' line 9) and 'what-we-know' ('your wife's (p)assing' lines 9–10). Given that the Family Support Coordinator is a stranger, she cannot be heard to be calling simply to offer condolences or notify the family of the death. Therefore, this sequence is designed to establish that the recipient has a spouse (or other family member) who died, making a discussion of some aspect of the family member's passing relevant.

Extract 2

C: Mister Sierr:a ↑my name is Do::nna and I'm a Family
Support Coordinator with First Regional ↑Donor
↑Service::s,
A: Ye:s Ma'am-
C: An: Sir the ho:spital informed us of your wife's
(p)assing and I wanted ta offer my (.) sis- h (0.1)
sincere condolences to you and your fa::mily,
(0.4)
A: Thank you,=
C: =You we::lcome an Sir I'm sorry to be calling you at
this difficult ti::me, the reason I need (.) ta speak
with you (.) .hh your wi:fe ha:s the ability to
donate corneas >to restore vision< ta o::thers .hh
and I wanna check with ya sir if that might have been
in her wi:she::s?
(0.2)

Citing knowledge of the death of the decedent gained from a valorized healthcare institution (line 9) further establishes the legitimacy of the call. This helps to deal with the delicate issue of calling a family's home at a time when phone calls, particularly from unacquainted parties or strangers, may be an intrusion. Citing an institutional source of information regarding the death also reflects that this is a business rather than a personal call.

Note that the epistemic display is completed at the start of line 10, but not in a way that allows for acknowledgement, as such displays often do. Instead, the Family Support Coordinator continues with an 'offer' of 'condolences' (lines 10–11).

How-are-you versus condolence sequence

In this collection of tissue donation solicitation calls, there are also no '*how-are-you?*' exchanges as are typical following the greeting in ordinary call openings (Schegloff 1986b). Instead, given that the Family Support Coordinator has now established through the epistemic display sequence that she knows of the family member's death, the context-sensitive initiation of a condolence is made relevant.

There is a parallel, however, between 'condolence' and 'how-are-you (h-a-y)' sequences. Just as h-a-y sequences make the current state of the other party a matter of joint concern (Schegloff 1986b), a condolence sequence presumes the current state of the call recipient to be one of grieving and proposes it as a matter of joint concern to be addressed sympathetically by the Family Support Coordinator (Maynard and Weathersbee 2006).

Regularly in the tissue donation solicitation calls, the condolence offering (lines 10–11, Extract 2) initiates an 'adjacency pair' turn (Schegloff 2007) whose second pair part is the recipient's gratuity (line 13), followed by an additional turn ('You we::lcome', line 14) that ends the sequence. This 'minimal post-expansion', an addition to the sequence after its second pair part, is designed to propose sequence closing and is in fact referred to as a 'sequence-closing third' turn (Schegloff 2007: 118). The call opening and closing are important in both ordinary and institutional talk as they provide an anchor position for the introduction of the first topic, something that is readily identifiable as the 'reason for the call' (Schegloff 1986b: 116).

Delaying the move to the reason for the call

Though the parties in Extract 2 have agreed on the closure of the condolence sequence, the Family Support Coordinator delays moving to the reason for the call and instead apologizes for the timing of the call ('an Sir I'm sorry to be calling you at this difficult ti::me,' lines 14–15), elaborating on the epistemic display and the condolence sequences by claiming to relevantly assess this as a 'difficult time'. The recipient withholds acknowledgement or acceptance of this further offering, which may resist the Family Support Coordinator's claim or, at the very least, work to maintain the formal or business nature of the call.

It should be noted that the assessment of a 'difficult time' is somewhat more presumptive than the caller's initial and formal condolence. This assessment embodies what Labov and Fanshel (1977) call a 'b-statement' about a state of being to which the recipient has primary access and the initiator has only secondary and, in this case, inferential access. The epistemic rights to make such assessments can be very contentious territory (Heritage and Raymond 2005).

Given the possibility of less presumptive courses of action, the caller may be initiating this apology and assessment of a 'difficult time' in anticipation of the call recipient's complaint that this is not a good time for a stranger to be calling. As more than one Family Support Coordinator observed, 'you do a lot of apologizing [in this job]' (Weathersbee, interview). This suggests that the potentially contentious course of action is motivated by the Family Support Coordinator's own need to maintain a positive self-evaluation or 'face' (Lerner 1996). The caller's 'face' being threatened first by calling to perform a dispreferred action (a request) and, second, by intruding on a grieving family with a request that is 'treated in the official culture as delicate' (Schegloff 1986a: 132). In addition to maintaining 'face' for the Family Support Coordinator, these apologies and assessments also serve to delay the move to the 'reason for the call', another indication of the dispreferred status of the social action to come (Schegloff 2007), the tissue donation solicitation.

And, in fact, this tissue solicitation call ends with the family member declining to donate. It may be that a less presumptive course of action in the call opening or less work on the part of the Family Support Coordinator to maintain her own 'face' in the interaction would have resulted in consent to donation.

Reason for the call-requesting

By adulthood we have myriad ways in which to make and understand requests in social interaction (Schegloff 1979, 1986b; Wootton 1981, 1997) and across a variety of work and life settings such as medical interactions (Curl and Drew 2008; Gill 2005; Gill et al. 2001; Lindström 2005; Robinson 2001; Stivers et al. 2003), the survey interview (Maynard et al. 2008; Maynard and Schaeffer 1997), and ordinary conversations (Davidson 1984; Heinemann 2006; Schegloff 2007). Across these various work and life settings, we can observe that interlocutors generally prefer to entirely avoid overt requesting (Curl and Drew 2008; Maynard and Schaeffer 1997) since making a direct request of a party risks rejection of the request – a potentially disaffiliative action in both ordinary conversation (Schegloff 2007) and institutional talk (Gill 2005; Maynard et al. 2008).

Reason for the call-requesting in ordinary conversation

Competent adult speakers use a variety of devices in ordinary conversation designed to avoid direct requesting and instead elicit an offer from the other party. These devices include prefacing the request with some preliminary matters termed 'pre-requests'; and adding 'preliminaries to the preliminaries' ('pre-pre's') or 'pre-pre-requests' (Schegloff 2007: 44–45) to project that a request is in the offing. These conversational turns are shaped as dispreferred social actions and therefore may be 'masked' as offers; accompanied by accounts and mitigations; or found late in the conversation rather than in the first topic position, where the reason for the call is usually initiated (Schegloff 2007: 84).

Notice in Extract 3, an example from ordinary conversation, that after an initial 'pre-pre-request' is started at line 1, it is followed by a 'pre-request' at lines 3 and 5–6 as Fred moves, in a step-wise fashion, toward the projected request. Laurie, however, pre-empts the request at line 7 with an offer to 'do the buttonholes' (Schegloff 2007: 44–45).

Extract 3

Fred: Oh by the way ((sniff)) I have a bi:g favor to ask ya.
Laurie: Sure, go'head.
Fred: 'Member the blouse you made a couple weeks ago?
Laurie: Ya.
Fred: Well I want to wear it this weekend to Vegas but my mom's buttonholer is broken.
Laurie: Fred I told ya when I made the blouse I'd do the buttonholes.
Fred: A ((sniff)) but I hate ta impose.
Laurie: No problem. We can do them on Monday after work.
Fred: Ya sure ya have time?
Laurie: I'm sure.
Fred: Gee, thanks.
Laurie: Okay well listen...

The tissue donation solicitation uses these 'context-free' practices along with 'context-sensitive variations' specific to the Tissue Centre (Weathersbee and Maynard 2009) such as assessing the call recipient's emotional state, and informing of the potential to donate tissue.

Reason for the call-requesting and the tissue donation solicitation

Family Support Coordinators, like members of any work setting, do not stop being generically competent social actors when they go to work (Garfinkel 1967). They have, consequently, already embodied the rules of making a request in daily life before joining the Tissue Centre. Unlike most call centres, the Tissue Centre does not provide Family Support Coordinators with official rules such as scripts for the tissue donation solicitation calls. Instead, Family Support Coordinators learn to make donation solicitation calls by listening to archived, audio-recorded calls and then role playing with the Tissue Centre Director. After a few weeks, they are allowed to make their own calls and encouraged to 'act natural' as they 'adapt the calls to their own personalities' (Weathersbee, interview).

Family Support Coordinators follow a tacit, indirect approach to requesting, similar to the ordinary conversation requesting in Extract 3 but with 'context-sensitive' variations specific to the Tissue Centre. In the next sections, I briefly describe two variations on the 'pre-pre-' and 'pre-requests' used to elicit an offer of the tissue donation.

ASSESSING THE CALL RECIPIENT'S EMOTIONAL STATE

In Extract 4, at lines 13–14, the Family Support Coordinator travels again into contentious territory with a 'pre-pre request' shaped as an assessment of the call recipient (and her family's) emotional state ('I kno::w it's gonna be >ha:rd on you and your< fa:mily').

Extract 4

C: =I kno::w it's gonna be >ha:rd on you and your< fa:mily
ri:ght no::wuh?
A: >~uh- ye:s< ma'am?
C: Uh (.) the reason I'm ca::lling you <is that> (.) she
do::es have po↓tential (0.4) ta donate corneas
[°an- ( )
A: [NO MA'AM WE NOT DONATIN ANYTHING HONEY ↑THANK YA
((clicking sound))
C: Tha:t's okay th-
((beeping busy signal sound))

The Family Support Coordinator's turn at lines 13–14 does 'double duty' (Schegloff 2007), as she works to save 'face' and delay the move toward the reason for the call, a very indirect hint at the dispreferred social action to come. Note, however, how this contrasts with the more direct 'pre-pre request' Fred uses in the ordinary conversation Extract 3. There he formulates the reason for the call as informing Laurie, 'I have a bi:g favor to ask ya' (line 1), a 'preliminary to the preliminary' that projects a request is in the offing and also delays the move toward the reason for the call.

In Extract 4, the family member's turn at line 15 is delivered quickly, with an affirmative continuer, and again, with the deferential address term 'ma'am' common in this region of the United States. The hesitation and rising intonation at the end of the turn, however, though it displays alignment with the caller's prior turn, continues to hint at trouble.

INFORMING OF THE POTENTIAL TO DONATE

In the Family Support Coordinator's next turn at line 16, she initiates a 'pre-request', masking the donation solicitation as an informing ('she do::es have po↓tential (0.4) ta donate corneas °an-'), which is shaped to elicit an offer from the call recipient. This shares the generic features of Fred's informing at lines 5–6 in Extract 3 ('Well I want to wear it this weekend to Vegas but my mom's buttonholer is broken'). The tissue solicitation interaction turn, however, has strong features of a dispreferred in that it is delivered with hesitations, sound stretches, and a significant pause after the falling intonation on 'potential'. This also aligns with the trouble projected by the call recipient at line 15.

Not surprisingly, this pre-request does not elicit an offer of the tissue donation. Instead, the family member of the deceased – in overlap with the Family Support Coordinator's very quiet, clipped continuer ('an-') at line 18 – initiates a strong blocking move that, when coupled with a terminal token such as '↑THANK YA' (line 19) and a hanging up of the phone (line 20), represents an 'impolite declination' in that the call recipient hangs up the phone and 'unilaterally disable[s] pursuit of the interview' (Maynard and Schaeffer 1997: 53). The recipient does, however, show some orientation to the dispreferred status of this impolite call-closing as she uses both formal and informal address terms ('MA'AM' and 'HONEY'), an account for why they are not donating corneas ('WE NOT DONATIN ANYTHING'), and a gratuity token ('↑THANK YA'), social actions that at least partially embody practices from polite telephone call closings (Schegloff and Sacks 1973). This may be a similar face-saving move for the call recipient as she does the dispreferred call-closing action.

Future directions

The call recipient's blocking move in the last extract (4) demonstrates that the pre-request shaped as an informing of the 'potential to donate' is hearably a request. This finding is compatible with Searle's (1975) discussion of 'indirect speech acts', that is, 'cases in which one illocutionary act is performed indirectly by way of performing another' (60). This linguistic approach, and speech act theory more broadly, are certainly complementary to Conversation Analysis (CA) though CA focuses more on sequential analyses of naturally occurring conversation as it unfolds in interaction. As this chapter so poignantly demonstrates, the donation decision reflects the outcome of an interaction between Tissue Centre personnel and a surviving family member who makes the final determination in real time and with an anonymous but concerned other, whose skills at requesting in talk-in-interaction deserve more attention in future research.

The conversation analytic approach to donation solicitation demonstrates why actual donation consent rates have failed to correlate with the results of attitudinal surveys on the topic of organ and tissue donation; and the number of driver's license donor designations or other advance directives to donate, distinct phenomena in their own right that cannot, however, be used to predict donation solicitation outcomes. As this chapter has demonstrated, the outcome of the donation solicitation has a local context, the generic practices of requesting in ordinary conversation, and the conversational turn-by-turn unfolding through the interaction that must be considered if we are to ever increase donation consent rates. Future studies should look closely at the various formulations of the reason for the call that exist across Family Support Coordinators, to identify if one approach leads to more consents to donation than another. It is possible that the instruction to make the interaction 'as natural as possible' may hew too closely to the ordinary practices for requesting, and consequently be so indirect that family members are not entirely aware of what is being requested and therefore more likely to decline to donate.

It is also clear from my interviews and observations that the Tissue Centre staff believe 'families are already either going to donate or not' (Weathersbee, interview) and there is nothing the tissue requesters can do to influence that decision. Of course, this belief runs contrary to the Tissue Centre management's desire to increase consent rates. Using the job title 'Family Services' or 'Family Support' *Coordinator* may help Tissue Centre personnel work to resist the notion that what they are doing is making an actual *request* for the tissue donation. Clearly, Family Support Coordinators, who are hired for their professional counseling and healthcare backgrounds, do not consider themselves to be in the business of requesting or soliciting donor tissue. One instance particularly highlights this disconnect between the notion of coordinating and supporting families and soliciting a donation when – at the beginning of one telephone interaction – the family member demands to know 'Is this a soliciting call?' and the Family Support Coordinator responds in a slightly indignant and bewildered tone, 'No ma'am, my name is Deb Torkelson I'm a Family Services Coordinator' (call transcript). Rather than thinking of themselves as telephone solicitors, Family Support/ Family Service Coordinators consider themselves part of the end-of-life team which is there to facilitate the procurement of tissues in cases where the family has already decided to donate. From this perspective, there is nothing the caller can, or perhaps should, do to encourage families to donate.

These multiple pressures make it more difficult for Family Support Coordinators to pursue consent to donation and somewhat easier to accept, and at times even encourage, declination. Workshops and training that discuss the concept of 'saving face' in solicitation interactions, outline the practices of requesting in ordinary conversation and tissue donation solicitation, and identify solicitation formulations and ways to tailor the call to the unfolding interaction should be developed, in conjunction with campaigns to educate the public that putting a dot on your driver's license and discussing your donation wishes with your family will not necessarily ensure that your wishes will be carried out.

Related topics

Tissue donation; organ donation; conversation analysis; talk-in-interaction; donation solicitation.

Notes

1 Call centre staff are allowed to refer to themselves as they choose. Though most use the title 'Family Support Coordinator', some choose to identify as 'Family *Service* Coordinators' or to switch between the two as they choose.

2 This data collection protocol was approved by the University of Wisconsin (UW) Institutional Review Board (IRB), conditioned on preserving confidentiality for all participants and, additionally, providing pseudonyms for any geographical references in research reports.

Further reading

Childress, J. F. and Liverman, C. T. (2006) *Organ Donation: Opportunities for action*, Washington, DC: National Academies Press. (Institute of Medicine's meta-analysis of organ donation.)

Healy, K. (2006) *Last Best Gifts: Altruism and the market for human blood and organs*, Chicago, IL: University of Chicago Press. (Excellent organizational analysis of organ procurement organizations.)

Schegloff, E. A. (2007) *Sequence Organization in Interaction: A primer in conversation analysis*, Cambridge: Cambridge University Press. (Foundational handbook for conversation analysis of ordinary conversation.)

References

Barnett, A. H. and Kaserman, D. L. (2000) 'Comment on "The shortage in market-inalienable human organs" faulty analysis of a failed policy', *American Journal of Economics and Sociology*, 59: 335–349.

Bellali, T. and Papadatou, D. (2007) 'The decision-making process of parents regarding organ donation of their brain dead child: a Greek study', *Social Science & Medicine*, 64: 439–450.

Callero, P. L. (1985) 'Role-identity salience', *Social Psychology Quarterly*, 48: 203–215.

Callero, P. L., Howard, J. A., and Piliavin, J. A. (1987) 'Helping behavior as role behavior: disclosing social structure and history in the analysis of prosocial action', *Social Psychology Quarterly*, 50: 247–256.

Childress, J. F. and Liverman, C. T. (2006) *Organ Donation: Opportunities for action*, Washington, DC: National Academies Press.

Clayman, S. E. and Gill, V. T. (2004) 'Conversation analysis', in M. Hardy and A. Bryman (eds) *Handbook of Data Analysis,* 589–606, London: Sage.

Curl, T. S. and Drew, P. (2008) 'Contingency and action: a comparison of two forms of requesting', *Research on Language and Social Interaction,* 41: 129–153.

Davidson, J. (1984) 'Subsequent versions of invitations, offers, requests, and proposals dealing with potential or actual rejection', in J. M. Atkinson and J. Heritage (eds) *Structures of Social Action: Studies in conversation analysis,* Cambridge: Cambridge University Press.

Donate Life America (2012) *Statistics*. Online. Available HTTP: <http://donatelife.net/understanding-donation/statistics/> (accessed 2 April 2012).

Epstein, R. (2006) 'Kidney beancounters', *Wall Street Journal,* May 15, A.15.

Gallup Organization, The (2005) *National Survey of Organ and Tissue Donation Attitudes and Behaviors,* Rockville, MD: Health Resources and Services Administration.

Garfinkel, H. (1967) *Studies in Ethnomethodology,* Englewood Cliffs, NJ: Prentice Hall.

Gill, V. T. (2005) 'Patient "demand" for medical interventions: exerting pressure for an offer in a primary care clinic visit', *Research on Language and Social Interaction,* 38: 451–479.

Gill, V., Halkowski, T., and Roberts, F. (2001) 'Accomplishing a request without making one: a single case analysis of a primary care visit', *Text,* 21: 55–81.

Haddow, G. (2004) 'Donor and nondonor families' accounts of communication and relations with healthcare professionals', *Progress in Transplantation,* 14: 41–48.

Healy, K. (2004) 'Altruism as an organizational problem: the case of organ procurement', *American Sociological Review,* 69: 387–404.

——(2006a) 'Do presumed consent laws raise organ procurement rates?' *DePaul Law Review,* 55: 1017–1043.

——(2006b) *Last Best Gifts: Altruism and the market for human blood and organs,* Chicago, IL: University of Chicago Press.

Heinemann, T. (2006) '"Will you or can't you?" Displaying entitlement in interrogative requests', *Journal of Pragmatics,* 38: 1081–1104.

Heritage, J. and Raymond, G. (2005) 'The terms of agreement: indexing epistemic authority and subordination in talk-in-interaction', *Social Psychology Quarterly,* 68: 15–38.

Kaserman, D. L. and Barnett, A. H. (2002) *The US Organ Procurement System: A prescription for reform,* Washington, DC: AEI Press.

Koh, H. K., Jacobson, M. D., Lyddy, A. M., O'Connor, K. J., Fitzpatrick, S. M., Krakow, M., et al. (2007) 'A statewide public health approach to improving organ donation: the Massachusetts organ donation initiative', *American Journal of Public Health,* 97: 30–36.

Kurtz, S. F., Strong, C. W., and Gerasimow, D. (2007) 'The 2006 revised Uniform Anatomical Gift Act – A law to save lives', *Health Law Analysis,* February, 44–49.

Labov, W. and Fanshel, D. (1977) *Therapeutic Discourse,* New York: Academic Press.

Lee, L., Piliavin, J. A., and Call, V.R.A. (1999) 'Giving time, money, and blood: similarities and differences', *Social Psychology Quarterly,* 62: 276–290.

Lerner, G. (1996) 'Finding "face" in the preference structures of talk-in-interaction', *Social Psychology Quarterly,* 59: 303–321.

Lindström, A. (2005) 'Language as social action: a study of how senior citizens request assistance with practical tasks in the Swedish home help service', in A. Hakulinen and M. Selting (eds) *Syntax and Lexis in Conversation: Studies on the use of linguistic resources in talk-in-interaction,* Amsterdam: Benjamins.

May, T., Aulisio, M. P., and DeVita, M. A. (2000) 'Patients, families, and organ donation: Who should decide?' *Milbank Quarterly,* 78: 323–336.

Maynard, D. W. (2003) *Bad News, Good News: Conversational order in everyday talk and clinical settings,* Chicago, IL: University of Chicago Press.

Maynard, D. W. and Schaeffer, N. C. (1997) 'Keeping the gate: declinations of the request to participate in a telephone survey interview', *Sociological Methods & Research,* 26: 34–79.

Maynard, D. W. and Weathersbee, T. E. (2006) 'An initial investigation on the use of condolences in ordinary conversation and in telephone requests for tissue donation', paper presented at the annual meeting of the American Sociological Association, Montreal, Quebec, August.

Maynard, D. W., Freese, J., and Schaeffer, N. C. (2008) 'Requesting as a social action: implications for nonresponse and "Leverage-Saliency" in the survey interview', paper presented at the annual meeting of the American Sociological Association, Boston, MA, August.

Morgan, S. E. (2004) 'The power of talk: African Americans' communication with family members about organ donation and its impact on the willingness to donate organs', *Journal of Social and Personal Relationships*, 21: 112–124.

Muyskens, J. L. (1978) 'An alternative policy for obtaining cadaver organs for transplantation', *Philosophy and Public Affairs*, 8: 88–99.

National Conference of Commissioners on Uniform State Laws (2012) *Anatomical Gift Act (2006)*. Online. Available HTTP: <http://www.uniformlaws.org/Act.aspx?title=Anatomical Gift Act (2006)> (accessed 21 November 2012).

Peters, D. A. (1986) 'Protecting autonomy in organ procurement procedures: some overlooked issues', *Milbank Quarterly*, 64: 241–270.

Piliavin, J. A. and Callero, P. L. (1991) *Giving Blood: The development of an altruistic identity*, Baltimore, MD: Johns Hopkins University Press.

Robinson, J. (2001) 'Asymmetry in action: sequential resources in the negotiation of a prescription request', *Text*, 21: 19–54.

Rodrigue, J. R., Scott M. P., and Oppenheim, A. R. (2003) 'The tissue donation experience: a comparison of donor and nondonor families', *Progress in Transplantation*, 13: 258–264.

Rodrigue, J. R., Cornell, D. L., and Howard, R. J. (2006) 'Organ donation decision: comparison of donor and nondonor families', *American Journal of Transplantation*, 6: 190–198.

Sacks, H., Schegloff, E., and Jefferson, G. (1974) 'A simplest systematics for the organization of turn-taking for conversation', *Language*, 50: 696–735.

Satel, S. (2006) 'Death's waiting list', *New York Times*, May 15, A.21.

Schegloff, E. A. (1979) 'Identification and recognition in telephone conversation openings', in G. Psathas (ed.) *Everyday Language: Studies in ethnomethodology* (23–78), New York: Irvington Publishers.

——(1986a) 'Preliminaries to preliminaries: "Can I ask you a question?"' *Sociological Inquiry*, 50: 104–152.

——(1986b) 'The routine as achievement', *Human Studies*, 9: 111–151.

——(2007) *Sequence Organization in Interaction: A primer in conversation analysis*, Cambridge: Cambridge University Press.

Schegloff, E. A. and Sacks, H. (1973) 'Opening up closings', *Semiotica*, 3: 289–327.

Searle, J. R. (1975) 'Indirect speech acts', *Syntax and Semantics*, 3: 59–82.

Siminoff, L. A., et al. (1995) 'Public policy governing organ and tissue procurement in the United States: results from the national organ and tissue procurement study', *Annals of Internal Medicine*, 123: 10–17.

Siminoff, L. A., Gordon, N., Hewlett, J., and Arnold, R. M. (2001) 'Factors influencing families' consent for donation of solid organs for transplantation', *Journal of the American Medical Association*, 286: 71–77.

Stivers, T., Mangione-Smith, R., Elliott, M., McDonald, L., and Heritage, J. (2003) 'Why do physicians think parents expect antibiotics? What parents report vs. what physicians believe', *Journal of Family Practice*, 52: 140–148.

ten Have, P. (1999) *Doing Conversation Analysis: A practical guide*, London: Sage.

Titmuss, R. (1971) *The Gift Relationship: From human blood to social policy*, New York: Vintage.

Verble, M. and Worth, J. (2000) 'Fears and concerns expressed by families in the donation discussion', *Progress in Transplantation*, 10: 48–55.

Weathersbee, T. E. (2006) Field interview manuscripts.

Weathersbee, T. E. and Maynard, D. W. (2009) 'Dialling for donations: practices and actions in the telephone solicitation of human tissues', *Sociology of Health & Illness*, 31: 803–816.

Whalen, M. and Zimmerman, D. H. (1987) 'Sequential and institutional contexts in calls for help', *Social Psychology Quarterly*, 50: 172–185.

Whalen, M. R. and Zimmerman, D. H. (1990) 'Describing trouble: practical epistemology in citizen calls to the police', *Language in Society*, 19: 465–492.

Wootton, A. J. (1981) 'The management of grantings and rejections by parents in request sequences', *Semiotica*, 37: 59–89.

——(1997) *Interaction and the Development of Mind*, Cambridge: Cambridge University Press.

Zink, S. and Wertlieb, S. (2006) 'A study of the presumptive approach to consent for organ donation: a new solution to an old problem', *Critical Care Nurse*, 26: 129–136.

Appendix 40.1: Transcription conventions

Adapted from Paul ten Have (1999).

Sequencing

[	A single left bracket indicates the point of overlap onset
=	Equal signs, one at the end of one line and one at the beginning of a next, indicate no gap between the two lines. This is often called 'latching'.

Time intervals

(0.0)	Numbers in parentheses indicate elapsed time in silence by tenth of seconds, so (7.1) is a pause of 7 seconds and one-tenth of a second.
(.)	A dot in parentheses indicates a tiny gap within or between utterances.

Characteristics of speech production

word	Underscoring indicates some form of stress, via pitch and/or amplitude.
::	Colons indicate prolongation of the immediately prior sound. Multiple colons indicate a more prolonged sound.
-	A dash indicates a cut-off.
.,?	Punctuation marks are used to indicate characteristics of speech production, especially intonation; they are not referring to grammatical units.
.	A period indicates a stopping fall in tone.
,	A comma indicates a continuing intonation, like when you are reading items from a list.
?	A question mark indicates rising intonation.
	The absence of an utterance-final marker indicates some sort of indeterminate contour.
↑↓	Arrows indicate marked shifts into higher or lower pitch in the utterance-part immediately following the arrow.
WORD	Upper case indicates especially loud sounds relative to the surrounding talk.
°	Utterances or utterance parts bracketed by degree signs are relatively quieter than the surrounding talk.
< >	Right/left carets bracketing an utterance or utterance-part indicate slowing down.
> <	Left/right carets bracketing an utterance or utterance-part indicate speeding up.
.hh	A dot-prefixed row of h's indicates an in breath. Without the dot, the h's indicate an out breath.
w(h)ord	A parenthesized h, or a row of h's within a word, indicates breathiness, as in laughter, crying, etc.
~	A tilde indicates creakiness or crackling, as in crying, etc.

Transcriber's comments

(( ))	Double parentheses contain transcriber's descriptions rather than, or in addition to, transcriptions.

Index

Note: page numbers in **bold** refer to tables; page numbers in *italics* refer to figures.